D0435039

Advance Praise for *Caring for the Heart: Mayo Clinic and the Rise of Specialization*

"This book describes the intersection of two of the greatest success stories in twentieth century medicine: the evolution of the subspecialty of cardiology, responsible for the greatest prolongation of life in industrialized nations, and the development and growth of the Mayo Clinic, the largest and arguably the finest high quality health care system in the United States. Fye is a highly respected consultant cardiologist at Mayo and an equally distinguished medical historian who has risen to the top of both of these fields. He has produced a lively, insightful book that should be of interest to health care professionals, cardiac patients, their families and all who are interested in the evolution of medical care in the United States."

> —*Eugene Braunwald, MD, Distinguished Hersey Professor of Medicine,*
> *Harvard Medical School*

"In his latest book Bruce Fye tells the story of how the Mayo Clinic has, through the years, been a valuable contributor in the fight against heart disease and stroke. The American Heart Association is devoted to building healthier lives, free of cardiovascular disease and stroke, and allies like the Mayo Clinic are essential to achieving this mission."

> —*Nancy Brown, CEO, American Heart Association*

"The Mayo Clinic has long epitomized the development of cardiovascular care, cardiology practice, and medical technology in the United States. Dr. W. Bruce Fye vividly recounts the history of this world-renowned, yet uniquely American, medical center. As a cardiologist and historian, he provides unique insights into the Mayo model of care, the growth of medical specialization, and the evolution of diagnostic and therapeutic techniques. He also presents fascinating glimpses into American society and culture. The personal stories about patients and physicians are particularly compelling. This scholarly yet engaging book deserves a broad audience of both medical and lay readers."

> —*Denton A. Cooley, MD, founder and president emeritus,*
> *Texas Heart Institute*

"Millions of people owe their lives and health to the rise of cardiac specialization and the remarkable personalities who made it happen. Bruce Fye, MD, has written a frank, fast-moving, and thoroughly readable account of this scientific revolution as it occurred at Mayo Clinic, Cleveland Clinic, and elsewhere. Those of us who played some small role in the events described can only thank Dr. Fye for his honest and generous history."

> —*Delos M. Cosgrove, MD, CEO and President,*
> *Cleveland Clinic*

"American health care is so often portrayed as a problem that it's easy to overlook the pioneers and visionaries whose remarkable advances have saved and improved millions of lives. With a focus on heart care, the rise of specialization, and the application of new technologies and protocols pioneered by the Mayo Clinic, Dr. Bruce Fye brings these remarkable achievements to life. He has written a scrupulously researched yet thoroughly readable book for experts and non-experts alike. *Caring for the Heart* is a compelling story and readers will be in awe of how far we have come in so short a time."

> —*Thomas J. Donohue, President and CEO,*
> *US Chamber of Commerce*

"Bruce Fye's *Caring for the Heart: Mayo Clinic and the Rise of Specialization* is a unique and brilliant platform to understand the complex interplay of medical, scientific, technological, social and economic forces that over a century have shaped the practice of medicine and cardiology. The author is a cardiologist and historian of international reputation who has produced a highly stimulating, pragmatic, didactic and easy to read book for the general public, health care professionals and policy makers. It portrays beautifully more than a century of cardiovascular science, sophisticated technology, and humanistic medicine. Mayo Clinic has been an American phenomenon for over 100 years. Whether the reader is concerned about the development and future of medicine in general, or heart disease in particular, or about integration of the best care on a technological or human basis, he or she must read this unique and brilliant book.

—*Valentin Fuster, MD, PhD, Physician-in-Chief, The Mount Sinai Medical Center, and Editor-in-Chief,* Journal of the American College of Cardiology

"There are many scholarly books about cardiology. This volume is unique as its focus is on the emergence and development of an institution whose goal is to do the very best that cardiology offers, and to apply this knowledge to patient care. Reading through the chapters, one becomes quickly aware that the Mayo Clinic has successfully implemented a partnership between the management of the institution, the clinical and scientific faculty, and the patients—including both their physical and emotional care and well-being. The best illustration of this is shown by the development of open-heart surgery beginning in the 1950s. The story of this advance of cardiology at the Mayo Clinic is unique and fascinating, but so is what it has done to extend or improve the lives of thousands of patients. Reading about this is an experience that no one should miss."

—*Claude Lenfant, MD, former Director, National Heart, Lung and Blood Institute*

"This well-written and thoroughly researched book is very timely and deserves wide readership. The chapter on Franklin Roosevelt's hypertensive heart disease is outstanding. Bruce Fye provides convincing evidence to support his argument that a few White House insiders conspired to mislead the press and the public about the president's health. While this precise and clear history recounts events occurring over seventy years ago, its lessons should be carefully studied by our leaders in the medical and public arenas; indeed by all Americans concerned about the need for honest politics."

—*Walter F. Mondale, former Vice President of the United States*

"Who other than the uniquely talented Bruce Fye could have written such a magnificent narrative of the development of cardiology and its growth at the pioneering Mayo Clinic? This beautifully researched volume is panoramic while meticulously informative; scholarly while engrossingly literate; historic while of the moment—it is vintage Fye at his very best. Here he has created the template on which subsequent such treatises should be based."

—*Sherwin Nuland, MD, emeritus clinical professor of surgery, Yale University*

"Bruce Fye is a magnificent storyteller. I had a hard time putting this book down."

—*William C. Roberts, MD, executive director, Baylor Heart and Vascular Institute and Editor-in-Chief of the* American Journal of Cardiology

"It is impossible to think of anyone else with the experience and passion to write this extraordinary book. Bruce Fye is a cardiologist who has lived through many of the changes he describes, and a historian who is well recognized in both careers."

—*Rosemary A. Stevens, PhD, emeritus professor, History and Sociology of Science, University of Pennsylvania*

"W. Bruce Fye uses his unique background as a cardiologist and historian-writer to charm and educate a broad audience. He weaves the history of the Mayo Clinic and its world class surgical and cardiovascular programs with the worldwide historical advances in heart disease diagnosis and treatment. The pages seem to turn themselves, as the text is readable, entertaining, and educational."

—*Myron L. Weisfeldt, MD, professor of medicine and former Director, Department of Medicine, Johns Hopkins Medical Institutions*

Caring for the Heart

MAYO CLINIC AND THE RISE OF SPECIALIZATION

W. Bruce Fye

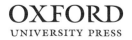

OXFORD

UNIVERSITY PRESS

OXFORD

UNIVERSITY PRESS

Oxford University Press is a department of the University of
Oxford. It furthers the University's objective of excellence in research,
scholarship, and education by publishing worldwide.

Oxford   New York
Auckland   Cape Town   Dar es Salaam   Hong Kong   Karachi
Kuala Lumpur   Madrid   Melbourne   Mexico City   Nairobi
New Delhi   Shanghai   Taipei   Toronto

With offices in
Argentina   Austria   Brazil   Chile   Czech Republic   France   Greece
Guatemala   Hungary   Italy   Japan   Poland   Portugal   Singapore
South Korea   Switzerland   Thailand   Turkey   Ukraine   Vietnam

Oxford is a registered trademark of Oxford University Press
in the UK and certain other countries.

Published in the United States of America by
Oxford University Press
198 Madison Avenue, New York, NY 10016

© Mayo Foundation for Medical Education and Research 2015

All rights reserved. No part of this publication may be reproduced, stored in
a retrieval system, or transmitted, in any form or by any means, without the prior
permission in writing of Oxford University Press, or as expressly permitted by law,
by license, or under terms agreed with the appropriate reproduction rights organization.
Inquiries concerning reproduction outside the scope of the above should be sent to the
Rights Department, Oxford University Press, at the address above.

You must not circulate this work in any other form
and you must impose this same condition on any acquirer.

Library of Congress Cataloging-in-Publication Data
Fye, Bruce, author.
Caring for the heart : Mayo Clinic and the rise of specialization / W. Bruce Fye.
p.; cm.
Includes bibliographical references and index.
ISBN 978–0–19–998235–6 (alk. paper)
I. Title.
[DNLM: 1. Mayo Clinic.   2. Cardiology—history—Minnesota.   3. Academic Medical
Centers—history—Minnesota.   4. Cardiovascular Diseases—history—Minnesota.
5. Coronary Care Units—history—Minnesota.   6. Diagnostic Techniques,
Cardiovascular—history—Minnesota.   7. History, 19th Century—
Minnesota.   8. History, 20th Century— Minnesota.
9. History, 21st Century—Minnesota.   10. Specialization—history—Minnesota.
WG 11 AM6]
RC681
616.'2—dc23
2014016050

5 7 9 8 6 4
Printed in the United States of America
on acid-free paper

Dedication

For Lois Baker Fye

{ CONTENTS }

SECTION III **Technologies Transform Heart Care
and Stimulate Subspecialization**

{ LIST OF FIGURES AND TABLES }

Figures

Tables

{ FOREWORD }

A vigorous life: the steady beating of a healthy heart. *An unsatisfactory one*: the heart is physically sick (or even mentally sick when "heart" acts, as it often does, as metaphor: heartsick, heartbroken, heartless). *The heart stops* and cannot be revived: that is death. The doctor who chooses cardiology as a field of study and practice takes on a vital mission. In turn, *Caring for the Heart* offers a poignant window into the broader, idiosyncratic history of American medicine from the early twentieth century into the twenty-first.

It is impossible to think of anyone else with the experience and passion to write this extraordinary book. Bruce Fye is a cardiologist who has lived through many of the changes he describes, and a historian who is well recognized in both careers. His former book, *American Cardiology: The History of a Specialty and Its College* (1996) explored the history of cardiology as an organized professional field in the twentieth century, including the politics that made this possible and the transformation of cardiology, by the 1970s, from a technologically oriented to a technology-dominated field. *Caring for the Heart* is broader and more ambitious. Here is the history of cardiology writ large.

Several kinds of medical history are involved here. The human element is a constant presence through stories of patients as well as practitioners, managers, technology innovators, and researchers. Case illustrations of individual patients include some whose names are otherwise unknown; some who became known through press reports on their last-ditch efforts to stave off death through agreeing to procedures that were then experimental, such as Barney Clark, recipient of an artificial heart; and some with international reputations, including Presidents Franklin D. Roosevelt and Lyndon B. Johnson, both of whom suffered from heart disease. Fye takes the reader through the history of scientific and technological change in approaches to heart disease; the specialization and now the sub-sub-specialization of cardiac fields that accompanied such changes; and the organizational and economic contexts in which cardiology has developed with its sister fields in cardiac surgery, radiology, and bionic medicine.

By centering his sight on the Mayo Clinic, his professional home, Fye provides a steadying base for studying the dizzying shifts, complexities and tussles over control inherent in the invention of modern medicine. Nevertheless, the result is more John Dos Passos than a straightforward narrative account.

One chapter may return to an earlier period than the chapter before in order to fill in gaps. But that is how American medicine has evolved, not on a straight line but in reconfigurations and bumps. For though, as always, medicine is a creature of its time, different times involve shifting sets of participants, each bringing in or rearranging the resulting strands of history. Nurses come to the fore in cardiology in the 1960s as essential technical experts in the care of patients in the new coronary care (intensive care) units, though of course nurses, including nurse-anesthetists, had long been a vital force at Mayo. Cardiologists and radiologists negotiate the question of who "owns" cardiac angiography in the 1960s. Interventional cardiologists use balloon catheters to treat coronary blockages. Cardiologists and cardiac surgeons negotiate their respective roles vis-à-vis angioplasty. All of which is to say that medicine is as political as any other field.

The Mayo Clinic has been an American phenomenon since Doctors Will and Charlie Mayo joined their father's practice in the 1880s on the cusp of a revolution in American surgery, borne along by new antiseptic techniques and by the general use of anesthesia. For patients surgery became not only safe, relatively speaking, but also painless. New hospitals opened with modern surgical operating rooms. Though it would be decades until surgery would be ventured on the heart, the abdomen was soon open for investigation and soon other parts of the body would be, too, including the brain. In the early twentieth century the Doctors Mayo and the organization they put together were as triumphant and successful a symbol of modernity as the automobile, aircraft, and mass production. Americans boasted of their surgeries with the same enthusiasm with which they downed pills.

While the Mayo Clinic drew difficult surgical cases to Minnesota by train from far and wide, at the same time the medical part of the clinic evolved through its early focus on getting an accurate diagnosis as part of each patient's surgical plan. No one wanted a patient to die of heart failure or a heart attack on the operating table. With amazing speed Mayo developed its own medical production machine, a highly organized set of services specialized, coordinated, and tailored for the individual patient. "Henry Ford could not improve on it," a former US Secretary of the Interior remarked after his evaluation for chest and abdominal pain in Rochester in 1920.

From today's perspective, these organizational features are of special interest for two reasons: first, because the successes of the clinic in later years in cardiac treatment and research (and in other fields) were based on its industrial-type efficiency, first-rate salaried staff, standard records system, and coordination of increasingly diverse services; second, because with a few exceptions, this model of modernity did not become the standard form for American medicine as a whole. Specialization of medicine and across the health professions is here to stay—indeed it is needed. Yet for at least a hundred years it has been self-evident that specialization of function in any domain must be accompanied by coordination of the specialized parts if the full advantages of specialization are to be gained. At one and the same time, then, this book elicits admiration and congratulations to the American medical profession and its allies on how far the diagnosis and treatment of heart disease has come in the past century, and especially in the past few decades, *and* provokes questions about the best methods of making these advances (and other advances in medicine) effectively available across the population.

The heart is no longer a mystery but a pump with chambers throbbing away from birth to death, serviced by pipes that sometimes get clogged. A diagnosis of heart disease is no longer a death sentence. Problems can be fixed. Not all of them, but many. We are blessed to live in such a time. But still, we are not machines. A great strength of this book is that it makes the science and technology of medicine human, reminding us that we cannot escape death, but with the help of dedicated researchers, inventors, and practitioners we may extend life and face death down.

Rosemary A. Stevens
Emeritus Professor, History and Sociology of Science
University of Pennsylvania
Philadelphia, PA

{ PREFACE AND ACKNOWLEDGMENTS }

This book is the final volume of an unplanned trilogy that began with the publication of *The Development of American Physiology: Scientific Medicine in the Nineteenth Century* in 1987. Nine years later, *American Cardiology: The History of a Specialty and Its College* told the story of a professional society for physicians whose careers focused on the care of patients with heart disease.[1] The idea for the present book arose in 2000, when I joined the staff of the Mayo Clinic. A. Jamil Tajik, who chaired the Cardiovascular Division, encouraged me to write a history of cardiology at Mayo. I agreed because it seemed to be a logical extension of my previous research and writing, as well as a good way to learn about the institution I was joining.

I had no idea that this project would evolve into such an exhaustive (and at times exhausting) endeavor. But it soon became apparent that I had a unique opportunity to produce something much more interesting and significant than a standard celebratory history of an institution or a medical specialty. My new goal was to write a book that explained how and why the care of patients with heart disease changed so dramatically during the twentieth century. Although I would emphasize events at the Mayo Clinic in Rochester, Minnesota, I decided to place them in a larger medical, scientific, and social context. Above all, I wanted to write a series of interconnected stories that would appeal to a broad audience including general readers. I also wanted this book to interest and inform individuals who are in positions to influence the future of health care delivery and biomedical innovation.

I reviewed more than fifteen thousand published and unpublished documents during the dozen years that I researched and wrote this book on the history of heart care, the Mayo Clinic, and specialization. This arduous expedition through a mountain of potentially relevant sources reflects my personality and an unlimited photocopying budget; but there is something more. It is hard to predict where a historical gem—a valuable insight or very compelling sound bite—may be discovered. That is the fun of the hunt! My search for material about Mayo's history and its role in heart care was especially exciting because I had access to a treasure trove of minutes, memos, reports, and letters that other historians have not seen.

At the other end of what might be termed the access spectrum, I found fascinating material in sources that millions of general readers have seen, such as the *New York Times*, the *Saturday Evening Post*, and *Life* magazine. Newspaper and magazine articles provided valuable perspectives that complemented those published in journals produced by and for medical professionals. When journalists report heart care innovations, they often translate medical jargon into words and phrases that the public can understand. In several instances, I have used their popular descriptions of technologies and new diagnostic and therapeutic procedures in order to help make this book more accessible to a general audience. I also provide brief explanations of key concepts to help guide readers through thickets of medical jargon. Fortunately, in this age of the Internet, it is easy for individuals to find straightforward definitions and illustrations of medical conditions, technologies, and procedures.

Quotations from participants in (and observers of) the events and developments that I discuss enliven my narrative. Most of their words were drawn from articles and editorials in medical journals or from stories in newspapers and magazines. I also interviewed sixty-three individuals, including physicians, surgeons, scientists, nurses, and technicians. Oral histories provide personal perspectives—memories—that complement contemporary printed and manuscript sources. The interviewees were divided almost equally between Mayo insiders and individuals from elsewhere. I have also included several patient stories that enable readers to hear directly from men and women who have had various types of heart disease. Their unique experiences illustrate how diagnostic approaches and treatment strategies have changed over time in response to new knowledge, technologies, and techniques.[2]

General readers should not be put off by the voluminous endnotes. In fact, the book can be read without looking at them. They document my sources and serve as a guide for individuals seeking additional information on a specific subject. For each major topic or theme, I have included references to what I consider the most useful secondary (historical) sources. These, in turn, usually contain lists of relevant primary (contemporary) sources that illustrate how several individuals or groups of workers contributed to developments that are often attributed to one physician, surgeon, or scientist. There are many challenges associated with trying to assign priority in terms of discoveries and innovations. In general, I emphasize individuals who functioned in a dual innovator-promoter role.

This book benefits from the fact that I have been a practicing cardiologist and medical historian for almost four decades. From this clinician-historian perch, I have watched health care change through two distinct but complementary lenses. I entered the Johns Hopkins University as a premedical student in 1964 and graduated from the Johns Hopkins Medical School eight years later. After spending three years as a resident at the New York Hospital-Cornell Medical Center in Manhattan, I returned to Hopkins where I completed a cardiology fellowship, was a Robert Wood Johnson Clinical Scholar, and was awarded a master's degree in the history of medicine. I left Baltimore in 1978 and spent the next twenty-two years at the Marshfield Clinic in Wisconsin. In 2000 I joined the staff of the Mayo Clinic in Rochester, Minnesota. This position has provided me with access to remarkable archival materials and firsthand knowledge of how patients are cared for there. It is important to emphasize that my academic independence has been respected throughout the research and writing of this book. The contents have not been subjected to any editorial oversight or institutional review.

During the four decades since I began my cardiology fellowship at Johns Hopkins, I have helped provide care to thousands of men and women with heart disease and have marveled at the many innovations that have revolutionized diagnosis and therapy. My understanding of changes in health care delivery has been enriched by a broad range of experiences inside and outside the four institutions where I have worked. For example, I chaired the Cardiology Department at Marshfield Clinic for eighteen years and served on the Board of Trustees of St. Joseph's Hospital in Marshfield for a decade.

At a national level, I have been a member of more than two dozen committees of the American College of Cardiology and the American Heart Association. Those opportunities exposed me to many perspectives on a broad range of issues, including specialty training, physician supply, research funding, the diffusion of innovations, practice guidelines, and health care policy, among many others. I interacted with hundreds of professionals who worked in different fields in many contexts and several countries when I served as president of three organizations: the American College of Cardiology, the American Association for the History of Medicine, and the American Osler Society.[3]

Medical history, the other half of my professional life, has informed my clinical practice as well as my administrative and organizational roles. Historians may perceive trends that individuals caught up in the present do not recognize. Rather than following a predictable path from the past to the present, history is like a meander: a twisting and turning stream shaped over time by a combination of obvious and imperceptible forces. I do not know who coined the phrase "history teaches humility," but I like it very much, and this book includes examples that support the notion. The Mayo Clinic, widely perceived as an innovative and admired institution, has thrived for more than a century. But I describe some missed opportunities and identify factors that contributed to programmatic failures as well as successes.

In terms of acknowledgments, I thank the Mayo Clinic Center for the History of Medicine's Executive Committee and the three sequential chairs of Mayo's Cardiovascular Division, A. Jamil Tajik, David L. Hayes, and Charanjit (Chet) Rihal, for granting me time to research and write this book. I am grateful for two years of support provided by a National Library of Medicine Grant for Scholarly Works in Biomedicine and Health (1-G13-LM007922-01A1). I also thank Myron Weisfeldt, who was the cardiology fellowship director at Johns Hopkins when I began my subspecialty training, for helping to arrange a unique cardiology-medical history program. That experience, which ignited my passion for historical writing and research, placed me on a path toward a very rewarding career.

It is impossible to list all of the individuals at the Mayo Clinic who facilitated this project, but I especially thank Janice Aaker, Elve Albrecht, Cynthia Allen, LaVonne Beck, Renee Benson, Carol Beyer, Terrence Cascino, James Gaffey, Kaye Halstead, John Joyce, Jane Juenger, Shannon Meier, Helen Mundahl, Paul Scanlon, Charlene Tri, Mark Warner, Sister Ellen Whelan, Sister Lauren Weinandt, and Douglas Wood. A few staff members of the Mayo Clinic Library and the Mayo Historical Unit deserve special thanks: Nicole Babcock, Patricia Erwin, Michael Homan, Karen Koka, Hilary Lane, Kristen Van Hoven, and Renee Ziemer. Mayo cardiologist John Callahan shared material with me in 2000 that he had collected for a brief history of cardiology at the clinic.[4]

During this book's long gestation, I benefited from conversations about it with several historians, especially Michael Bliss, Christopher Crenner, Jacalyn Duffin, Jennifer Gunn, Bert Hansen, Joel Howell, Peter Kernahan, Kenneth Ludmerer, Charles Roland, Charles Rosenberg, Rosemary Stevens, and Keith Wailoo. I also thank each of the individuals whom I interviewed for this book. Their names appear in the appendix.

I am grateful to individuals who provided feedback after reading drafts of one or more chapters: Pamela Abrams, Kenneth Berge, Henry Blackburn, John Bresnahan, Howard Burchell, Gordon Danielson, David Driscoll, Robert Frye, Elizabeth Fye, Katherine Fye, Lois Fye, Bernard Gersh, George Gura, David Hayes, Arthur Hollman, Arlene Keeling, Thomas Killip, Paul Kligfield, Verghese Mathew, Ronald Menaker, John Merideth, Drew Meyers, Walter Mondale, Steven Peitzman, James Pluth, Guy Reeder, David Rhees, David Rosenwaks, Kathy Cramer Walsh, and Allen Weisse. A few individuals read many chapters, and I thank them for their valuable suggestions: James Broadbent, Vincent Gott, Sandra Moss, Ronald Numbers, Craig Panner, William Roberts, Marni Rolfes, Ronald Vlietstra, and Jacqueline Wehmueller. Caroline Hannaway read early and final drafts of every chapter. An accomplished historian and very experienced editor, she provided much useful feedback.

I have published two articles based on research for this book: W. B. Fye, "The Origins and Evolution of the Mayo Clinic from 1864 to 1939: A Minnesota Family Practice Becomes an International 'Medical Mecca,'" *Bulletin of the History of Medicine*, 2010, *84*: 323–357; and W. B. Fye, "Resuscitating a *Circulation* Abstract to Celebrate the 50th Anniversary of the Coronary Care Unit Concept," *Circulation*, 2011, *124*: 1886–1893. I thank those journals for granting me permission to incorporate some material that appeared in those articles in this book. Several archival sources are cited in the notes, but I especially want to thank the staff of organizations that provided substantial help in identifying and providing copies of materials in their collections: the Alan Mason Chesney Medical Archives of the Johns Hopkins Medical Institutions, the American Heart Association, the Cleveland Clinic Archives, the Francis A. Countway Library of Medicine, the Franklin D. Roosevelt Library, the Mayo Historical Unit, the National Library of Medicine, and the University of Minnesota Archives.

{ INTRODUCTION }

Why is a book that weaves together histories of heart care, a celebrated medical center, and specialization important? And why should it interest general readers as well as health care professionals, historians, social scientists, and policymakers? First of all, most individuals living in industrialized countries have or will develop cardiovascular disease during their lifetimes. And most of them have already seen coronary heart disease alter or end the lives of family members and friends. Despite astonishing developments in diagnosis and treatment in recent decades, cardiovascular disease still kills more Americans than any other cause. Its economic implications are staggering. In the United States alone, medical costs and productivity losses related to cardiovascular disease are approaching $500 billion annually.[5]

Second, the Mayo Clinic is the world's oldest and largest multispecialty group practice. There is value in understanding why this institution has been a national leader in health care since the early twentieth century. Unlike traditional academic medical centers, Mayo did not grow up around a medical school. And patient care, rather than research or education, has always been its main mission. The research and educational programs that complement the practice of medicine and surgery at Mayo have emphasized clinical investigation and the training of specialists. Ever since *U.S. News & World Report* published its first annual survey of hospitals and specialty care in 1990, the magazine has ranked Mayo's cardiology–heart surgery program as one of the top two in the nation. In its inaugural survey report, the magazine named the Mayo Clinic "The Best of the Best" because it ranked first in more medical and surgical specialties than any other institution.[6]

Specialization is the book's third major topic. I agree with historian Rosemary Stevens's assertion that "specialization is the fundamental theme for the organization of medicine in the twentieth century."[7] In the United States today, most patients with serious heart disease receive some of their care from a cardiologist—a medical specialist whose practice focuses on the diagnosis and treatment of cardiovascular disorders. This book explores how and why new technologies and procedures encouraged specialization in cardiology (and eventually subspecialization within cardiology). It also describes the development of cardiac surgery, cardiology's twin discipline.[8] Although the book focuses on cardiovascular disease, many of the forces that shaped heart care during the twentieth century also influenced the development of other medical and surgical specialties.

This book is organized by topic. There is a general chronological flow, but some overlap in time frames is inevitable. The first three chapters explain the origins and early growth of the Mayo Clinic. Then, the focus shifts to cardiovascular disease. Each of these latter chapters serves two purposes. Taken together, they reveal how the care of patients with heart disease changed during the twentieth century—in general and at the Mayo Clinic. Each chapter is also designed to be read separately, as a self-contained study of a specific theme, technology, or cluster of related techniques.

This is mainly a twentieth-century story, but it begins earlier—before there were cardiologists and when medical specialization was just emerging in America's largest cities. It ends in the early twenty-first century—when there is serious and growing concern about health care costs and the various factors that have contributed to their steady increase.

The Mayo Clinic has its origins in the 1880s, when William and Charles Mayo joined their father's general practice in Rochester, Minnesota. The brothers, known as Dr. Will and Dr. Charlie, wanted to become specialists in surgery. They benefited from a unique set of circumstances that catapulted them from a small Minnesota town into an international orbit in two decades. Their success as surgeons owed much to the Franciscan sisters who opened and staffed St. Mary's Hospital in Rochester in 1889. After a trip to the town in 1905, Johns Hopkins surgeon Harvey Cushing told his physician-father that the Mayo brothers "have built up a wonderful operative clinic and are well protected by an able staff of internists, specialists, etc. and are little likely to make mistakes. They do as good and as much surgery in their own particular lines as any other two men in the world. It has become worthily quite a Mecca for medical men."[9]

The growing outpatient practice moved into a custom-designed five-story outpatient building named "Mayo Clinic" in 1914, the same year the group acquired an electrocardiograph. This new diagnostic instrument, one of the first installed in the Midwest, traced the heart's electrical signal and catalyzed the creation of cardiology as a specialty.

More doctors decided to become specialists after World War I. As specialization grew in popularity, residency training began to shape a physician's professional identity more than his or her medical school experiences. Despite this, historians have devoted very little attention to this critical part of a doctor's career path. This book describes some of the major contributions that the Mayo Clinic made to the development of postgraduate specialty training. By the time Will and Charlie Mayo died in 1939, their institution had trained about 1,500 residents, far more than any other medical center in the United States.

Cardiology gained momentum as a specialty during the 1940s, but physicians who cared for patients with cardiovascular disease had very few effective treatments. The case of Franklin Roosevelt, which is detailed in Chapter 7, exemplifies this shortcoming. Uncontrolled severe hypertension contributed to his death at the age of sixty-three, just five months after he had won re-election to a fourth term. When his successor Harry Truman signed the National Heart Act in 1948, federal funds began flowing to academic institutions to support cardiovascular research and the training of heart specialists.

New Technologies Transform Heart Care

During the second half of the twentieth century, several new technologies and therapeutic procedures revolutionized the care of patients with heart disease. The organization of this book reflects this fact. More than one-half of the chapters are devoted to specific innovations, such as cardiac catheterization, open-heart surgery, coronary angiography, coronary artery bypass surgery, and echocardiography.[10] Each of these topics could be the subject of a book-length history, so I had to be very selective in choosing what to include in the technology-themed chapters. Generally, I focused on a few key individuals and institutions that played major roles in the late-stage development and diffusion of innovations that resulted in new approaches to heart care.

Technologies that transformed patient care were the end products of decades of discoveries, inventions, and innovations that involved countless individuals working in many countries and institutional contexts. The paths that innovations follow on their way to becoming the standard of care are often steep and winding. To show how some key breakthroughs successfully completed the journey, I discuss the dynamics surrounding their acceptance and application in patient care. Cardiology and cardiac surgery provide many compelling examples of innovators and pioneers who became missionaries on behalf of a specific technology or technique. These individuals broadcast their messages at medical meetings and in professional journals. The media, always eager to report medical breakthroughs, amplified their voices. I emphasize the interplay between the profession, the public, and the medical-industrial complex to demonstrate how socioeconomic factors (such as the high prevalence of heart disease, the federal funding of biomedical research, the expansion of health insurance, entrepreneurism, and consumerism) contributed to the rapid growth of cardiology and heart surgery during the last half-century.

To provide insight into how significant innovations were introduced into clinical practice, I look beyond the Mayo Clinic. This strategy provides a comparative framework for understanding when, why, and how Mayo's medical and surgical heart specialists adopted specific diagnostic techniques and therapeutic interventions. For example, the University of Minnesota is highlighted in Chapter 10, which describes the advent of open-heart surgery. In 1955 open-heart operations were performed on a regularly scheduled basis at just two institutions in the world: the University of Minnesota and the Mayo Clinic. The chapters on coronary angiography and coronary artery bypass graft surgery describe the Cleveland Clinic's pioneering role in developing diagnostic and treatment approaches that have been applied to millions of patients.

The final chapter, which brings the story into the twenty-first century, addresses a range of issues in health care delivery. Mayo's enviable reputation has been maintained for more than one hundred years. In 2009 Harvard surgeon and popular author Atul Gawande described Mayo as having "fantastically high levels of technological capability and quality" in a much-cited article on health care costs in the *New Yorker* magazine.[11] But he and others emphasize that some of the diagnostic and treatment technologies that are synonymous with state-of-the-art cardiology and heart surgery contribute significantly to the ever-rising costs of health care. It is important, especially in this era characterized by the "technological imperative," to reflect on whether an individual patient is likely to benefit from diagnostic tests and therapeutic procedures that are possible but may, in fact, produce harm. Likewise, it must be acknowledged that when we speak of caring for the heart, the ultimate goal should be preventing heart disease in the first place.

{ ABBREVIATIONS AND ACRONYMS }

ACC	American College of Cardiology
AHA	American Heart Association
BMI	Body mass index
BOG	Board of Governors
BOT	Board of Trustees
CABG	Coronary artery bypass graft surgery
CASS	Coronary Artery Surgery Study
CCU	Coronary care unit
CPC	Clinical Practice Committee
CPR	Cardiopulmonary resuscitation
CT	Computerized tomography
CV	Cardiovascular
DSR	Dynamic spatial reconstructor
EC	Executive Committee
ECG	Electrocardiogram (or electrocardiograph)
FDA	Food and Drug Administration
ICD	Implantable cardioverter defibrillator
ICU	Intensive care unit
LVAD	Left ventricular assist device
MC	Mayo Clinic
MICU	Medical intensive care unit
MRI	Magnetic resonance imaging
NHLBI	National Heart, Lung, and Blood Institute
NIH	National Institutes of Health
PTCA	Percutaneous transluminal coronary angioplasty
SMH	St. Mary's Hospital and Saint Marys Hospital (after ca. 1940)
TEE	Transesophageal echocardiogram
WPW	Wolff-Parkinson-White (syndrome)

Journal titles in the notes are abbreviated using the National Library of Medicine's format; see http://www.nlm.nih.gov/tsd/serials/lsiou.html.

Inventing the Mayo Clinic and Cardiology

The Nineteenth-Century Origins
of the Mayo Practice

In 1883 a deadly tornado destroyed much of Rochester, Minnesota. The disaster brought together two immigrants whose collaboration resulted in the construction of St. Mary's Hospital and the creation of the Mayo Clinic. In less than a quarter of a century, these interdependent institutions would become known internationally for providing safe and successful surgical care to thousands of patients each year. Despite Rochester's small size and rural location, it provided fertile soil for the development of what would become America's largest and most influential medical group practice.[1] Several factors contributed to the Mayo Clinic's creation and success, but three key ingredients intersected at a specific time and place: a family of ambitious doctors, an order of Catholic sisters, and hospital-based antiseptic surgery.

William Worrall Mayo, founder of the practice that would evolve into the Mayo Clinic, was born near Manchester, England, in 1819.[2] He studied privately with chemist John Dalton and had limited exposure to medical teaching in Manchester and elsewhere in England. In 1846 Mayo spent a month on a sailing ship with 250 men, women, and children crossing the Atlantic Ocean. Settling first in New York City, he worked at Bellevue Hospital preparing medicines. It was a dreary and deadly place, staffed by a single resident physician and six assistants. One doctor complained in 1846, "Fully two-fifths of all cases sent to the hospital are pronounced incurable before they are sent, and are received in a dying state."[3] Mayo left New York the following year.

Like many mid-nineteenth-century immigrants, William Mayo moved west, settling first in Lafayette, Indiana, where he became an apprentice to Elizur Deming, one of the state's leading doctors. Deming taught at two medical schools, and Mayo earned degrees from both of them. He graduated from the Indiana Medical College in La Porte in 1850 and the University of Missouri in St. Louis four years later. Because the medical school terms were just four months long, the English immigrant spent most of his time practicing medicine with his mentor in Lafayette.[4] During his brief stay in La Porte, thirty-year-old William Mayo met twenty-three-year-old Louise Wright. They were married in 1851 in Lafayette, where Louise would open a hat shop, the New York Millinery, to help support the couple.[5]

Doctor Deming stimulated Mayo's interest in medical organizations and microscopy. When Deming was president of the Indiana State Medical Society, he encouraged his protégé to present a paper at its annual meeting. Mayo spoke on the value of using chemical tests and microscopy to study a patient's urine—topics that reflected his respect for new diagnostic methods.[6]

In 1854 Doctor Mayo and his wife moved to Minnesota. The territory's population had quadrupled in the preceding four years as settlers took over land that the government had acquired from the Dakota Indians.[7] The Mayos settled in St. Paul, a flourishing city of 9,000 on the Mississippi River. One of the city's physicians had just published an article on Minnesota's doctors, diseases, and climate in the *Boston Medical and Surgical Journal*. After boasting that Minnesota was located in "the healthiest portion of our country," he conceded that "disease and death are here; and the true physician can find problems enough to solve, and subjects enough for patient study and investigation."[8]

It is unclear how difficult it was for Doctor Mayo to establish a practice in St. Paul, but he drifted away from medicine. "Those were very hard times," his wife Louise recalled, "particularly hard for a physician."[9] She opened a new millinery shop to help support the family while her husband traveled around the region trying to earn money as a prospector, riverboat captain, territorial agent, and veterinarian. As the decade came to a close, he decided to try to launch a medical practice once again—this time in a less competitive context. In 1859 the struggling doctor built a house, which included a small office, in the village of Le Sueur in southern Minnesota. Louise delivered William James (Will) Mayo there on June 29, 1861, shortly after the outbreak of the Civil War.

The Civil War Leads Doctor Mayo to Rochester, Minnesota

The Civil War, centered a thousand miles from the new state, shifted Doctor Mayo's career path. After Congress passed the Conscription Act in 1863, President Lincoln appointed him examining surgeon for southern Minnesota's enrollment board, which was located in Rochester.[10] When Mayo began practicing medicine there in 1864, the ten-year-old town had a population of about 3,000.[11] Further growth was assured because two major transportation routes intersected in it. Many wagons carrying goods and people passed through the community each day on a trail that stretched between the Mississippi River towns of St. Paul, Minnesota, and Dubuque, Iowa. The Winona & St. Peter Railroad reached Rochester in 1864, linking it to North America's rapidly expanding rail network. A steady stream of pioneers populated the region as train tracks spread westward and fertile lands yielded impressive harvests of wheat, corn, and other crops.[12] The Mayos would spend the rest of their lives in Rochester, where Louise delivered their last child, Charles Horace (Charlie) Mayo, on July 19, 1865.

Doctor Mayo was forty-nine years old in 1868, when New York City physician-editor George Shrady praised established "country practitioners" who sought to enhance their skills and reputations by enrolling in "metropolitan" medical schools. "There is hardly a medical class in our colleges which cannot number among its devoted students many a gray-haired veteran."[13] Shrady noted the older doctors' special interest in courses on practical surgery, microscopy, and use of the stethoscope. Balding but not yet gray, Mayo made a pilgrimage—the first of many—to metropolitan hospitals in 1869. The *Rochester Post* informed readers that he would spend the winter in New York City attending lectures and "perfecting himself, especially, in the practice of surgery." Noting that Doctor Mayo already had "a large practice and a high standing in the profession," the writer predicted that he would "return in the spring with still better claims upon the confidence of his patients."[14]

Surgery, a special interest of Doctor Mayo, would be the centerpiece of the practice that his two sons would build in Rochester in the 1890s. Surgery had been revolutionized by the discovery of ether anesthesia a few weeks after his arrival in the United States in 1846. This breakthrough set the stage for the expansion of surgical territory and the introduction of new operations during the second half of the nineteenth century. In a semi-centennial tribute to anesthesia, a St. Paul medical editor reminded doctors what patients had experienced before ether and chloroform were used to numb their senses:

> Then a surgical operation was a matter that was looked forward to with dread for months and even for years before it was performed, a dread felt not only by the unfortunate sufferer but by the surgeon himself, to whom the infliction of unavoidable suffering of an operation was a veritable ordeal. What wonder is it then that operations were deferred to the last moment.... Think of the contrast between one of these preanesthesia operations, with the patient strapped to the table and rending the air with his shrieks, as compared with an operation of today with the patient lying in a quiet slumber and nothing to break the stillness of the room.[15]

Doctor Mayo operated more often than most general practitioners and developed a regional reputation for his surgical skills. Usually the procedures were performed to treat traumatic injuries, such as large cuts or broken bones. But sometimes they were done to deal with chronic problems, such as hernias. Mayo's practice grew by word of mouth among patients and doctors. He enjoyed participating in professional organizations that provided

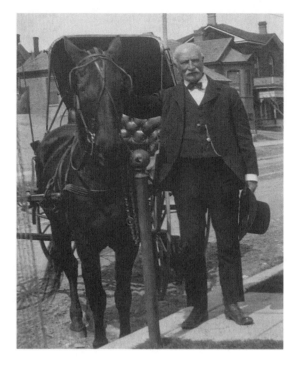

FIGURE 1.1 *William Worrall Mayo (1819–1911) in Rochester, Minnesota, ca. 1900.*
Used with permission of Mayo Foundation.

him with educational and social opportunities. When he was president of the Minnesota State Medical Society in 1873, he challenged his peers not to be satisfied with mediocrity.[16] Mayo (Figure 1.1) was a small man (five feet four inches tall) from a small town, but he impressed Minnesota's doctors with his ambition—for himself, for them, and for their profession.

The Mayo Boys Become Doctors and Join Their Father's Practice

As Doctor Mayo's practice grew in the late 1870s, his sons Will and Charlie reached adolescence and became his apprentices. He had a very large library, so the boys grew up surrounded by books on medicine and other subjects. They learned to prepare medicines in a drugstore located under their father's office. Although Will and Charlie attended local academies to supplement their high school educations, they did not enroll in college. In this era, no American medical school required an applicant to have attended college. Will Mayo was nineteen in 1880 when he matriculated at the Medical Department of the University of Michigan, one of the nation's best medical schools.[17]

When Will entered medical school, surgery was being transformed by refinements in antiseptic techniques that Joseph Lister had invented a dozen years earlier. The British surgeon used carbolic acid as an antiseptic to destroy minute organisms in the air that could settle in wounds and cause infections, which, in turn, could lead to disability and death. Will watched surgery professor Donald Maclean operate in a new amphitheater that was attached to the University of Michigan's sixty-bed hospital. The Canadian-born, Scottish-trained professor used Lister's antiseptic system, which included spraying carbolic acid over an anesthetized patient. Mayo later credited Maclean with stimulating his interest in surgery.[18] Will was ambitious and eager to enter medical practice. Just before graduating in 1883, he told his sister, "Don't let father work too hard.... I am anxious to get out and put my shoulder to the wheel for the common good. I am in love with my profession and with hard study and work, with plenty of time, hope to make a success."[19]

Charlie Mayo matriculated at the Chicago Medical College in 1885. Affiliated with Northwestern University, it was among America's best medical schools. Like his older brother, Charlie was attracted to surgery. He was able to watch some of Chicago's leading surgeons operate because his school was located near the 300-bed Mercy Hospital and the 550-bed Cook County Hospital.[20] Before the Mayo boys graduated from medical school, they had helped their father perform procedures, such as amputations and hernia repairs, on a portable operating table that he used in his office, in patients' homes, in local hotels, and a in small private home-hospital in Rochester run by a nurse.[21]

The Mayo brothers joined their father's busy practice immediately after graduating from medical school. As was typical at the time, neither one did an internship. They were privileged, however, because they returned home to a well-established practice and a very experienced mentor. Will and Charlie also took advantage of a new academic model designed to help practitioners supplement a standard medical school education, which consisted almost exclusively of lectures. Will enrolled in the New York Post-Graduate Medical School in the fall of 1884 and graduated three months later. The following year, he spent several weeks at the New York Polyclinic, where he saw surgeons operate and physicians visit hospitalized patients.[22]

Very few American doctors considered themselves specialists when the country celebrated its centennial in 1876. During the next decade, however, some of those who lived in the nation's biggest cities began gravitating toward specialty practice. These centers of population provided aspiring specialists with a critical mass of patients seeking their care and general practitioners soliciting their opinions. Doctors who were attracted to specialty practice cited the growth of knowledge and the invention of diagnostic tools as major factors in their decision. They also thought that specialization would enable them to provide better care, contribute more to their profession, earn more money, and have a better lifestyle.[23]

Specialization was gaining momentum when the Mayo brothers joined their father's practice in the 1880s. Mary Putnam Jacobi, who taught at the New York Post-Graduate Medical School when Will studied there, had discussed the social dynamics of specialization in 1882. Practicing in America's biggest incubator of specialists and specialty societies, she was impressed by the attitudes of affluent patients: "Every sick person who can pay for it begins to expect to divide up his body among a cluster of 'eminent specialists' before any positive diagnosis of his case can be reached.... The laity are very ready to infer not only that specialism is good, but that the more of it the better."[24] When Jacobi made these observations, surgery was just beginning to emerge as a viable specialty in some large cities.

The "New Surgery" and the Hospital Movement in the United States

Surgery was changing rapidly when Will Mayo joined his father's practice in 1883 and Charlie joined them five years later. The new science of bacteriology, with its implications for understanding the causes of life-threatening postoperative wound infections, catalyzed surgery's sudden expansion in the late nineteenth century.[25] New York surgeon Steven Smith stressed the significance of the recent changes in a textbook published when Charlie was in medical school: "Within the period 1879–86 the principles and practice of operative surgery have undergone so complete a revolution, that the term, 'the new surgery,' applied to the present practice is not inappropriate."[26] This sudden shift, due mainly to the advent of antiseptic techniques, affected both patients and practitioners. "Not only have the principles governing the treatment of wounds been so modified as to render operations, formerly very fatal, safe and expedient," Smith explained, "but the field has been so extended as to embrace a wide range of successful procedures for the cure of injuries and diseases hitherto regarded and treated as necessarily incurable."[27]

Before the advent of antiseptic practices, a surgeon's knife that could cure one disease might carry another one. From a patient's perspective, antisepsis was not about seeing bacteria through a microscope or smelling the acrid odor of carbolic acid; it was about avoiding pus-draining surgical wounds and death. Minneapolis surgeon James Dunn made this point to members of the Minnesota State Medical Society in 1887. He had recently returned to Minneapolis after a year of postgraduate training in Berlin and Vienna, where he saw antiseptic surgery "in its full glory." Dunn acknowledged that excellent antiseptic surgery was being performed in some parts of his state, but he demanded that all doctors condemn the "dirty methods" of pre-antiseptic surgery that harmed patients: "The unfortunate are sacrificed upon altars of the reputations of the men who refuse to believe in what they do not comprehend, and who rest upon laurels won decades ago."[28] This was a stinging indictment of doctors who remained wedded to old doctrines and practices as the new surgery gained momentum.

During the 1890s, Lister's cumbersome and controversial antiseptic system was replaced by so-called aseptic techniques and technologies that were designed to prevent bacteria from entering a surgical wound in the operating room. The advent of asepsis emboldened some doctors to push surgery's boundaries into regions of the body that had been too dangerous to enter because of the risk of infection and death. Claudius Mastin of Alabama celebrated surgery's rapid territorial expansion in 1891:

> It was but yesterday when the closed cavities of the body were held as sacred; the organs within the abdomen, the lungs and heart within the thorax, the brain and spinal cord cased by the skull and vertebral column, were each surrounded by a dead-line which none dared to cross. To-day, they have each become the legitimate fields into which the surgeon has carried his knife.[29]

During the final decade of the nineteenth century, the Mayo brothers would practice the new surgery, inserting scalpels into each cavity mentioned by Mastin. They were able to do this because they operated in a new state-of-the-art hospital where they used antiseptic and aseptic techniques. Hospitals were the centerpiece of the new surgery and the training ground for the first generation of full-time surgeons. Antisepsis and asepsis encouraged them to enter the abdomen and other territories that were previously out of bounds, but the modern hospital, with its trained nurses and technological assets, was equally important. Between 1873, when Will reached adolescence, and 1911, when his father died at age ninety-one, the number of hospitals in the United States exploded from fewer than 200 to more than 4,000.[30] In 1894 a Massachusetts doctor attributed the hospital movement to the new "germ-defying régime" (which required special technology) and compared a modern operating room to a "fully equipped machine shop."[31] Meanwhile, the focus of surgical treatment shifted gradually from emergency operations done when and where the need arose to elective procedures performed in hospitals.

The hospital movement also reflected America's romance with technology. During the last third of the nineteenth century, an avalanche of new technologies transformed life in the United States. Some of the most impressive culture-changing inventions involved communication (telephones, typewriters, and phonographs) and transportation (expanding rail networks, turbine-powered steamships, bicycles, and automobiles). Electricity, another breakthrough technology that ran machines and lit dark spaces, was also touted as a therapeutic tool.[32] Hundreds of thousands of individuals attended huge international exhibitions that showcased technology and modernity. The Mayo brothers would embrace both. By constructing St. Mary's Hospital in Rochester, the Sisters of St. Francis gave them an alternative to operating in patients' homes or hotel rooms, as their father had done.[33]

A Hospital Rises in Rochester after a Deadly Tornado

"THE CYCLONE": These two words stretched across the front page of the *Rochester Record & Union* on August 24, 1883. The story described the devastation: "Last Tuesday at seven o'clock Rochester was one of the loveliest cities in the west. Ten minutes later its beauty had disappeared, and in parts of the city ruin and desolation reigned. A terrible cyclone visited us, leaving death and destruction in its track.... To describe it is impossible. It must be seen for the mind to grasp its terrible destruction."[34] The tornado destroyed or damaged hundreds of buildings, killed more than twenty persons, and injured dozens more, many seriously.

Will Mayo and his eighteen-year-old brother were driving a buggy through town when the tornado struck, and they barely escaped harm. Their father and other doctors treated the injured in two hotels and a makeshift hospital set up in a dance hall. Some of the injured were taken to the Academy of Our Lady of Lourdes, a private school run by the Sisters of St. Francis. Mother Alfred Moes, the leader of the local congregation of sisters, looked past the immediate disaster and proposed building a hospital in Rochester.[35]

Born in Luxembourg, Maria Moes was twenty-three years old when she sailed to the United States in 1851. She decided to devote herself to service as a sister in the Catholic Church and made her final vows with the Sisters of the Holy Cross seven years later. In 1865 Sister Alfred was appointed first Mother General of the Franciscan sisters and was placed in charge of a convent in Joliet, Illinois. Mother Alfred's biographers describe personality clashes and political intrigues that eventually resulted in her relocation to Minnesota. Shortly after she arrived in Rochester in 1877, Mother Alfred bought land and oversaw construction of the Academy of Our Lady of Lourdes, a school that would provide education to about two hundred children through the twelfth grade.[36]

As Rochester recovered from the tornado, Mother Alfred told Doctor Mayo that her sisters would raise money to build a hospital if he would agree to be in charge of it. The sixty-four-year-old general practitioner hesitated, but she persisted. Catholic sisters were busy building hospitals across the country, and Mother Alfred could point to the local educational academy as proof that her congregation could plan and complete big projects.[37] A decade after the disaster, Doctor Mayo recounted their conversation:

> Some weeks after the…temporary hospital closed, the Mother Superior came down to my office and in the course of her visit asked, "Doctor, do you not think a hospital in this city would be an excellent thing?" I answered, "Mother Superior, this city is too small to support a hospital."

I told her too that the erection of a hospital was a difficult undertaking and required a great deal of money, and moreover we had no assurance of its being a success even after a great deal of time and money had been put into it. "Very true," she persisted; "but you just promise me to take charge of it and we will set that building before you at once. With our faith, hope and energy, it will succeed." I asked how much money the Sisters would be willing to put into it, and her reply was, "How much do you want?" "Would you be willing to risk forty-thousand dollars?" I said. "Yes," she replied; "and more if you want it. Draw up your plans. It will be built at once."[38]

Doctor Mayo's reluctance to accept Mother Alfred's offer is understandable given the time and place. When the tornado devastated Rochester, there were only six general hospitals in all of Minnesota. Five were in the Twin Cities (of Minneapolis and St. Paul).

It took the sisters five years to raise enough money to buy nine acres of land in Rochester and to begin construction of what would be named St. Mary's Hospital. Meanwhile, Doctor Mayo and Will toured East Coast hospitals in order to help a local architect develop the plans.[39] As carpenters and bricklayers worked on the building, Charlie, who had just graduated from medical school in Chicago, visited hospitals equipped with the latest paraphernalia of antiseptic surgery. The Mayos imported ideas, techniques, and technologies that would help make St. Mary's Hospital a state-of-the-art institution for patient care when it opened in September 1889 (Figure 1.2). The forty-by-sixty-foot, three-story brick structure contained

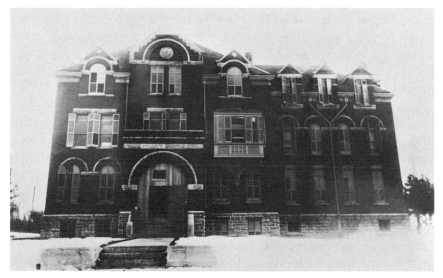

FIGURE 1.2 *St. Mary's Hospital, Rochester, Minnesota, 1889.*
Used with permission of Mayo Foundation.

an operating room and forty-five beds (divided among three ten-bed wards and small private rooms). A local newspaper boasted that the building was "designed for convenience in caring for the sick" and incorporated the latest technologies.[40]

Alfred Worcester of Waltham, Massachusetts, published a book on small hospitals in 1894, eleven years after he had graduated from Harvard Medical School. Like the Mayo brothers, Worcester had returned to his hometown to practice. This keen observer of hospital politics and procedures proclaimed:

> The large hospitals have still the prestige of years of splendid service; they also have the curses of self-satisfaction, of red tape in profusion, of sluggishness in adopting improvements. In them the individuality of the patient is lost sight of.... True, on the staff of the large hospitals are the ablest physicians and surgeons of the city and of the state. But in reality the direct immediate care of the patients is in the hands of the "house officers," who are either still students of medicine or at best graduates having no acquired skill in the art of healing. In the smaller hospitals, on the other hand, there is no prestige, no red tape, no self-satisfaction; instead there is an immediate, eager readiness to adopt every improved method.... The patient's individuality is not lost...he is under the care of his own physician or surgeon, who...will devote his whole attention to his patient, and who would not, even if he could, surrender the care of him to unskilled hands.[41]

Patients who had surgery at St. Mary's Hospital did not have to worry about confronting unskilled hands. The Mayo brothers performed all of the operations at the small hospital for more than a decade. Other caring hands touched the patients. Alfred Worcester attributed much of a hospital's success to its medical and surgical staff, but he emphasized that "even more does it depend upon its nursing service."[42]

The Franciscan sisters who founded St. Mary's Hospital had been teachers, so they had to be trained to be nurses. A few months before the hospital opened, the Mayos hired Edith Graham, who had grown up around Rochester, to do this. The daughter of a midwife, she had recently completed nurse's training in Chicago. Edith worked in the Mayos' office and taught the sisters how to care for hospitalized patients.[43] The Mayos were the only doctors to care for the inpatients. Shortly after St. Mary's Hospital opened, the sisters decided that any patient seeking admission had to be examined by one of the Mayos. This so-called closed-staff model—impractical in most contexts for social, economic, or political reasons—was a key part of the sisters' and the Mayos' strategy to coordinate and enhance patient care.[44]

The Mayos' Surgical Practice and St. Mary's Hospital Grow

St. Mary's Hospital was a success from the start. Statistics from its first report, published in 1893, show that two-thirds of the patients admitted since it opened four years earlier had surgery. Those who had an operation had a 98 percent chance of surviving. Will or Charlie Mayo performed each of the 655 operations. More than 200 separate categories of surgery were listed in the first report; almost fifty of them were intra-abdominal procedures. Less than a decade after the senior Doctor Mayo had resisted Mother Alfred's offer to build a hospital, he and his sons asked the sisters to expand it. They wanted a second operating room, more beds, and more staff to accommodate increasing patient demand.[45] The first addition, opened in 1894, increased the hospital's capacity to seventy-five beds. One-third of them were in private rooms, and the rest were in large and small wards. That year 509 patients were admitted, including 158 Catholics, 137 Lutherans, 54 Methodists, and 73 who identified with other faiths.[46]

The minister of Rochester's Universalist Church, one of the speakers at the dedication of the 1894 addition, boasted about the hospital's regional reputation. Reverend Boynton recounted a recent conversation he had had with one of the oldest and most respected physicians in Minneapolis. The big-city doctor had told the small-town minister that if he ever needed "a difficult operation" he would go to Rochester rather than to Chicago or Philadelphia and would "ask Dr. Mayo (pardon me, not old Doctor Mayo) to hold the knife."[47] Boynton's quip about Will Mayo triggered prolonged applause. The elder Doctor Mayo, now seventy-five years old, sometimes assisted his sons in surgery, but he never operated independently in the hospital.

Reverend Boynton emphasized the interdependence of the Mayo brothers, who operated on patients, and the Franciscan sisters, who operated the hospital that made their surgical practice possible: "Someone has said this evening that St. Mary's Hospital has made the reputation of these men. I said Amen to that, but might there not have been added with equal truth that the skill of these physicians has made the fame of St. Mary's Hospital?"[48] Will Mayo told the well-wishers, "All the credit for the successful treatment of patients at the hospital here, is due to the ministrations of the devoted, skillful Sisters in charge. We are but the Sisters' agents."[49] The symbiotic relationship between the Mayo brothers and the Franciscan sisters would continue to be central to the success of their joint venture, which transformed Rochester into a destination for patients seeking surgical care and cures.

The opening of the hospital addition in 1894 coincided with the advent of newer aseptic techniques and technologies designed to further reduce the risk of infection and death. The Mayo brothers read about these developments and saw surgeons implementing them during their travels to urban hospitals. In 1895, for example, Will Mayo attended a postgraduate course at the Johns Hopkins

Hospital, where he watched surgeons William Halsted and Howard Kelly operate. The huge Baltimore institution, which opened the same year as St. Mary's
Hospital, was been made possible by a Quaker merchant's $3.5 million bequest.[50]
Will's diary documents his impressions of the state-of-the-art system of aseptic
surgery that he observed at Johns Hopkins: "Rubber sole shoes. Operating suits.
Iodoform, Boric Acid & Bismuth. Sterilize by steam. Circle tables for instrument trays. Rubber gloves. Mattress stitch. Subcuticular stitch."[51]

Will and Charlie Mayo helped pay for the aseptic surgery apparatus that was
installed in the new operating rooms that were part of the addition to St. Mary's
Hospital. The institution's 1894 annual report boasted that they were equipped
with white enameled iron operating and dressing tables, sterilizers, and instrument cases. Tables of surgical statistics were supplemented by statements about
postoperative care. One goal of these annual reports was to assure referring
physicians that their patients would receive excellent care at St. Mary's. Thanks
to new technology, a sister-nurse was never far away from her patients: "An
important feature of the hospital is its electrical annunciator system, connected
with all the beds, by means of which patients are at all times in direct communication with the nurses."[52] This was reassuring to patients who were used to being
cared for at home, surrounded by family and friends. The sisters sought to blend
hominess with modernity at St. Mary's Hospital (Figure 1.3).

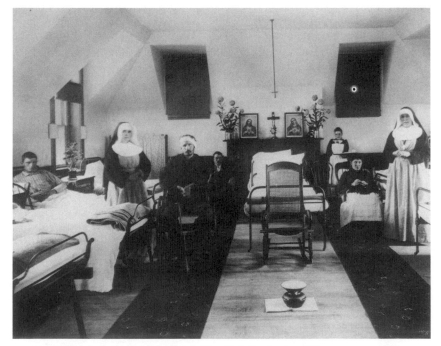

FIGURE 1.3 *Ten-bed ward at St. Mary's Hospital, Rochester, Minnesota, ca. 1890.*
Used with permission of Mayo Foundation.

Doctors learned about the Mayo brothers' accomplishments through standard professional channels. Participation in local, regional, and national medical societies was an effective way for ambitious doctors to accomplish three goals: listen to presentations to expand their knowledge and learn new techniques; report their personal experiences; and build and maintain social networks. The Southern Minnesota Medical Association was organized in 1892. One of the founders explained that doctors in Rochester and nearby towns thought "it would be a good thing if an organization could be effected which would enable the physicians of the towns along the line of the Winona and St. Peter railroad to get together for the purpose of becoming better acquainted with each other and participating in the presentation of papers."[53] Will, who helped organize the society, was one of five doctors who spoke at the first meeting.

Will Mayo was elected president of the Minnesota State Medical Society in 1894, just eleven years after he received his medical degree. In a commencement address the following year, he urged graduates of the University of Minnesota Medical School to avoid complacency and take "a conscientious interest in the welfare of those who entrust themselves to your care." Will described his philosophy of patient care in this 1895 address to the new Minnesota medical graduates. He stressed the importance of careful physical examinations, and he cautioned against jumping to conclusions. Performing a thorough examination on every patient benefited two individuals: "The mental effect on the patient is good, the practical knowledge to yourself is better."[54] He also argued that repeated examinations would result in fewer unexplained problems. This philosophy was a major factor in the Mayo brothers' decision to begin building a group practice around the turn of the century. It would include doctors who specialized in the diagnosis of disease in order to help the Mayo brothers decide which patients were likely to benefit from surgery.[55]

The Mayos Add Partners Who Focus on Preoperative Diagnosis

Will and Charlie Mayo were committed to becoming specialists in surgery, and their strategy included regular trips to urban hospitals to watch renowned surgeons operate. In terms of travel, they had a distinct advantage over solo practitioners, who lost patients and income when they were away. The Mayo brothers, realizing that they needed help to meet the demand for their services and to achieve their surgical ambitions, decided to bring another doctor into their practice. Rather than recruiting a recent medical graduate, they turned to an experienced and respected local practitioner.

Augustus Stinchfield had practiced in a village fifteen miles from Rochester for almost two decades when the *Rochester Post* reported his return in 1891 from a short postgraduate medical course in Chicago: "It is

gratifying to the people of Eyota to know that they have a physician who
will not permit cobwebs to accumulate on him, but who will keep abreast
of the times."[56] Fifty years old when he joined the Mayo family practice
the following year, Stinchfield was about two decades younger than the
patriarch of the practice and about two decades older than Mayo's sons.
In addition to being experienced, he was popular with his patients—something that mattered to the Mayo brothers as they sought to expand their
surgical practice.[57]

Stinchfield focused on diagnosis after he joined the Mayo practice. His
case notes provide insight into the types of patients he saw and his conclusions. They were very brief (usually five to ten lines) and included just a few
words about the patient's main complaint, current symptoms, past history,
family history, physical findings, diagnosis, and prescriptions. Short notes
were standard at the time because they were created for an individual practitioner's personal use. Doctors did not need to document the care they provided in order to justify a fee.[58]

Stinchfield saw some patients with symptoms of heart disease. Shortly
after he joined the Mayo practice, he recorded a fifty-two-year-old man's case
in telegraphic style: "Sick 10 years. Pain in left chest. Short breath. Can't
work. Nervous. Bowels costive. Old chronic diarrhea. Loud heart murmur.
Cascara at night. Nitro-Glycerine pill after meals 1/50. Urine acid 1015. All
good. Nov. 28th Returned much improved. Continue."[59] Three years later,
Stinchfield saw a fifty-four-year-old man with serious heart disease complicated by a stroke: "Been well until last two years. Began with palpitation of
heart. Had rheumatism about twenty years ago. Difficulty of breathing has
been quite marked. Jan 95 had an aphasia lasting a short time with marked
relief. April had hemiplegia from which he has not fully recovered. Heart
hypertrophied and later dilated." Stinchfield prescribed nitroglycerine and
digitalis, standard cardiac remedies.[60]

The number of patients seeking surgical care from the Mayo brothers
continued to grow after Stinchfield joined their practice. St. Mary's Hospital
witnessed a 50 percent increase in admissions and operations between 1893
and 1895, when Will and Charlie did 762 operations on 640 patients, including 95 intra-abdominal procedures.[61] They added a second diagnostician to
the practice in 1895. Christopher Graham had much more formal education
than the Mayo brothers, holding a bachelor's degree from the University
of Minnesota and veterinary and medical degrees from the University of
Pennsylvania. Although Graham lacked Stinchfield's practical experience,
the 1894 medical graduate was more knowledgeable about newer disease concepts, laboratory tests, and treatment strategies. Moreover, he had served as
the first intern at St. Mary's Hospital in 1894. Another thing distinguished
Graham from other potential partners—he was a relative. His sister Edith,
the Mayo's nurse, had recently married Charlie.[62]

During the late 1890s, Will and Charlie relied increasingly on Stinchfield and Graham to see new patients. After these diagnosticians completed their initial evaluation, one of the Mayo brothers saw each patient to make a final decision regarding surgery. Will wrote about reducing the risks of elective operations in 1897. Citing the problem of missed diagnoses, such as acute bronchitis or chronic kidney disease, he emphasized that it did not matter if an operation was successful if the patient died during recovery from a problem unrelated to the surgery. Will explained that "unfortunate experience[s] of this character, days of anxiety, and final disappointments" had convinced him "of the absolute necessity of a more thorough preliminary examination." Specific goals included "fitting the operation to the patient" and being sure not to overlook contraindications.[63] This pragmatic approach contributed to the Mayo brothers' low surgical mortality rates.

Will and Charlie Mayo (Figure 1.4) had established reputations as surgeons by the beginning of the twentieth century, when fewer than 2 percent of US doctors were identified with that specialty.[64] Word continued to spread about the brothers' superior surgical skills and the sisters' compassionate care—provided to all, regardless of religion or financial resources. Men and women traveled to Rochester from ever greater distances as train

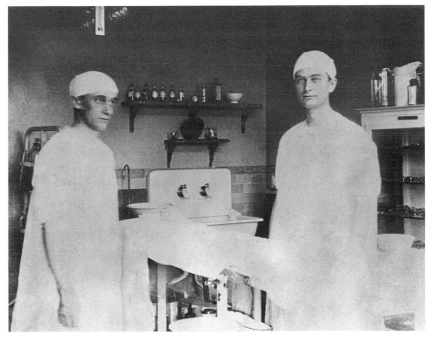

FIGURE 1.4 *Charles H. (Charlie) Mayo and William J. (Will) Mayo in an operating room at St. Mary's Hospital, Rochester, Minnesota, ca. 1895.*
Used with permission of Mayo Foundation.

tracks fanned out across the continent, linking cities, small towns, and villages.[65]

Growing and Restructuring the Mayo Outpatient Practice

Between 1895 and 1905, the Mayo practice would add almost a dozen doctors, mainly to increase its capacity for evaluating new patients. Meanwhile, a new specialty—internal medicine—was beginning to gain momentum in large cities and leading medical schools. Doctors who identified with internal medicine focused on medical diagnosis and non-surgical treatment. William Osler, one of the specialty's pioneers and physician-in-chief of the Johns Hopkins Hospital, had difficulty defining its boundaries. In an 1897 address on internal medicine as a vocation, he tried to explain what it was by saying what it was not. It was the "wide field of medical practice which remains after the separation of surgery, midwifery, and gynecology."[66]

Christopher Graham functioned as the Mayo practice's first internal medicine specialist (internist). The second one, Henry Plummer, would play a key role in expanding the diagnostic arm of the practice after he was hired in 1901. Plummer had grown up in a village twenty miles south of Rochester, where his father was a successful general practitioner. After two years of college at the University of Minnesota, he entered Northwestern University Medical School in 1894.[67] Plummer's professor of medicine, Frank Billings, was a pioneering Chicago internist who had equipped his office with new diagnostic technologies, such as bacteriological apparatus, to differentiate himself from the city's general practitioners.

Frank Billings spoke on the relationship of general practice to the specialties in 1898, the year Plummer received his medical degree. Themes from this talk would resonate in Rochester a few years later, as the diagnostic part of the Mayo practice grew in size and sophistication. Billings predicted progressive specialization in medicine and surgery, especially in larger cities. The internist warned, however, that excessive specialization might result in a situation where "one finds specialists of the kidneys who do not treat diseases of the cardiovascular system or of the digestive system."[68]

Billings caricatured a situation that some affluent patients confronted when they saw a cadre of specialists: "It is not unusual to find an invalid whose suffering depends upon one principal thing visiting an oculist, a stomach specialist, a dermatologist, a urinalysist and several other specialists, at one and the same time, acting independently of one another, while the family physician, the general man of the constellation stands by as umpire, occasionally throwing in an anti-constipation pill."[69] Billings also thought that medical students should be taught to think of the specialties as secondary to general medicine and surgery. The question of how an ever-expanding number of specialties should interrelate would continue to generate controversy in the United States.[70] In Rochester, Henry Plummer would help the Mayo brothers coordinate the introduction of specialties and the rules that governed the doctors who practiced them.

Plummer joined his father's rural practice after he graduated from medical school in 1898. Sickness and serendipity brought the young doctor and Will Mayo together two years later. Henry's father had asked the Rochester surgeon to accompany him to a patient's home to provide a consultation. When Mayo arrived, the senior Doctor Plummer was ill, so he sent his son along. Years later, Will recalled spending two hours in a carriage with the twenty-six-year-old doctor. The patient was thought to have a blood disease, and Mayo was very impressed by young Plummer's knowledge about this type of disorder.[71]

Will Mayo was not especially interested in blood diseases, but he knew that they sometimes made surgery riskier. In 1897 he had predicted that "blood study as a part of the preliminary examination of surgical cases will soon be as common as examination of the urine."[72] Surgeons saw blood all the time, but they were now urged to pay attention to its invisible attributes. In addition to a microscope, this required a growing number of laboratory tests that could help make a diagnosis or assess a patient's operative risk. Hiring Henry Plummer was also a business decision. Will told his brother that the new doctor would help the practice see more patients and update its laboratory procedures.[73]

Plummer joined the firm known as "Drs. Mayo, Stinchfield, and Graham" in 1901, the same year the doctors moved their offices into the first floor of the Masonic Temple building. Their office practice was located in the center of Rochester, about a mile from St. Mary's Hospital, which was on the edge of town. The group's custom-designed space included offices, examination rooms, a clinical laboratory, and a darkroom for an X-ray machine. When patients entered the office, they saw modern medicine in action as diagnosticians used various technologies to examine them and their bodily fluids. Plummer introduced new laboratory tests and ran the X-ray apparatus that the Mayos had purchased in 1900. (Previously, independent Rochester practitioner Grosvenor Cross had taken X-rays for them.) X-ray machines produced still pictures as well as fluoroscopic images that revealed the motion of a patient's heart, lungs, and other internal organs. This remarkable technology, which rendered clothing, skin, and soft tissues transparent, mesmerized the public and the medical profession.[74]

Philadelphia surgeon William Keen, who wrote early and often about the new surgery, summarized his experience with X-rays just three months after German physicist Wilhelm Röntgen reported their discovery in December 1895. Emphasizing their value in surgical diagnosis, Keen predicted that improvements in the technology would make X-rays even more useful to doctors.[75] Charlie Mayo published a case report in January 1897 that described their role in a surgical success story. He asked Doctor Cross to X-ray a three-year-old boy's chest in order to see a belt buckle he had swallowed.

Charlie used the image to plan an operation. The child did well, and Mayo reported the case to demonstrate the usefulness of X-rays in surgery.[76]

The Mayo Brothers' Reputations and Distinctive Personalities

Building a successful surgical practice required more than technologies. Regional general practitioners had to perceive the Mayo brothers more as collaborators than competitors. And patients had to be willing to travel to Rochester for care. Both things happened. As the Mayo brothers built their surgical practice at St. Mary's Hospital during the 1890s, they traveled farther and more often to participate in medical meetings. They also became better known to the profession through a steady stream of journal articles; more than seventy-five papers appeared during the decade. By 1900, they were recognized nationally because they performed so many major operations with so few deaths. More and more doctors traveled to Rochester to watch them operate. Stories of what the visitors saw—circulated by word of mouth and published in medical journals—accelerated the growth of the Mayo practice in the new century.

Patients, visiting physicians, and almost everyone else who interacted with the Mayo brothers noticed how different they were in many respects. Will Mayo, four years older than Charlie, was always the dominant figure in their family and in the group practice they established.[77] Harry Harwick, their long-time business manager, characterized him as the group's mastermind and visionary leader. Will's colleagues called him "Chief" to acknowledge his dominant position. Some visiting doctors compared him to J. Pierpont Morgan, Theodore Roosevelt, and other powerful and influential Americans of the Progressive Era. Harwick, like others who knew Will and Charlie very well, was impressed by the brothers' devotion to one another.[78] Charlie's son Charles W. (Chuck) Mayo, who later would join the practice as a surgeon, described his uncle as a man with "an aristocratic face and the bearing of a general." He explained that Will spoke distinctly and dressed impeccably, whereas his father "mumbled and drawled his words" and "could look disheveled in a freshly-pressed suit."[79]

Will's demeanor and attitudes influenced the Mayo Clinic's atmosphere. Harwick explained: "Professional dignity was a religion with Dr. Will. If he saw a young man without clean linen, or unshaved, without his shoes shined, or in any sort of unconventional clothing, or showing facetiousness toward a patient he would call him in and talk to him."[80] William Braasch, a surgeon who joined the Mayo practice in 1907, recalled that all staff members were expected to conduct themselves in ways that "conformed to his ideas of decency, decorum, and dignity." The contrast between Will's formality and his brother's informality was striking. Braasch described Charlie as being humorous, with an engaging "homespun manner of speaking."[81] By the dawn of the twentieth century, Will and Charlie Mayo, with their complementary surgical skills and personalities, were eager to expand their practice and their influence in medical circles.

The Mayos' Invention of Multispecialty Group Practice

The Mayo brothers' surgical practice was already very large by 1900, and it continued to grow rapidly. Their excellent surgical outcomes were the result of accurate preoperative diagnosis, strict adherence to antiseptic and aseptic techniques, manual dexterity, a small, established team of operating room assistants, enormous experience, and expert postoperative care provided by the sister-nurses. Trains arrived in Rochester full of patients who were seeking surgery or a second opinion. They also contained doctors who wanted to see how Will and Charlie Mayo performed so many major operations with so few deaths. Canadian physician Ernest Hall coined the phrase "The Clinic in the Cornfields" in 1906 to describe what he had found in a small Minnesota town surrounded by farms. He considered the Mayo practice to be "the most unique, elaborate and scientific clinic in the history of medicine."[1] Many visiting doctors used superlatives in their published accounts, which detailed key features of the emerging group practice.

The trend toward specialization in diagnosis and treatment accelerated in the early twentieth century. In this context, the Mayo brothers took advantage of their fame and fortunes to invent and invest in the multispecialty group practice model of surgical and medical care. To expand the scope of the services they provided to patients and referring physicians, they kept adding doctors who devoted their time to diagnosis.

The Mayo Brothers Achieve International Reputations

St. Mary's Hospital had been open little more than a decade in 1902, when Chicago surgeon Albert Ochsner told a group of Minneapolis doctors: "Several years ago I visited the medical Mecca of Southern Minnesota, and found Dr. [Will] Mayo busily engaged in removing gall-stones from many patients."[2] Several doctors would use the Mecca metaphor to describe a phenomenon that was unique in the history of American medicine. Nicholas Senn, another Chicago surgeon, published a series of reports of his visits to hospitals in several countries. "The Mayo Brothers at Rochester control the lion's share of the surgery of the west," he wrote in 1904. "Their hospital in the little prairie city of not more than 5,000 inhabitants has become a Mecca for surgeons not only from this country but from abroad. There is no other hospital on this side of the Atlantic in which so many important operations are performed daily."[3]

The annual reports of St. Mary's Hospital documented the size, scope, and safety of the Mayo brothers' surgical practice. In 1903, for example, Will and Charlie performed 2,640 operations (including 1,302 intra-abdominal procedures) on 2,300 patients. The number of patients who died (69) was remarkably low, and 84 percent of those who died had undergone abdominal operations, acknowledged as a risky type of surgery.[4]

Experienced and aspiring surgeons visited Rochester to watch the Mayo brothers operate and to learn how they did so much surgery with such excellent results. The Society of Clinical Surgery was formed in 1903 to encourage group excursions by its members to observe prominent surgeons perform operations in their own hospitals rather than listen to them lecture at meetings. Will Mayo had discussed creating such a society with Chicago surgeon Albert Ochsner and Johns Hopkins surgeon Harvey Cushing three years earlier, when they were attending the International Medical Society Congress in Paris. Cushing recalled that they were "completely fed up with listening to a succession of papers presented in polyglot we could ill understand."[5] The new society got off to a good start, holding four meetings (in Baltimore, New York, Cleveland, and Boston) before going to Chicago and Rochester in 1905.

After the special two-city meeting, Cushing informed his physician-father: "I did not come away [from Chicago] with a very high opinion of their work particularly as regards their thoroughness. They seem to bite off more than they can chew—a penalty of having too much business possibly. Rochester on the other hand had no defects, at least none apparent on one short visit and of course their best foot was forward." Cushing concluded that the Mayo brothers "have built up a wonderful operative clinic and are well protected by an able staff of internists, specialists, etc. and are little likely to make mistakes.... They do as good and as much surgery in their own particular lines as any other two men in the world." The Johns Hopkins surgeon declared that Rochester "has become worthily quite a Mecca for medical men."[6] Will and Charlie Mayo had accomplished this in less than two decades since they began operating at St. Mary's Hospital (see Figure 2.1).

Cushing described one end of the surgical spectrum—very experienced surgeons operating in well-equipped hospitals—but most patients undergoing surgery in the early twentieth century had a different experience. The

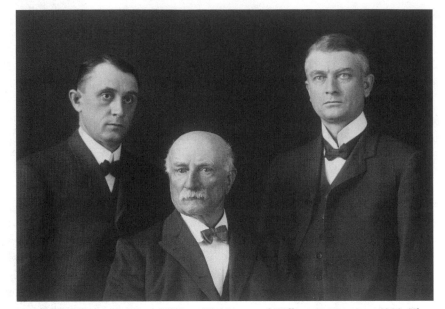

FIGURE 2.1 *Charles H. Mayo, William W. Mayo, and William J. Mayo, ca. 1900. The*
men were standing, which illustrates why W. W. Mayo was sometimes referred to as the
"Little Doctor."
Used with permission of Mayo Foundation.

number of operations skyrocketed as more and more general practitioners
began performing surgery in small hospitals that were springing up in towns
and cities across America. Richard Beard, a Minneapolis physician and
physiology professor at the University of Minnesota Medical School, discussed the implications of the phenomenon in 1905. The sudden expansion of
surgery's boundaries and the potential for high fees had resulted in the field
being "invaded by a great army of operators who are not surgeons." Beard
claimed that doctors were not the only ones alarmed by the situation: "The
public is growing as fearsome of the ready and familiar knife of the modern operator as it was of the slow, reluctant, and stranger instrument of his
fathers."[7] A few months later, a popular periodical delivered the same disturbing message.

In 1905 *McClure's Magazine* published an article entitled "Scientific
Surgery" in which journalist Samuel Hopkins Adams contrasted the present
and recent past. With a circulation of 400,000, the illustrated monthly reached
a large number of potential patients. "Of the major operations now fearlessly
undertaken every day," Adams declared, "ninety percent would have been
considered by the surgeon of the last generation extremely hazardous, if not
actually murderous."[8] This sudden shift was due mainly to the introduction
of aseptic surgical techniques that reduced the risk of postoperative infection

and death. But, Adams warned, "[u]nbridled enthusiasm for the new worlds thrown open to their conquering progress carried the great body of surgeons too far. They operated wherever operation was remotely indicated and, in many cases, where it wasn't indicated at all."[9] When Adams made this pronouncement, he was one of America's most prolific muckrakers—journalists and writers who sought to stimulate cultural changes by exposing greed and deceit in various industries and institutions.[10]

Surgery might harm rather than heal a patient, depending on who did what to whom and where. Adams sounded alarms, but he devoted most of his article to advances that offered patients hope. For example, he listed several procedural innovations and cited the surgeons who had pioneered them. In one part of his article, Adams described the Mayo brothers as "the surgeon's surgeons" and St. Mary's Hospital as "the most remarkable surgical institution of its kind." He remarked that the hospital in the "little city" of Rochester, Minnesota, "handles more surgical cases annually than any institution in the United States, including the great Johns Hopkins Hospital."[11] Data published in the two institutions' annual reports supported his claim, which seemed incredible because Rochester was a town of 7,000 and Baltimore had a population of half a million.[12]

The American Medical Association Showcases Will Mayo

When physicians and the public read about surgical successes in Rochester just after the turn of the century, Will Mayo was scaling organized medicine's highest peak. The forty-five-year-old surgeon became president of the American Medical Association in 1906, and the honor accelerated the growth of the Mayo practice. More than 4,000 doctors who gathered in Boston that year for the association's annual meeting heard him speak on challenges confronting the profession. His presidential address reached the desks of ten times as many physicians when it was published in the *Journal of the American Medical Association.*

In his speech, Will Mayo promoted an educational philosophy that would later be termed "continuing medical education" or "lifelong learning." The small-town surgeon who had achieved international fame argued that medical school graduation was "merely a commencement of a life study of medicine." He also expressed frustration with the lack of educational opportunities for aspiring surgeons: "Young men without special training under competent teachers should not be encouraged in wanton assaults on major surgical diseases unless justified by necessity." Will predicted that "the future will demand schools for advanced training for those who desire to do special work." But in 1906, postgraduate training for most physicians meant brief trips rather than prolonged study. He advised his audience: "The practitioner must make frequent trips away for the purpose of observation. In no other way can he avoid the rut of self-satisfied content, which checks advancement and limits usefulness."[13] Quite a few doctors interpreted Will's remarks as an invitation to visit Rochester.

When Will Mayo's term as American Medical Association president ended in 1907, most doctors in North America knew his name and hundreds rode trains to Rochester each year to watch him and his brother perform surgery. A New York physician described his experience to a group of nurses in 1908. He was impressed by the Mayo brothers' demeanor in the operating room, where they would "talk to the doctors about them in an easy, friendly way, always ready, even anxious, to impart knowledge, but never showing egotism or assuming superiority." Instead of "operating to the gallery," they exhibited concern for "the patient's best good." In Rochester, the patient, rather than a performing surgeon, was the center of attention.[14] A South Carolina doctor reported that there was "no hurry about anything during an operation" and emphasized that procedures were performed quietly with "the precision of clock-work."[15] The operations may have been unhurried, but the Mayo brothers certainly did a lot of them. Another surgeon marveled that he saw 104 operations performed during a six-day visit in 1906.[16]

Professional visitors, many of whom had attended surgical teaching sessions in large amphitheaters in urban hospitals, were impressed by the intimacy of the operating rooms at St. Mary's Hospital. Rutherford Gradwohl of St. Louis described these extremes in 1908: "The onlooker at most surgical clinics has a beautiful view of the tops of the heads of the assistants and occasionally sees a bloody sponge or a gaping wound, but he seldom really sees the various steps of an operative procedure." The situation was different at St. Mary's, where "each brother has but one assistant or actual helper." A second assistant or nurse stood back, stepping forward to exchange instruments, provide sutures, or perform another specific task. Gradwohl concluded that the Mayo brothers "have apparently found that one highly-trained assistant is better than a half-dozen poorly trained ones."[17] In fact, Sister Joseph had been Will's first assistant in surgery for fifteen years when a Canadian doctor described her as "so proficient that when he stops operating to talk to the doctors the sister goes on with the operation, half unconsciously perhaps."[18]

The turnover of assistants typical of teaching hospitals did not take place at St. Mary's, where staff stability contributed to superior surgical results. In 1904 a Chicago doctor complained to members of the American Surgical Association about the challenges of working with rotating residents: "We have a different set of assistants at the end of every three months, and by the time one set is broken in, so to speak, they have to give way to another."[19] There were only two interns and two residents at St. Mary's Hospital at this time, and their main responsibility was postoperative care. Fifteen years after the hospital opened, Will and Charlie were still the only surgeons on its staff. Moreover, every other member of the professional staff was part of the Mayo practice.[20]

Visiting Doctors Marvel at the Mayo System of Diagnosis

"Patients operated on by the Mayos scarcely ever die," declared a St. Louis surgeon after a 1906 trip to Rochester. Augustus Bernays attributed the Mayo brothers' low mortality rates to their surgical skills and to the fact that they had "learned to select their cases and not operate unless they see a fair chance of success." Their patients also benefited from a "more scientific [pre] operative examination and diagnosis than at any other place in America."[21] Preoperative diagnosis was a vital part of the brothers' surgical practice. When they added physicians to meet patient demand, Will and Charlie chose individuals with interests and skills that augmented their integrated program of preoperative diagnosis and surgical treatment.

Most doctors who described their visits to Rochester during the first decade of the twentieth century emphasized what they observed in the operating rooms, but some wove non-surgical strands into their stories. For example, Rutherford Gradwohl explained that all new patients were examined by "special diagnosticians." This division of labor allowed the Mayo brothers to spend most of their time operating while each patient got "a close, careful and exhaustive examination at the hands of men specially trained for their work."[22] These evaluations could be exhausting for patients, who usually spent several days undergoing a series of tests. In 1909 a South Carolina doctor described the detailed diagnostic process that Christopher Graham supervised:

> He and his immediate assistants pass upon the circulatory system, lungs, nervous system, digestive apparatus, etc., all of which is noted upon the history blank and then the patient is passed on perchance to the eye man, or the nose and throat man, or to the cystoscopist; or maybe he must be subjected to the X-ray, or the medical chemist must examine his urine, his stomach contents, or his feces; or the pathologist and bacteriologist must pass upon his blood or sputum, until the patient is thoroughly gone over and, by exclusion or otherwise, a positive or tentative diagnosis is made.[23]

This rigorous system of diagnosis was just one element that impressed Canadian physician Ernest Hall, who used a mechanical-military metaphor to describe the efficiency and effectiveness of the care he observed: "All parts of this vast Mayo machine move with the regularity and precision of well-disciplined troops."[24]

Patients sensed that they were in a special place when they arrived in Rochester, and their postcards to family and friends provide candid snapshots of their impressions and experiences. In 1909 a woman told a friend in Iowa: "I came up last Wed. but can't get into the hospital before a week yet. Everyone is so *nice*. I have been examined and they say appendix & perhaps gall stones. They'll see when they take the appendix out. But I don't dread it much. The Drs. are so far ahead of them there that it don't amount to much. They take from 4 to 6 minutes to operate for appendix alone."[25] This woman's comments reflected the perception that patients who had surgery in Rochester did well. Physicians read published reports that confirmed this impression. The year the woman's postcard traveled across the state line, more than 7,000 operations were performed at St. Mary's Hospital, and almost 20 percent were associated with a diagnosis of appendicitis. Every patient with chronic appendicitis survived, and less than 1 percent of 524 patients operated on for acute or so-called suppurative appendicitis died.[26]

The delay in hospital admission that the woman awaiting surgery described was not unusual. Crowded waiting rooms and congested operating schedules were the norm in the Mayo practice. Patients often waited days to complete their diagnostic evaluation and even longer to be admitted to St. Mary's if surgery was recommended. One reason was that there were no scheduled appointments. A patient named Ollie informed a friend in Iowa in 1909, "I was examined again yesterday by Dr. Mayo. He said the same thing as the other one." Next came news of the delay. "I hate to wait so long but it can't be helped. There were over one hundred in the office at one time. There are 150 beds at the hospital and all full."[27] No one could claim that this part of a patient's experience was efficient. But many patients and visitors applauded the methodical evaluations. In an attempt to meet patient demand, the Mayo practice kept adding doctors and office space. The Franciscan sisters approved an addition to St. Mary's Hospital in 1909 that increased its capacity to 280 beds. Reflecting the nature of the Mayo practice, their institution was devoted exclusively to surgery. Almost five thousand patients were admitted that year, and all but four had an operation.[28]

Group Practice as a Model to Coordinate Specialty Care

The main purpose of the Mayo's office-based practice was to decide whether a patient was likely to benefit from an operation. This decision was made jointly by one or more diagnosticians and a surgeon. Individuals thought not to need surgery were sent back to their hometown doctors for ongoing care. In 1908 Chicago physician Wallace Abbott attributed the "remarkable success" of the Mayo practice "to the wonderful organization of its clinical and diagnostic staff." For patients, this meant that "guesswork is eliminated so far as this is possible, *before* the operation instead of *after* it. In other words this institution is a triumph of co-operation." He thought that the Mayo model of care should be replicated in other contexts: "What this group of physicians has succeeded in doing by working together to a common end, other physicians can do, even on a smaller scale." Abbott argued that the profession must acknowledge the merits of "medical partnership."[29] Two years earlier, Canadian physician Ernest Hall had pinpointed and promoted the main organizing principle that differentiated the Mayo practice from all others: "Specialization and cooperation, with the best that can be had in each department, is here the motto. Cannot these principles be tried elsewhere?"[30]

In 1910 Will Mayo delivered a commencement address at Chicago's Rush Medical College in which he discussed factors that contributed to the trend toward specialization. He also promoted group practice as a way to provide coordinated patient-centered care:

> The sum-total of medical knowledge is now so great…that it would be futile for one man to attempt to acquire…a good working knowledge of any large part of the whole. The very necessities of the case are driving practitioners into cooperation. The best interest of the patient is the only interest to be considered, and in order that the sick may have the benefit of advancing knowledge, union of forces is necessary. The first effort made to meet the situation was in the development of clinical specialties. Man was divided for treatment into parts, as a wagon is divided in the process of manufacture. Each part of man was assigned to those who could devote special attention to their particular portion, giving the benefit of superior skill in treatment. Unlike a wagon, man could not be treated in parts, but only as a whole…[so] it became necessary to develop medicine as a cooperative science; the clinician, the specialist, and the laboratory workers uniting for the good of the patient, each assisting in the elucidation of the problem at hand, and each dependent upon the other for support.[31]

Will told the new medical graduates that this patient care model need not be confined to big cities. Even a country doctor "must be allied with a group of associated workers and no longer thrown upon his own resources." Technologies, some of them new, were spreading and could help connect doctors at a distance: "By means of the rural free delivery, telephone, automobile, trolley, and steam-lines, quick communication will aid the new order of things and help make possible such association."[32] Augustus Bernays of St. Louis, who portrayed the Mayo brothers as group practice pioneers, argued in 1906: "We can have nothing but pity and sympathy for our poor colleague who, be it in the country or in a city, practices medicine or surgery on his own hook. He, poor soul, is consequently obliged to keep up the appearance of knowing it all to the public."[33]

Specialization and cooperation, which Ernest Hall had praised when he visited Rochester in 1906, would be the centerpiece of the group practice model that the Mayo brothers and their first partners were inventing. Many visiting physicians considered the small Minnesota town an unlikely place for such a successful surgical practice, but Rochester offered some advantages. Specialization was an urban phenomenon because large cities provided the critical mass of patients necessary to develop a practice that focused on an organ system or a disease. On the other hand, big cities encouraged competition rather than cooperation. Baltimore physician Daniel Cathell had published a book when Will Mayo was in medical school that gave doctors advice about how to build and maintain a successful practice. The 1903 edition, revised by his son, explained that the "constant and sharp rivalry" among physicians in many contexts was due to the fact that "the demand for medical and surgical services is limited."[34] On the other hand, the demand for these services seemed almost limitless in Rochester.

Chicago ophthalmologist Casey Wood wrote an article in 1909 on the advantages and disadvantages of cooperative practice and business partnerships among physicians. He argued that teamwork was much better than "undisciplined play" and that partnerships benefited patients, physicians, and the community. Patients received better care when "a number of specialists" worked together. Wood used an example that physicians surely understood to suggest how they could benefit from cooperative practice. A doctor could "take a vacation without feeling that his practice is not being properly attended to or, worse than all horrors, falling into the hands of that dreadful competitor in the next block."[35] Physicians competed for patients in most contexts, and many of them struggled financially.[36] Members of the Mayo practice cooperated, and the group thrived.

Some Physicians Express Frustration About High Surgical Fees

Tensions surrounding doctors' fees were chronic, but the problem became acute after the advent of the so-called new surgery. Although many general practitioners did some surgery, very few attempted complex operations—especially intra-abdominal procedures. A doctor from a rural community near Rochester explained in 1900 that a surgeon who operated inside a patient's abdomen "gets the credit for doing a brilliant thing and pockets a generous fee." Then he complained: "In the quiet room of some patient ill with typhoid fever, in the lying-in-room or even at his office the general practitioner does work requiring perhaps a greater profundity of thought, brilliancy of mind or the use of a much larger amount of gray matter. He gets a nominal fee and a proportionate amount of credit."[37]

A committee of the South Dakota Medical Association published a list of recommended fees in 1908. The suggested charge for an office visit was one dollar, whereas charges for operations (especially major ones) were much higher. For example, the fee for removing a prostate gland was $100, and the fee for removing a uterus or operating on a kidney was $150. The article included a disclaimer: "These are all minimum charges. You are at liberty to go as much higher as you like."[38] For most doctors though, the issue was not how much to charge a patient; it was how much he or she could afford to pay.

America's leading surgeons attracted wealthy patients seeking expert care for serious and life-threatening illnesses, and many of them charged fees based on an individual's ability to pay. One extreme example involved William Halsted, the chief of surgery at Johns Hopkins, who charged a wealthy Cleveland industrialist $10,000 for a gall bladder operation in 1900. He added $1,000 because he spent the first night after surgery at the hospital rather than sleeping at home. In current dollars, Halsted's fee was about $270,000 for the case.[39] This type of surgery was one of the most common procedures the Mayo brothers performed. They did 1,000 operations for gall bladder disease between June 1891 and the end of 1904.[40] But most of their patients were ordinary citizens rather than prominent capitalists.

The Mayo brothers did attract wealthy patients from across the continent and beyond, especially after Will was president of the American Medical Association. "Speculation is rife among the doctors as to the amount of the Mayos' income," wrote one visiting surgeon in 1906, who concluded that "it must be very large."[41] Will and Charlie would exhibit their wealth by building large homes and spending in other ways that reflected personal success. But they also used a significant portion of their incomes to subsidize the care of poor patients, the salaries of staff, the construction of facilities, and the acquisition of equipment (some of which was placed in St. Mary's Hospital).

Doctors Visit to Satisfy their Curiosity and to Get Care

New York physician James Walsh told Will Mayo in 1910, "I am not at all interested in surgery, but I am very much interested in the history of medicine." Walsh, whose recent book *Makers of Modern Medicine* dealt with the eighteenth and nineteenth centuries, thought that twentieth-century medical history was being made in Rochester. Amazed that America's "best surgical clinic" was in such a small town, he wanted to see it for himself.[42] Walsh published his perceptions of the Mayo practice shortly after returning to New York City. Noting the profession's fascination with what took place at St. Mary's, he remarked that there were thousands of American hospitals that were "of absolutely no interest to any except townspeople and to some medical statisticians."[43]

Discussing the social aspects of what he saw during his visit, Walsh considered the relations between patients and doctors in Rochester "in many ways ideal." The philosophy about fees surprised him: "Poor or rich, they are all examined thoroughly, their cases carefully studied, their conditions elucidated just as far as possible, and the suggestions as to the treatment necessary made." The fee scale was based on a patient's ability to pay. "While handsome fees are collected from the rich, no one is turned away because of poverty." Most of the patients in Rochester were from Minnesota and neighboring states, and many were farmers. But Walsh was impressed that physicians and wealthy patients came "from all over the country" to see or to seek surgery.[44]

Prominent surgeons also got sick, and some joined the throngs of patients traveling to Rochester for treatment. Published accounts describe the circumstances surrounding operations that Will Mayo performed on two world-renowned doctors. In 1910 Philadelphia surgeon William W. Keen considered the history of his own illness so instructive that he asked Will to allow visiting surgeons to watch his operation.[45] Keen had developed persistent diarrhea while vacationing in Rhode Island and had sought medical attention before a planned trip to Europe. He traveled to Boston to see Reginald Fitz and to New York City to see Edward Janeway. Unimpressed with those experiences, Keen explained, "Neither of them made a physical examination but both prescribed medicines, which I took without benefit."[46] These doctors were not ordinary practitioners. Fitz was a prominent Boston internist and Harvard professor who had recommended early surgery in patients with symptoms suggesting appendicitis, a term he had coined. Janeway, one New York's leading internists, was a recent president of the Association of American Physicians.

William Keen's symptoms persisted while he was in Europe, and he sought additional opinions. George Gibson, one of Scotland's leading internists, examined him and discovered a mass in his lower left abdomen. Keen also saw London internist William Hale-White, who examined his colon with a sigmoidoscope. Hale-White concluded that the prominent American surgeon had "an inoperable cancer of the bowel," but he did not share his impression with his patient. Keen subsequently saw a surgeon in Berlin, who told him that the abdominal mass was probably malignant. Right after this consultation, Keen wrote to Will Mayo, "asking for an exploratory operation as soon as I could get to Rochester." The Philadelphia surgeon crossed the Atlantic and bypassed every major East Coast and Midwest medical center. Two days after reaching Rochester in November 1910, he had surgery. Finally, there was good news. The mass was due to inflammation; it was diverticulitis, not cancer. Keen explained, "I left the hospital in three weeks and have been entirely well since. As the tumor was not malignant, there is no fear of its return."[47] He lived for three decades after some doctors concluded that he had incurable cancer.

Will Mayo operated on the gynecologist-in-chief of the Johns Hopkins Hospital in 1911. Howard Kelly thought he had gall bladder disease and wanted an operation, but his surgical colleagues William Halsted and John Finney were away. Kelly's protégé Thomas Cullen was unwilling to operate on his friend, but he accompanied him on the train trip to Rochester.[48] The English-speaking world's leading internist William Osler, now the Regius Professor of Medicine at Oxford University, reassured his former Johns Hopkins colleague, "The Mayos have great success with their professional brethren."[49] Osler meant what he said. In a 1909 talk, he boasted that the brothers had built up "one of the largest and in some respects the most important surgical clinic in the world."[50] While recuperating after surgery, Kelly confided in his diary: "Will Mayo told me he informed any inquirers that I came here because of the season and that my Baltimore colleagues were away. I told him . . . that he was my preference under all circumstances."[51] Newspaper reports of national leaders in medicine, politics, and business having operations in Rochester sent a message to patients who led ordinary lives.

The Mayo brothers' surgical outcomes were usually excellent, but this was not always the case. A well-known Minnesotan had four operations in Rochester over a dozen-year period.[52] John Johnson was a newspaper editor and aspiring politician when Will removed his appendix in 1897. Two subsequent surgeries went well. Johnson was in his third term as governor (and a potential presidential candidate) when he had a fourth operation in September 1909, following months of episodic abdominal pain. Visiting doctors watched Will and Charlie struggle to get their patient through a long and complex operation for intestinal obstruction caused by adhesions. The governor's death six days after surgery sent a shock through the state and the nation. He was among the 1.7 percent of patients who died after undergoing abdominal surgery at St. Mary's Hospital in 1909, when 3,746 operations of that type were performed there.[53] Still, these odds of survival after surgery were very favorable, and more and more patients came to Rochester.

Planning and Constructing a Very Large Outpatient Building

The Mayos hired doctors and staff at an accelerating rate during the first decade of the twentieth century to meet growing patient demand and to incorporate new diagnostic technologies and techniques into their practice. One hundred and ten doctors and non-physician staff were scattered in several downtown Rochester locations in the fall of 1912, when the cornerstone of a new building was laid.[54] Internist Henry Plummer, who had joined the Mayo practice eleven years earlier, developed a detailed floor plan for the structure with the St. Paul architectural firm of Ellerbe and Round. The five-story building would include more than thirty combination office-examination rooms and dozens of rooms for laboratories and for special examinations.

The new building would also contain space for the practice's expanding academic infrastructure. Plummer's plan for the third floor included a large library and reading room, a studio for medical artists, and two editorial offices. Will Mayo informed Johns Hopkins medical illustrator Max Brödel in 1913: "We are putting up a new building which will contain our offices, X-ray, blood, chemical and clinical laboratories and all of our work for expert examinations, and on the roof we shall have the quarters for the animal experimentation which we have been carrying on for about three years." Turning from facilities to people, he boasted, "The best of it is that we have a large number of clever young men who are turning out good work not only in surgery but in the other departments."[55]

Evidence of the good work that Will mentioned was appearing in a wide range of regional and national medical journals. But these articles were scattered, so the Mayo brothers arranged for W. B. Saunders, a prominent Philadelphia medical publishing firm, to produce annual compilations of them. The first volume, *Collected Papers by the Staff of St. Mary's Hospital, Mayo Clinic* (hereafter *Collected Papers*) was published in 1911. It contained articles coauthored by twenty staff members and illustrations by Dorothy Peters and Eleanora Fry, medical artists who had studied with Max Brödel in Baltimore.[56] Having artists produce stunning illustrations to accompany articles written by Mayo staff members was part of a strategy to showcase the group's contributions to knowledge and practice.

Articles conveyed information and established academic reputations. The Mayo brothers wanted to ensure that their group's publications were well written. Maud Mellish was editing the writings of Chicago surgeon Albert Ochsner when Will offered her a job as a medical librarian and editor in 1907: "Dr. Charles and I . . . want you, and want you badly, and the sooner the better." Mellish, who accepted their offer of a permanent position to "run the literary end of the business," would play a major role in helping to enhance the institution's academic image.[57] Harold Foss, who started his surgical training in 1913, told Will three years later: "I followed your suggestion and wove a paper about the material I gathered in connection with the errors in surgical diagnosis. . . . I sent a copy to Mrs. Mellish for her blue pencil and scissors and I trust, after sufficient censoring, she will think it worth printing with the papers of the Mayo Clinic."[58]

The *Collected Papers* series included a retrospective two-volume compilation of almost 150 articles that Will and Charlie had published between 1884 and 1909. A reviewer in the *Bulletin of the Johns Hopkins Hospital* proclaimed in 1912 that the thick books provided "splendid evidence of the constant activity, thoughtfulness and broad interest of these most remarkable men, who in their joint work, remind one somewhat of the Wright brothers, devoted to each other, and working with the highest of principles."[59] This analogy resonated with readers because of the rapid development of aviation that had followed the Wright brothers' first successful flight a decade earlier.

The "Mayo Clinic" Building: A Showcase for Group Practice

On March 6, 1914, more than fifteen hundred individuals attended the opening of the large new building (Figure 2.2) that symbolized the Mayo brothers' success as surgeons and showcased their homegrown multispecialty group practice. Richard Beard of the University of Minnesota described the structure in a long article that included several photographs of interior spaces and floor plans depicting more than 300 rooms. Beard boasted that the Mayo Clinic building "as a work of art, science, and service, is as complete as anything that modern medicine has yet achieved."[60]

The structure reflected Henry Plummer's desire to organize the outpatient diagnostic portion of the practice as well as his passion for technology.

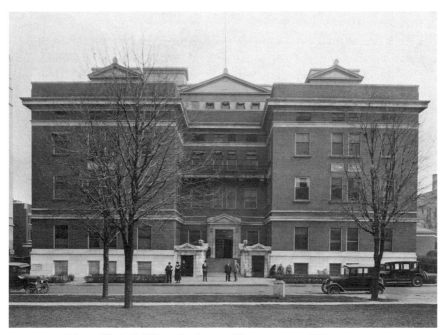

FIGURE 2.2 *Mayo Clinic Building, Rochester, Minnesota, ca. 1925.*
Used with permission of Mayo Foundation.

A newspaper reporter emphasized that electricity played a major part "in making this building unusual," but he concluded that "an adequate description would be too technical for the casual reader."[61] Will Mayo was not a casual reader, but he could not comprehend some of the technologies that Plummer had incorporated into the structure. Frederic Washburn, the administrator of Boston's Massachusetts General Hospital, had requested details about the building's signal system, which was designed to indicate when a patient was ready to be examined and whether a physician was in the room. At Will's request, Plummer replied to Washburn's letter: "I regret to say that it is too complicated for me to write you regarding it at the present time. I would gladly do so if I had the time at my disposal."[62]

Washburn, frustrated by Plummer's curt response, complained to Will, who replied: "I very much regret the letter Dr. Plummer sent to you and my only explanation is that he is a genius with the usual eccentricities. We are so used to it here that we take no notice, but not knowing, I don't wonder that you were a little disturbed." Pivoting from apology to technology, Will mentioned Plummer's design for the telephone system. "The General Electric Company at first stated his ideas could not be carried out, but finally he convinced them by a very elaborate series of plans and drawings, which appeared so complex that I refused to inspect them. Frankly, they made me dizzy." Hoping to smooth feathers in Boston, Will ruffled some in Rochester when he sent Plummer a draft of his reply to Washburn. Plummer penciled in the margin, "Let the letter go, though [I] do not like to be maligned by being called a genius."[63]

Like it or not, many of Plummer's colleagues considered him a genius— and attributed episodes of odd behavior to his brilliance. For example, urologist William Braasch, who joined the practice in 1907, described Plummer decades later as an able, restless genius.

> I can see him yet, striding through the Clinic halls looking neither to the right nor left, intent on completing some line of thought. If questioned, he might pay no attention to you and continue on his way. He might come back, however, and answer your question an hour or more later. He had a complex personality. The casual observer would gain the impression that he was an eccentric, absent-minded person. However, his apparent diffidence was usually explained by complete absorption in solving some problem of the moment, so that when spoken to he often made no reply.[64]

Fredrick Willius, who worked with Plummer for more than two decades, titled his biography *Henry Stanley Plummer: A Diversified Genius*. After describing his mentor's many contributions to the Mayo practice and his "amazing mind," Willius acknowledged that Plummer was "frequently recollected by comic incidents related to so-called eccentricities."[65]

The Development of Mayo's Unified Medical Record System

Henry Plummer invented, imported, and improved several systems to enhance efficiency and encourage collaboration in the practice. One of his most significant innovations was a unified medical record system designed to help coordinate patient care. Like many doctors, the Mayo brothers and their first associates used standard business ledgers to record clinical histories. Their entries were brief and lacked consistency. The editor of the *St. Paul Medical Journal* complained in 1902: "Too many physicians, some from pure carelessness, some because they are too busy, and some from a failure to appreciate the importance do not keep records of their cases. Careful case taking and record keeping is a duty which the physician owes to his patient as well as himself."[66] By this time, the case records at St. Mary's Hospital were tabulated and indexed so the Mayo brothers could report the results of large series of patients who had undergone specific operations. But there was no similar system in the office-based outpatient portion of the practice.

In 1904 Plummer designed a printed form for documenting a patient's evaluation that included sixteen sections: case number, date, name, residence, age, sex, civil state, occupation, family history, personal history, previous diseases, subjective symptoms, objective symptoms, laboratory findings, diagnosis, and operation. There were also six anatomical cartoons for depicting abnormal physical examination findings. Separate color-coded printed slips were used to report test results, such as urinalysis and gastric fluid analysis.[67] Mayo's unit record system, which became more sophisticated during the second decade of the century, impressed visiting doctors. Boston internist Reginald Fitz, who was on the Mayo Clinic staff briefly in the early twenties, wrote later in the decade: "The experience of many observers has shown that a uniform type of case history for all patients examined is highly desirable.... In my opinion, the Mayo Clinic General History Form offers an excellent outline for a thorough and satisfactory case record, and I have no hesitation in recommending it to any doctor or group of doctors as a good working model."[68]

In 1907, three years after Plummer began using standardized history forms, he introduced a sequential numbering system for all new patients who were "registered" by the practice. Number 000-001 was assigned to the first patient seen on July 1, 1907, a Canadian from New Westminster, British Columbia's oldest city. Thereafter, all notes and reports pertaining to a patient evaluated in the clinic or cared for in the hospital would be kept together. This innovation, which medical technology historian Stanley Reiser considers a breakthrough, facilitated communication among the doctors who participated in a patient's care. A parallel indexing system was introduced to identify similar cases seen by various members of the practice. This index of diagnoses and procedures was useful for research and for preparing lectures and publications.[69]

The "Mayo Clinic" Building Exemplifies the Efficiency Movement

"The watchword of the age is efficiency," proclaimed Assistant Surgeon General Colby Rucker in an article published in *Public Health Reports* on March 6, 1914, the day the Mayo Clinic building opened.[70] The timing was a coincidence, but efficiency was very much on Henry Plummer's mind when he designed the building. Philadelphia engineer and efficiency expert Frederick Taylor had published his bestselling book on scientific management shortly before the Rochester project got underway. Although Taylor focused on manufacturing, he described organizational principles that were pertinent to other segments of society, including medical practice.[71] Taylor and others laid the foundations of the efficiency movement in the late nineteenth century, but medical historian George Rosen emphasizes that "it was not until 1910–1911 that the notion of efficiency caught the American imagination and spread like wild fire."[72] Plummer was consumed by the flames before most physicians smelled the smoke.

Henry Plummer was not alone in his desire to enhance the efficiency of the practice. The Mayo brothers encouraged the division of labor and hired staff with complementary interests and skills. In 1905 they hired University of Minnesota medical graduate Louis Wilson to improve the laboratories at St. Mary's Hospital. He had served as an assistant to the professor of pathology and bacteriology at the university and as assistant bacteriologist at the Minnesota State Board of Health for almost a decade.[73] Wilson argued in a 1913 article on laboratory efficiency that a "non-medical technician" could do work that many institutions assigned to medical students or interns. The rationale for the status quo was that the experience was "supposed to be a good thing for the embryo doctor" and "their labor is cheap." But Wilson considered the problems associated with using "shifting, imperfectly trained assistants" so serious that he insisted the "arrangement should not be considered for a moment if the highest efficiency is to be expected from the laboratory." Wilson's prescription reflected contemporary stereotypes. He recommended training and hiring female high school or college graduates because "women will do routine technical work more accurately and conscientiously than men."[74]

The Mayo practice was dedicated to patient care, but it had become a big business by the turn of the century. William Graham had been hired in 1900 as the group's first business manager. Although he had relevant experience, he was chosen mainly because he was Christopher Graham's brother and Charlie Mayo's brother-in-law. In fact, several of the Mayo brothers' early partners were related by marriage. The 1914 building focused attention on the practice's apparent profitability. Louis Wilson informed a physician two years after it opened that "practically all of the patients coming to the Clinic are referred cases, and consequently more or less complicated." Charges depended to a large extent on an individual's income. Thirty percent of the 35,000 patients evaluated in the clinic in 1915 paid nothing, and 25 percent "paid less than the cost of examination." The remaining 45 percent "supported the institution," according to Wilson.[75]

"Better Doctoring for Less Money" was the title of a 1916 magazine article written by Richard Cabot, a prominent Boston internist who was chief of a medical service at the Massachusetts General Hospital. He explained that "when a patient visits the world-famous Mayo Clinic at Rochester, Minnesota, he is often examined not merely by the surgeon who may eventually operate on him but by other specialists representing the different fields of medicine." Cabot, who was interested in the social and economic aspects of medical care, applauded the arrangement. "For the patient the special point of excellence is this: He pays a certain fee, and for that lump sum gets *whatever examinations he may need* from any or all of a group of specialists there assembled and working on salary."[76]

Many doctors denounced any system that threatened the traditional fee-for-service arrangement. For example, Chicago surgeon Arthur Bevan argued that "compensation for the peculiarly personal and individual services rendered by the medical man to his patient should be paid to the individual rendering those services and not to anyone else or to any institution." He considered it unethical to interfere with this custom.[77] But Will and Charlie Mayo did not grow up in a traditional urban or academic medical environment. They oversaw the development of a group practice that established several precedents.

The new Mayo Clinic building contributed to a change in the profession's perception of the Mayo practice. Seattle surgeon Tate Mason called it "the greatest medical building in America" in a 1914 article describing his recent visits to various "surgical clinics" around the country.[78] When Mason entered the structure, he walked under a limestone lintel with "MAYO CLINIC" carved in large capital letters. This simple two-word phrase signaled a shift in the name of the practice. It also represented a new definition of the word "clinic," which had been in the medical lexicon since the early nineteenth century.

Traditionally, the word "clinic" referred to a recurring hospital-based teaching event. It followed the name of a specific doctor who taught in a ward or an amphitheater. Turn-of-the-century examples included the Murphy Clinic at Mercy Hospital in Chicago and the Osler Clinic at the Johns Hopkins Hospital.[79] In these teaching clinics, a surgeon would demonstrate a procedure on a cadaver or would operate on an anesthetized person, and a physician would interview or examine a patient. The audience of students, residents, or practitioners varied in size from a few to a few hundred, depending on the institution, the session's purpose, and the professor's popularity.[80]

Doctors who visited Rochester before the new building opened in 1914 used the term "Mayo Clinic" in its traditional sense—to describe a teaching event. Standing in a small operating room gallery at St. Mary's Hospital (see Figure 2.3), they watched Charlie or Will perform surgery and listened to them explain what they were doing and why. After the big outpatient building opened, the phrase "Mayo Clinic" that emblazoned the entryway no longer referred exclusively to such events. It now identified a special place that embodied a novel concept—a group practice that united patients with several types of specialists and a large support staff.

The phrase "Mayo Clinic" replaced names that had been used to describe the practice or "firm," as the early partners called it. By 1913, the firm known as "Drs. Mayo, Stinchfield, and Graham" had evolved into "Drs. Mayo, Graham, Plummer, and Judd."

E. Starr Judd had joined the practice in 1904, and the Mayos' first partner, Augustus Stinchfield, had retired two years later. Starr Judd and Henry Plummer married sisters Helen and Daisy Berkman, who were nieces of Will and Charlie Mayo. In 1913 an assistant in the business office, in correspondence

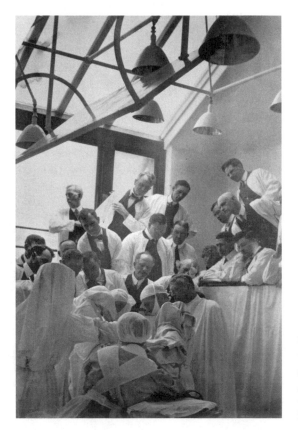

FIGURE 2.3 *Visiting doctors watching Charles H. Mayo operate at St. Mary's Hospital, ca. 1920.*

Used with permission of Mayo Foundation.

with a Chicago printing firm, described ongoing discussions about changing the name of the group practice to Mayo Clinic.[81] Will Mayo initially resisted having the group practice identified with his family name. Several years later, he explained that the phrase Mayo Clinic "was not chosen by us but was given to us by our friends throughout the country, and as we became known by that name, it seemed expedient for us to adopt it eventually ourselves."[82]

Shortly after the growing practice settled into the Mayo Clinic building in 1914, another name would be associated with the Rochester group. The Mayo Foundation for Education and Research, created the following year, signaled a major new academic initiative that would complement the clinical programs of outpatient diagnosis and inpatient surgical care. The creation of the foundation also led some physicians in the Twin Cities and elsewhere in Minnesota to vocalize their frustrations about the growing regional influence of the Mayo Clinic and the competition this represented.

The Development of an Academic Medical Center in Rochester

The Mayo Clinic building, which opened in 1914, showcased the success of the multispecialty group practice that Will and Charlie Mayo had developed in Rochester since the turn of the century. Although the brothers' main focus was patient care, they had become increasingly interested in grafting programs of postgraduate specialty training and research onto their thriving surgical practice. During the second decade of the twentieth century, the Mayo Clinic was transformed into an academic medical center as the result of an affiliation with the University of Minnesota. The Progressive Era movement to reform American medical education had gained momentum, but it focused on changing the medical school experience rather than hospital-based postgraduate training.[1] The Mayo Clinic made major contributions to the training of specialists, which have been underappreciated by historians.[2]

Contrasting Visions of Postgraduate Surgical Training

William Osler, physician-in-chief of the Johns Hopkins Hospital, was the master of ceremonies at a 1904 banquet honoring eye and ear specialist Daniel Roosa, the founder of the New York Postgraduate Medical School, which had opened two decades earlier. Will Mayo, who had studied there, was one of five individuals who spoke at the celebration. Osler introduced Mayo as the "teacher of teachers," high praise for the forty-two-year-old surgeon, who did not teach at a medical school or have an academic appointment.[3] Will's prominent place on the program reflected the role that he and his brother played in creating a unique educational environment at St. Mary's Hospital in Rochester.

Will Mayo told the two hundred doctors assembled at Delmonico's Restaurant in New York City that postgraduate training was assuming ever greater significance in terms of a doctor's career path. Applauding the "university plan of instruction" that was "cultivating broad scholarship," he argued that "the spirit of science, which today is German, must in the years to come call itself American."[4] Although medical education in the United States had improved dramatically during the two decades since the Mayo brothers had joined their father's general practice, chauvinism and turn-of-the-century optimism contributed to Will's charitable assessment of its status in 1904.

William Halsted, surgeon-in-chief of the Johns Hopkins Hospital, heard Will Mayo claim that "every growing city of 5,000, or even less, has its hospital equipped on modern lines and its surgeon, young, ambitious and capable."[5] But Halsted did not share the Midwesterner's positive opinion of America's surgeons. During a speech at Yale University four months later, he declared that "the problem of the education of our surgeons is still unsolved" and described the present methods of training them as inadequate.[6]

Will Mayo and William Halsted, both world-famous surgeons, had very different backgrounds and day-to-day experiences. Will had spent a few months studying at two postgraduate medical schools in New York City and had traveled regularly to watch other surgeons operate. Halsted, a decade older than Mayo, was a graduate of Yale who had received his medical degree from the College of Physicians and Surgeons in New York City. He then spent two years in Europe, where he studied with some of the German-speaking world's leading surgeons. After practicing and teaching surgery in New York for six years, Halsted's career went off track. He was hospitalized for cocaine addiction, a consequence of self-experimentation with the new local anesthetic. William Welch, a close friend from New York who was pathologist-in-chief of the Johns Hopkins Hospital, offered him a position working in his Baltimore laboratory. Halsted's narcotic addiction (controlled but never cured) was kept secret, and he was appointed as the first surgeon-in-chief at Hopkins.[7]

Halsted and Mayo viewed patients very differently. Harvey Cushing, Halsted's most successful protégé, recalled that the Johns Hopkins surgeon "spent his medical life avoiding patients—even students, when this was possible."[8] Meanwhile, the Mayo brothers spent their lives with patients and welcomed visiting doctors into their operating rooms at St. Mary's Hospital. Will Mayo had been very impressed by the technical skills of German surgeons during a visit to Europe in 1900, but their priorities troubled him: "Science was the center of German surgery, and around this revolved the patient, the surgeon and the student. The typical feature of American surgery is that the patient is the center and around him revolve science, the surgeon and the student."[9] When the Mayo brothers decided to develop a structured surgical training program at St. Mary's Hospital during the first decade of the twentieth century, it would be framed around patients.

In 1904, when Will Mayo and William Halsted spoke on separate occasions, about half of American medical graduates completed internships. This twelve-month experience had become increasingly popular since St. Mary's Hospital and the Johns Hopkins Hospital had opened fifteen years earlier.[10] Medical graduates who hoped to perform some surgery as part of a general practice were attracted to these hospital-based positions. Hospital administrators liked the idea because interns provided various services, such as administering anesthesia, performing laboratory tests, and substituting for a staff doctor, in exchange for room and board.

The training program that Halsted had inaugurated at the Johns Hopkins Hospital produced few surgeons because it was structured like a pyramid, and some individuals were dropped each year. In 1904, for example, there were twelve interns, three assistant resident surgeons, and one resident surgeon. One or two interns were chosen to be assistant residents for a term that might last six years, but only one assistant resident was selected to serve a two-year term as a chief resident. The goal of this very competitive system was to produce a few highly skilled surgeons to fill positions at progressive medical schools where they would focus on teaching and research.[11]

Halsted knew that hundreds of American hospitals trained general practitioners who did some surgery, but he looked to select institutions to set new standards: "Reforms, the need of which must be apparent to every teacher of surgery in this country, must come on the side both of the hospital and of the university, and it is natural to look to our newer institutions, unhampered by traditions and provided with adequate endowment, for the inception of such reforms."[12] St. Mary's Hospital was not bound by traditions or burdened by bureaucracies, and Will and Charlie Mayo controlled access to it. The hospital, run by the Franciscan sisters, was totally dependent on the Mayo brothers' practice for patients, so cooperation was beneficial to both institutions.[13]

A Pathologist Organizes Mayo's Specialty Training Program

The Mayo brothers sponsored a postgraduate training program in Rochester during the second decade of the twentieth century that was designed to produce surgeons for private practice as well as academic posts. They had hired Louis Wilson in 1905 to improve the laboratories at St. Mary's Hospital and further develop its small internship program. A University of Minnesota medical graduate, Wilson had spent the previous decade as an assistant to Frank Wesbrook, the professor of pathology and bacteriology at the university and the assistant director of the bacteriology laboratory at the Minnesota State Board of Health.[14] Wilson's focus shifted from bacteriology to surgical pathology when he moved to Rochester. Shortly after joining the Mayo practice, he described a diagnostic technique that established his reputation as a surgical pathologist.

Wilson froze tiny pieces of tissue removed during surgery, which he then sectioned and stained for microscopic examination. The entire process, done while the patient was anesthetized on an operating table, took less than two minutes. Surgeons at the Johns Hopkins Hospital and in Europe had developed similar techniques during the previous decade, but Wilson's approach attracted more attention because it was published in the *Journal of the American Medical Association*.[15] In 1906 a visiting surgeon from St. Louis praised Wilson's "beautiful demonstration" of the "art of freezing, cutting, and staining fresh tissues."[16] From a patient's point of view, the frozen section technique meant that his or her surgeon was better equipped to perform a curative operation if a microscopic examination of the tissue revealed a malignant tumor. Wilson ridiculed the standard practice of sending the pathology report to a surgeon several days after an operation: "The patient is dead or well before any diagnosis is rendered."[17]

Wilson's original role in Rochester was to enhance and direct the laboratories, but soon he would devote considerable energy to developing a formal postgraduate training program. When he arrived in 1905, there were two interns and two clinical assistants at St. Mary's Hospital. Five years later, there were eighteen trainees: four interns, seven clinical assistants, four assistants in pathology, and three first surgical assistants. The names of these positions reflected a progression from intern to junior staff status.[18]

Will Mayo as President of the American Medical Association

Will Mayo began his term as president of the American Medical Association in 1906, the year after the organization's Council on Medical Education published its first annual report. In his presidential address, the Minnesota surgeon praised the association's commitment to educational reform, proclaiming that "no more important work has ever been taken up by the profession." Will argued that "the profession owes it to itself to investigate in some manner what the schools are actually doing and to make it known whether or not they fulfill their obligations to the student."[19]

There were no medical students in Rochester, but Will would soon have reason to take a personal interest in the University of Minnesota College of Medicine and Surgery. In 1907 Governor John Johnson appointed him to the University of Minnesota's Board of Regents. Johnson knew Will Mayo and St. Mary's Hospital very well, having undergone three abdominal operations in Rochester during the previous decade.[20] An editorial in the state medical journal applauded Will's appointment, boasting that his wisdom, experience, and fame ensured that his advice would "carry weight with his fellow regents

and with the teaching faculty."[21] Will would use his position to influence policies and faculty appointments at the medical school in Minneapolis and to
promote clinical opportunities in Rochester.

Will Mayo became involved in the policies and politics of the University of
Minnesota at a tumultuous time in the history of American medical education. Several individuals and groups seeking to improve physician training
came together after the turn of the century. An influential coalition of scientifically oriented physicians, biomedical scientists, educators, and philanthropists prescribed tonics to strengthen the nation's better medical schools
and poisons to kill the worst ones. The reformers wanted to place a new generation of well-trained medical scientists and physicians in institutions that
provided ample space, supplies, and support staff for basic research and clinical investigation. They argued that this would benefit society and patients by
producing new knowledge and better-trained doctors.[22]

Abraham Flexner's 1910 Report on American Medical Education

Abraham Flexner's 1910 report *Medical Education in the United States and
Canada*, sponsored by the Carnegie Foundation for the Advancement of
Teaching, attracted the attention of the profession and the public. The former schoolteacher (whose brother was a Hopkins-trained pathologist who
directed the Rockefeller Institute for Medical Research in New York City)
dissected every North American medical school in his widely circulated
346-page report. For example, Flexner described Chicago as "the plague spot
of the country" in terms of medical education and judged just three of the
city's fourteen schools fit to train doctors.[23]

The Mayo brothers' home state, with just one medical school, the University
of Minnesota College of Medicine and Surgery, fared well in Flexner's report.
"Minnesota is perhaps the first state in the Union that may fairly be considered to have solved the most perplexing problems connected with medical
education and practice," he wrote.[24] Flexner praised the medical school's laboratories and predicted that better hospital and outpatient facilities for clinical teaching would be available soon. An editorial writer in the state medical
journal boasted, "Minnesota's scientific competition, as is clearly shown by
the Flexner report, is not with the low-grade schools but with Johns Hopkins,
Harvard, and other schools of that type."[25]

Flexner's focus was on medical schools; he devoted just four pages of his
1910 report to postgraduate training. There were thirteen postgraduate medical schools in the United States. The New York Postgraduate Medical School,
whose founding William Osler and William Mayo had celebrated six years
earlier, was one of the best. On the other hand, Flexner described the Brooklyn
Postgraduate Medical School as a commercial institution with a half dozen

students who had access to "a wretched hospital, really a death-trap, heavily laden with debt, and without laboratory equipment enough to make an ordinary clinical examination."[26] Looking ahead, he predicted that improvements in medical schools would result in more advanced and intensive postgraduate instruction. In keeping with his report's prescriptive tone, Flexner concluded that "postgraduate schools of the better type can hasten this evolution by incorporating themselves in accessible universities, taking up university ideals, and submitting to reorganization on university lines."[27]

Louis Wilson Becomes a Vocal Critic of Postgraduate Training

Louis Wilson shared Abraham Flexner's passion for reforming the training of physicians, but his focus was different. Working with the Mayo brothers in Rochester, he became very interested in the postgraduate training of surgeons and other specialists. Wilson debuted as an educational reformer in 1912, when he spoke to members of the Minnesota Academy of Medicine. He told them that he had recently surveyed the opportunities for postgraduate training in the United States and Europe. Sounding very much like Flexner, Wilson pilloried America's private postgraduate medical schools. He claimed that many of these small schools were staffed by second-rate teachers who were more interested in collecting students' fees than in dispensing knowledge. Complaining that most were no better than the proprietary medical schools that Flexner had denounced two years earlier, the pathologist rendered his verdict: "When they are dead we will be better off."[28] A tough judge, Wilson also criticized well-endowed private and state supported medical schools for their half-hearted approach to postgraduate education.

Shifting his gaze to Rochester, Wilson emphasized that the Mayo practice focused almost exclusively on surgery. He described three categories of doctors who visited the city for educational purposes: "We have frequent requests from men who wish to come to our clinic for a few weeks' work to aid them in their general practice, from a few who wish to come for two or three years' work as a preparation for a surgical career, and from a very few who wish to come for research work pure and simple."[29] Wilson was especially interested in enhancing opportunities for the middle group—recent medical graduates seeking structured specialty training. He envisioned a comprehensive program that combined two years of diagnostic and surgical experience with one year of pathology.

The editor of the *St. Paul Medical Journal* praised Wilson's proposal for improving postgraduate training. Applauding the focus on surgery, he argued that major operations should "be entirely in the hands of those whose special training has rendered them specially fit to do it."[30] Meanwhile, men and women who might be touched by a surgeon's hands were becoming better informed: "The amateur surgeon and the pseudo-surgeon will disappear because people will not trust themselves to them."[31] Still, most patients had no reliable way to distinguish between an adequately trained surgeon and a general practitioner who simply claimed to be a surgeon. One approach, favored by the editor, was to award a postgraduate degree in medicine or surgery to individuals who completed a rigorous training program. This degree would help patients choose a properly trained surgeon.

A New President Shakes Up the University of Minnesota

Faculty members of the University of Minnesota College of Medicine and Surgery were pleased that Flexner praised their institution, but they had little time to celebrate before an ambitious new president shook things up. George Vincent, the son of a Methodist bishop, brought missionary zeal to Minnesota when he took charge of the university in 1911.[32] A sociologist who had been dean of the faculties at the University of Chicago, Vincent saw an opportunity to create a unique program for training specialists by forging a link between the University of Minnesota and the Mayo Clinic. He discussed the notion with Frank Wesbrook, dean of the medical school and Louis Wilson's friend and former mentor. Vincent also had many conversations with Will Mayo, who chaired the Medical Committee of the university's Board of Regents.[33]

President Vincent urged Dean Wesbrook to make deep cuts in the clinical faculty, almost all of whom were unpaid private practitioners. Understandably, the proposal upset those doctors who would lose their teaching positions and academic titles. After all, Abraham Flexner had just held their institution up as a national model. When George Vincent arrived, the university had the highest combined standards for granting a degree of any medical school in the United States. Before a person could earn a medical diploma from the University of Minnesota he or she (a few women were enrolled) had to have completed two years of college, four years of medical school, and an internship. They also had to pass an examination at the end of their hospital experience.[34]

After George Vincent and Will Mayo discussed the reorganization plan with the faculty in 1913, murmurs of discontent grew louder. "Things have become very strenuous here," Wesbrook informed a friend. "It is a very serious thing...to reorganize a medical college in the middle of the school year when teachers, who have been faithful and earnest in their work for twenty or thirty years, are succeeded by younger men."[35]

George Vincent's plans for reforming medical education extended to Rochester. In March 1913, two weeks after Wesbrook resigned as dean to become president of the University of British Columbia, Vincent told the medical faculty in Minneapolis that their institution must develop a more sophisticated program of clinical research. In revealing his "plan for cooperation with the Mayo Clinic," he argued that an affiliation with the Rochester group practice would offer "new opportunities for scientific work."[36] This frustrated some clinical faculty members, who also were annoyed by the process for selecting Dean Wesbrook's successor. Charles Greene, a highly regarded internist and the chief of medicine, seemed destined for the position, but George Vincent had other ideas. He gave the job to physiologist Elias Lyon, his friend and former colleague at the University of Chicago, who was the dean of the St. Louis Medical College.[37] When Lyon arrived in Minneapolis in August 1913, he entered a hostile environment. In addition to local disappointment that Greene was not selected, more than 100 doctors had lost their part-time teaching appointments as a result of the faculty reorganization.[38]

As Elias Lyon settled into his job in Minneapolis, discussions about a possible affiliation between the University of Minnesota and the Mayo Clinic were going on behind the scenes. James Moore, the university's chief of surgery, informed Will Mayo in February 1914: "The idea in brief is this, that instead of doing ordinary postgraduate work, which I believe does more harm than good, we as a university do real graduate work and offer a school for the education of specialists. This will do a great deal to forward your scheme at Rochester, and will have much to do with amalgamating that institution with the University. With your help we are already in a position to offer men courses in all of the recognized specialties."[39] Moore told Mayo that in addition to George Vincent and Elias Lyon, Guy Ford, the recently hired dean of the Graduate School, was very interested in the idea.[40] The scheme at Rochester that Moore referred to was a novel three-year program to train surgeons, which Louis Wilson and the Mayo brothers had launched on a small scale two years earlier.

Several doctors in the state worried that an affiliation between the University of Minnesota and the Mayo Clinic would hurt their practices. In an attempt to address this concern, George Vincent encouraged Will Mayo to create a new entity in Rochester that would be distinct from the clinic. Just after Thanksgiving in 1914, Will informed the university president that he and his brother had agreed to establish the Mayo Foundation for Medical Education and Research: "It gets away from all connection with the Mayo Clinic and furnishes a reasonable method of taking care of those particular activities which are essentially outside the scope of the clinic itself."[41] Will and Charlie Mayo decided to make a major financial commitment to postgraduate training and research. George Vincent told Will in December that creating the foundation would "mark an important epoch in the development of your work as well as in the growth of American medicine generally."[42]

Building a Medical Research Program at the Mayo Clinic

The 1914 Mayo Clinic building provided much needed room for the practice's growing diagnostic arm. It also contained research laboratories for medical scientists. Will and Charlie Mayo, unlike their surgeon friends George Crile in Cleveland and Harvey Cushing in Boston, had no training in research, nor did they have any interest in doing research themselves.[43] Nevertheless, they understood the vital role that research played in expanding the scope and safety of surgery. Will Mayo had defended animal experimentation, vivisection, in his 1912 Ether Day Address at the Massachusetts General Hospital. Acknowledging the half-century campaign against the controversial research method, he declared, "More humane and highly scientific methods of investigation have gradually brought the fair-minded individual to view vivisection as a legitimate and, at present, the only sure means of obtaining certain important truths to aid in the preservation and prolongation of human life."[44]

Will articulated a philosophy in his Boston speech that helps to explain why he and his brother decided to add scientists to their group practice: "Medicine must no longer be practiced individually, but by groups of men, each one bringing the results of his work and studies to bear upon the case. In no other way can the patient receive the benefits to which he is entitled."[45] Scientists with specific skills could work on clinically relevant projects that complemented the activities of the diagnosticians and surgeons. In 1914 the Mayo brothers hired Frank Mann to develop and direct an experimental surgery laboratory on the top floor of the new clinic building. A recent medical graduate of Indiana University who had spent two years as assistant in physiology, Mann was eager to assist staff members and trainees in performing animal experiments designed to help answer clinical questions or improve operative procedures.[46]

Adding a physiologist to the Mayo staff seemed logical in terms of the role that such a person would play in developing a program of experimental surgery. The decision to hire a biochemist was driven by a clinical problem that was a prominent part of the Mayo practice. The surgical treatment of goiter, an enlarged thyroid gland, was one of Charlie Mayo's main interests, and patients with the disorder flocked to Rochester for treatment. By July 1914, almost 7,000 operations for goiter had been performed at St. Mary's Hospital during the previous two decades. Most of them were done to treat "hyperthyroidism," a term that Charlie had coined seven years earlier.[47] Henry Plummer oversaw thorough diagnostic examinations of the patients Charlie operated on for thyroid disease, and Louis Wilson subjected the tissue that was removed to a detailed pathologic examination. These three men shared a deep interest in thyroid disorders, and they were enthusiastic about adding a scientist to the staff whose research focused on this endocrine gland.

Biochemist Edward Kendall was hired in 1914 to establish a research laboratory where he could continue his investigations into an iodine-containing substance produced by the thyroid.[48] A PhD graduate of Columbia University, Kendall had worked briefly for a pharmaceutical firm, where he tried to isolate the substance. Charlie Mayo, Henry Plummer, and Louis Wilson were eager to have Kendall continue this research, so he was allowed to begin working in the new building before it opened. "For six weeks," the biochemist recalled, "I climbed over piles of plaster and building debris, the only member of the staff in the new building."[49] The Mayos' investment and Kendall's persistence paid off. On Christmas Day 1914 he isolated in crystalline form the biologically active iodine-containing substance secreted by the thyroid gland, which he named thyroxin.[50] Hiring Kendall and Mann demonstrated that the Mayo Clinic was about science as well as surgery. This commitment to research impressed the University of Minnesota's new leaders who supported the affiliation.

The Mayo Foundation for Medical Research and Education

President George Vincent initially envisioned an affiliation between the Mayo Clinic and his university's medical school, but intense criticism from some clinical faculty members and practitioners stimulated a series of strategic decisions. The creation of the Mayo Foundation was designed to address some concerns raised about the Rochester end of the arrangement. In Minneapolis, Vincent decided that the proposed postgraduate program should be linked to the university's Graduate School rather than to the College of Medicine and Surgery.

Hoping to advance the affiliation plan, Graduate School dean Guy Ford visited Rochester in January 1915 to survey the facilities and potential faculty. A historian who was the son of a general practitioner, Ford found "a research and teaching staff, available and at work, sufficient to do its full part" in achieving the goal of training about three dozen medical school graduates for specialty practice or academic careers. He was also impressed by the academic apparatus incorporated into the new Mayo Clinic building: "I found what I was looking for in the laboratories, [pathological] museum and library of the upper floors, and in the countless case records in the basement." The University of Minnesota dean saw a solid scientific foundation for building an innovative postgraduate training program in Rochester: "The richness of this material, not seen by the casual visitor, furnishes opportunities for graduate medical work in certain lines such as can be found nowhere else on this continent, nor probably in the world."[51]

On February 8, 1915, shortly after Ford's visit, Will and Charlie Mayo signed the articles of incorporation for the Mayo Foundation for Medical

Education and Research (Figure 3.1). This legal document stated that the "general purposes of this corporation shall be educational, scientific, medical and surgical, and to establish, maintain, and operate clinical, pathological, medical and surgical research laboratories."[52] Ten days later, Louis Wilson went to Minneapolis to speak to the University of Minnesota General Alumni Association about the benefits of the proposed affiliation between their university and the new Mayo Foundation. The pathologist told his well-educated audience that specialization had become an "inevitable necessity," but he argued that the training of specialists was one of the biggest problems in medical education.[53]

Wilson complained that the traditional path to specialty practice was much too easy to traverse. Experienced general practitioners—even new medical graduates—could pronounce themselves specialists after a few weeks or months of casual observation or unsupervised training. "Like the hurried business man," these doctors "rushed to the European lunch counters, bolted 'ready-to-serve' specialties, keeping one hand on their pocketbook and both eyes on the clock and then rushed home again hoping to digest the meal on the return trip." Mocking the situation, Wilson declared, "Usually they have regurgitated these meals undigested, rarely have they assimilated them."[54] He shifted from disparaging this shortcut scenario to describing the sophisticated thirty-six-month postgraduate training program developed in Rochester during the previous three years.

One distinctive feature of Mayo's specialty training program was that each doctor accepted into it was required to spend several months working in areas

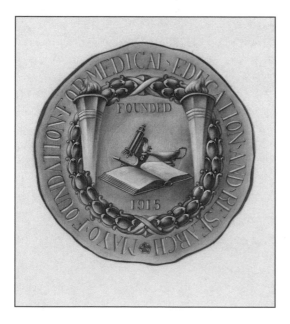

FIGURE 3.1 *Seal of the Mayo Foundation for Medical Education and Research, 1915.*
Used with permission of Mayo Foundation.

complementing his or her chosen field. For example, aspiring surgeons spent up to two years in pathology and general diagnosis. They were also expected to participate in research. Wilson told the Minnesota alumni that demand for these positions in Rochester was high, in part because they provided a significant stipend, in contrast to traditional residencies. A decision had been made to call these postgraduate students "fellows" to distinguish the Mayo Clinic's training program from standard hospital-based residencies. The term "fellow" was already used at leading universities, such as Johns Hopkins and Harvard, to describe postgraduate students in non-medical departments.[55] Meanwhile, the Mayo Clinic would benefit from a larger training program, which would function as an incubator for future staff members who could help the group practice meet growing patient demand and develop emerging specialties.[56]

In March 1915, one month after Wilson spoke in Minneapolis and the Mayo brothers incorporated the foundation, any doctor interested in the proposed affiliation could read a detailed report about it. Most institutional committee reports are internal documents, but this one was published in the *Journal-Lancet*, the official journal of the medical associations of Minnesota, North Dakota, and South Dakota. It was signed by university president George Vincent, the dean and assistant dean of the medical school, and the chiefs of surgery and obstetrics-gynecology. These men supported the proposed Mayo affiliation and proclaimed that a better program for training specialists was desperately needed. For a generation, they argued, some ambitious doctors had spent one or two years in Europe to acquire the knowledge and skills of a specialist. But for each person willing to devote years to achieve this goal, many burst "into full bloom during a summer's junket to the Old World."[57]

The Mayo-University Affiliation Comes Under Attack

The proposed affiliation offered advantages to aspiring specialists and their future patients, but it threatened the status quo for Minnesota's practitioners, some of whom viewed the Mayo Clinic as a great and growing competitor. Charles Greene, the chief of the Department of Medicine who had expected to become dean when Frank Wesbrook resigned, took up their cause. The *Journal-Lancet* published his six-page point-by-point rebuttal to the university committee's report on the affiliation. Greene argued that the arrangement would award the Mayo Foundation, which he considered a private corporation, "an amount of prestige, power, authority, rights, and privileges such as are without modern precedent."[58]

Greene complained that the new foundation was controlled by the leaders of the Mayo Clinic, which, in turn, was "inseparable from the firm of

Drs. Mayo, Graham, Plummer, Judd, and Balfour, all of whom are related through ties of blood or marriage." The affiliation, Greene fumed, was "being pressed despite the opposition of at least 80 percent of the clinical staff of the medical school, the protest of various medical societies, including the two largest in the state, and the emphatic disapproval of medical alumni and of the great body of Minnesota physicians." When he claimed that the Mayo practice would enjoy an enormous potential financial advantage as a result of the affiliation, Greene spoke for many of the region's doctors.[59]

In 1912, three years before the proposed affiliation was publicized, Benjamin Randall, a general practitioner in a small Minnesota town near the South Dakota border, had written to St. Louis physician George Broome. Broome published the letter two years later in his book *Rochester and the Mayo Clinic: A Fair and Unbiased Story Calculated to Aid Physicians to Greater Cures and Larger Incomes*. Randall claimed:

> The attitude of the profession in Minnesota is not entirely friendly towards the Mayo corporation, and I believe the main reason is the same as that which prejudices the general merchants against the big department stores. Prices are cut in a way that is annoying to the surgeons of the Minnesota cities, but they have a graduated scale of fees and no doubt make adequate charges to the rich. Personally, I cannot complain of lack of ethical treatment, tho I have heard charges of this character.... The amount of money accruing to this medical firm must be very large; the statement that they take in more than a million a year might easily be true, and their donations are also very large; that they have contributed to the building of St. Mary's Hospital is not unlikely.[60]

Broome's book, unlike most publications about the Mayo practice, included many criticisms based on his three-week visit to Rochester.

Will and Charlie Mayo committed $1.5 million to endow their namesake foundation in 1915. This huge gift (equivalent to about $34 million in 2015) placed them in the company of other philanthropists seeking to reform medical education.[61] In fact, it matched the $1.5 million grant that the Rockefeller-endowed General Education Board gave to the Johns Hopkins Medical School in 1913 to launch the full-time salary system for the chiefs of three clinical departments (medicine, surgery, and pediatrics). The purpose of that salary plan was to encourage research and teaching by prohibiting those professors from earning money from private practice. But the scheme was very controversial before and after it was implemented.[62]

William Osler, the former chief of medicine at Johns Hopkins, had warned the university's president in 1911 that adoption of a full-time salary plan might encourage "the evolution throughout the country of a set of clinical prigs, the boundary of whose horizon would be the laboratory, and whose only human interest was research."[63] The contentious debate surrounding the full-time salary experiment in Baltimore was irrelevant in Rochester. Will and Charlie Mayo had implemented a version of it a decade before the Rockefeller-sponsored plan debuted at Johns Hopkins. Every doctor in the Mayo group practice (except the brothers and their four relative-partners) was paid a salary. The Mayo Clinic was unique; it did not conform to any contemporary model of patient care or physician training. Will and Charlie, who profited from the practice and funded its growth, were not bound by the weight of tradition, the fear of competition, or the demands of philanthropic foundations.

World War I Disrupts Overseas Specialty Training

Events in Europe imparted momentum to the Minnesota-Mayo affiliation plan to develop a rigorous postgraduate training program for aspiring specialists in Rochester. The assassination of the heir to the throne of the Austro-Hungarian Empire in June 1914 triggered a complex series of political and military reactions. By year's end, more than a million soldiers and civilians were dead as a result of the European conflict, which at the time was called the Great War. President Woodrow Wilson pursued a policy of neutrality, but the escalating war affected United States citizens.[64] This was highlighted in May 1915, when a German submarine sank the British ocean liner *Lusitania*, killing more than one thousand men, women, and children, including more than one hundred Americans. Two days later, the Mayo brothers' longtime friend Harvey Cushing passed the wreckage when he was returning from Europe. "Steamer chairs, oars, boxes, overturned boats—and bodies" is how he described the scene in his diary.[65] Transatlantic travel for recreation or education came to a standstill. A month after Cushing passed the traumatic scene, the Mayo brothers took a decisive step that had profound implications for the future of their growing group practice.

On June 9, 1915, Will and Charlie Mayo signed a formal agreement approving a six-year trial affiliation between their new foundation and the University of Minnesota. Although many of the state's doctors opposed the arrangement, St. Cloud physician Warren Beebe applauded it. He urged members of the Minnesota Medical Association to "make most respectful bows whenever the names are mentioned of the greatest medical organizers on this green footstool of the Almighty—Drs. W. J. and Charles H. Mayo."[66] The enormous amount of money that the Mayo brothers invested in the affiliation attracted widespread attention. A New York newspaper, *The Sun,* printed their pictures with a headline "The Mayo Brothers, Who Have Given $2,000,000 for Science." Horatio Alger, who once wrote for that paper, could have crafted the subtitle: "Remarkable Careers of Two Country Surgeons Who Built America's Greatest Clinic in the Little Minnesota Town of Rochester." The writer praised the Mayo brothers' success and philanthropic spirit:

> The world, in wearing a beaten path to their door, rewarded them with fame and wealth. Year after year they have been setting aside a large part of their income toward the establishment of an endowment fund and now comes the announcement that the Mayo Foundation of Rochester, comprising the physical plant, equipment and staff at Rochester, has made an arrangement whereby the University of Minnesota comes into absolute possession of $2,000,000 or more and an equipment for medical research said to excel any other in the world.[67]

He also emphasized that a patient's wealth, celebrity, or social position made no difference in Rochester, where a man or woman without money received the same care as a millionaire.

Doctors from urban teaching hospitals had been visiting Rochester for more than a decade, but news of the affiliation piqued their interest. It promised to transform the Mayo Clinic into a major academic medical center. One thing distinguished the Rochester-based program from traditional teaching institutions. It was devoted exclusively to postgraduate education; there were no medical students. Moreover, candidates for a Mayo Foundation fellowship must have completed an internship elsewhere before they could begin their training. Research, a key ingredient in the evolving definition of an academic medical center, would be a priority in Rochester. Louis Wilson, who directed the expanded fellowship program, informed Francis Peabody, a leading Boston internist and clinical investigator, in 1916: "We thoroughly believe that neither research nor routine diagnosis and treatment can reach high-water mark without the other."[68] By this time, Mayo employed more than 250 individuals to meet patient demands and to contribute to an expanded academic mission. Their responsibilities are summarized in Table 3.1.

A Renewed Attack on the Mayo-University Affiliation

Smoldering cinders of discontent surrounding the Mayo-university affiliation burst into flames in 1917, when seventy-eight doctors signed a petition urging state government representatives to support pending legislation that would end it. The *Minneapolis Tribune* reprinted the petition, which contained a long list of philosophical and financial concerns. For example, the antagonists argued that the affiliation "placed too much emphasis on research and graduate work at the expense of undergraduate work which is the main duty

TABLE 3.1 Mayo Clinic Personnel and Patient Volumes, 1916[a]

Total members of the "permanent staff" of the Mayo Clinic	46
Physicians engaged in general clinical diagnostic work	14
Physicians engaged in special clinical diagnostic work (e.g., diseases of the urinary organs or ear, nose, and throat)	9
Physicians engaged in general surgery	8
Physicians engaged in special surgical work (e.g., orthopedic surgery, otolaryngology, or thoracic surgery)	3
Physicians engaged in special laboratory diagnostic work (e.g., pathology, bacteriology, or radiology)	6
Physicians engaged entirely in laboratory research (e.g., pathology, bacteriology, biochemistry, or experimental surgery)	5
Veterinarian in charge of the farm for experimental animals	1
Fellows [residents] enrolled in the three-year postgraduate training program	48
"Professional" employees (e.g., editors, librarians, artists, or nurse anesthetists)	28
Laboratory technicians	29
Clerks and stenographers	77
Miscellaneous (e.g., engineers, mechanics, janitors, or gardeners)	30
Patients who had clinical examinations in 1915	35,417
Patients who had surgery in 1915 (each one was "thoroughly examined by clinicians before [being] seen by a surgeon," except in emergency cases)	13,574

[a] Adapted from Louis B. Wilson to Richard Cabot, May 24, 1916, MCA.

of the state medical school and the chief reason for its existence."[69] There was also resentment about Will Mayo's role as an influential member of the University of Minnesota's Board of Regents. Above all, there was tremendous frustration about the financial success of the Rochester-based practice: "This corporation is an immense business concern engaged in money making and is attempting to make the State of Minnesota its agent to further these plans."[70]

The Mayo Clinic building was just one visible sign of the brothers' wealth. Charlie had recently built a thirty-eight-room home on his 3,000-acre farm outside town. When the new assault on the affiliation was launched in 1917, Will had just taken delivery of a luxurious 115-foot paddleboat to use on the Mississippi River. He was also constructing a forty-seven-room mansion between the new clinic building and St. Mary's Hospital.[71] Louis Wilson, aware of perceptions about the Mayo brothers' wealth, informed a Boston physician that a large part of their fortunes had come from investment income. He explained that their assets represented "a great excess over the fees actually collected" over the three decades they had been in practice.[72]

Leaders of the national movement to reform medical education rallied to defend the Minnesota-Mayo affiliation against this new and potentially lethal attack. A St. Paul newspaper published excerpts from letters that several of them (including Abraham Flexner) sent in the spring of 1917. Subheadings set the tone: "Clinic Held Vital...Pride to Country...National Calamity...Profound Misfortune...Better than Harvard...Mayos' Fame World-Wide...Repeal Seems Incredible...Opportunity Is Unique."[73] Former Johns Hopkins Medical School dean William Welch, the national reform movement's maestro, declared, "The unequaled opportunity for graduate medical training and work accorded by the affiliation of the University of Minnesota with the Mayo Foundation has made your graduate school the envy of other institutions as well as a source of pride to the country. I cannot believe that the experiment will be interrupted by adverse legislative action."[74]

Theodore Janeway, the chief of medicine at Johns Hopkins, expressed outrage that the university might be forced to "throw away not merely $2,000,000, but the center which attracts more physicians and graduate students than any other hospital in the United States."[75] State legislators defeated the bill on April 4, 1917, but any celebration was short-lived. President Woodrow Wilson signed a declaration of war against Germany two days later.

When the United States entered World War I, most individuals who had been following the affiliation fight lost interest, assuming that the issue was resolved. But the Mayo brothers and their confidants at the University of Minnesota were not complacent. They worked on a new agreement during the summer of 1917 that would lengthen the term of the affiliation from six to twenty-five years and would grant control of the endowment to the university's Board of Regents. An editorial in the *Journal-Lancet* outlined the presumed terms and applauded the Mayo brothers "for their generous and liberal proposals."[76] Will and Charlie Mayo signed the new agreement on September 13, 1917.[77] Will explained the rationale to reporters:

> Why do we do this now? What has led us to the offer of the affiliation in the first place and to a change of terms that modifies materially the relation? My brother and I are at a time of life when we see things as clearly as we may ever be able to see them.... We are in our fifties, and we don't want to take a chance on what the future may bring. We are at war. My brother and I expect that next year when the recruits go over one or the other will go too.... War is serious business, especially to men of our years.... If I should not come back, I shall be satisfied. I have done the thing in life that I wanted to do.[78]

Will was fifty-six years old when he made this public statement. A few months earlier, Charlie reminded American Medical Association members during his presidential address that a doctor's average life expectancy was fifty-eight years.[79] Soon, Will and Charlie would confront their own mortality—not from enemy action but from potentially fatal illnesses (Figure 3.2).

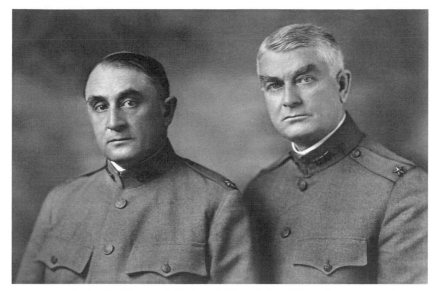

FIGURE 3.2 *Charles H. Mayo and William J. Mayo in World War I military uniforms, 1918.*

Used with permission of Mayo Foundation.

Confronting Mortality and Ensuring Institutional Survival

During World War I, the Mayo brothers' main military responsibility was to co-chair the General Medical Board of the Council of National Defense. They took turns working at the Surgeon General's Office in Washington and operating at St. Mary's Hospital in Rochester. Will was in the capital in August 1918 when he developed severe jaundice. He told the clinic's long-time business manager Harry Harwick that he thought he had liver cancer, a fatal disease.[80]

Will Mayo was wrong. On Christmas Eve, six weeks after the war ended, he informed a surgeon friend still on duty in France that he had "felt very miserable for two or three months" but was better. Now his brother was sick. "Charlie got a cold and bronchitis of the general nature of an influenza-pneumonia, raising a large amount of frothy blood. He arrived from Washington Sunday morning and is just getting around."[81] Will's matter-of-fact tone does not reflect the context or possible consequences of his brother's illness. Men and women who had worried about war-related deaths and devastation now faced an invisible foe. A deadly influenza pandemic racing around the world would kill millions. In fact, ten times more Americans died from the flu than from battle injuries. In Rochester, 16 percent of 734 patients hospitalized with influenza between September 1918 and April 1919 died.[82]

Will and Charlie Mayo survived scary sicknesses, and World War I was over. In this context, Will began to focus on the "study of agencies that would safeguard the future of the institution," according to chief administrator Harry Harwick.[83] This resulted in profound changes in the Mayo Clinic's ownership, legal status, and organizational structure. On October 8, 1919, Will and Charlie transferred all of the clinic's buildings, equipment, and endowments to a new entity, the Mayo Properties Association. The legal document they signed explained that the association's mission was "to aid and advance the study and investigation of human ailments and injuries, and the causes, prevention, relief and cure thereof, and the study and investigation of problems of hygiene, health, and public welfare, and the promotion of medical, surgical, and scientific learning, skill, education and investigation, and to engage in and conduct and to aid and assist in medical, surgical, and scientific research in the broadest sense."[84] The Mayo brothers had presided over the birth and adolescence of a unique and expanding multispecialty group practice. Now, they wanted to ensure its future as a major academic medical center where the main focus was on patient care.

A few hours after Will and Charlie signed the legal document that established the Mayo Properties Association, they spoke to former residents who had assembled in Rochester for their second annual alumni meeting. Will explained:

> It has been our desire to maintain at Rochester an institution in which medical and surgical treatment may be had by anyone, without regard to financial status, race, color or creed, all meeting on a common level. A prominent feature of the work of the Clinic in the future as in the past will be scientific research into the causes of disease, its prevention and cure, and not least, advanced education for physicians and surgeons and the furnishing of opportunities for study for the exceptional man of medicine in the various specialties.[85]

By creating the Mayo Foundation for Medical Education and Research in 1915 and the Mayo Properties Association four years later, Will and Charlie used their wealth and influence to establish a self-perpetuating academic program that would complement their group practice's patient care activities. There is no doubt that their main motive was altruism, but the institution of a federal income tax in 1913 and the dramatic increases in the tax after America entered World War I surely influenced their decisions.[86]

A Salary System to Encourage Cooperation, Not Competition

The salary system that the Mayo brothers had instituted in the early twentieth century contributed to their clinic's stability because it encouraged collaboration rather than competition. In 1921, Will informed his longtime friend Victor Vaughan, dean of the University of Michigan Medical School, "An adequate salary is given each man, not based on whether he earns or spends money, but on the value of his services to any or all the objects of the Clinic, the patient, education, research, etc. Earnings are not personal, but the result of the work of all the men."[87] This salary model succeeded at the Mayo Clinic, where staff members were chosen, and chose to stay, because they embraced the ideals of multispecialty group practice. The postgraduate training program, already producing more specialists than any other American institution, provided a pool of potential staff members imbued with the values that Will Mayo had articulated.

The creation of the Mayo Properties Association ended an arrangement whereby the Mayo brothers had a controlling interest in the clinic (in partnership with four relatives: internists Christopher Graham and Henry Plummer and surgeons Starr Judd and Donald Balfour). Will told Vaughan, "The Mayo Clinic has passed out of the hands of my brother and myself and has been turned over to trustees in perpetuity by a deed of gift. The trustees hold all the physical properties, equipment, endowments, etc. for medical education and research in the future, amounting to about five million dollars."[88] This gift (worth about $67 million in 2015 dollars) was separate from the money the brothers had given to create the foundation and establish the affiliation with the University of Minnesota. The transition also involved a new system of governance.

Will summarized the new organizational plan that was implemented in 1921: "The permanent staff elect a chairman, vice chairman, and secretary, and the executive committee of five. The faculty chairman and the executive committee with five members of the board of governors form the council, which controls the affairs of the clinic. We have in this way established a medical democracy."[89] Although some power was spread among other committees and individuals, much of it remained in the hands of the Board of Governors, a small self-perpetuating group led by Will Mayo. This seemed to be the surest way to maintain the principles that had proved so successful since the turn of the century. Meanwhile, the controversy over the affiliation continued to smolder in Minneapolis.

In 1921 Lotus Coffman, the new president of the University of Minnesota, appointed an external committee to review the history of the affiliation conflict, as well as to assess the current status and future prospects of the Minneapolis-based medical school and the Rochester-based Mayo Foundation.[90] Victor Vaughan, Frank Billings, and Johns Hopkins surgeon John Finney produced a report that was published in the *Journal-Lancet*, the region's leading medical journal. These three men rejected the charge that Will Mayo, in his role as a university regent, consistently favored the Rochester end of the affiliation rather than the medical school in

Minneapolis. They applauded his "unselfishness, breadth of mind, [and] excellent judgment."[91]

Former chief of medicine Charles Greene and other doctors who had tried to destroy the affiliation surely bristled at this conclusion because they knew that the three men whom Coffman had selected were longtime friends of the Mayo brothers. Looking beyond the state's borders, the consultants from Ann Arbor, Baltimore, and Chicago concluded that "the University of Minnesota possesses in the Mayo Foundation an asset which is not equaled in any other university in the world."[92]

No one could dispute the fact that the specialty training program in Rochester was thriving. Louis Wilson prepared the first annual report of the Mayo Foundation for the university's Board of Regents in 1924. During the first nine years of the Minnesota-Mayo affiliation, 432 post-graduate trainees had devoted themselves to clinical fields. He also applauded the productivity of the research laboratories in Rochester that focused on experimental physiology and surgery (Frank Mann), experimental biochemistry (Edward Kendall), and experimental bacteriology (Edward Rosenow). Wilson pointed to the thick annual volumes of the *Collected Papers of the Mayo Clinic* as evidence of the staff members and trainees' non-clinical productivity. Wilson described the postgraduate training program that had been developed as an attempt to supplement the best features of the old apprenticeship system with the best features of graduate education.[93]

Louis Wilson, the postgraduate training program's chief architect, concluded his report: "Without boasting it may be stated that during the past two years numerous commissions and individual investigators who have studied the Foundation have said in effect that the University of Minnesota has in the Mayo Foundation and the Graduate Department of its Medical School the most effective working graduate school of medicine in the world and one of the best, if not the best, organized, manned and most productive departments of medical research."[94] Louis Wilson was boasting, but it would have been difficult for anyone to dispute his claims.

Patient Care and Clinical Research in the 1920s

Will Mayo informed a Milwaukee internist in 1918, "The war as never before has shown us how dependent we are on scientific medicine."[1] There was no standard definition of scientific medicine, but Will was eager to infuse its essence into Rochester's atmosphere. The creation of the Mayo Foundation for Medical Education and Research and the affiliation with the University of Minnesota in 1915 signaled a significant expansion of Mayo's mission. Prior to World War I, the practice had focused almost exclusively on surgery. During the 1920s, the clinic would hire and train more specialists in internal medicine, including several who were interested in clinical research. The experiences of patients who came to Rochester during this decade were influenced by the increasing size and sophistication of the group practice.

A Tennessee physician claimed in a 1919 editorial that almost every medical graduate wanted to do surgery and that surgeons ran most hospitals. This disgruntled doctor declared, "Are our 'internists' and general practitioners failures? Is there nothing worthwhile in medicine except through surgery? Oh, for an Osler or two, if two there could be, to demonstrate the possibilities for real scientific and beneficial work in the field of general medicine!"[2] William Osler, the English-speaking world's most influential internist, responded in a letter to the editor: "Surely you have misjudged the situation in internal medicine. As I see it, the outlook in the United States has never been so hopeful."[3] Osler proclaimed, "The surgeons have had their day—and they know it! The American St. Cosmas and St. Damien—The Mayo Brothers—have made their clinic today as important in medicine as it ever was in surgery. Wise men! They saw how the pendulum was swinging."[4]

Will Mayo did not disagree with William Osler. In fact, he told the president of the Tennessee State Medical Society in 1921 that "a large number of the brightest young men are now taking up internal medicine."[5] Some of the excitement that had surrounded surgery for a generation was now shifting to internal medicine thanks to new discoveries, diagnostic techniques, and treatments. "Medicine has been in a state of flux," Mayo explained, "and is now rather definitely passing from the stage of pills and powders into a new conception of internal therapy based on physiologic processes, biochemistry and physics."[6] When Will Mayo wrote this, the clinic was actively adding staff and developing programs devoted to basic medical research and clinical investigation involving patients. Increasingly, Rochester would provide an environment that encouraged the integration of patient care with clinical and laboratory research.

Clinical Investigators Complement Internist-Diagnosticians

During the first two decades of the twentieth century, Christopher Graham and Henry Plummer had led a growing team of internist-diagnosticians at Mayo. But Graham, who was Charlie Mayo's brother-in-law and a partner in the practice, opposed the creation of the Mayo Properties Association. He resigned in 1919. Meanwhile, Plummer had been the main person responsible for developing the comprehensive approach to outpatient diagnosis that impressed patients and visiting doctors.[7] The main goal of this process was to identify patients who would benefit from surgery. Plummer did some clinical research related to thyroid disease, but it was not his passion. He did appreciate the increasing importance of organized clinical investigation involving patients as a tool to decipher disease mechanisms and develop new and better treatments.

In 1920 Will Mayo hired internist-investigator Leonard Rowntree to develop a major hospital-based program of clinical research. Rowntree, in many ways Plummer's polar opposite, was gregarious, a gifted speaker, prolific author, and active participant in several professional organizations. During the 1920s, he played a major role in transforming the Mayo Clinic from a surgically oriented group practice into a patient-centered academic factory that produced medical knowledge and clinical investigators. "My first concern in joining the clinic," Rowntree recalled, "was to find a productive staff—men with both clinical and laboratory training who would be interested in teaching and research as well as in the care of the sick."[8] He was well prepared to accomplish these goals when he arrived in Rochester.

A Canadian who had received his medical degree in 1905, Rowntree then spent seven years working with pharmacologist John Jacob Abel at the Johns Hopkins Medical School. During this time, he published more than two dozen scientific papers, some of which described new kidney and liver function tests that changed medical practice. Rowntree also coauthored two papers describing an "artificial kidney" for use in animal research. It was a precursor of human hemodialysis, which was introduced decades later to treat patients with acute kidney failure.[9] The launch of the full-time salary system at Johns Hopkins in 1913 led to resignations that allowed Rowntree to shift from experimental pharmacology into clinical medicine. Theodore Janeway, the new professor of medicine at Hopkins, invited him to join his department as an associate professor.[10]

Rowntree moved to Minneapolis in 1916, when he was hired by the University of Minnesota to replace Charles Greene, who had been forced to resign as chief of medicine because of his aggressive campaign to end the Mayo-university affiliation.[11] In a letter of recommendation, Janeway described Rowntree as "a very remarkable man, with a genius for fruitful research."[12] Although Rowntree was based in Minneapolis, he interacted regularly with the Mayo brothers, Louis Wilson, and others in Rochester as a result of the affiliation. On the basis of his training, experience, and passion for research, Rowntree seemed to be the perfect person to develop a productive program of clinical investigation at the Mayo Clinic.

When Rowntree moved to Rochester in the spring of 1920, the staff was informed that he had come "to work in the graduate school of medicine, to participate in the work of the clinic, and to carry on research . . . in the field of internal medicine, especially in connection with vascular, renal, and metabolic diseases."[13] Rowntree coordinated the creation of research laboratories at St. Mary's Hospital that were designed to support an inpatient program of clinical investigation. His group of internist-investigators devoted time to routine diagnosis, but they were expected to develop new or improved treatments for specific diseases, such as diabetes and kidney failure.[14] When Will Mayo informed his longtime friend Chicago internist Frank Billings that Rowntree had accepted a full-time position in Rochester, he explained that they were also recruiting "one or two other high grade men in physiology and biochemistry who will help in building up the scientific work on the clinical side."[15]

In the fall of 1920, the Mayo brothers and Rowntree tried to recruit Walter Cannon, the head of physiology at Harvard Medical School. Although the Wisconsin-born scientist seriously considered the opportunity, he decided to stay in Boston. Cannon informed Rowntree that he was concerned that the "emphasis would be on applied physiology" in Rochester.[16] Having succeeded Henry Bowditch, Harvard's first full-time physiologist and a key figure in the professionalization of the field, Cannon emphasized that he was committed to mentoring medical scientists. In a letter to Charlie Mayo, he explained, "There is a great dearth of trained physiologists. It was this fact which really settled my determination to stay on my present job."[17]

Will Mayo, informing Cannon that he was disappointed but not surprised by his decision, wrote, "I believe that physiology should be brought directly into contact with the sick man instead of being kept at a distance, because it . . . will do much to elucidate problems which hamper the clinical man in his efforts to care for the sick, as well as to advance the science and art of medicine."[18] The sixty-year-old surgeon's response reflected the fact that he envisioned research programs in Rochester as an important adjunct to the Mayo Clinic's main mission of patient care.

Shortly after Leonard Rowntree joined the Mayo Clinic, he became president of the prestigious American Society for Clinical Investigation.[19] When he delivered his presidential address in 1921, the audience included many leaders of academic internal medicine. Rowntree challenged them to help convince the public and the profession that research was vitally important—that the "routine practice of today is based on the investigation of yesterday."[20]

The recent European war had devastated some of the world's most productive medical research centers and had disrupted the traditional career path of aspiring clinical investigators. Reminding his audience that "much of the sowing and early cultivation" of clinical investigators had been done abroad before the war, Rowntree argued that America must assume those responsibilities. His metaphorical seeds were recent medical graduates with the potential to mature into productive clinical investigators. But these scarce hybrids, part physician–part scientist, required a special milieu: "Environment is all important and includes subsidiary factors necessary for production, such as time, space, facilities for work, inspiration, guidance, criticism, advice, and access to literature."[21] Rowntree did not boast about his new institutional context in Rochester, but he knew that the Mayo Clinic provided all of these things.

The Kahler: A New Combination Hospital-Hotel Building

Downtown Rochester's skyline changed in 1921, when a hybrid hospital-hotel named the Kahler opened across the street from the seven-year-old Mayo Clinic building (Figure 4.1).[22] Will Mayo, explaining the Kahler concept to members of the American College of Surgeons, said that some beds would be set aside for "borderline cases in which the diagnosis is doubtful or in which the indications for treatment are not clear, in order that a joint attack may be made on disease."[23] Clinical research was part of the plan: "One group of cases may be treated surgically, and another similar group medically, and direct comparison made from a noncompetitive standpoint." This strategy would encourage "scientific co-operation for the welfare of the sick."[24] When the American Congress of Internal Medicine met at the Mayo Clinic in 1922, Will welcomed the internists and predicted that collaboration between physicians and surgeons would increase in the future: "In no sense is the surgeon an independent worker, but rather the 'chief carpenter' while the internist and the diagnostician are the 'architects.' "[25]

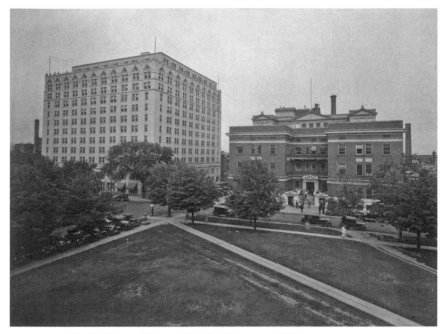

FIGURE 4.1 *The Kahler and Mayo Clinic buildings, ca. 1925.*
Used with permission of Mayo Foundation.

The twelve-story Kahler served several purposes. The first four floors functioned as a hotel for patients undergoing outpatient diagnostic evaluations at the clinic and their families. Three middle floors were a convalescent unit with 150 beds for postoperative patients. The top floors were a hospital containing 210 beds for medical and surgical patients, laboratories, and operating rooms. Two of these floors were reserved for patients with a goiter, a thyroid disease that especially interested Charlie Mayo, Henry Plummer, Louis Wilson, and Edward Kendall.[26] Plummer's team of internist-diagnosticians cared for some of the patients admitted to the Kahler. He supervised research there, which resulted in his recommendation that patients with hyperthyroidism be given iodine (in the form of so-called Lugol's solution) before a surgeon operated on the overactive gland. This intervention significantly reduced the risk of surgery.[27]

Physiologist Frank Mann, who oversaw Mayo's busy laboratory of experimental surgery, spoke to members of the American Congress of Internal Medicine when they met at the clinic in 1922. Anti-vivisection sentiment was smoldering at the time, and he implored the visiting internists to "educate the patients of today and those of the future with regard to the necessity of experimental investigation."[28] When Mann spoke, the new Institute of Experimental Medicine was nearing completion on eighty acres of land that Charlie Mayo had donated. One reason for moving Mayo's research facilities to the nearby countryside was that the new Kahler towered over the clinic building with its rooftop animal pens. The rural site provided much more space, and the animals were invisible to individuals sympathetic to the anti-vivisectionist movement.

The president of the American Congress of Internal Medicine, Johns Hopkins internist Sydney Miller, asked Will Mayo to "thank all the members of the clinic for their untiring efforts to make the recent meeting in Rochester so successful."[29] Most of the doctors who visited the Mayo Clinic during the 1922 congress also attended the annual meeting of the American College of Physicians in Minneapolis the next day. College president James Anders was impressed by what he had seen in Rochester. In his speech to college members, the Philadelphia internist praised two institutions that were producing a new type of physician: "The University of Pennsylvania and the Mayo Foundation are offering courses at present that qualify men and women for the ranks both of 'internists' and scientific research workers."[30]

The annual volumes of the *Collected Papers of the Mayo Clinic* provided evidence that the institution was producing new knowledge and well-trained specialists. The 1922 edition was impressive by any measure. Eighty-five authors contributed almost 150 papers to the 1,408-page book, which weighed more than five pounds. Most of the authors were surgeons, but internists and scientists were becoming increasingly visible in these annual compilations of published articles.[31]

The Mayo Clinic's reputation as a major academic medical center grew as a result of publications and presentations by its staff and trainees. If regional or national societies asked for speakers, Will Mayo thought that only those "of known ability should be sent and that only papers well worthwhile should be presented."[32] Eager to showcase his institution's commitment to research, he told Mayo's Board of Governors in 1923 that it was "very important for the clinic to maintain at all times a group of what might be called 'window dressers'... investigators who would always have something new and interesting to present to the profession and to show visiting men."[33] Will and Charlie Mayo had used a similar strategy to build their surgical practice in the late nineteenth century. Now, it was employed to promote Mayo's image as a well-rounded academic medical center.

Internists Require Hospital Beds for Clinical Research

Leonard Rowntree injected a big dose of medical science into Rochester's atmosphere after his arrival in Rochester in 1920. One of the world's best trained pharmacologists and a committed clinical researcher, he assembled a group of internist-investigators that complemented Henry

Plummer's team of physicians, who devoted most of their energy to diagnosis. Members of Rowntree's group spent a significant part of their time working in the hospital, but these internists' needs were different from those of the surgeons who had previously dominated the inpatient environment. Surgeons worked in operating rooms, where their scalpel- and suture-based therapeutic acts took a few minutes to a few hours. On the other hand, internists involved in clinical investigation needed a different kind of space and much more time (usually several days to a few weeks) to treat patients medically and to monitor their progress as part of a research program.

St. Mary's Hospital opened a new surgical pavilion in 1922 that contained ten operating rooms, a 200-seat amphitheater, and 300 beds. The building it replaced was renovated for medical patients who would be cared for by the internist-investigators that Rowntree had recruited and trainees who were assigned to their hospital services. A booklet published that year to celebrate the growth of St. Mary's Hospital proclaimed, "The heads of the Medical Department and their associates are picked men of splendid abilities, commanding the choicest advantages of science, art and experience. Opportunity is now afforded them to carry on their work under favorable conditions and to duplicate, if not to surpass, the record made by the Surgical Department in the past." Rowntree's team, with access to almost 150 beds, would "receive from the hospital administration the same support and co-operation that made possible the great success of surgery at St. Mary's."[34]

The first patients were admitted to the new medical unit in September 1922. The annual report listed Rowntree as head of the Medical Department, which included four other staff members, each of whom was in charge of a hospital service devoted to patients with a specific type of disease: Russell Wilder (diabetes), Norman Keith (kidney disease), George Brown (vascular disease), and George Eusterman (gastrointestinal disease). These internist-investigators, along with the fifteen trainees assigned to work with them, had access to special hospital-based laboratories, including one designed for small animal experiments.[35]

Rowntree was an influential member of a national group of therapeutic reformers that advocated for basic research to discover new drugs and for clinical studies to test promising ones on patients.[36] As chair of the American Medical Association's Section on Pharmacology and Therapeutics in 1921, Rowntree argued that "experimental therapy and access to wards would accomplish much for the advancement of medical treatment." He was also concerned about patient safety: "The welfare of the public demands preliminary experimentation and adequate controls. The results in ten well-controlled cases are of more value than the haphazard impressions from a thousand cases."[37]

Insulin Therapy of Diabetes Exemplifies the Value of Research

Three months after Rowntree's paper on drug therapy was published in the *Journal of the American Medical Association*, he and his Mayo colleague Russell Wilder heard University of Toronto physiologists Frederick Banting and Charles Best lecture during the annual meeting of the American Physiological Society.[38] The Canadians described their preliminary research on a pancreatic gland extract that reduced blood sugar levels. This work led to one of the biggest therapeutic breakthroughs in the history of medicine— the discovery of insulin treatment for diabetes.[39]

Wilder was interested in diabetes before he joined the Mayo Clinic in 1919. His prior training and experience, combined with the clinic's reputation and expanding research infrastructure, led to his selection as one of six doctors who were given pre-market samples of insulin for human studies in December 1922. The following month he was the first of the six to submit a manuscript to the *Journal of Metabolic Research*, which was assembling a special issue containing the earliest reports of the use of insulin in patients.[40] Wilder and his Mayo coauthors were convinced of insulin's "great value in the treatment of severe forms of diabetes and in the emergencies of this condition (acidosis, infection, and so forth)."[41] Insulin's life-saving potential was impossible to ignore.

Traditionally, doctors had come to Rochester to learn, but after the formalization of the postgraduate training program and the affiliation with the University of Minnesota, academic physicians and scientists visited the city to lecture. In February 1923 Frederick Banting and John Macleod, professor of physiology at the University of Toronto, spoke at the clinic about the recent discovery of insulin and its role in treating diabetic patients. Macleod emphasized that animal experiments had been indispensable in the discovery of insulin—a compelling example of how research could advance patient care.[42]

Insulin's ability to restore weight and save lives amazed patients, physicians, and the public. Historian Michael Bliss produced a vivid word picture of its power: "The most spectacular of insulin's triumphs came when comatose diabetics were virtually resurrected by the injections."[43] Frederick Gates, a Baptist minister who became John D. Rockefeller's main philanthropic adviser, was among the first patients to receive insulin. Gates described his initial dose as "simply magical" and marveled that it instantly restored his sense of well-being.[44]

Russell Wilder supervised forty patients with diabetes on the new medical service at St. Mary's Hospital. He opened his 1923 article "How Is the Overworked General Practitioner to Use Insulin?" by acknowledging that community physicians and specialists in academic medical centers worked in very different worlds: "In his enthusiasm for elevating medicine to a high scientific plane, the specialist, surrounded by elaborate hospital and laboratory facilities, often fails to realize that the general practitioner, omniscient and omnipotent though he must be, is becoming bewildered in the maze of new and rapidly multiplying technical procedures."[45] But there was hope for the busy practitioner with minimal laboratory facilities. Wilder explained that most patients with diabetes could be managed without a specialist's help. In fact, about 7,000 American doctors were prescribing insulin to more than 20,000 patients in September 1923.[46]

Will Mayo spoke at the dedication of Boston City Hospital's Thorndike Memorial Laboratory in November 1923, fourteen months after Rowntree's medical unit opened at St. Mary's Hospital. He considered the new Massachusetts facility especially noteworthy because it represented "the first recognition by a municipality of the practical value of research." Adopting the rhetoric of educational reformers, Will linked the mission of academic medical centers to better patient care: "A hospital which functions as a school for graduates in medicine, giving advanced scientific training, will enlist the best efforts of the highest type of recent graduates in medicine, and automatically give to its clientele the great advantage of a young, intelligent, and enthusiastic junior staff."[47] Shortly after he returned to Rochester, Will wrote to his friend Harvey Cushing, who had been in Boston for a decade: "While it is idle to say that surgery has reached its height, many conditions which have been treated surgically have gone back to medicine, or will do so. When the great cures for tuberculosis, cancer, and so forth, come—and come they must—they are sure to be medical."[48]

Will recognized the Mayo Clinic's shifting image and expanding mission. He told the Board of Governors in 1924 that their institution occupied "the prominent position that it does by reason of its investigative and educational program rather than by its clinical work."[49] The Progressive Era educational reformers had witnessed major improvements in the quality of medical schools and hospitals during the first quarter of the twentieth century. Emphasizing the dynamic national context and its implications for clinical and academic programs in Rochester, Will warned the board: "While excellent clinical and surgical results are necessary to the successful operation of the clinic, good work along these lines is also being done all over the country and what constantly brings the spotlight on the clinic is its investigative and educational program rather than its routine clinical and surgical work."[50]

The Interurban Clinic Club, an organization of academic internists who shared an interest in clinical research, met in Rochester in 1925. After the meeting, Chicago internist Joseph Miller informed Will: "We were all greatly interested in the work going on there. The thing that impressed me most was that you are obtaining the problems for investigation from your daily work, just the things that come up in the ordinary course of examining patients. Consequently all these problems were of interest to the clinician. This seems a much better method for carrying on investigation than to get hold of a theory and then try to produce evidence to support it."[51] Will responded that he was glad that Miller valued the "practical application of scientific research."[52]

James Anders, a recent president of the American College of Physicians, praised the Mayo Clinic in 1926 for providing laboratories for internists interested in clinical research. In a talk on "Idealism in Internal Medicine," he cited the Johns Hopkins University, the Rockefeller Foundation, and the Mayo Clinic for having "potently fostered the movement for higher medical research in this country."[53]

Shaping Staff Attitudes and Patient Experiences

London surgeon Rickman Godlee wrote to Will Mayo in 1923, a decade after he had visited Rochester: "Are you still ruling over your little kingdom with the same beneficent autocracy, and does it function in the same harmonious way which was so striking to me and others of my compatriots?"[54] In fact, the little kingdom Godlee referred to had grown tremendously. Around the time his letter arrived, the Mayo Clinic's daily bulletin challenged staff members to reflect on their unique environment:

> There are nearly 800 persons in the clinic including the professional members of the staff. How many of them do you know? Do you know enough about the workings of the clinic to explain it to someone who wants to know? What is the work of each section? What is the routine of the clinic? Who is doing the unusual and striking work? What are all the other 799 doing, and how does their work affect you? We are all here together working for the same thing, some in big ways, some in little ways, but consciously or unconsciously we share a common objective.[55]

These Mayo staff members were part of a huge workforce that operated Rochester's massive medical and surgical machinery. The city's hospitals employed more than a thousand other men and women in dozens of job categories. And more than 400 students were enrolled in nursing schools sponsored by St. Mary's Hospital and the Kahler Hospital.[56]

As Rickman Godlee suggested, Will Mayo did rule over the clinic. Urologist William Braasch, who had joined the staff in 1907 and was a long-time member of the Board of Governors, recalled that Will "laid down definite standards of conduct for members of the staff."[57] If he thought that a staff member's behavior at (or even outside) work was unacceptable and a warning did not result in change, dismissal was a distinct possibility. Rather than relying on disciplinary measures, however, the main method of maintaining decorum was to create a culture of respect.

Will Mayo and chief administrator Harry Harwick dealt with most behavioral issues that involved doctors, but occasionally the Board of Governors

got involved. In 1923, for example, the board discussed tensions in the operating rooms at Colonial Hospital, which had opened seven years earlier and
was staffed exclusively by Mayo doctors. They were concerned that "several
of the surgeons operating there act very temperamentally," which was making it "difficult to keep competent [nurse] anesthetists and operating room
technicians." After discussing these dynamics, the board agreed that surgeons "must conduct themselves so as to win the respect and confidence of
their operating room staff. This cannot be accomplished by 'prima donna
temperament,' cursing, nagging, or displaying irritation while operating."[58]

Employees were coached on conduct and were reminded about rules. The
Mayo Clinic Desk Book, a comprehensive policy manual, contained chapters
describing the facilities, functions of various sections, and operational procedures. Its first portion included aphorisms designed to shape attitudes and
behaviors: "*Remember*: A call from a patient takes precedence over personal
engagements. Neglect of a patient means that you are in the wrong profession. A smile at the right time can often alleviate the sting of a bad prognosis.
Taking a personal interest in each patient is good for the patient, the clinic
and yourself."[59]

Will told the Board of Governors in 1924 that "the clinic should aim at all
times to deliver to each patient the same type of service that a member of the
staff would desire and insist upon for his own family." In response, the board
charged each clinical section head with making sure that "patients registered
in his section are rendered a type of personal service that will satisfy and
please them and will be a credit not only to the section but to the institution."[60] The daily *Clinic Bulletin* reminded the staff that "each patient is a
private case, and that while the patients are here in large numbers, each must
be treated as an individual with every courtesy possible."[61]

The same philosophy of patient care was evident at St. Mary's Hospital,
run by the Franciscan sisters, and at Rochester's other hospitals, all staffed
exclusively by Mayo doctors.[62] Treating all patients respectfully contrasted
with the situation in other settings, such as some urban teaching hospitals.
Historian Rosemary Stevens explains: "For some patients, particularly those
of lower social class, the teaching hospital was a terrifying place before World
War I (and later). Chicago reformer Jane Adams remarked caustically that
the patient was not the chief concern of those hospitals at all. Training the
intern seemed to come first; then came the visiting staff of physicians; third,
the training of the nurse; and, only last, the comfort of the patient."[63] In
Rochester, the activities in the hospitals centered on the patients who had
chosen to come to the city for care.

Contemporary cultural norms in the United States did affect local attitudes
and actions. For example, they influenced which applicants were accepted
into Mayo's postgraduate training programs. Once again, Rosemary Stevens
provides perspective on the national situation: "Through the educational

system white medical students were socialized into a profession whose model of quality was the white (preferably WASP) male."[64] In 1927 Louis Wilson explained to the director of the Rockefeller Foundation's Division of Medical Education why the Mayo Foundation Graduate Committee had decided not to offer a fellowship to a Haitian doctor: "All of our patients are 'private.' Though one-third of them are actually charity patients in the sense that they pay nothing to the clinic, they are all treated as though they were pay patients. You will thus see that we do not have any charity-patient group who might be willing to be under the care of a colored physician."[65]

Louis Wilson cited a single experience in an attempt to justify the Graduate Committee's decision: "Several years ago we had one very able physician from India here, to whom a great deal of objection was raised by patients. Since then we have had several Japanese fellows. They do excellent research work but have never had duties bringing them into contact with patients." Wilson closed, "I greatly regret that it seems impossible for us to do this."[66] The Rockefeller Foundation official responded: "I feared the difficulty you mention might arise. I felt, however, that in view of the many advantages possible for [the doctor] in Rochester, I should at least make an attempt to secure an opening for him in your clinic before approaching other institutions."[67]

Mayo's leaders were products of and participants in American culture. Their words and actions must be viewed in the context of their time rather than through a present-day lens.[68] Racial, ethnic, and religious prejudices were ubiquitous in the United States when Louis Wilson wrote to the Rockefeller Foundation official. Minnesota, especially outside the Twin Cities, was very homogeneous in terms of race. The 1930 census of Olmsted County (where Rochester is located) recorded only 38 African Americans and one Mexican among a population of more than 35,000. Compared to urban settings, Rochester's medical workforce was also very homogeneous. A majority of employees were descendants of Northern European immigrants, and many of them lived (or had been raised) on farms in the region.[69]

Each person who traveled to Rochester for care found himself or herself in the center of several personal interactions involving family members, doctors, nurses, and countless other clinic and hospital employees. Hundreds of men and women worked in town to provide lodging, food, transportation, and a host of other services to about one thousand patients who arrived each week. Regional American and international accents attested to the Mayo Clinic's enormous geographic reach. A newsstand in the clinic building sold newspapers from more than two dozen cities across the country. These papers arrived on the same trains that brought most patients to the city.[70]

Trains were the main mode of public transportation to Rochester throughout the 1920s. By the end of the decade, some affluent patients and visitors had another option. Charles Lindbergh, who had grown up on a Minnesota farm, heightened awareness about the potential of commercial air travel with his 1927 transatlantic flight. One year later, a Minneapolis-based company inaugurated scheduled flights between Minneapolis and Rochester in a new Ford Trimotor, which the local newspaper described as "the safest aircraft flying."[71] The first flight, which carried thirteen passengers, landed at Rochester's fairgrounds on July 13, 1928. Soon, the city would have a real airport. The *Minneapolis Evening Tribune* reported that "a completely equipped airport and bus terminal to cover 284 acres is to be established at Rochester... by the Mayo Properties Association at a cost of $150,000." Scheduled air service between Rochester and Chicago began in November 1928.[72]

Making a Patient's Mayo Clinic Experience More Personal

Most patients who came to the Mayo Clinic were used to getting their medical care from a local general practitioner. Henry Plummer and Will Mayo developed a system before World War I that forged a personal doctor-patient relationship in the context of their large group practice. The plan was simple: "The physician who originally examines a case shall hold himself entirely responsible for the patient's care."[73] The internist-diagnostician who filled this role also ordered tests and requested consultations from one or more specialists. A patient's diagnostic evaluation, referred to as "going through the clinic," usually took several days. It often included a consultation with a surgeon and culminated in a return visit to see the coordinating internist, who discussed diagnoses that had been made and outlined a treatment plan. Almost all patients who were felt not to require surgery were returned to the care of their local doctor.

The Mayo Clinic's success as a specialty care center depended, in part, on building and maintaining good relations with referring physicians. At a Board of Governors meeting in 1928, Charlie Mayo emphasized that it was important "to please country doctors and general practitioners who refer patients to the clinic."[74] Letters that about fifty Mayo doctors sent to small town general practitioner Frank Brey in the 1920s exemplify this strategy. The authors of a review of the correspondence concluded that the letters "were invariably gracious and usually began with an expression of thanks for the referral. Brief and to the point, they contained all essential information."[75]

It was also important to project an image of competence and collegiality. A notice in the *Clinic Bulletin* reminded staff doctors that casual comments could resonate locally or at a distance: "Great care must be taken that the opinion of other men in the clinic or that of the home physicians are not belittled by word or look. A word dropped in conversation may destroy confidence in the opinion given by another consultant."[76] The use of the term "consultant" to refer to members of the clinic's professional staff sent a signal to hometown doctors that the Rochester group practice was not trying to take over the care of their patients. It reinforced the notion that Mayo staff members provided expert opinions and short-term problem-focused treatment, rather than ongoing care. The goal was to complement rather than compete with actual or potential referring physicians.

Many patients welcomed the very thorough diagnostic evaluations that were a central part of the Mayo Clinic experience, especially if their hometown doctor had been unable to identify a cause for their symptoms or to provide an effective treatment. Some postcards sent from Rochester recounted personal health care experiences. One patient told a friend in Minneapolis, "They have smart doctors here. This p.m. one found out what may be the cause of my embarrassing ailment. I will have to stay more than a week, but I'd better...let them do a thorough job."[77]

Not every patient welcomed Mayo's intensive and time-consuming evaluations. One woman, Martha, was disgruntled about her husband's protracted diagnostic workup. "Charles got his evaluation," she told a friend in Iowa. "They sure take their time up here getting ready to do anything. I am more disgusted with them than ever."[78] Another patient informed a friend in Illinois, "I really do not know any more yet than when I left home. I have finished going through the clinic today at two o'clock. Tomorrow morning at nine I will know what I have to do. So many have to go through more than once, so I may have several days yet but I hope not."[79] Individual experiences and attitudes varied, but the clinic was committed to trying to achieve complete and accurate diagnoses.

The 1924 booklet *Compend of Clinical Examinations at the Mayo Clinic*, which was circulated to the fellows and medical staff, provides insight into the philosophy and procedures designed to decipher clues that could help a doctor make diagnoses. After opening with a statement about the value of the history and physical examination, the tone became prescriptive:

> An accurate history of the present complaint and a history of previous accidents or acute illnesses is [*sic*] of distinct value. The printed outline on the history sheet should be followed. When the patient presents himself, evidence a friendly interest in him. If at the start his confidence is gained, the true facts may be obtained much more easily and accurately. Take time to listen to his story and then question as you need, inviting replies about the various systems, such as cardiovascular, gastro-intestinal, et cetera. A patient who is of the neurotic type and who has many complaints is likely to be labeled a "neuro." One is prone to discount his statements. This to some extent may be necessary in their proper evaluation but care must be taken not to overlook a diseased condition which may be obscured by the many and varied symptoms. It takes tact and persistence and a broad general knowledge of medicine

in many instances to elicit points in the general history which may lead to the diagnosis.[80]

The booklet's introduction placed diagnostic technologies and procedures in perspective, and Mayo doctors were advised to "make judicious use of the various laboratory aids to diagnosis, including the X-ray and special examinations."[81] The text was divided into twenty parts that mirrored the clinic's sectional structure: esophageal, gastric and abdominal, intestinal, chest, anemias, heart and circulation, thyroid gland, hypertension and arteriosclerosis, nephritis, urology, glycosuria (diabetes), gynecology, obstetrics, orthopedics, otolaryngology and rhinology, ophthalmology, neurology, psychiatry, syphilology, and dermatology.[82] The diagnostic approach detailed in the document helps to explain why evaluations at the Mayo Clinic took so long and were viewed as exhausting by many patients and exhaustive by most visiting physicians.

A New Building for More Patients, Staff, and Technologies

Henry Plummer had designed the 1914 Mayo Clinic building to facilitate the methodical system of diagnosis that he had been largely responsible for developing. By the middle of the next decade, however, several factors undermined efficiency and contributed to the frustration that some patients expressed during their evaluations. Although more and more patients sought care in Rochester, this was not the main reason for a decline in efficiency. A more important factor was the growing number and complexity of diagnostic procedures and technologies used to investigate a patient's symptoms and abnormalities detected by physical examination or basic laboratory tests. Marie wrote in a 1924 postcard: "Was at clinic today from 7:30 to 10:25. Have to report again at 3:30. There are so many divisions at the clinic that it is somewhat confusing."[83] By this time, more than 100 rooms devoted to the outpatient practice were located in an annex attached to the main Mayo Clinic building or were scattered in other downtown sites.[84]

Will Mayo and Henry Plummer discussed the need for a new outpatient diagnostic building with the Board of Governors in 1925. They had high expectations for such a structure and the opportunities it would afford for reorganizing the clinic's work and workers. Early the following year, Will told the board that a new building must result in "more compactness and centralization, particularly of laboratories, and should do away as much as possible, with the duplication of personnel, both professional and non-professional, the duplication of equipment, and should provide better and more frequent contacts between the clinical and research men." The building should also make it easier for "clinical men" to do research and "permit better and more efficient work in every department of the clinic."[85]

Two months later, Plummer told the board that the building he envisioned might cost $3 million. The board minutes document Will's concern about this grandiose plan: "Dr. Mayo stated he felt it would be a mistake to invest so much money in a new building as it would constitute too large an amount in proportion to the endowments of the clinic." But after Plummer "went into the needs of the clinic exhaustively," the board agreed "to ascertain the opinion of the general staff as to such an investment."[86] The professional staff expressed enthusiasm for the plan, which emboldened the clinic's leaders.

In May 1926 the board discussed the building proposal in detail: "The great increase in the number of patients at the Mayo Clinic has made it impossible, with our present quarters and facilities, to give that prompt service to which patients are entitled and which they demand and must have if they are to continue to come." If these concerns were not addressed soon, "patients will become dissatisfied and not remain for examination and treatment." Recognizing that this dissatisfaction would resonate far beyond Rochester, the board concluded, "The only way to prevent a decrease in the business is to be prepared to properly care for it."[87]

Turning from patient care to Mayo's academic mission, the board concluded that the crowded conditions "made it difficult to carry on the [postgraduate] medical education and research. . . . The faculty is working under adverse and disheartening conditions, which should be alleviated if we are to continue to have an efficient and loyal organization." There was only one choice: "We are at a point where we cannot stand still; we must either go forward or drop backward, and we are of the opinion that the future welfare, success and usefulness of the clinic depends upon its ability to meet conditions as they arise and care for patients efficiently and promptly, and this cannot be done under present conditions."[88]

The Mayo Clinic Board of Governors sent a document to the Mayo Properties Association justifying the expenditure of more than $2 million. Created seven years earlier when Will and Charlie donated all of the clinic's assets, valued at $5 million, the association controlled all decisions about facilities. Approval of the request was assured, however, because there was so much overlap between the boards of the clinic and the property association.[89]

Henry Plummer unpacked his architect's tools in 1926, when he began working with the Ellerbe firm of St. Paul to plan a new Mayo Clinic building. Like the earlier one, he designed it to encourage efficiency and collaboration. Fredrick Willius, Plummer's protégé and biographer, said that his colleagues saw little of the senior internist for the next two years "except for occasional glimpses, carrying large rolls of blueprints under his arm."[90] In his own compulsive way, Mayo's chief diagnostician and systematizer designed, redesigned, and refined plans for an ornate but functional structure that would eventually bear his name. Although not tall by New York City standards, it was visible from miles around when it opened in 1928 (Figure 4.2). It was the state's tallest structure until a bigger one was completed in Minneapolis the following year. The twenty-floor Art Deco building incorporated more than three thousand tons of steel and was faced with limestone and more than 1.5 million bricks. Patients, visitors, and staff appreciated the fact that it contained more than 2,000 radiators to combat Rochester's long and bitter cold winters.[91]

The number of telephone calls passing through the Mayo Clinic's switchboard in 1928 is another indicator of the institution's size and complexity. Telephone technology had spread rapidly in rural America after World War I. Several clinic operators controlled communication through an extensive internal telephone system and lines that linked the practice to the outside world. When the number of calls grew to the point that they threatened efficiency, employees were told: "Telephones in the clinic building are for business calls only. Due to the fact that there are between 8,000 and 9,000 calls daily it is requested that absolutely no social calls be put through between the hours of 8:30 am and 5:30 pm."[92] Mayo's leaders continued to develop policies to shape behaviors and control technologies.

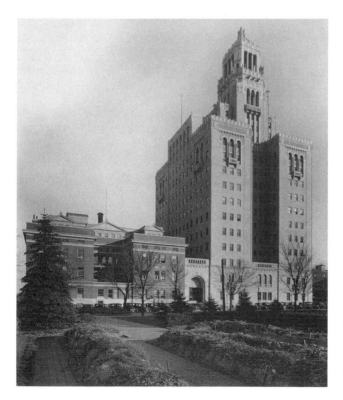

FIGURE 4.2 *The 1914 and 1928 Mayo Clinic buildings.*
Used with permission of Mayo Foundation.

Ten thousand people gathered in Rochester on September 17, 1928, for the dedication of a twenty-three-bell carillon that topped off the towering new edifice. Charlie Mayo told the crowd, "Because of the great necessity of using the new clinic building as rapidly as the floors are completed there will be no formal opening, and this day of dedication must serve. The clinic is declared now open."[93] Henry Plummer choreographed a staged move that took seven months.

The Mayo Clinic's new building exemplified the mismatch between the number of doctors in Rochester and the town's population. The 1929 *American Medical Directory* reported that Minnesota had 3,084 doctors and a population of 2.7 million; Minneapolis had 847 doctors and a population of 455,900; and Rochester had 397 doctors (almost all of them employed by the clinic) and a population of only 17,700.[94] These ratios of physician per capita reflected the Mayo Clinic's geographic reach. Since the turn of the century, several hundred thousand patients had chosen to travel to Rochester based on some combination of their personal concerns, their family's encouragement, or their local doctor's advice.

The Electrocardiograph and the
Birth of Cardiology

The opening of the Mayo Clinic building in 1914 reflected the success and growing sophistication of the group practice.[1] This five-floor facility included space for an electrocardiograph, a new technology that would contribute to the creation of cardiology as a specialty around World War I.[2] Before the war, the Mayo practice focused almost exclusively on surgery. Patients came seeking help for a range of health problems, but their hometown doctors would not have referred them to Rochester for evaluation of heart disease. The main job of Mayo's internist-diagnosticians, led by Henry Plummer, was to sort out a patient's symptoms and signs of disease in order to help a surgeon decide whether an operation was indicated and if it was safe to perform it.

Men and women with known or suspected heart disease were considered to be at increased risk for an operation. Will Mayo had warned at the turn of the century that the first clue of heart disease might be "sudden death of the patient upon the operating table or shortly afterward."[3] He urged caution if surgery was being considered in patients with signs or symptoms of heart muscle disease, such as an irregular pulse, chest pain, or shortness of breath with activity. Plummer, whose team of diagnosticians sought to identify such patients, was among the first American physicians to use the electrocardiograph as a tool to help detect and characterize heart disease. In the decade after World War I, Mayo would establish a cardiology program that attracted national attention as a result of the academic activities of a few of its staff members whose interest centered on the heart and cardiovascular system.

The Advent of the Electrocardiograph: Tracing the Heartbeat

The electrocardiograph, invented by Dutch physiologist Willem Einthoven in 1902, produced a tracing of the heart's electrical impulse (see Figure 5.1). It provided physicians and medical scientists interested in the heart with unique

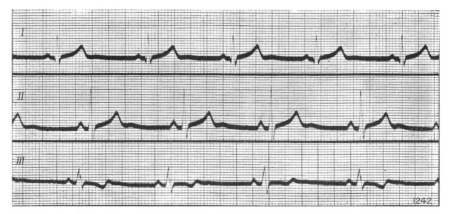

FIGURE 5.1 *Three-lead electrocardiogram recorded with Cambridge Electrocardiograph Apparatus, 1915.*

Original printed advertisement in the author's possession.

information that led to a new understanding of the organ and its diseases.[4] The Johns Hopkins Hospital installed an electrocardiograph, one of the first in the United States, in the fall of 1909. Chief of medicine Lewellys Barker and his associate Arthur Hirschfelder were enthusiastic about the new instrument's potential. The following year they predicted that "this new method will enable us to penetrate one step further into the problems which cannot be solved by older procedures and will bring us closer to a perfect understanding of what goes on in a diseased heart."[5]

In 1910 Hirschfelder published *Diseases of the Heart and Aorta*, a 632-page book filled with physiological data and diagrams that represented a dramatic departure from earlier textbooks.[6] He highlighted the origins and implications of this shift the following year in an article on the electrocardiograph. One word was repeated six times in the first sentence: "New methods lead to the discovery of new facts, new facts to new doctrines, new doctrines to new lines of treatment."[7] In addition to celebrating the notion of new, Hirschfelder linked research to theory and theory to practice. The editor of a 1911 book, *Recent Studies on Cardiovascular Diseases* (which reprinted Hirschfelder's article), explained in his introduction: "Throughout the field of internal medicine, the work of the investigator, in clinic and in laboratory, is producing profound changes in our outlook as practical physicians. In none of its subdivisions are these changes more fundamental than in the field of cardio-vascular disease."[8]

Hirschfelder left Johns Hopkins in 1913 to become the head of the new Department of Pharmacology at the University of Minnesota. Shortly after arriving in Minneapolis, he published a second edition of his book on heart disease. The section on electrocardiography was now much longer because the new test had "become a procedure of routine examination of heart cases in many medical clinics."[9] Thomas Lewis, a London-based clinical investigator who was the English-speaking world's most influential electrocardiographer, went further. In his book *Clinical Electrocardiography*, also published in 1913, he proclaimed: "This new method of examination has become essential to the modern diagnosis and treatment of cardiac patients."[10]

Hirschfelder and Lewis exaggerated the use of the technology they were pioneering and promoting. In fact, very few institutions possessed an electrocardiograph in 1913. When Hirschfelder moved to Minnesota that year, the only electrocardiograph in the state was located at new Elliott Memorial Hospital in Minneapolis.[11] A survey of American hospitals conducted five years later revealed that fewer than 10 percent possessed the technology.[12] Several factors contributed to the slow diffusion of the electrocardiograph during the second decade of the century. The instruments were expensive (almost three times the cost of a Model T Ford), large, complex to operate, and difficult to maintain.

Henry Plummer was what sociologists would describe as an "early adopter" of technology, and the Mayo Clinic's diagnostic arm reflected this.[13] When Plummer began planning the big Mayo Clinic building in the fall of 1912, he wrote to the Cambridge Scientific Instrument Company in England about their electrocardiographic apparatus (see Figure 5.2). The firm had sold about fifty units by this time, the majority to physiologists for use in animal

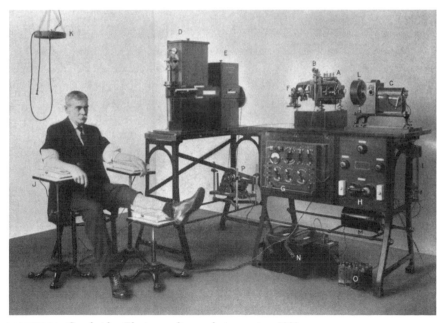

FIGURE 5.2 *Cambridge Electrocardiograph Apparatus, 1915.*
Original printed advertisement in the author's possession.

research.[14] Plummer, eager to incorporate new diagnostic methods into the Mayo practice, faced a challenge with the electrocardiograph. Responding to an inquiry from the Rochester group, the director of the Cambridge-based company stressed that the instrument of precision was very vulnerable to vibration. To minimize vibration, which "depends so much on the proximity of the roadway, and on the weight and amount of traffic which is passing," the company representative recommended mounting the electrocardiograph on "an independent concrete pier."[15] The letters were exchanged in 1912, but the installation of the electrocardiograph had to wait until the new Mayo Clinic building was finished two years later.

The first electrocardiogram at the Mayo Clinic was recorded on August 1, 1914.[16] Plummer asked John Blackford, a medical fellow who functioned as his assistant, to operate the instrument and interpret the tracings it produced. Patients seen the day before and the day after the debut of Mayo's electrocardiograph in the summer of 1914 were no different, and their doctors had no new heart treatments.[17] Cardiac diagnosis was different, however, because the novel technology complemented a patient's history, physical examination, X-ray, and laboratory findings. During the first seventeen months that the apparatus was in operation at Mayo, about 900 electrocardiograms were performed (exclusively on outpatients). This number of tests is impressive, considering the fact that very few hospitals possessed the technology at this time.[18]

In 1916, when about 1,200 patients had electrocardiograms at the clinic, Plummer assigned medical fellow Fredrick Willius to help Blackford record, process, and interpret them. A University of Minnesota medical graduate, Willius had begun his fellowship in Rochester one year earlier.[19] Blackford and Willius showcased Mayo's electrocardiograph in 1916, when the Interurban Clinical Club met in Rochester. Membership in the club was limited to thirty internists; most of whom were affiliated with prestigious medical schools in the Northeast.[20] Shortly before Christmas, twenty of its members watched surgeons operate at St. Mary's Hospital and listened to physicians and scientists lecture in the new Mayo Clinic building. Blackford and Willius discussed heart block, a disturbance in the electrical conduction system that could cause a slow pulse, fainting, or death. They coauthored the first article from the clinic to include electrocardiograms in 1917. It reported their experience with administering Mayo biochemist Edward Kendall's thyroid extract to patients with heart block in an attempt to speed up their pulses.[21]

Blackford moved to Seattle in 1917, and under normal circumstances Plummer might have assigned another physician to help Willius. But the United States was involved in the European war, and many of the clinic's doctors were in the service. Willius trained a technician, Julia Fitzpatrick, to record and process electrocardiograms. Since the late nineteenth century, the Mayo practice had trained nurses and technicians to do work that doctors did in most other institutions. In response to the war and the influenza epidemic of 1918, this staffing model was expanded in Rochester. Will Mayo explained the philosophy shortly after the war: "Positions as technicians of various sorts are now held by highly trained nurses, which gives the physician an opportunity to do other work."[22] Additional technicians would be trained as the volume of electrocardiograms grew.

Fred Willius was appointed to a junior staff position in 1920. Two years later, he published his book *Clinical Electrocardiography*, which he wrote in response to the "constantly increasing use of the electrocardiograph among clinicians, especially in hospitals and clinics."[23] Will Mayo, aware of the individual and institutional benefits of authorship, congratulated Willius: "It is a fine thing and a distinct addition to the books which have originated in the clinic."[24] Advertisements for *Clinical Electrocardiography* drew attention to Mayo's emerging cardiology program. For example, the front cover of several issues of the *Boston Medical and Surgical Journal* included a half-page advertisement for the book by the W. B. Saunders Company. It boasted that the volume documented "the clinical accomplishments of the electrocardiograph and particularly the work being done in this field at the Mayo Clinic."[25]

A Prominent Patient's Symptoms, Evaluations, and Treatments

Initially, the electrocardiograph was used mainly to evaluate abnormal heart rhythms. Willius was among the first cardiologists in the United States to study its role in other types of heart disease. His interest in one specific electrocardiographic pattern, abnormal T waves as a clue to coronary artery disease, influenced the management of a prominent patient who came to the Mayo Clinic in 1920.[26] This man's story, told in a series of letters, details the care he received in Rochester and elsewhere. In addition to highlighting some of the difficulties involved in the diagnosis and treatment of coronary heart disease at the time, this case history illustrates how new technologies and unproven theories may influence treatment strategies.

Fifty-six-year-old Franklin Lane had served under Presidents Theodore Roosevelt, William Howard Taft, and Woodrow Wilson. A writer in the *New York Times* claimed that no other member of Wilson's administration "enjoyed a larger circle of friends among people of all political opinion in all walks of life."[27] The letters that the former secretary of the Department of the Interior sent to friends were enlivened by witty comments. They detail his search for health—an expedition that took him from the East Coast to Rochester to the West Coast and back to Rochester.[28] During 1920, Lane became progressively disabled by chest pain that occurred with activity and at rest. He informed a friend in the fall: "My nights are so unforgivably bad, wakened up two or three times, always with this Monster squeezing my heart in his Mammoth hand."[29] Lane also had recurring upper abdominal pain that did not improve despite various dietary regimens and a rest cure at Dr. John Gehring's health retreat in Maine.[30]

After an East Coast doctor diagnosed gall bladder disease, Lane decided to go to Minnesota, "where the Mayos will take me in hand . . . to see if it is true that my stomach and my gall bladder have become too intimate. Rochester is the Reno where such divorces are granted."[31] Writing from Rochester on New Year's Eve in 1920, he told Dr. Gehring: "I am being ground and wound and twisted and fed into and out of the Mayo mill, and a great mill it is."[32] Four days into his diagnostic evaluation, Lane informed a friend:

> Slowly I am doing the stations of the Cross in this most thorough institution. I am delighted with my experience. . . . This is the most scientifically organized organization of scientists there ever was. Henry Ford could not improve upon it. Combine him with M. Pasteur, add a touch of one Edison, and a dose of your friend, Charlie Schwab, and you have the Mayo Clinic, big, systematized, modernized, machinized, doctorial plant, run by a couple of master workmen. I am seeing it all, and am prepared for any fate. . . . Tomorrow I am to be photographed and fluoroscoped—and then will come the verdict. If it is the guillotine I shall go gaily. . . . What I fear is an order to "rest," on a new diet. But I guess whatever is said will be the last word—the Supreme Court decision.[33]

As Lane was making his way through Mayo's maze of diagnostic procedures and consultations in preparation for abdominal surgery, he had an episode of chest pain. In a letter to Gehring, Lane expressed his frustration with Willius, who recorded an electrocardiogram when he was having pain:

> After I had practically been declared one hundred percent pluperfect I gave the electric cardiograph [*sic*] man a picture or exhibition performance under an attack. This revealed to him a change in polarity in the current passing through which signified something, but what that something was, other than that I was having a spasm, I don't know. . . . The smug, mysterious gentleman who made this picture was much pleased, apparently at nothing more than that he had proved that I had a clutch of the heart, which I had announced, by wire, before arriving here.[34]

Describing his episodes of exertional chest pain to Gehring, Lane explained that he could not "walk half a block without that trigger being pulled. . . .

If I walk half a dozen blocks I stop a half a dozen times, and once or twice nibble at a precious pellet of nitro."[35]

Lane was describing typical "angina pectoris," a term coined by eighteenth-century British physician William Heberden, who described what a person felt and feared during an attack: "Those, who are afflicted with it, and seized, while they are walking, and more particularly when they walk soon after eating, with a painful and most disagreeable sensation in the breast, which seems as if it would take their life away, if it were to increase or to continue: the moment they stand still, all this uneasiness vanishes."[36] Lane's "precious pellet of nitro" was nitroglycerin, the only drug that predictably relieved anginal pain. It acted immediately, but there was no effective long-term treatment or cure for the distressing symptom.[37]

Lane's caricature of Willius and his cynical comment about the cardiologist's excitement when he recorded the abnormal electrocardiogram are significant. As a patient, Lane was uninterested in the intellectual aspects of the finding. But he was very concerned about how it might affect his care. Willius thought about both things. Although the cardiologist was eager to correlate the electrocardiographic and clinical findings in patients with angina, he recognized his responsibility to Lane and to the other Mayo doctors who were involved in his care. The abnormal electrocardiogram contributed to a shift in strategy. Will Mayo would not operate on Lane's abdomen. Another surgeon would take out his tonsils. *Take out his tonsils?*

The former interior secretary retraced the steps to his tonsillectomy in another letter: "After peering into, and probing, all known and unknown parts of the Mortal Man, they found the heart in one part changed its polarity,—turned over, by George, or tried to,—hence the Devil's clutch." He was referring to the T wave abnormality that Willius recorded during an attack of angina. Lane joked about the presumed cause of this finding and its implications for his care: "Why did it do this vaudevillian act? Bugs, bugs, of course. But where? So they chased them to their lair in that wicked, nasty-named and most vulgar organ known as the gall bladder. Damn the gall-bladder! Out it must come! On with the knifing! But soft, not so swift. Suppose the heart should try to play its funny stunt in the midst of the operation?"[38]

After noting that Mayo surgeons had performed 8,000 gall bladder operations with excellent results, Lane revealed his doctors' concerns and their new treatment strategy: "Hearts that do somersaults and lungs that choke up fill us with fear. So out with the tonsils where bugs accumulate and men decay, and then off with you to California where bugs degenerate and men rejuvenate." So, the middle-aged man with severe angina pectoris and persistent abdominal pain had his tonsils taken out and traveled to the West Coast to recuperate.[39]

Focal Infection: An Example of Theory Influencing Therapy

The decision to perform a tonsillectomy in a patient with angina pectoris and abdominal pain was based on the focal infection theory, which was proposed in an era when doctors thought bacteria might cause some non-contagious diseases. Frank Billings, a leading Chicago internist and longtime friend of the Mayo brothers, was the theory's chief champion. The concept was that a localized area of infected tissue could cause chronic diseases of various organs distant from the site of focal infection. Billings argued that tonsils could harbor a chronic infection that was not evident clinically. Pertinent to Lane's case, some physicians thought that focal infection involving the gall bladder and appendix could cause or worsen certain types of cardiovascular disease.[40]

Edward Rosenow, a proponent of the focal infection theory, had arrived in Rochester in 1915, when he was hired to organize a laboratory of experimental bacteriology. Before then, he had worked with Billings, who boasted that "the broad significance of focal infection to systemic disease has been made definite by the brilliant work of Edward C. Rosenow."[41] The Mayo brothers accepted the theory, and Charlie Mayo wrote several articles about it.[42] Will Mayo postponed Lane's abdominal operation, hoping that a tonsillectomy would improve his angina, making subsequent surgery safer. William Thayer, the former chief of medicine at Johns Hopkins, speculated that "many instances of angina may be fundamentally dependent on general infection arising from some unsuspected focal infection." He advised searching for and removing focal infections, which might predispose a patient to anginal attacks.[43] Lane informed a friend that his Mayo doctors had taken out his tonsils, but they would do nothing else until spring.[44]

Lane spent several weeks in California, but at the end of April he was back in Rochester "going through the grinding of the Mayo mill."[45] After a week of examinations, Lane was happy that the plan was to remove his gall bladder and appendix. Then came the bad news: "They say that my heart has grown much worse in the last three months, but that I probably have four chances out of five of pulling through, which is more chance than I ever had in politics in California."[46] On May 5, 1921, Lane informed Eleanor Roosevelt that Will Mayo would operate on him the next day: "I find myself quite serene about the matter, although I believe my heart is so bad that they fear giving ether and will keep me conscious if they can, applying only a local anesthetic."[47]

Several visiting doctors (including Frank Billings) watched the world-renowned surgeon prepare to open Lane's abdomen. The plan to avoid ether anesthesia was abandoned when he developed severe chest pain on the operating table. The former interior secretary survived the operation. Five days after having his gall bladder and appendix removed, he reported: "I am doing well, cared for well, as happy as can be; have had none of my angina pains since the operation."[48] He expected to spend three more weeks in St. Mary's Hospital.

A dozen days after surgery, Lane's recovery suddenly veered off track. A newspaper headline announced: "Former Secretary of Interior in Wilson Cabinet Victim of Heart Disease Following an Operation."[49] He had died suddenly at 6:10 a.m. after an hour-long episode of severe chest pain. Another newspaper reported: "A post-mortem examination late today revealed that death had been caused from sclerosis of the coronary artery of the heart. He had practically recovered from his operation...and the heart attack was unexpected."[50] Statistics from St. Mary's Hospital for 1921 show that only twelve of 774 patients who had their gall bladders removed did not survive.[51]

In 1925, four years after Franklin Lane died, Willius published an article on the relationship between chronic gall bladder infection and cardiovascular disease. He summarized the cases of seventy-nine patients with various types of cardiovascular disease who had gall bladder surgery, and noted that there was only one death. Although the patient was not identified, the clinical features suggest that it was Lane. Willius explained that his study did not prove that chronic gall bladder infections caused cardiovascular disease, but he thought they might contribute to its progression. He was impressed that there was "distinct improvement in the cardiac condition in more than half the cases following operation."[52] By this time, however, enthusiasm for the focal infection theory was waning.

Charlie Mayo admitted in 1927, "I have always taken an interest in the down and out, and I don't know anything that is nearer down and out just now than focal infection."[53] The rise and fall of the focal infection theory in one generation exemplifies a phenomenon that Will Mayo discussed with a group of surgeons four years later: "As I see the younger men picking up the torch and carrying it on, I realize that scientific truth which I formerly thought of as fixed, as though it could be weighed and measured, is changeable. Add a fact, change the outlook, and you have a new truth. Truth is a constant variable. We seek it, we find it, our viewpoint changes, and the truth changes to meet it."[54]

The Mayo Clinic Creates a Cardiology Section

The electrocardiograph was central to Fred Willius's identity as a heart specialist. It was also a catalyst for the development of cardiology as a specialty around World War I. In 1917 New York internist Lewis Conner was appointed chief of the Army Medical Corps Division of Internal Medicine, which included a Cardiovascular Section. To qualify as a "cardiovascular specialist" an internist must have had "adequate training in the modern

aspects of cardiac diagnosis." He also had to know how to use the electrocardiograph and the polygraph, a small instrument for recording arterial and
venous pulse wave forms.[55] Willius remained in Rochester during the war, but
an Anglo-American network of doctors that formed in Europe influenced his
career by promoting the development of cardiology as a specialty.[56]

Mayo's Board of Governors established a "separate section for diseases
of the heart" on October 25, 1923, and appointed Willius to lead it. Henry
Plummer made the recommendation, which acknowledged the "rapidly
increasing practice in diseases of the heart" at their institution. The board
also gave the cardiologist two rooms in the new Kahler hospital-hotel for a
second electrocardiograph and "a sufficient number of beds there to carry
on his work."[57] Although the phrase "separate section" implies autonomy,
Willius remained in Plummer's general diagnostic section. In 1924 the clinic's
outpatient General Diagnostic Medical Services included ten separate general
medicine sections that were staffed by twenty-six internist-diagnosticians,
eleven first assistants (junior staff members), and twenty-six fellows (residents).[58] At the beginning of the decade, Willius devoted most of his time to
general diagnosis, but gradually his work shifted toward the evaluation of
patients with known or suspected heart disease.

The first annual report of the cardiology section, which Willius prepared
in December 1924, revealed a striking increase in the number of electrocardiograms performed since the technology had been introduced at the
clinic a decade earlier. During the year, technicians recorded electrocardiograms on 4,369 outpatients, 709 patients hospitalized at the Kahler, and 560
patients hospitalized at St. Mary's. Willius and his half-time assistant Arlie
Barnes (an Indiana University medical graduate who had almost completed
his fellowship) provided "cardiac consultations" on 4,695 patients.[59] Barnes
would become the Mayo Clinic's second cardiologist when he joined the
staff in 1925.[60]

One patient hospitalized at the Kahler in the spring of 1924 was of special
interest to Willius. The cardiologist was using the electrocardiograph to try
to clarify the relationship of coronary artery disease to clinical situations that
ranged from brief bouts of angina to severe and prolonged spells of chest pain
that might lead to shock and sudden death.[61] Willius published the story of a
forty-seven-year-old man who was in Rochester with his wife. She was awaiting surgery, but her husband suddenly became the center of attention. After
eating a large breakfast at their hotel, he developed severe chest and left arm
pain. A half hour later, he was being examined in the Mayo Clinic building,
where a nitroglycerin tablet was put under his tongue.[62]

Because of persistent severe chest pain, the man was "immediately hospitalized on the cardiologic service" in the Kahler building across the street.
His face reflected "extreme suffering, and he had a pasty pallor." A morphine
injection did not relieve his pain. His heart rate and blood pressure were

normal. An electrocardiogram recorded fifteen minutes after hospital admission revealed "exaggeration of the T wave." Despite three more morphine injections, the pain lasted almost eight hours.[63] Willius, who concluded that his patient had an acute occlusion of a coronary artery caused by a thrombus (blood clot) that had formed in the vessel, described the therapy in just two sentences: "Treatment consisted of complete rest in bed and a restricted low protein diet. No medication was given after the first day, when nitroglycerin and morphine sulfate were administered."[64]

Although the middle-aged man did not receive any medicines after the first day, he did have twenty-one electrocardiograms recorded during his month-long hospitalization. Those serial electrocardiograms, which Willius summarized in a table, did not influence treatment. The cardiologist followed the conventional wisdom that prolonged bed rest was necessary to allow the damaged heart muscle to heal. After two weeks of strict bed rest, the patient was permitted to sit in a chair for fifteen minutes a day. By the time he was discharged, he was allowed to sit up for eight hours a day. But the man was not well when he went home. He had symptoms of severe heart failure, becoming very short of breath with the slightest exertion.

Willius recommended that the forty-seven-year-old man's activities be "rigidly restricted" indefinitely and that his local doctor consider administering digitalis, an eighteenth-century remedy.[65] This case report, together with the Mayo cardiologist's other publications, reveals that he was concerned mainly with diagnosis rather than treatment. Willius's reluctance to prescribe digitalis during the hospitalization reflected contemporary debate about its indications and adverse effects. Some (but by no means all) first-generation heart specialists would have given the drug to a patient who had obvious signs and symptoms of heart failure after a myocardial infarction.[66]

When Willius published his patient's story in 1925, more hospitals were acquiring electrocardiographs. Some physicians warned about overreliance on the technology, but others considered it indispensable. Henry Christian, the chief of medicine at Boston's Peter Bent Brigham Hospital, was an experienced clinician and electrocardiographer. He claimed that a physician could usually diagnose an acute myocardial infarction without an electrocardiogram and disparaged the practice of moving a patient from his or her bed to record one: "Rest is more important to the patient than an electrocardiogram. A live patient with a probable diagnosis of cardiac infarction is by far preferable to a dead one, definitely diagnosed by finding a typical electrocardiogram, and the moving of the patient may make the difference between recovery and death."[67] Willius's patient remained in bed for each of his electrocardiograms at the Kahler because wires connected each hospital room with the instrument, which was installed in a special laboratory.

What explains the huge gap between zero and twenty-one electrocardiograms? Christian was speaking of standard care, while Willius was conducting clinical research in an attempt to expand knowledge about a deadly condition that doctors were just beginning to diagnose with regularity. Warfield Longcope, the chief of medicine at Johns Hopkins, emphasized the importance of clinical investigation in a 1922 article on angina pectoris and coronary thrombosis: "Since pain in the region of the heart is a symptom that quickly attracts the attention of the patient, and frequently arouses, not only his anxiety, but that of his physician, it behooves us to take stock from time to time of our knowledge of this condition; to realize our limitations in interpreting the symptoms and to add what grains of information that we may possess in an effort to elucidate more clearly its causes or its meaning."[68] Willius's case report revealed his passion for electrocardiography and his intellectual interest in coronary artery disease.

Organizing Regional and National Professional Societies

Fred Willius, who by 1922 had published a book on electrocardiography and sixteen articles, was gaining recognition as an American pioneer of cardiology. That year he was among four dozen doctors who attended an invitation-only luncheon at the American Medical Association meeting to hear a proposal to establish the "National Association for the Prevention and Relief of Heart Disease." This luncheon meeting was a critical first step in the creation of the American Heart Association (AHA), which was incorporated two years later.[69]

One of the AHA's original goals was to encourage the establishment of local heart associations, and Willius led the effort to bring his state's few cardiologists together. In December 1924 he hosted an organizational meeting in Rochester of the Minnesota Cardiologic Club, which one of its founders described as "an informal group composed of men intensively interested in heart and circulation."[70] The founders, who practiced in Duluth, Minneapolis, St. Paul, and Rochester, were all partial specialists. Like Willius and his associate Arlie Barnes, they blended general internal medicine with heart-related work that emphasized electrocardiography. The club members met quarterly to discuss interesting patients, recent publications, and new concepts about heart diseases.[71]

The name of the Minnesota Cardiologic Club was changed to the Minnesota Heart Association in 1925, when it became affiliated with the AHA. Willius, the first president of the newly named state association, reminded members that it had been organized "for the study of the problems of heart disease and the coordination of efforts to solve them." Although he identified its main object as "the study of scientific cardiology," Willius argued for expanding the association's agenda: "The time has arrived when, as physicians intensely interested in heart disease, we are obligated to extend our efforts in the great cause of preventive cardiology." He suggested promoting the prevention of heart disease among physicians and the public using the state medical journal, local newspapers, and the new technology of radio.[72] Willius, eager to inform doctors about developments in his specialty, published "The Progress of Cardiology during 1924: A Review of the Works of Clinicians and Investigators in the United States" in *Minnesota Medicine*, a monthly journal.[73]

Willius explained why he published the review: "In this age of scientific progress, in which the cogs of clinical and laboratory investigations grind ceaselessly, it seems appropriate to record the achievements in diseases of the heart and circulation during the year just past." His words suggested action, accomplishment, and anticipation. But many challenges remained because heart disease was "the greatest single factor in causing disability, dependence and death." It caused about 155,000 deaths annually in the United States, more than any other disease, and was responsible for the "more or less continuous disability of 2.5 million people."[74] These statistics challenged the lingering perception that tuberculosis and other communicable diseases posed the biggest threat to a person's life and livelihood. Public health lawyer James Tobey opened a 1925 article in the popular magazine *American Mercury* with a warning: "A generation ago tuberculosis was the captain of the men of death in this country. Today heart disease is."[75] The founders of the AHA repeated this message regularly to draw attention to the problem, to the importance of research, and to the need to establish community clinics for patients with heart disease.

Willius, in addition to founding the Minnesota Heart Association, was very active in the national organization. He coauthored one of the nine papers presented at the AHA's first annual meeting held in Atlantic City, New Jersey, in 1925.[76] When Willius was not elected to the American Society for Clinical Investigation the following year, Leonard Rowntree gave him a boost. A recent president of that prestigious organization, Rowntree informed New York City internist Emanuel Libman: "Willius is a fine man, has done splendid work, and I feel that he is the type for which this society is intended." He asked Libman, one of the society's founders, to "drop a line to the council, asking them for favorable consideration of his nomination."[77] This old boy network approach worked—and quickly. Willius informed Libman one month later that he was very pleased to have been elected to the society, which was "molding the younger men of this country."[78]

In 1925 Willius took the lead when Rowntree wanted to create a regional organization patterned after the American Society for Clinical Investigation. He and George Brown, who worked mainly with Rowntree, met with eight internists (two each from Chicago, Iowa City, Minneapolis, and St. Louis) who came to the Mayo Clinic to help organize the club. But it got off to a slow start; the first meeting of the Central Society for Clinical

Research was held three years later in Rochester. Willius was appointed temporary chair of the society, and twenty-one Mayo doctors joined as charter members. Several of them lectured at the first meeting.[79]

Networking at local, regional, and national medical society meetings was a well-established method for building individual and institutional reputations. Mayo's Executive Committee had agreed earlier in the decade that "representatives from the specialties must be allowed considerable flexibility in order that they may attend such meetings as will naturally increase their volume of business."[80] Willius took advantage of the opportunity. In 1928, for example, he spoke at medical meetings in Illinois, Indiana, Iowa, Minnesota, North Dakota, and Washington, D.C. An Indiana newspaper described him as "one of the foremost authorities on the human heart in this country" in its announcement of his talk at the Terre Haute Academy of Medicine.[81]

The significance of the Mayo Clinic's cardiology program was underscored in 1927, when Willius profiled it in the Rockefeller Foundation's *Methods and Problems of Medical Education* series.[82] Twenty-one volumes, published between 1924 and 1932, included hundreds of articles that described "clinics, laboratories, and methods of teaching in different parts of the world" in the hope that they might "be of assistance to those planning improvements in buildings and methods."[83] Mayo was one of only four institutions in the United States whose cardiology or electrocardiography programs were described in separate articles. The others were the Massachusetts General Hospital and the Peter Bent Brigham Hospital in Boston and the University of Michigan Hospital in Ann Arbor. Each of these institutions had a world-class electrocardiography laboratory as the centerpiece of its cardiology practice.[84] Willius explained in the Rockefeller publication that cardiology at the Mayo Clinic included three parts: a diagnostic and consultation service, a hospital service, and an electrocardiography service. At the time, he and Arlie Barnes were engaged in clinical research relating to electrocardiography, angina pectoris, myocardial disease, and aortic valve stenosis.

Leonard Rowntree's Group and Cardiovascular Disease

Willius's article in the Rockefeller Foundation's series did not mention Leonard Rowntree's cardiovascular group at St. Mary's Hospital. This omission reflected the distinction between cardiology, which emphasized electrocardiography and heart disease, and disorders of the *cardiovascular system*, which were the focus of some of Rowntree's associates. The vascular system, comprised of arteries and veins, was peripheral not only to the heart but also to the professional interests of Willius and almost every other first-generation cardiologist.

When Will Mayo recruited Rowntree to Rochester in 1920, he gave him the authority to hire and direct a small group of internist-clinical investigators whose interests would complement those of Henry Plummer's large team of internist-diagnosticians. Within a year, Rowntree hired two men who would focus on the cardiovascular system. Norman Keith, with whom he had worked at Johns Hopkins, shared his interest in hypertension and kidney disease. George Brown had been an internist in Montana and had spent some time as a postgraduate student in biochemistry at Johns Hopkins before he joined the clinic. Brown, like Keith, was interested in hypertension, but he would devote himself mainly to peripheral vascular disease.[85]

Brown, by focusing on the body's blood vessels (including the microscopic capillaries), was exploring terrain far away from the heart, which Willius and Barnes studied with the electrocardiograph. This dichotomy was apparent to Mayo staff members and visiting doctors. Willius was put in charge of a new electrocardiograph that was installed at St. Mary's Hospital in 1922, when the Medical Department (which Rowntree ran) was established there. Norman Keith informed the staff: "Those who are working in the cardiovascular group are keenly looking forward to his cooperation and his newer interpretation of the electrocardiogram."[86] When members of the Mississippi Valley Medical Association met in Rochester that year, they heard Rowntree, Keith, and Brown lecture on "cardiovascular diseases" at St. Mary's Hospital as well as Willius discuss "electrocardiography and diseases of the heart" at the Kahler Hospital.[87]

The Mayo Clinic's reputation as an academic center grew after World War I as a result of its staff members' publications and presentations as well as its annual output of trained specialists. Rowntree, Mayo's most ambitious internist-investigator, sought new ways to draw attention to the institution's programs in internal medicine. Like the Mayo brothers, he understood the value of having well-known academic physicians and scientists visit Rochester, where they would see the facilities and meet the staff. In 1923, Rowntree, in his capacity as chair of the Committee on Medical Education, Research, and Scientific Progress, proposed that the institution invite an outside speaker every month to deliver a Mayo Foundation Lecture.[88] The plan was implemented, and a dozen individuals came to Rochester each year to lecture in the series.

Several prominent American and European physicians and medical scientists spoke on cardiovascular topics beginning in 1923. During the next two years, the lecturers (and topics) included Karel Wenckebach of Vienna on heart rhythm disorders and angina pectoris, Homer Swift of the Rockefeller Institute on rheumatic fever, Emanuel Libman of New York City on endocarditis, William Thayer of Johns Hopkins on endocarditis, and Ludwig Aschoff of Freiburg, Germany, on atherosclerosis.[89] A high point in the series was when Dutch physiologist Willem Einthoven spoke on electrocardiography in November 1924, less than two weeks after he was informed that he had won the Nobel Prize in Physiology or Medicine for his invention of the technology.[90]

Two Groups Care for Patients With Cardiovascular Disease

During the early 1920s, the number of patients hospitalized in Rochester for non-surgical problems such as arthritis, diabetes, and hypertension increased significantly. New buildings were constructed to accommodate the expanding inpatient medical practice. The Sisters of St. Francis had been stalwart supporters of the Mayo practice for three decades when the Kahler opened in 1921. Will Mayo told the Executive Committee the following year: "We must bear in mind that the hospitals are now in two groups and that great care and diplomacy must be used to prevent the development of a spirit of competition which may grow into antagonism." He knew that the success of the Mayo practice was due, in part, to a tradition of respect for the patient: "If patients wish to go to St. Mary's Hospital and it is possible to send them there, always acting in the best interest of the patient, they should be allowed to go. The men on the permanent staff understand this and exercise tact in explaining to patients why another hospital may be the right one under the circumstances."[91]

When the Medical Department opened at St. Mary's Hospital in 1922 and Willius was given beds in the Kahler Hospital the following year, a significant number of patients with disorders of the heart and cardiovascular system began being admitted for inpatient care. These men and women did not recognize the boundaries that specialty-oriented doctors and scientists assigned to different diseases or parts of their bodies. They might have problems involving their heart, kidneys, or blood vessels, along with other health issues. Although a patient's main reason for seeking medical attention, the so-called chief complaint, influenced his or her path through the Mayo Clinic, it was not the sole determinant. If a diagnostician thought that a patient with heart or blood vessel disease would benefit from hospitalization, he or she could choose to admit the individual to Willius's cardiology service at the Kahler, to the Rowntree's cardiovascular service at St. Mary's, or another inpatient medical service.

Tensions sometimes arose with respect to who should care for patients with heart disease and where they were hospitalized. For example, Willius and Barnes complained to the Board of Governors in 1926:

> All cardiac patients referred to us for treatment are hospitalized at the Kahler. We have received splendid support and cooperation from most

of the sections of the clinic, but we believe that this cooperation should be complete. In view of the fact that the treatment of diabetes, nephritis, thyroid disorders, blood dyscrasias, etc., are definitely assigned to specific sections we feel that the failure to apply this principle to the treatment of critically sick patients as most of the cardiac cases are, is an incongruity.[92]

Patients who required hospitalization for problems related to the four medical conditions the cardiologists mentioned were usually placed on the inpatient service supervised by members of the clinic's internal medicine section that focused on those problems.[93] This was not the case with patients who had cardiac problems. In 1926, for example, an almost equal number of patients classified as having heart disease were admitted to Willius and Barnes's cardiology service at the Kahler and to Rowntree's Medical Department at St. Mary's.

A comparison of Tables 5.1 and 5.2 reveals interesting patterns regarding the distribution of patients between the two main Mayo-staffed hospitals.

TABLE 5.1 Patients Admitted to Cardiac Service, Kahler Hospital, 1926[a]

TOTAL PATIENTS	294 (24 deaths)
CORONARY ARTERY DISEASE	
Angina pectoris	36
Coronary sclerosis	82 (9 deaths)
Coronary thrombosis	3 (3 deaths)
HYPERTENSIVE HEART DISEASE	
Hypertensive heart disease	70 (4 deaths)
HEART VALVE DISEASE	
Aortic insufficiency (regurgitation)	4
Aortic stenosis	4 (2 deaths)
Mitral insufficiency (regurgitation)	4
Mitral stenosis	49 (3 deaths)
ENDOCARDITIS	
Acute bacterial endocarditis	1 (1 death)
Subacute bacterial endocarditis	12
PERICARDIAL DISEASE	
Chronic adherent pericarditis	7 (2 deaths)
Subacute fibrinous pericarditis	1
MISCELLANEOUS CARDIOVASCULAR DIAGNOSES	
Cardiac neurosis	6
Paroxysmal tachycardia	4
Syphilitic aortitis	10
Thoracic aneurysm	1

[a] Adapted from F. A. Willius, Cardiology Section Report to MC BOG for 1926, MCA.

Caring for the Heart

TABLE 5.2 Patients Admitted to Medical Department, St. Mary's Hospital, 1926[a]

HEART DISEASE	315 total (32 deaths)
CORONARY ARTERY DISEASE	
Angina pectoris	12
Coronary embolus	1
Coronary sclerosis	13
HEART VALVE DISEASE	
Aortic insufficiency (regurgitation)	6
Mitral insufficiency (regurgitation)	8 (1 death)
Mitral stenosis	7
ENDOCARDITIS	
Acute endocarditis	2
Chronic endocarditis	11
Chronic mitral endocarditis	33 (4 deaths)
PERICARDIAL DISEASE	
Pericarditis	12 (3 deaths)
MISCELLANEOUS CARDIOVASCULAR DIAGNOSES	
Auricular (atrial) fibrillation	16 (3 deaths)
Cardiac decompensation	38 (6 deaths)
Cardiac hypertrophy	40 (3 deaths)
Cardiac insufficiency	6
Myocardial degeneration	94 (12 deaths)
Paroxysmal tachycardia	1
Other diagnoses (8 different)	15
VASCULAR DISEASES AND HYPERTENSION	906 total (27 deaths)
Arteriosclerosis	314 (14 deaths)
Hypertension (benign or essential)	375 (6 deaths)
Hypertension (malignant)	49 (3 deaths)
Thrombo-angiitis obliterans	61
Other diagnoses (20 different)	107 (4 deaths)

[a] Adapted from *Thirty-seventh Annual Report of St. Mary's Hospital* [for 1926] (Rochester, MN:
St. Mary's Hospital, 1927), 51, 54–55.

Most of the diagnostic terms attached to these patients are familiar to present-day readers with medical training, but some of them are obsolete or ambiguous.[94] Willius and Barnes cared for most but not all patients with coronary artery disease and heart valve disease (most of which was the result of earlier episodes of acute rheumatic fever). Although Willius was interested in heart rhythm disorders, very few patients with this problem were hospitalized because technology for continuous monitoring had not been invented and treatment was limited mainly to digitalis. Rowntree's group at St. Mary's Hospital cared for almost all patients admitted with a diagnosis of arteriosclerosis, hypertension, or peripheral vascular disease. In addition, they cared for essentially all patients who had evidence of heart failure, whether it was attributed to hypertrophy (thickening) or degeneration (weakening) of the myocardium (heart muscle).[95]

Defining and Debating Specialty Boundaries

The boundaries between established and emerging specialties were contested throughout the twentieth century as doctors defined and redefined their professional interests and identities. When cardiology was invented around World War I, a few individuals played key roles in shaping professional and public perceptions of the evolving specialty. The names they chose for the organizations and journals they founded were negotiated as part of the dynamic process of specialization.

Lewis Conner, the first president of the AHA and the founding editor of its official journal, informed Emanuel Libman in 1925 that the periodical's title would be the *American Journal of Diseases of the Heart and Circulatory System*.[96] When the first issue appeared a few months later, however, it was titled simply the *American Heart Journal*. Despite the periodical's organ-centered title, Conner explained in his inaugural editorial that it would cover "the field of diseases of the heart and circulation."[97] Leonard Rowntree was on the original editorial board of the journal, but almost all of the other two dozen members were interested in the heart alone, rather than the entire cardiovascular system.

By the end of the decade, the Mayo Clinic's complementary programs devoted to heart disease and disorders of the cardiovascular system had achieved national recognition. Willius and Barnes continued to emphasize electrocardiography in their research and writings. Rowntree's colleagues Norman Keith and George Brown were becoming acknowledged experts in hypertension and peripheral vascular disease, respectively. Willius had played a significant role in linking his state's cardiologists to the AHA, and Brown and Barnes would play major roles in the organization in the next decade.

The AHA's 1928 publication *A Directory of Heart Associations, Committees, Convalescent Homes and Cardiac Clinics in the United States and Canada* demonstrated dramatic differences between the organization of cardiology at the Mayo Clinic and other institutions. In a foreword, the directory's editor explained that there were three state associations, five local associations, and 185 cardiac clinics.[98] In 1928 there were only three state heart associations: California, Minnesota, and New York. Willius served as president and secretary of the Minnesota Heart Association, which he had founded three years earlier. One striking feature of the directory is the description of the hours of operation of the 185 cardiac clinics. Most of them were based in hospitals, and all but two of them had very limited hours. Their directors were office-based private practitioners who devoted just a few hours a week to the endeavor.

The Mayo Clinic and the Cleveland Clinic were the only institutions with all-day cardiac clinics each weekday. Paul Dudley White was in charge of the cardiac clinic at the Massachusetts General Hospital, which was open for four hours on Wednesdays and Thursdays. Samuel Levine was in charge of the clinic at Boston's Peter Bent Brigham Hospital, which was open for two hours on Thursdays. This does not mean that patients with known or suspected heart disease were seen just during these restricted hours. Many of them would have been evaluated in the hospital's general medical clinics. It does reflect, however, a different institutional philosophy. By the end of the decade, the Mayo Clinic's stature as a leading academic center was widely acknowledged. But its main mission was and would remain patient care.[99]

Challenges and Changes During the Depression

The Mayo Clinic, like many American institutions that thrived during the so-called Roaring Twenties, confronted significant challenges in the 1930s. America's economy was still booming in the summer of 1929. Will Mayo, supremely self-confident but chronically concerned about expenses, told the Board of Governors in August: "Professional salaries should not be increased beyond a reasonable amount in order that they may be maintained under all conditions.... The business should not be asked to carry a load of fixed overhead which would hazard its future stability."[1]

The stock market crash at the end of October was heralded by frantic selling on the twenty-fourth, Black Thursday. Word spread quickly that the financial markets were in chaos and the economy was headed for big trouble. Charlie Mayo expressed cautious optimism a month after the October 1929 crash. "Everything is going on fine," he told Will. "The work is keeping up pretty well. Four hundred and ninety-five registered Monday, and there is a fair amount of surgical work."[2] The Mayo brothers' statements bracketed the stock market plunge. In retrospect, Will's warning about overhead sounds prescient. Charlie's comments, on the other hand, minimized the magnitude of the financial landslide that had already crushed countless investors and would soon threaten the Mayo Clinic. The crash, in the words of business historian Maury Klein, "brought to a stunning halt a decade that had witnessed the greatest economic prosperity and most profound cultural changes yet known and ushered in a decade blighted by the longest and deepest depression Americans had ever endured."[3]

The Mayo Clinic Responds to the Depression

The Mayo Clinic and Rochester's many businesses that depended on it were caught in the downdraft caused by the falling economy. In January 1930 Mayo's Board of Governors approved borrowing $500,000 to meet expenses, as well as across-the-board salary cuts. It imposed additional salary reductions and restricted clinic-sponsored trips in July.[4] Will Mayo informed the staff the following month: "It is hardly necessary for me to call the attention of the faculty to the financial adjustments that are taking place in this country." But he refused to let these concerns undermine the institution's mission. The clinic, he said, "must operate more efficiently and reduce its overhead to as great an extent as possible without interfering with its usefulness."[5]

Some of the staff doctors listening to Will surely second-guessed the board's decision to erect the large and lavish diagnostic building that had opened two years earlier. But he reminded them that the building (in which they were sitting) had real benefits in terms of efficiency. The senior Mayo brother then turned from bricks and mortar to human beings: "In these hard times the medical profession has suffered perhaps to a greater extent than any other profession, for sickness is a misfortune, not something that the patient buys, and comparatively few people are able to prepare for sickness as they prepare to buy some form of merchandise."[6] Author and social critic H. L. Mencken expressed a similar view: "The medical brethren suffer from the Depression like the rest of us, and perhaps to a more painful degree, for doctors' bills, as everyone knows, are always the last to be paid."[7] Still, Mayo's physicians and surgeons were better positioned than most doctors to cope with the Depression because they were salaried and had no personal practice-related expenses.

When Will Mayo spoke to the professional staff in the summer of 1930, new patient registrations were only 2 percent below their peak. But the problem was getting paid for services the clinic provided to them. Addressing the plight of the patient, Will declared: "We must meet him half way, and not by more severe methods of collection add to his great distress. We must adjust accounts, both past and present, to his ability to pay. We must send out, not collectors, but adjustors. We must not sacrifice the ideals of the clinic because of temporary inconvenience to ourselves." Will assured his colleagues that their leaders would "in the future as in the past take such action as seems wise to them to maintain and protect the standards of the clinic and the well being of its staff. The maintenance of the present spiritual status of the Mayo Clinic is of the greatest importance. We must not permit the material side to encroach upon our ideals."[8] America had previously experienced economic recessions, some of them serious, but in 1930 no one could predict the length or severity of this new depression (Figure 6.1).

Harry Harwick, the clinic's longtime chief administrator, painted a grim picture of what happened to patient visits during the early 1930s: The number of new patients "dropped and dropped and kept on dropping—from 79,000 in 1929, to 75,000 in 1930, to 65,000 in 1931, to less than 50,000 in 1932."[9] Billed charges fell from $7.1 million 1929 to $4.3 million four years later.[10] The director of Mayo's collection department reported in 1931 that

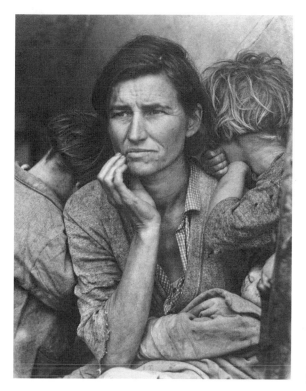

FIGURE 6.1 *Dorothea Lange, "Migrant Mother," 1936.*

Library of Congress, LC-USF34-T01-009058-C, in the public domain.

patients were "appreciative of the services received and many of them tell us they are grateful that we have not pressed them unduly for payment of their accounts."[11] St. Mary's Hospital, which relied on the Mayo Clinic for all of its patients, experienced a 50 percent decline in admissions between 1928 and 1931. The Kahler Corporation's hotel-hospital business also decreased dramatically.[12]

As the depression deepened, the clinic's receipts kept dropping and its leaders looked for more ways to cut expenses. The board had decided in December 1929 that "in view of the general economic outlook, no men should be added unless absolutely necessary."[13] Between that month and December 1931, the number of men and women on the clinic payroll fell by 13 percent (from 1,276 to 1,110). Because doctors generated income, most of the layoffs or terminations affected the support staff.[14] In the summer of 1932, Will wanted several chairs removed from each waiting room so those public spaces would not look so empty.[15] Meanwhile, there were periodic attempts to boost morale. For example, the *Clinic Bulletin* reported in August 1932 that during the prior month new patients had registered from every American state, six Canadian provinces, Mexico, Guatemala, India, China, and the Philippines.[16]

As economic conditions deteriorated, many of the nation's physicians struggled to maintain their practices. Between 1930 and 1933, the average income of American general practitioners fell from about $4,000 to $2,600. Specialists' incomes were higher, but they also dropped dramatically.[17] Scores of Mayo-trained specialists (mostly surgeons) had launched small group practices after World War I. The Depression stunted the growth of these practices and led to the dissolution of several of them. Robert Sanders, who had been a surgical fellow at Mayo before the war, informed Will in 1932 that he and his partners had dissolved their twelve-man group practice in Memphis: "The service we rendered was satisfactory, but it was a financial failure. I have not been able to make expenses out of it for a long while, as the overhead was too great."[18] Soon after the struggling surgeon wrote to Will Mayo, Americans elected a new president who pledged to revitalize the economy.

Two days before Franklin Roosevelt was inaugurated on March 4, 1933, Harry Harwick wrote to Will, who was vacationing in Tucson, Arizona. Citing the "banking collapse" that had begun in Michigan and was spreading across the nation, he described meeting with Minnesota bankers. Although Harwick thought the local situation was "in pretty good shape," he confessed that "checks are bouncing back at us from all parts of the country due to bank holidays."[19] Just after Roosevelt took office, he closed the nation's banks for four days and instituted a federal program to insure deposits. Harwick informed Will on March 9 that there was "very little hysteria locally" in response to the bank holiday and assured him that "things at the clinic have been moving very smoothly."[20]

Will expressed cautious optimism in a May 1933 letter to British surgeon Grey Turner: "As for the economic slump, of course America has been hit hard, and like England we seem to be lifting out of the depression." Turning to politics, he declared: "We have gained all the advantages of a dictatorship by peacefully passing the burdens into the hands of President Roosevelt, an excellent man, giving him the right to use various methods of starting the wheels going, and the general outlook at the present time is encouraging."[21]

The air in Rochester was saturated with patriotism fifteen months later, when President Roosevelt rode through town sitting beside the Mayo brothers in an open-top automobile (Figure 6.2). He had come to participate in an American Legion ceremony honoring their service to the nation. The *Washington Post* proclaimed, "Some 25,000 persons from all over the state gathered in the blistering sun at Soldier's Field for the ceremony."[22] Many attendees had another reason to celebrate. Business was picking up. For the first time in four years, the Mayo Clinic's charges had increased (from $4.3 million in 1933 to $5.5 million in 1934).[23]

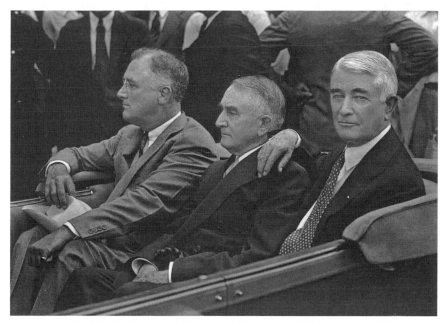

FIGURE 6.2 *Franklin D. Roosevelt, Charles H. Mayo, and William J. Mayo riding through Rochester, Minnesota, August 8, 1934.*
Used with permission of Mayo Foundation.

Reining in Leonard Rowntree and Clinical Research

The economic challenges that the Mayo Clinic faced at the beginning of the Depression contributed to the dissolution of Leonard Rowntree's Medical Department at St. Mary's Hospital. Duluth cardiologist Edward Tuohy had praised Rowntree in a 1928 letter to Will: "You have devoted your life to the problem of making surgery safe, and in so doing the Mayo Clinic has done yeoman service in making it popular. Now we see in the various intricate fields of medicine this same intensive endeavor, under the splendid guidance of such men as Rowntree and those with him."[24]

By the late 1920s, Rowntree's hand-picked group of internist-investigators were spending much of their time working in seven hospital-based specialty sections: Russell Wilder in diabetes; Norman Keith in kidney and vascular diseases; George Brown in vascular diseases; Charles McVicar and James Weir in gastrointestinal and liver diseases; Philip Hench in arthritis; Albert Snell in endocrinology; and Walter Alvarez in gastrointestinal physiology.[25] Suddenly, however, the stability of Rowntree's program seemed uncertain.

Rowntree informed Will in the summer of 1929 that he had been offered the position of professor of medicine at Northwestern University in Evanston, Illinois. He explained, "I will not make any decision, of course, without talking it over with you and getting your advice."[26] When Will shared this news with the Board of Governors three days later, he emphasized that the clinic must "constantly bring on trained young men so that as the older men left there would always be able men to succeed them." Thinking strategically, Will also "stressed the importance of the clinic maintaining an active medical education and research program as work of this character differentiates the clinic from the stereotype or commercial type of practice."[27] In fact, this had been the main reason for establishing the Mayo Foundation for Medical Education and Research in 1915. Expenses related to these programs were covered by profits from the Mayo practice and income from investments; they were not subsidized by any external sources.

Will Mayo wanted Rowntree to stay in Rochester. After a long conversation with the internist-investigator, he informed Harry Harwick in November 1929 that he thought things would "straighten out."[28] But much had changed in the two months since Rowntree first mentioned that he might leave. With the clinic confronting an unprecedented economic crisis, Will outlined a strategy to Harwick that would have important implications for the future of clinical research in Rochester. He wanted Rowntree to transfer his close-knit group of academically oriented internist-investigators from St. Mary's Hospital to the big new Mayo Clinic outpatient building:

> I talked to him about moving downtown, and I think he is willing to take all his laboratories down, his men, papers, and everything, so that he can work in harmony with the Sanford and Kendall laboratories. He and Brown and Keith have been discussing the matter, and evidently he wants to arrange it among them. My guess would be that Keith would take the Rowntree section and Brown another, leaving Rowntree as a sort of superconsultant for the two.... It will clean everything out at St. Mary's, which is what we have all wanted, except what is necessary to carry on the clinical work there and will bring about a definite relationship with the clinic, which has been lacking.[29]

A week later, board member Melvin Henderson, an orthopedic surgeon, informed Will that he planned to meet with Rowntree, who had decided to stay in Rochester: "He is a good man and as you say is valuable to us but not if he is looking for [a] chance to fly away to anything that looks for the moment better for him."[30] Loyalty mattered to Will, and it influenced his attitude about Rowntree, who had built a celebrated program of clinical research in Rochester.

Shortly before Thanksgiving in 1929, Will wrote to Henderson: "I hope that Rowntree will be satisfied, but I think we must insist on his coming downtown and bringing his work, as far as possible, downtown, rather than have the reduplication that we have had. It had led to a little high-hatting, which has irritated the men. Of course, we want to maintain the fine service at St. Mary's and carry on the clinical investigation and research there that is necessary, but I believe the bulk of it can be done at the Clinic and the Institute [of Experimental Medicine]."[31]

Will Mayo was the clinic's chief decision maker during the 1920s, but he and his brother had decided early in the decade to establish several committees to distribute certain responsibilities. The Council, which was charged with determining the clinic's general policies, consisted of the Board of Governors, the Executive Committee, and the chair of the faculty. In the context of concerns about the economy and the Rowntree situation, the Council appointed a three-man committee to review the functions, leaders, and locations of all of the Mayo's clinical and research laboratories. It included pediatrician Henry Helmholz and laboratory scientists Thomas Magath and Frank Mann. Laboratory diagnosis had grown dramatically since the turn of the century. By the mid-1920s, about 150 rooms in various clinic buildings, Mayo-affiliated hospitals, and the Institute of Experimental Medicine were used for laboratory purposes.[32]

When Mayo Foundation director Louis Wilson described the clinic's academic activities in 1928, he boasted, "Of the staff of 132 physicians, physicists, and chemists, eighteen are engaged wholly in research work and twenty-two in part-time laboratory research work. Most of the others are devoting a considerable portion of their time to clinical research. All the staff are on a 'full-time' basis."[33] Wilson's statement about the time devoted to research was a major exaggeration, and Henry Plummer's team of internist-diagnosticians, who were kept busy evaluating hundreds of outpatients every day, knew it.

The Depression influenced decisions about the fate of Rowntree's ambitious and semi-autonomous program of hospital-based clinical research. Will informed his brother in February 1930: "We had about 800 more new patients in January than a year ago, but collections have been very light. People simply do not have the money. I am insisting on moving almost everything connected with research at St. Mary's out to the Institute or down to the Clinic, to relieve the hospital of a burden which is a nuisance to them and an expense to us."[34] The following week the Board of Governors approved the Helmholz-Magath-Mann committee report. It recommended that all research projects have a formal budget, that clinical investigation be reorganized to make use of existing routine laboratories, and that all technicians be assigned to laboratories rather than to individuals. The board approved policies that were designed to introduce controls and eliminate duplication rather than cripple research at the Mayo Clinic. One goal was to provide more physicians with opportunities for clinical investigation. The board agreed that "the head of the laboratory and his associates [should] give full cooperation to all problems brought to the laboratory by members of the clinic staff."[35]

Leonard Rowntree made a half-hearted attempt to disguise his frustration with the decision to dismantle the infrastructure of his clinical research programs when he informed Will in February 1930: "If these changes are made, I will at least try them."[36] As part of the reorganization, the board changed Rowntree's title from "Chief of the Department of Medicine, the Mayo Foundation" to "Professor of Medicine, University of Minnesota; Senior Consultant in Medicine and Director of Clinical Investigation, Mayo Clinic."[37] Despite the impressive-sounding new titles, Rowntree had been demoted relative to Henry Plummer, and his research programs had been gutted. In September 1930, a few months after the changes were implemented, Rowntree informed his longtime friend and former Johns Hopkins dean William Welch:

> Since writing you in January much has happened that makes me eager to leave Rochester. The new titles and increased salary were accompanied by a demand that I must sign a "declaration of intention" or make a public statement that I would never leave the Mayo Clinic. This I refused to do and in consequence Doctor Mayo's attitude towards me has changed considerably. Research opportunity in medicine has been cut down materially, Dr. Will stressing more and more his desire for clinical work.... I fear that unless I acquiesce in this demand the great opportunity is past.[38]

One year later, in September 1931, Charlie Mayo welcomed former trainees back to Rochester during "hard times." Despite the grave economic situation, he was optimistic about the future of medicine because researchers were "never quite satisfied with the present." Ironically, Charlie praised Rowntree and two of the men who had helped to marginalize him:

> I have talked with medical men all over this country and all over Europe, and it seems to me that the men here have broader contact with scientific research than in any other place. I want to say that contact with my associates who are advancing medicine has done a great deal to keep up my interest in it. Rowntree has a research type mind which appeals to me...[Frank] Mann who directs the vision of many into practical channels is a most important member of our research department and one need hardly mention our Henry S. Plummer who has done so much to advance medicine.[39]

Charlie made no mention of the turmoil surrounding Rowntree and the new approach to clinical research.

The clinic's culture of collegiality impressed visiting physicians and patients, but tensions surrounding controversial individuals and decisions were inevitable in such a large institution. Serious interpersonal conflicts and other problems involving the physicians were handled discreetly, usually by

Will Mayo or Harry Harwick. Charlie, who tried to avoid contentious issues, warned the Board of Governors in November 1931 to "be very 'close-mouthed' about the affairs of the clinic, as often-times a big rumor will start from a small remark."[40]

Rowntree informed Will in December 1931 that he was leaving to become the director of the newly created Philadelphia Institute for Medical Research. "In resigning," he wrote, "let me express my deepest gratitude to you and Dr. Charlie, to the Board of Governors and to the staff of the Mayo Clinic, for the great opportunity you have given me here. The last twelve years represent days full of work, joy in labor and pleasure in accomplishment."[41] After Rowntree resigned, the institutional directory listed Plummer as Chief of Medical Staff. For the first time in a dozen years, he was in charge of all of Mayo's internists. Rowntree's research productivity plummeted after he left Rochester because the Philadelphia institute had almost no staff and had none of the Mayo Clinic's massive infrastructure.[42]

Two members of Rowntree's group published their impressions of the dynamics three decades later. Russell Wilder explained that Plummer's "disaffection for the Rowntree program at St. Mary's Hospital was widely known."[43] Walter Alvarez recalled frustrations shared by members of Plummer's team of internist-diagnosticians: "The coming of the new men into the place [in the early 1920s] caused tensions to build up, particularly in the hearts of some of the old-timers who had never done much writing or lecturing. With some justification, a number of them felt that they had been so swamped with clinical work they never had the time." These feelings intensified when members of Rowntree's academically oriented group achieved national recognition as a result of their research and publications. "An old-timer," Alvarez explained, "might feel that the young men were constantly going to meetings, and leaving him to see the patients and make the money for the clinic."[44]

The Local and National Ascent of Vascular Medicine

Rowntree, who had put clinical investigation on a firm footing at the Mayo Clinic, had mentored several individuals who continued to pursue patient-oriented research projects and to enhance the institution's academic image. For example, the dismantling of Rowntree's group at St. Mary's Hospital in the spring of 1930 boosted George Brown's career. It also resulted in the creation of a vascular section at the clinic in June. Given the opportunity to choose associates, Brown selected three men who had just completed medical fellowships in Rochester: Edgar Allen, Nelson Barker, and Bayard Horton.[45] Brown and Allen had coauthored a book on a rare form of peripheral vascular disease with the tongue-twisting title *Thrombo-Angiitis Obliterans* in 1928. Rowntree, in a foreword written in happier times, applauded the authors for inviting internists, surgeons, pathologists, physiologists, bacteriologists, and physicists to collaborate with them. He emphasized that this "group investigation" approach had led to "real progress" in the diagnosis, prognosis, and treatment of peripheral vascular disease.[46]

George Brown, Edgar Allen, and their associates made important contributions to the emerging field of vascular disease. Brown and Allen also played a critical role in convincing the American Heart Association (AHA) to expand its mission. In the mid-1930s they supported New York City vascular specialist Irving Wright's campaign to convince the association's leaders to look beyond the heart's boundaries—to blood vessel diseases. Irvine Page of the Rockefeller Institute Hospital in New York City contributed to the effort. Personal connections and proximity gave Wright and Page a platform. They had been classmates at Cornell University Medical College in Manhattan, where Lewis Conner was the chief of medicine. Conner, the AHA's first president, was editor of the *American Heart Journal* when the men lobbied on behalf of the peripheral circulation.[47]

Wright recalled that some "classical cardiologists" had reservations about expanding the AHA's focus to include the entire circulation.[48] In 1935 he asked its leaders to transform an independent group that he, Page, Brown, and Allen were planning to form into a standing committee of the association. The organization's leaders responded by establishing the Committee for the Study of the Peripheral Circulation and by asking Brown to chair it. These decisions had important implications for the AHA's identity and structure.[49] Later that year, Lewis Conner acknowledged this in an editorial celebrating the first decade of the *American Heart Journal*:

> This tenth anniversary is to be marked, also, by certain developments in the policy of the JOURNAL by which its scope will be widened and its usefulness, it is believed, much increased. The recent extraordinarily rapid growth of interest in the peripheral vascular disorders and their study has led to recognition by the workers in that field of the need of some form of organization and of some central outlet for their contributions. As the result of recent conferences between a representative group of workers in the field of peripheral vascular disease and the directors of The American Heart Association it has been decided to establish in The American Heart Association a standing committee, or special section, for the study of the peripheral circulation. It is expected that THE AMERICAN HEART JOURNAL will serve as the chief medium for the publications of this group.[50]

Conner also informed readers that the journal would double its publication frequency to monthly to accommodate an anticipated increase in articles. Wright was appointed one of three associate editors, and Allen was added to the editorial advisory board.[51]

George Brown's future seemed bright in 1935, when he was chosen to chair the AHA's new Section for the Study of the Peripheral Circulation. Two years later, William Middleton, the dean of the University of Wisconsin Medical School, explained that Brown's dynamic personality and boundless energy had made him a natural leader. Middleton painted a vivid word-picture of the Mayo vascular specialist in motion:

> If you can envisage the short, compact figure, the clear-cut features, the keen, blue-gray eyes (engaging in smile and intense in debate), the retreating hairline, the alert expression of the intent listener or the absorbed speaker whose abstraction took the form of toying with his horn-rimmed glasses, if you can see this short man rising to his toes habitually or lengthening his stride to match his taller companion, if you can sense the animation of his speech and movements, the cordiality of his spontaneous greeting and the warmth of his genial handshake, then, gentlemen, I have given you my friend, George Elgie Brown.[52]

There was a problem with Middleton's description of Brown's energy and ambition—it was part of a eulogy. Brown was only fifty years old when he died from pneumonia on Thanksgiving Day 1935.

Following Brown's unexpected death, Edgar Allen became head of Mayo's vascular section and chair of the AHA's Section for the Study of the Peripheral Circulation. The impact of Wright, Page, Brown, and Allen on the association was far out of proportion to the number of physicians who shared their interest. For example, they set a major precedent by establishing a new membership category that differentiated ordinary practitioners from academically oriented specialists. Any doctor could become a member of the AHA, but fellowship in its vascular section was "reserved for those particularly interested in peripheral circulation and who are actively engaged in research in this field." By 1938, six of the thirty-seven individuals who had been elected to fellowship in the vascular section of the AHA were from the Mayo Clinic.[53]

Willius Promotes Prevention and Cardiology as a Specialty

While George Brown and Edgar Allen were gaining recognition as vascular specialists in the late 1920s, Mayo cardiologists Fredrick Willius, Arlie Barnes, and their new associate Harry L. Smith were busy evaluating and managing patients with heart disease. Smith, who had joined the cardiology section in 1928 after completing his medical fellowship in Rochester, shared his colleagues' interests in electrocardiography and coronary artery disease. Willius, who led efforts to organize the state's cardiologists, had just been appointed chair of the Minnesota State Medical Association's new Heart

Committee. He promoted disease prevention as part of its mission. In a 1929 article on the subject, he emphasized that heart disease was the leading cause of death in America and listed factors thought to predispose to it, such as heredity, stress, and a diet with excessive "animal proteins."[54]

Physicians interested in disease prevention had begun promoting routine medical checkups as a strategy to help accomplish this goal around World War I. The notion that a healthy person should see a doctor regularly, even if she or he felt well, was a radical departure from standard practice for both patients and physicians.[55] Charlie Mayo, an advocate of routine checkups, spoke about prevention at Carleton College in Northfield, Minnesota, in 1930.

> If you read the papers...you cannot help but be impressed by the enormous number of sudden deaths which are laid to heart failure. It is true that the heart failed, but why? That old heart didn't just get tired all of a sudden and decide to quit: no sir, for years, perhaps ten or twenty, it might have been sending out SOS calls, which were unheeded, or indeed there may have been little apparent evidence of ill health during all these years. This makes it imperative for us to have periodic physical examinations.... It is difficult to draw the line between where prevention stops and where remedy or treatment starts, because treatment of a minor condition today is sometimes the most effective, or the only method of preventing some serious condition that otherwise would arise tomorrow.[56]

Charlie had mentioned treatment, which would be the subject of a lecture that Arlie Barnes delivered two years later in Seattle. There, the cardiologist urged doctors to choose "the most effective measure for the treatment of heart disease."[57] This statement implied that effective therapies were available and that doctors agreed about which ones worked best. But it was not that simple.

Boston cardiologist Paul Dudley White made comments in his 1931 book *Heart Disease* that revealed the challenges faced by physicians and their patients. Rheumatic fever was common, but he acknowledged that there was no specific treatment for its major long-term complications of mitral and aortic valve disease. Treating hypertension was "a difficult and almost hopeless task." Despite new insights into angina pectoris and myocardial infarction, White conceded that there was no specific treatment for coronary artery disease.[58]

Most patients who sought medical attention for heart disease symptoms received care from general practitioners who prescribed a range of treatments. These physicians attended medical meetings and read books and journals in an attempt to keep up with advances in diagnosis and therapy. Willius informed Mayo's Board of Governors in his 1934 report that he and Barnes "placed special emphasis on accepting invitations to county and district medical societies, fully appreciating the fact that personal acquaintance and contacts with the general practitioner of medicine means more patients for the clinic."[59] This was not a novel approach. The Mayo brothers had built their practice this way, beginning in the late nineteenth century.

In 1934 Willius inaugurated the "Cardiac Clinics" series in the *Proceedings of the Staff Meetings of the Mayo Clinic* (hereafter *Proceedings*). This weekly publication, launched eight years earlier, was sent free to thousands of doctors and medical libraries. Willius informed readers that the heart-related series would consist of short single-topic articles designed for busy practitioners who did not have access to or time to read "a host of journals devoted to the various phases of medicine."[60] His comment reflected the publication of more and more specialized periodicals. Although the *American Heart Journal* was the only English-language cardiology periodical at the time, many of its articles were too technical to interest general practitioners. Will Mayo congratulated Willius for the series of "very practical talks on cardiac subjects."[61] An internist in the US Army also thanked him for his efforts to transmit "modern views in cardiology" to general practitioners.[62]

Fred Willius knew that Mayo's leaders valued the opinions of referring physicians, and he tried to use this fact to advance his own agenda in the mid-1930s. The workload of the clinic's three cardiologists grew as patient volumes rebounded after the early years of the Depression. Their daily routine included seeing patients with known or suspected heart disease in the clinic, making rounds on the inpatient cardiology service (which moved from the Kahler to Colonial Hospital in 1932), interpreting electrocardiograms, and responding to requests for consultations in the clinic and Mayo's hospitals. They also shared responsibility for the large number of general diagnostic evaluations that were assigned to each medical section.

In 1934 Willius complained to the board about the distribution of "cardiac patients in various hospitals and on numerous services." Describing this situation as "unsatisfactory from every conceivable standpoint," he proposed that "patients as ill as most cardiac patients are should be cared for by the group specially trained and intensively interested in this field." Willius claimed that "the present indiscriminate management of cardiac patients has provoked considerable criticism from referring physicians." Displaying impatience and demanding action, he declared, "We suggest special consideration of this problem and will expect a definite opinion from the Board."[63]

Six of the eight members of Mayo's Board of Governors were surgeons, and they were unsympathetic to Willius's complaints. The clinic's highly structured system of diagnosis, in place for a generation, was considered vital to its reputation and financial success. Each internist was expected to function as a general diagnostician, mainly to help triage patients to surgery or back home to the care of their local physician. The recent integration of Leonard Rowntree's group of internist-investigators into the clinic's general diagnostic sections reinforced this notion. On the other hand, each of Mayo's four dozen diagnosticians also had a subspecialty focus, such as cardiology, gastroenterology, or hematology.

After discussing Willius's concerns, the board concluded: "There is danger in overspecialization in the clinic, every man in general medicine should be capable of advising and treating patients with many types of cardiac disease, particularly in view of the fact that special consultants are always available from the cardiac section." It saw another problem: "The insistence that practically all cardiac cases requiring hospitalization be placed on the cardiac service will lead to the demand that every local patient with a chronic cardiac complaint be cared for by the Willius section. This arrangement would become a tremendous and burdensome responsibility." The board's response was clever. The men knew that Willius did not want to see *more* patients—he wanted to shift the balance of the work in his medical section from general diagnostic evaluations to cardiology.[64]

Letters were the most common form of communication between Mayo doctors and referring physicians, and the printed stationery that Willius used attracted the board's attention in 1935. When the board debated the implications of progressive specialization and how to balance an individual internist's dual identity as a general diagnostician and a specialist in some medical field, it developed a policy for printed stationery:

> A number of letterheads indicating a specialty in some of the sections practicing general medicine were reviewed.... Such letterheads are apt to be confusing, particularly when used in writing about a patient whose trouble has nothing at all to do with the specialty; for example, a letter written about a patient with a pelvic tumor from the section in cardiology seems rather contradictory and is apt to be misleading. Similar difficulties may and do occasionally arise when the clinician writes about a case that would come under the specialty, for instance a patient with some heart trouble. Obviously it is unnecessary for the section on cardiology to see every heart case that comes to the Clinic.[65]

The board wanted to reserve specialty headings on letterheads for sections "in which the work is confined to a definite specialty." Willius's stationery posed a problem because it stated simply "Section on Cardiology." It did not mention internal medicine, and the board wanted it changed.[66]

The board's use of the phrase "definite specialty" in discussing stationery implied that there was general agreement about what clinical fields deserved this distinction. Mayo's leaders could adjudicate the issue in Rochester, but no entity was empowered to address it at a national level. The boundaries between several established and emerging specialties were contingent and contested—as exemplified by internal medicine and cardiology. Walter Bierring, an Iowa internist-cardiologist who had been a longtime national leader in medical licensing, told members of the American College of Physicians in 1934: "It seems unfortunate in some respects that heart diseases have become a highly specialized field of medicine, and to a large extent have been taken out of general practice."[67] With very few exceptions, America's first-generation cardiologists considered themselves general internists with a special interest in patients with heart disease. This model would be formalized in the mid-1930s, and Mayo played a role in the process.

Louis Wilson and the Movement to Regulate Specialization

Louis Wilson, who had been director of the Mayo Foundation for Medical Education and Research since its creation in 1915, played a key role in the reform of specialty training and the organization of specialties. Rosemary Stevens, in her classic book on the history of specialization in America, describes him as "a dominant figure in the structural emergence of specialist education in the 1920s and 1930s."[68] Wilson's role in Rochester and his knowledge of specialty training in North America and Europe positioned him to lead national reform efforts. He was an influential member of the American Medical Association's Council on Medical Education and Hospitals and was active in several other groups. Philadelphia surgeon Stuart Rodman, who was secretary of the National Board of Medical Examiners, informed Charlie Mayo in 1923 that Wilson would chair a committee charged with investigating how to "protect the public from the unqualified specialist."[69]

Discussions about reforming and regulating the process of specialization were often heated because egos and economics were involved. Philosophical differences also contributed to tensions around the subject. In a 1924 speech to members of the Southern Medical Association, Wilson declared that "the country suffers greatly from a host of self-announced specialists who are unqualified to do good work." He argued that this was due mainly to the lack of any means "for properly determining who is competent to practice in a special field."[70] In response, a North Carolina tuberculosis specialist protested: "Men like Dr. Wilson are so full of their ideals, which may someday be rendered practical, that they are trying to push forward the wheels of medical progress too fast. It will not do to tear down the existing fabric because we have a brilliant future."[71] This physician, who had trained at leading American and European institutions, understood the issues. Unlike Wilson, he was content with the status quo.

Cardiology provides compelling examples of how easy it was for a doctor to claim to be a specialist in this era. During the mid-1920s, a few academic medical centers began offering brief courses for practitioners interested in heart disease. For example, in 1925 Washington University School of Medicine in St. Louis advertised an "intensive" five-day course for ten dollars "for graduate students in Diseases of the Heart."[72] Wilson mocked this model four years later: "I often wonder what modicum of wisdom really remains in the head of a graduate man who has indulged in one of these six-day, dawn-to-midnight postgraduate lecture orgies which have recently become so popular." Proud of the rigorous specialty training program he had helped invent in Rochester, Wilson boasted that the Mayo Foundation accepted "superior graduates of the best American and European schools who have had an average of more than two years of hospital experience before coming to us." He argued that at least thirty more months of training were necessary before a doctor could "begin the practice of a clinical specialty in a scientific manner without supervision."[73] But almost no doctors had this much training when Wilson promoted Mayo's postgraduate model in 1929.

Louis Wilson knew that it was very difficult to achieve consensus about how to design, construct, and patrol paths to specialization. In a speech before the Annual Congress on Medical Education and Medical Licensure in 1932, he listed ten groups interested in the training of specialists: "patients, family physicians, physicians seeking to become specialists, medical schools, hospitals, clinical specialists, the American Medical Association, specialists' societies, state and provincial licensing boards, and the National Board of Medical Examiners."[74] Wilson's ordering of these groups was not arbitrary; he had worked at the patient-centered Mayo Clinic for almost three decades.

Wilson completed a two-year term as president of the Association of American Medical Colleges in the fall of 1933, when the organization met in Rochester and Minneapolis. Reporting on his role as its representative at a conference on the training and registration of specialists, Wilson explained that there was support for the notion that "each specialty group" should be granted authority to certify that a doctor was a qualified specialist. By this time, there were dozens of medical and surgical specialty societies in the United States, but almost none of them had developed a process for certifying specialists. Wilson said this was changing: "During the past fourteen years only three specialty boards have been organized until this year, when four such boards have been organized.... So the thing seems to be gathering some momentum."[75]

Stanford University president Ray Lyman Wilbur was chair of the American Medical Association's Council on Medical Education and Hospitals in 1933, when he spoke on "Order in the Specialties" at the Annual Congress on Medical Education and Licensure. Wilbur, a physician who had been dean of the Stanford Medical School for two decades, was very familiar with Mayo's rigorous program of specialty training. His son, Dwight Wilbur, had just joined the clinic staff after completing a four-year medical fellowship in Rochester.

The senior Wilbur complained to American Medical Association members that problems related to the education of medical students around the

turn of the century "are now showing themselves in nearly all of the specialties.... It has been frequent in recent years for self-anointed specialists
to present themselves to the public without adequate training and without
passing through a well-defined period of preparation." He argued that the
American Medical Association council, which he chaired, was in a position
to "control the important specialties" without interference from other entities. But some representatives of those other groups, seeking to protect their
interests and to influence the process of specialization, disagreed.[76]

After hearing Wilbur's 1933 speech, Walter Bierring of Iowa made
a motion that the American Medical Association Council on Medical
Education and Hospitals "carry forward its plan in developing control of
the specialties."[77] Wilson offered an amendment to Bierring's motion that
would have major implications for the future of specialization in America.
The Mayo pathologist-educator proposed convening "a conference of representatives of the groups concerned" before the council acted. "One of the
factors which prevents this movement from going forward at present," he
explained, "is the existence of just a little distrust of each other, because
we do not know what we are driving at." Wilson hoped to encourage collaboration rather than competition among the men representing the groups
seeking to control specialization: "If the Council would invite two representatives from each of the specialty societies, two from the Association
of American Medical Colleges, perhaps two from the National Board
[of Medical Examiners] and certainly two from the Federation of State
Medical Boards to come together and put their cards face up on the table
we would know what we are all aiming at. I believe the Council could then
proceed more intelligently."[78] The participants approved Wilson's amendment, which set the stage for a coordinated approach to defining specialties
and credentialing specialists.

Louis Wilson's amendment led to an unprecedented gathering of more
than one hundred physicians representing dozens of organizations at the
1933 American Medical Association meeting in Milwaukee. Seven years
later, he told historian Helen Clapesattle that it was a "dog fight" because
the participants were "full of hysterical prejudices."[79] Despite the drama,
the Milwaukee meeting resulted in the creation of the Advisory Board for
Medical Specialties. Historian Rosemary Stevens stresses Wilson's central
role in the establishment of this overarching board. As its first president, he
oversaw negotiations that resulted in what she describes as "a framework in
which new specialty boards might develop." This structure, Stevens explains,
"was significant in respect to the initial definition of a 'specialty.' It would be
difficult in the future for specialist pressure groups to gain approval as boards
on the basis of numerical strength alone."[80]

In 1934, during Wilson's term as the first president of the Advisory Board
for Medical Specialties, the new board defined minimum qualifications for

candidates who hoped to take a certifying examination. These tests would be offered in a dozen "branches of medicine at present...recognized as suitable for the certification of specialists."[81] They included internal medicine, surgery, pediatrics, obstetrics and gynecology, ophthalmology, otolaryngology, dermatology and syphilology, psychiatry and neurology, urology, orthopedic surgery, radiology, and pathology. The recommended length and content of specialty training mirrored Mayo's fellowship program. Among other things, candidates were expected to have completed "a period of study, after the internship, of not less than three years in clinics, dispensaries, hospitals or laboratories recognized by the same Council as competent to provide a satisfactory training in the special field of study."[82]

The Advisory Board for Medical Specialties influenced the future relationship of internal medicine and cardiology. In December 1935 Bierring submitted an application to the advisory board to establish an American Board of Internal Medicine. It approved the new board for certifying internists the following spring, and Bierring was chosen as the internal medicine board's first chair. He explained that it would develop "qualifications and procedures...for additional certification in certain of the more restricted and specialized branches of internal medicine [such] as gastroenterology, cardiology, metabolic diseases, tuberculosis and allergic diseases."[83] This strategy meant that cardiology would be a subspecialty—a branch—of internal medicine rather than an independent medical specialty. Doctors seeking board certification in cardiology (and the status this implied) would first have to be fully trained in internal medicine and to have passed the American Board of Internal Medicine's general medicine examination. The structure and philosophy of the Mayo Clinic had influenced Bierring's notion of the relationship of internal medicine and what he considered its more specialized branches.[84]

Bierring boasted to Wilson in 1936, "It now looks as if within the short period of three years since this movement had its real start at the Milwaukee session...certifying boards in the twelve recognized specialties will be established."[85] Wilson, whose support of the board was very apparent in Rochester, wrote to Bierring the following year: "I should like to send a copy of the handbook of the American Board of Internal Medicine to each fellow appointed in that field in the Mayo Foundation. Would it be asking too much to suggest that you let me have fifty copies?"[86]

Wilson retired as director of the Mayo Foundation for Medical Research and Education in 1937. During his more than two-decade tenure as director, he had overseen the postgraduate training of more than 1,200 fellows who had spent three or more years in Rochester.[87] Tulane University professor of medicine John Musser, a former president of the American College of Physicians, proclaimed in 1938: "A fellow who has completed three years at the Mayo Foundation has obtained, as far as I know, the most complete formal training in graduate work available in this country."[88] It would have been difficult for anyone to dispute this statement.

The Mayo Brothers Die, and Their Friends Respond

Will Mayo was seventy-seven years old in August 1938, when he gave a speech explaining the decision that he and his wife had made with respect to the disposition of their forty-seven-room mansion located halfway between the clinic and St. Mary's Hospital. Will believed that "it is a man's duty to provide moderately for his family, but anything beyond this may be a detriment to his descendants." After discussing the importance of education to society, he explained that they were donating their home to the Mayo Foundation so it could be become "a meeting place where men of medicine may exchange ideas for the good of mankind."[89] When he spoke, Will had no way of knowing that he and his brother would die in less than a year.

Charlie Mayo, who had survived a series of small strokes in the 1930s, was in Chicago when he developed pneumonia and died in May 1939. Cleveland Clinic cofounder George Crile wrote to Will to express his feelings. The surgeon, who had been the brothers' friend for a half-century, declared, "I would never have dreamed... that there would be such an institution as the Mayo Clinic, the greatest achievement that has been made in the world of medicine. It was your unique, penetrating certainty of prevision that led to this final achievement."[90] When Will received this letter, he knew that he was dying of stomach cancer. He succumbed to the disease in July 1939. The Mayo brothers' deaths, just two months apart, triggered a flood of tributes in medical journals, magazines, and newspapers. In the half-century since Will and Charlie had joined their father's general practice in Rochester, they had created a stunningly successful, self-sustaining center for patient care, postgraduate training, and medical research.

In a eulogy titled "The Mayo Brothers and Their Clinic," Will and Charlie's longtime friend Harvey Cushing proclaimed: "Not since the somewhat mythical attachment of those fifth-century physicians, Cosmas and Damien, both of whom in due time came to be sanctified, has there been anything like it."[91] The world-renowned neurosurgeon had written more than a dozen books and three hundred articles when his tribute to the Mayo brothers appeared in the September 8, 1939, issue of *Science*. It would be his last publication.

Two weeks later, Cushing began having recurrent bouts of chest and upper abdominal pain. After a severe episode that lasted all night, he was admitted to the New Haven Hospital where he was placed in an oxygen tent and given a narcotic that relieved his pain. Cushing's deterioration and death were described by the pathologist who performed his autopsy: "Twenty-four hours after admission the patient was in great distress, his color was grayish rather than cyanotic and rales appeared in the bases of both lungs. On the 6th an electrocardiogram revealed complete A-V [heart] block.... At about 2 a.m. on October 7, the heart rate, which was 30 per minute became irregular and stopped altogether 45 minutes later."[92]

The autopsy revealed that the seventy-year-old surgeon had severe coronary artery disease. The mid-portion of his left coronary artery had a "pinpoint lumen," and his circumflex coronary artery was also severely narrowed. But the third major coronary artery had caused Cushing's heart attack: "The right coronary artery contains a fresh subintimal hematoma which bulges into the lumen of the vessel and deforms it into a mere semilunar slit. Immediately below this point the entire lumen is occluded by a fresh thrombus."[93] This blood clot triggered a myocardial infarction that was complicated by heart block, which caused his death. There was no accepted treatment for blood clots in the coronary arteries when Cushing died in 1939. But Canadian physiologist Charles Best and his associates at the University of Toronto were performing animal experiments to study whether the anticoagulant heparin could prevent clots from forming in the coronary arteries and inside the heart's chambers.[94]

Mayo's Role in Attacking Blood Clots With Anticoagulants

Charles Best's heart-related heparin research did not have immediate clinical relevance, but his group's experiments relating to the prevention of postoperative pulmonary emboli did. A pulmonary embolus is a life-threatening problem that usually begins with blood clots that had formed in larger veins in the legs or pelvis. These clots can break off and travel through the right side of the heart and into the pulmonary arteries, where they block the flow of blood flow through the lungs. Mayo cardiologist Arlie Barnes described how patients with a major pulmonary embolus felt and looked in a 1937 article. They become suddenly short of breath, feel faint, are pale or cyanotic (a blue-purple skin color), and have a rapid pulse. Their blood pressure falls dramatically, and they may go into shock. Barnes estimated that about 34,000 Americans died of pulmonary embolism each year. A significant percentage of these individuals were recovering from surgery, a fact that had stimulated interest in the complication at Mayo for a quarter-century.[95]

Barnes provided perspective on the problem in the opening sentence of his article on pulmonary embolism: "An operation in which the patient has weathered all other hazards, a fracture that is healing satisfactorily, a puerperium in which all appears to go well, a thrombophlebitis in which the patient is well on the way to recovery or a minor sprain or bruise may be the setting for death from pulmonary embolism. The great tragedy of such a death is that in almost every such case the accident of pulmonary embolism was the sole barrier that stood between the patient and recovery."[96] Local research traditions, individual interests, and personal contacts facilitated early heparin research in Rochester.

The anticoagulant heparin had been discovered at Johns Hopkins during World War I, but the original substance was too toxic for clinical use. In the mid-1930s, Charles Best's group developed a purified product in crystalline form that was suitable for use in patients. Best gave Toronto surgeon Gordon Murray samples of purified heparin for a clinical trial in postoperative patients who were considered to be at high risk for pulmonary emboli.[97]

In June 1937 Mayo physiologist Hiram Essex informed Best that James Priestley, one of the clinic's surgeons, "has been particularly interested in the problem of postoperative embolism." Essex explained that he and Priestley planned to visit Toronto after the "summer rush" of patients in order to "get all the information we can from you" about heparin. They wanted to learn about the anticoagulant before beginning animal experiments and conducting a "thorough trial" in patients. Best responded that he would be happy to have them visit in the fall.[98] Best and Murray published an article in August that reported their initial results administering heparin to patients.[99]

In October 1937 Essex and Priestley visited Toronto and returned to Rochester with a small supply of purified heparin. Priestley administered it to a patient at St. Mary's Hospital the following month. This was the first time that purified heparin was given to a patient in the United States. Essex informed Best in mid-November, "Just after Priestley returned one of the patients he operated on before leaving showed symptoms of pulmonary embolism. She came through the first episode but had a second to which she almost succumbed. He came out to my laboratory and told me about the case, and I suggested that he take the heparin you gave us and use it which he did. She has been getting along splendidly since.... We feel that heparin is clearly indicated and should be given at once when such symptoms appear."[100] The Canadian physiologist responded, "I was very pleased to hear about Priestley's case. I have sent you off some more heparin so that you would have some for experimental work."[101]

Just after Christmas, Priestley told Mayo's Board of Governors that Best had "kindly supplied gratuitously a limited amount of heparin for experimental studies which Doctor Essex and I are now conducting." Based on his visit to Best's laboratory and his experience with one patient, Priestley was "convinced that the postoperative use of heparin merits clinical trial here." The surgeon sought institutional support for the study because he considered it "unfair to charge the patient" for heparin until its effectiveness was established.[102] The board asked Barnes to meet with Priestley and to make a recommendation regarding his request. As a heart specialist and board member, Barnes was a logical choice. He had recently told the staff that patients with pulmonary emboli often have "so many profound circulatory changes that it falls to the cardiologist to see many of them."[103] The board approved using $400 from the Emergency Fund for Clinical Investigation to support the heparin project.

Best came to Rochester in October 1938 to deliver a Mayo Foundation Lecture on heparin. He summarized experimental work on the substance that had been done in his laboratory and clinical trials that were underway in Toronto and Stockholm, Sweden. Noting that experience with more than 400 patients had shown that heparin could be "given safely to human subjects," the Canadian physiologist "hoped that by pushing ahead with more studies along physiological and experimental pathologic lines the clinical applications will become more obvious."[104]

By this time, a Mayo team (led by Priestley, Essex, and vascular specialist Nelson Barker) was evaluating heparin's value in the prevention and treatment of postoperative venous thrombosis and pulmonary embolism. In January 1941 they reported gratifying results in more than fifty-five patients who were thought to have had pulmonary emboli while recovering from surgery. If heparin was administered to such a patient, the likelihood of another pulmonary embolus was low. The Mayo investigators argued that heparin was of "definite value" in this situation and predicted that the anticoagulant would be used to treat many other thromboembolic disorders if its cost came down and if an alternative to intravenous administration could be developed.[105]

In June 1941, five months after Priestley, Essex, and Barker's article on heparin was published in the *Proceedings*, Mayo internist Hugh Butt, vascular specialist Edgar Allen, and experimental pathologist Jesse Bollman coauthored a preliminary report on a substance derived from spoiled sweet clover that inhibited blood coagulation. Their title included its complicated chemical name: 3,3'-methylene-bis-(4-hydroxycoumarin).[106] Three months later, the London-based *Lancet* published an editorial entitled "Heparin and a Rival." Citing the Mayo report, the writer was enthusiastic about the substance that appeared to be non-toxic, was less expensive than heparin, and had "the enormous advantage of being active when given by mouth in gelatin capsules." He had one request: "Let us hope its discoverers will think of a shorter name for it, preferably one that will recall its pastoral origin."[107]

The synthesis of the first oral anticoagulant was the end result of a discovery that veterinarians had made in the 1920s, when they were trying to figure out why cows sometimes bled to death for no apparent reason. They found that blood from cows that had eaten spoiled sweet clover hay did not clot normally. During the next decade, University of Wisconsin biochemist Karl Link led a team that studied the problem. In 1940 his group isolated and synthesized the "hemorrhagic agent" that caused "sweet clover disease."[108] This discovery fascinated Mayo internists Hugh Butt and Albert Snell, who had been conducting a clinical trial of vitamin K to reduce the bleeding tendency of patients with jaundice. When Snell reported the results of their research to the staff in 1941, he said that he and his co-investigator were grateful for "the enthusiastic cooperation of some of our colleagues and the healthy skepticism of others; both attitudes are equally necessary for sound clinical investigation."[109] Butt soon turned his attention from a vitamin that could help stop bleeding in one specific situation to a substance that could keep blood from clotting in any situation.

Hugh Butt told Edgar Allen about Karl Link's research at the University of Wisconsin in March 1941. Allen immediately contacted the biochemist because he thought the "hemorrhagic agent" that had been isolated and synthesized in Madison might be an oral alternative to intravenous heparin. Link sent the Mayo investigators samples of the novel anticoagulant known as 3,3'-methylene-bis-(4-hydroxycoumarin). After administering it to dogs over a three-week period, Allen gave it to a nineteen-year-old man with thrombo-angiitis obliterans on May 9, 1941. There was no obvious therapeutic benefit. When Butt, Allen, and Bollman published their article in the *Proceedings* five weeks later, they explained that the anticoagulant had been given to a total of six individuals, including volunteers. They acknowledged that their study of the substance in animals and humans "is very incomplete and much work, now underway, must be finished before conclusions can be drawn relative to the usefulness of the preparation in clinical practice."[110]

The Mayo researchers had a unique opportunity to compare the new compound (named dicumarol) with heparin because both anticoagulants were available in Rochester before almost any other clinical investigators had either one. Based on their experience with these drugs, they cited three advantages of dicumarol over heparin: oral administration, prolonged action, and lower cost. Commercialized versions of heparin and dicumarol (and a similar drug that would be named warfarin) would become mainstays of therapy to prevent acute and chronic thrombosis and embolism.[111] The ability of these drugs to prevent blood from clotting made them indispensable for the development of technologies that revolutionized treatments after World War II, such as kidney dialysis and open-heart surgery.

Karl Link delivered his first lecture on dicumarol outside Madison in Rochester on March 12, 1942. The Mayo chapter of Sigma Xi, a national honor society for research scientists, sponsored the talk. Link's audience knew that he was a last-minute substitute. The February 21 issue of the *Clinic Bulletin* had announced that French physicist Léon Brillouin, a visiting professor at the University of Wisconsin, would deliver the Sigma Xi lecture five days later. Brillouin, who had left his Nazi-occupied homeland, was scheduled to speak about "very short radio waves...now being used effectively in airplane detection and location," and his lecture would be "open to all those interested."[112] One day before the French physicist was supposed to speak, the *Clinic Bulletin* announced that his lecture had been "postponed indefinitely."[113] This is not surprising, considering the topic and the wartime context. Soon,

Brillouin would be working on radar with the National Defense Research Committee.

Radar had been a decisive factor in the Royal Air Force's September 1940 victory over the German Luftwaffe in the hard-fought Battle of Britain. Obviously, someone decided that Brillouin should not speak publicly in Rochester about strategic military technology in February 1942, just a month after the first American troops arrived in England. Edgar Allen, who was president of Mayo's Sigma Xi chapter, asked Link to substitute for the French physicist. A lecture about dicumarol's ability to prevent potentially lethal blood clots made more sense than a talk about radar's ability to pinpoint enemy planes.[114] The sudden switch of speakers at the Mayo Clinic was just one example of World War II's profound impact on the countries that were involved in the conflict.

Early in 1942 Arlie Barnes informed the Board of Governors that "members of our staff do not grasp as yet the changes that this present war is going to impose upon them. Somehow or other it is going to be necessary to get across to our staff that research as usual cannot go on. In general, only such research as has a fairly direct bearing on problems of war can be legitimately pursued or supported.... Men will have to be told in no uncertain words that they will have to forego time spent on research and devote exclusively to the care of patients."[115] The Mayo Clinic had survived the Depression, but there was much uncertainty in the air in the early 1940s.

Developments in the Diagnosis and Treatment of Heart Disease

President Roosevelt's Secret Hypertensive Heart Disease

A few days before the 1944 presidential election, Mayo cardiologist Arlie Barnes almost stumbled onto the national political scene because of casual comments he had made in Rochester, Minnesota, about Franklin Roosevelt's cardiovascular health. Barnes never provided medical care for the president, but his words mattered. He was recognized as one of America's leading heart specialists, and he worked at a world-renowned institution. Stephen (Steve) Early, Roosevelt's press secretary, was eager to silence Barnes and a few of his associates who had been discussing rumors about the president's health that had been circulating at the Naval Medical Center in Bethesda, Maryland. During the closing days of the 1944 campaign, Early and other White House insiders also orchestrated campaign events designed to project an image of a healthy commander in chief. Stifling speculation about Roosevelt's heart health was part of their strategy to keep Thomas Dewey from winning the election.[1]

Arlie Barnes, Electrocardiography, and the American Heart Association

Arlie Barnes's professional reputation resulted mainly from his publications on electrocardiography.[2] He was an early advocate of using a fourth electrocardiographic lead (placed on the chest), which had been developed to supplement the three leads attached to a patient's arms and left leg. Unlike those limb leads, a precordial (chest) lead could identify myocardial infarctions that involved the heart's anterior wall. When the fourth lead was introduced in the 1930s, Barnes considered it a major advance, analogous to giving an artist "an additional pigment with which to paint a richer and more significant picture."[3] An American Heart Association committee, composed of Barnes and electrocardiography pioneers Harold Pardee, Paul Dudley White,

Frank Wilson, and Charles Wolferth, published guidelines for using multiple chest leads in 1938. To standardize recording and reporting, they defined six specific chest wall locations and named them V_1 through V_6.[4] Two years later, Wolferth described Barnes as a "seasoned veteran in clinical electrocardiography" and one of the field's "foremost investigators."[5]

In the late 1930s, some cardiologists expressed concern that electrocardiography was diffusing too rapidly as companies marketed cheaper and more portable machines. For example, Boston heart specialist Samuel Levine complained in 1940 that "many inadequately trained physicians have assumed the responsibility of interpreting the tracings and the result is that there is a danger of prostituting the entire work."[6] Two factors contributed to this situation: there were no national standards for training heart specialists, and there was no way to control the diffusion of technologies that could increase the prestige and incomes of the doctors who used them. To help address these concerns, a certification examination in cardiovascular disease was introduced in 1941. Paul Dudley White was president of the American Heart Association two years later, when he appointed Arlie Barnes to the four-person Cardiovascular Subspecialty Board. This group decided who was eligible to take the certification examination. Its strict criteria excluded most self-proclaimed cardiologists.[7]

Barnes remained in Rochester during World War II, where he was kept busy seeing patients, while many of his associates were in the armed forces. Mayo's staff shortage was significant. In 1944 a man sent a postcard from Rochester to a friend in Virginia: "Went out to the Mayo Clinic today.... Five hundred doctors work at clinic now—nearly 1000 before the war."[8] Barnes, despite his responsibilities at the clinic, was willing to take on more work for the American Heart Association. He accepted an invitation to edit its monthly bulletin, *Modern Concepts of Cardiovascular Disease*, in 1944. "I pleaded that I lacked time," he told Mayo's Board of Governors, "but they were very anxious that the Mayo Clinic be represented." Barnes, who was a member of the board, explained that the editorial position would allow him "to introduce some younger men of the clinic in that field."[9] Two other wartime appointments reflected and reinforced Barnes's stature as a cardiologist. He was elected to the American Heart Association's Board of Directors as a representative of the Great Lakes region, and he was appointed to the National Research Council's new Subcommittee on Cardiovascular Diseases.

Barnes seemed destined to become president of the American Heart Association when H. M. (Jack) Marvin, chair of the organization's Executive Committee, raised a cautionary flag in the spring of 1944. The New Haven cardiologist informed White: "I shall not ask your pardon for writing perfectly frankly about the work of the Nominating Committee since I know this is what you would want me to do. Geographical considerations and regional jealousies unfortunately have to be considered, and I am not certain that Arlie Barnes should be put in line for the presidency, since this would mean that three consecutive presidents had come from the middle west or far west."[10] White, who had known Barnes for two decades, replied that it was "as reasonable to have a president from that region as from one of the eastern cities."[11] The Mayo cardiologist would become president of the association three years later.

In August 1944 Marvin asked Barnes to assist the American Heart Association in collecting information about cardiovascular research in the Great Lakes region. The survey was the result of a new law, which President Roosevelt explained gave the US Public Health Service the "authority to make grants-in-aid for research to public or private institutions for investigations in any field related to the public health."[12] Barnes asked officials at the University of Minnesota Medical School to summarize how much money their institution budgeted for cardiovascular research and how they might use additional federal funds if they became available.[13]

Physiologist Maurice Visscher responded, "As you know, we have always had considerable work going on in the Department of Physiology bearing on the problem of cardiovascular disease." He estimated that $8,000 was spent annually and thought that his department could use twice that amount. Considering how many deaths cardiovascular disease caused, Visscher was frustrated "that so little money is available for its investigation." He informed Barnes that an annual federal allocation of $1 million, distributed among laboratories across the country, would be "a very modest beginning toward adequate support."[14] Armed with information he had gathered for the American Heart Association, Barnes traveled to Washington for a meeting of the National Research Council Subcommittee on Cardiovascular Diseases that was held on October 18, 1944.[15]

Conversations About President Roosevelt's "Heart Ailment"

While Arlie Barnes was in the capital for the subcommittee meeting, he visited Howard Odel, a member of his five-man Mayo medical section who was stationed at the Naval Hospital during the war. Shortly after Barnes returned to Rochester, he discovered that he had trespassed on treacherous political terrain when he and Odel had chatted about Franklin Roosevelt's heart health in Bethesda. Neither man had provided care for the president, but that did not matter. They were affiliated with the prestigious Mayo Clinic, and the outcome of the election, less than three weeks away, was far from certain.[16]

On October 27, 1944, less than a week after Barnes returned to Rochester from the Washington meeting, two Federal Bureau of Investigation (FBI) agents interrogated him. FBI director J. Edgar Hoover wrote to presidential press secretary Steve Early (Figure 7.1) on November 1, explaining that his agents had interviewed doctors at the Mayo Clinic and the Bethesda Naval Hospital. Hoover concluded that there had been "a lot of loose conversation and talk, all predicated upon the supposition that the President was suffering from some heart ailment."[17] One of the FBI agents recalled that he had been sent to Rochester "in what proved to be an attempt to prevent the information on FDR's circulatory disease from becoming public knowledge."[18] The media had made no mention of the casual conversations in Rochester and Bethesda, and Steve Early wanted to keep it that way. Roosevelt's chief image shaper knew that some voters—perhaps many—might shift to Thomas Dewey if credible reports surfaced that the president had persistent severe hypertension and had experienced an episode of heart failure.

Steve Early understood the power of the press and had experience breaking big stories. Working for the Associated Press in 1923, he scooped fellow reporters by revealing that President Warren Harding had died suddenly in a San Francisco hotel at the age of fifty-seven.[19] Early had first met Franklin Roosevelt at the 1912 Democratic National Convention. They developed a personal relationship during the 1920s that became very close over time.

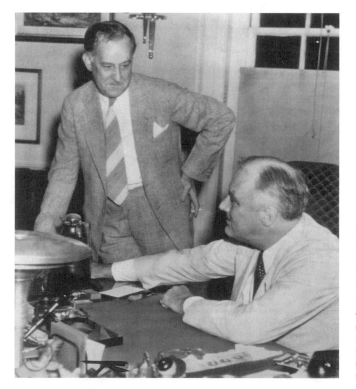

FIGURE 7.1
Stephen (Steve)
Early with
President Franklin
Roosevelt, August
25, 1939.

Original Associated Press (AP) wire photo in the author's possession, used with permission of AP.

After Roosevelt appointed him press secretary in 1933, the former reporter was in a position to shape or stifle news stories.

Early exploded in 1937 when *Life* magazine published a picture of the president that revealed his post-polio disability. He complained to White House physician Ross McIntire, "Here is a picture of the President in his wheelchair—a scene we have never permitted to be photographed. The photographer evidently made his way into the Naval Hospital grounds to do his job or someone at the Hospital made the picture for him.... I do think this should be investigated and steps taken to prevent any repetition."[20] For Early, investigation was part of a deliberate process designed to suppress stories that White House insiders did not want made public. He and Ross McIntire built and maintained a high and thick wall of secrecy around Roosevelt's health status.

During World War II, the media and the public accepted the government's position that it was critical to restrict information that might aid enemies. *Life* magazine published an article "Have You Heard?" in the summer of 1942. It was Steve Early's idea, and the editors asked Alfred Hitchcock to produce the "photo-dramatization." Published two months after the director's movie *Saboteur* premiered in Washington, the article, subtitled "The Story of Wartime Rumors," conveyed a clear message. A series of staged photographs with captions showed "how patriotic but talkative Americans pass along information, true or false, until finally deadly damage is done to their country's war effort. One false rumor is silenced by a man of goodwill who later is unwittingly responsible for starting a true rumor which ends in a great catastrophe. Moral: Keep your mouth shut."[21]

American military personnel were fighting on several fronts when the Office of War Information published posters warning that "Loose Lips Might Sink Ships." Loose lips might also sink political careers. Steve Early knew that what J. Edgar Hoover described as "loose conversation" about Roosevelt having heart disease was true. This was not the first time that concerns about the president's heart had been raised. But now, just days before the 1944 election, they came from credible sources.

The Roosevelt Family's Respect for the Mayo Clinic

The public knew that Franklin Roosevelt had great respect for the Mayo Clinic. He had visited Rochester in 1934 to participate in an American Legion ceremony honoring Will and Charlie Mayo. Speaking to a crowd of several thousand, the president praised the Mayo brothers' half century of "tireless, skillful and unselfish service" and proclaimed that they were "beloved at home and abroad."[22] Admiral Cary Grayson, who had been Woodrow Wilson's White House physician and had chaired Roosevelt's Inaugural

Committee, informed the Mayo brothers that the president "was delighted with his visit.... Ever since then he has been strong in his praise of you both and of the whole clinic."[23] Roosevelt would not receive care at the Mayo Clinic, but he and several of his friends and associates had great confidence in the institution.

James Roosevelt was working as his father's assistant in the White House in the spring of 1938, when his persistent abdominal pain led to an evaluation at the Mayo Clinic. The conclusion was that he had a benign stomach ulcer. Despite a special diet and medications, his symptoms persisted and an operation was advised. The president, Steve Early, and White House physician Ross McIntire were among those on a special train that arrived in Rochester on September 11. James Roosevelt's wife Betsey and his mother were already in town. Betsey's father, Harvey Cushing, a surgical pioneer and longtime close friend of the Mayo brothers, reassured the president: "Jimmy could not be in better hands, and I feel sure he will come through with flying colors."[24]

The *Rochester Post-Bulletin* reported that the president went straight from his train to St. Mary's Hospital, where he spoke with gastroenterologist George Eusterman, surgeon Howard Gray, and radiologist Byrl Kirklin to get "last minute information on the condition of his son" just before James was taken to the operating room.[25] *Time* magazine reported: "Afterwards, because of the public importance of the patient, surgeon Gray consented to a thing unprecedented at Mayo Clinic: a press conference." Ross McIntire was with Howard Gray when he reported that the president's son did not have cancer.[26]

Periodically, the public would be reminded that medical news from the Mayo Clinic was not always good. New York Yankee first baseman Lou Gehrig was one of baseball's biggest stars in 1938, having won three Most Valuable Player awards and having been in six consecutive All-Star games. The following year he became progressively weak and had to stop playing. Seeking an explanation, Gehrig flew to Rochester, where he spent a week being examined. Reporters hounded the thirty-six-year-old celebrity for answers, and he released a letter written by Harold Habein, the Mayo physician who supervised his evaluation. It read, in part, "After a careful and complete examination, it was found that he is suffering from amyotrophic lateral sclerosis. This type of illness involves the motor pathways and cells of the central nervous system and in lay terms is known as a form of chronic poliomyelitis (infantile paralysis). The nature of this trouble makes it such that Mr. Gehrig will be unable to continue his active participation as a baseball player."[27]

The Yankees announced that "Lou Gehrig Appreciation Day" would be held at their stadium in the Bronx on July 4, 1939. More than 60,000 fans attended the ceremony that was held between the games of a double-header.

Mayor Fiorello La Guardia and Babe Ruth spoke before Gehrig stepped up to the microphone to say a few words. Most newspapers published photographs of the American hero, whose Mayo press release had explained that he had a "form of chronic poliomyelitis." That phrase reminded some readers of another famous American who had continued to work almost two decades after he had contracted polio. Many published photographs showed Lou Gehrig standing in Yankee Stadium on the Fourth of July. Five years later, *Life* magazine and several newspapers printed a photograph of Franklin Roosevelt seated in a railroad car. The president's past history of polio was well known, but his wartime cardiovascular problems were top secret.

A Photograph Leads to Speculation About Roosevelt's Heart

Life magazine photographer George Skadding took several pictures of Roosevelt on July 20, 1944, as he was reading a speech to attendees at the Democratic National Convention in Chicago. Roosevelt expressed his willingness to be their presidential candidate in the fall election. But the president was not physically present at the convention. His address was broadcast live over the radio from a West Coast naval base to the Chicago Stadium audience and to citizens across the continent. The president was in California preparing to sail to Hawaii to discuss Pacific war strategy with General Douglas MacArthur and Admiral Chester Nimitz.

Roosevelt explained that he had accepted the nomination for a fourth term despite his "desire to retire to the quiet of private life." The president also lowered expectations in terms of public appearances during wartime: "I shall not campaign, in the usual sense, for the office. In these days of tragic sorrow, I do not consider it fitting. And besides, in these days of global warfare, I shall not be able to find the time." Stressing the significance of continuity, the commander in chief proclaimed, "The people of the United States will decide this fall whether they wish to turn over this 1944 job—this worldwide job—to inexperienced or immature hands... or whether they wish to leave it to those who saw the danger from abroad, who met it head-on, and who now have seized the offensive and carried the war to its present stages of success."[28]

One of George Skadding's photographs was circulated widely, and it upset White House insiders. Roosevelt's speech writer and trusted advisor Samuel Rosenman considered it "most unfortunate" that the picture was published because it depicted his boss as "a tragic-looking figure... [who] looked weary, sick, discouraged, and exhausted."[29] Steve Early complained to Roosevelt's personal secretary Grace Tully, "I was terrifically disappointed, let down to a new low, when I saw the photograph of the President delivering his speech of acceptance. I can't imagine what was wrong with Skadding, or his camera, or his subject. But something was decidedly wrong.... The rumor factory is working overtime—making all it can out of the rumors and lies about the President's health. That is why some of the photographs I have seen caused me much concern at this time."[30]

Early's concern that this picture of the president would fuel the "rumor factory" was well founded. Skadding, frustrated and fearing retribution, wrote to the press secretary:

> I'm sure you must have cussed as much as I did when LIFE came out with that terrible picture of the Boss last week. I feel like apologizing, but the dam [sic] picture [has] been used. When I brought the pictures in from San Diego it was extremely late—the A.P., Acme and INP were holding their wires open overtime. I turned the negatives over to them to rush through...and before I knew it they had this particular bad shot on the wires....To make sure my outfit [*Life* magazine] would not use the same picture I sent them only the better shots. And then they turned around and used the lousy one sent out by AP and the others....I have already griped like hell to my office—That kind of a shot certainly does not do me any good. And to try and make up for this, I'm going to personally supervise the next ones made and show the boss as he really is.[31]

The text that accompanied Skadding's photograph in the July 31, 1944, issue of *Life* magazine explained that the president was in "an old observation car on a railroad siding.... The shades were drawn, making secrecy complete." Although the location was secret, a few doctors recognized someone in the picture whose presence suggested that President Roosevelt had a heart problem.[32]

The *Life* magazine photograph (Figure 7.2) depicted Roosevelt, his chief of staff Admiral William Leahy, three family members, a radio announcer, and an unidentified naval officer. One week after the picture appeared in *Life*, Washington-based reporter Walter Trohan of the anti-Roosevelt *Chicago Tribune* published a story "Disclose Heart Specialist Is With Roosevelt." He explained that "Howard Gerald Bruenn, a New York City heart specialist, who was commissioned in the navy...was identified by friends here as the naval officer shown in photographs of the President delivering his radio address from his private railroad car.... It was reported in capital circles that Bruenn had been commissioned to look after Mr. Roosevelt." Trohan reminded readers that the wartime president had taken a month-long vacation at the "regal South Carolina plantation of Bernard M. Baruch" in the spring. Noting Roosevelt's obvious weight loss, the reporter ended his story with a quote from Ross McIntire. When the president returned to Washington in May, the White House physician had claimed that his health was "excellent

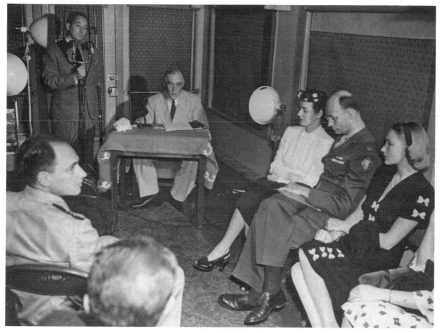

FIGURE 7.2 *Roosevelt delivering Democratic nomination acceptance speech over the radio from a railroad car on the West Coast, July 20, 1944. The man whose face is shown in profile in the lower left is cardiologist Howard Bruenn.*
Life, July 31, 1944, 13. Photograph by George Skadding, used with permission of Getty Images.

in all respects."[33] McIntire was lying. In fact, he had been concerned about Roosevelt's heart for more than a year.

Secret Knowledge About Roosevelt's Heart and Hypertension

When Warner Brothers released the motion picture *Casablanca* starring Humphrey Bogart and Ingrid Bergman on January 23, 1943, Roosevelt was in that North African city for a top-secret meeting with British prime minister Winston Churchill.[34] The president and a team that included close personal friend and top advisor Harry Hopkins, Admiral William Leahy, and Ross McIntire had crossed the Atlantic in a Boeing 314 Clipper. On January 11, shortly after the trip began, Roosevelt informed his cousin, confidante, and frequent companion Margaret "Daisy" Suckley that he "felt the altitude at 8 or 9,000 feet."[35] Harry Hopkins wrote in his diary that day: "Dr. McIntire was worried about the president's bad heart—nothing happened."[36] The next day he noted that "McIntire was quite disturbed about the President, who appeared to be very pale at times" as the plane reached an altitude of 9,000 feet.[37]

Howard Bruenn, who would become the president's cardiologist the following year, had coauthored a prewar article describing how a low blood oxygen level could cause cardiac pain. It contained a warning: "Persons known to have cardiac disease due to an affection of the coronary arteries should not be permitted to ascend to high altitudes. If such a flight is imperative, provision must be made for supplying the necessary concentration of oxygen."[38] Once Roosevelt's party reached Gambia in West Africa, they transferred to a C54 military transport plane that would carry them north toward Casablanca, Morocco. Two days after McIntire had expressed concern about the president's pale appearance at high altitude, Roosevelt wrote to Daisy Suckley: "We flew over a pass 10,000 ft. & I tried a few whiffs of oxygen."[39]

In November 1943 Roosevelt was in Tehran, Iran, for his first joint meeting with British prime minister Winston Churchill and Soviet leader Joseph Stalin. They would discuss a future invasion of Europe, a top-secret mission code-named Overlord. After returning to America, the president became sick with a cough, fever, and fatigue. He complained to his cousin Laura Delano two months later, "This 'flu' is Hell, as you know. I am not over mine yet."[40] On February 2, 1944, Daisy and Anna Boettiger, the president's daughter, accompanied him to the Bethesda Naval Hospital for treatment—not for the flu but for a lump on the back of his head.[41] At a press conference two days later, Roosevelt confirmed that surgeons had removed a large sebaceous cyst under local anesthesia.[42] Two Mayo Clinic doctors who were assigned to the hospital during the war participated in the procedure.

Mayo anesthesiologist John Pender recalled making a startling discovery in the Naval Hospital's operating room: "Had him sitting in his wheelchair with his arms resting on the anesthesia table, and of course I checked his blood pressure. And that was when I found out he had terrific hypertension. This was when he was running for his third [read: fourth] term so it was sort of political dynamite that some of my friends afterwards said that I should have divulged, but I didn't."[43] Mayo neurosurgeon Winchell Craig, who was chief of surgery at the Naval Hospital during the war, performed the operation with the assistance of a plastic surgeon. He removed a one-and-a-half-inch long egg-shaped mass from the back of the president's head, which the pathologist described as a benign epidermoid cyst "with no evidence of malignancy."[44]

Pender's discovery of severe hypertension would not have caused Craig to cancel the minor operation. On the other hand, the anesthesiologist almost certainly mentioned it to his Mayo colleague and to Ross McIntire who was with them in the operating room. Craig was an expert in sympathectomy, an operation on the sympathetic nervous system that a few surgeons performed in selected young patients with severe hypertension. He had opened a prewar article on the procedure with a grim observation: "Hypertension, or persistent elevation of the blood pressure, may produce progressively severe symptoms and in spite of all types of treatment it may terminate fatally."[45]

Daisy Suckley, who was outside the operating room, wrote in her diary: "The wen came out like a bantam's egg—There were no complications of any kind & Dr. McIntire said it was a perfect performance in every way."[46] During the next six weeks, Roosevelt continued to hold regular press conferences. By mid-March, his chronic sinus condition had worsened, and he had developed a fever. His daughter Anna, who had moved into the White House a few months earlier, insisted that McIntire call in other physicians to examine her father, who seemed to be getting sicker and had a persistent cough.[47]

A Cardiologist is Called in to Examine the Commander in Chief

On March 24, 1944, Roosevelt responded to a reporter's question about the critical shortage of civilian workers caused by a twenty-fold increase in military personnel in the past four years: "I haven't done anything on it in the last few days because I have had a cold."[48] Four days later, another reporter asked him about his health: "In view of a lot of stories that have appeared, would you like to tell us how you feel?" Roosevelt, aware that he had been seen in Bethesda, explained: "I was out to the Naval Hospital this afternoon—went out after lunch, to get a thing called X-rays taken; and I have—I have had for probably a couple of weeks—between two and three weeks, a touch of bronchitis. It isn't very—(coughing involuntarily)—serious."[49] The commander in chief did not reveal that a cardiologist had examined him that day, and the cardiologist did not reveal his findings to the public for a quarter century.

During Howard Bruenn's initial examination of Roosevelt, the cardiologist noted that the president coughed frequently, was slightly cyanotic (consistent with a low blood oxygen level), and that movement "caused considerable breathlessness." White House physician Ross McIntire, an ear, nose, and throat specialist, had attributed all of this to bronchitis, but the heart specialist found compelling evidence of cardiovascular disease. Roosevelt's blood pressure was high (186/108), and his eye examination showed arteriovenous nicking (blood vessel changes consistent with significant hypertension). When the cardiologist listened to the president's chest, he heard abnormal lung sounds and a heart murmur, which he attributed to a leaking mitral valve. Fluoroscopy revealed an enlarged heart and plump pulmonary vessels consistent with congestive heart failure. An electrocardiogram demonstrated dramatic T-wave inversions, a worrisome finding.[50] New York cardiologist Harold Pardee had written three years earlier: "Follow-up reports of the Mayo Clinic show that when associated with other abnormalities of the cardiovascular system, T wave abnormality added considerably to the gravity of the prognosis, such patients having a shorter average duration of life than those with normal T waves."[51]

Bruenn concluded that Roosevelt had "hypertension, hypertensive heart disease, cardiac failure (left ventricular), and acute bronchitis." He sent McIntire a detailed report with specific recommendations, including one to two weeks of strict bed rest with nursing care, an easily digestible low-salt diet, and gradual weight loss. Bruenn thought the president should receive digitalis for heart failure, codeine for cough, and a sedative "to ensure rest and a refreshing night's sleep." The cardiologist later explained that the White House physician rejected the regimen "because of the exigencies and demands on the President." McIntire, after consulting with three other Naval physicians, agreed to a modified plan that did not include digitalis.[52]

After Roosevelt returned from the Naval Hospital, he called Daisy Suckley, who wrote in her diary: "He said they took X-rays & all sorts of tests, found nothing drastically wrong, but one sinus clogged up. But they are going to put him on a strict diet."[53] He called her a week later to explain that he had been told to postpone a trip so two more doctors could evaluate him. "I'm worried," wrote Daisy, "for there must be something definitely wrong."[54] McIntire, concerned about the cardiologist's conclusions and their implications for the president's activity level and schedule, asked Atlanta internist James Paullin and Boston surgeon Frank Lahey to examine Roosevelt and review Bruenn's recommendations. They saw the president at the White House on March 31, 1944. Paullin was initially opposed to digitalis, but Bruenn convinced him that the president had congestive heart failure. Digitalis tablets were begun that day.[55]

Ross McIntire misled reporters about the president's recent medical evaluations during a press conference on April 4. Describing Roosevelt's "very complete" physical checkup as "satisfactory," he explained: "The only thing that we need to finish up on is just the residuals of this bronchitis and one of his sinuses; and they are clearing very rapidly. He is feeling quite well this morning." Continuing his pattern of partial disclosure, the White House physician informed the reporters that the evaluation "was thorough. It covered everything. And when we got through, we decided for a man of 62-plus that we had very little to argue about, with the exception that we had to combat the influenza, plus the respiratory complications that came along after."[56] McIntire made no mention of hypertension or heart failure.

The Challenges of Treating Heart Failure and Hypertension

Mayo cardiologist Thomas Dry had written in 1942 that congestive heart failure "represents, with few exceptions, a serious phase of heart disease."

This pronouncement was no secret; it appeared in the *Journal of the American Medical Association*.[57] His article on the prognosis of heart failure included a survival graph showing that two-thirds of patients were dead five years after their first episode. "The prolongation of life," Dry declared, "seems to depend on a systematic therapeutic program which calls for close cooperation between the patient and his physician."[58] The nation's commander in chief would follow his doctors' orders.

Several of Roosevelt's associates and appointees had health problems, and he encouraged them to follow their doctors' orders. This is exemplified by the case of Joseph Eastman, who was the same age as the president. Roosevelt had appointed the longtime member of the Interstate Commerce Commission to be director of the wartime Office of Defense Transportation. Steve Early informed the press on March 15, 1944, that Eastman had died earlier that day. He recounted a conversation he had had with Eastman one month earlier: "Joe called me on the telephone and said that, 'As you know, I have been in the hands of my doctors for about two years with angina trouble, and now they haven't asked me they have told me that I must go to a hospital for at least two months' rest.... If the President would like me to do so, because I shall be away from my office, I will offer my resignation."[59]

The same day that Early conveyed this information to Roosevelt, the president wrote to Eastman: "Dear Joe, "I am so sorry to hear that you are feeling somewhat below par. Your health is the prime concern and must receive every consideration. Follow strictly the doctor's orders, and take that much needed rest. Do not think of resigning. Get yourself back in good form, for the job needs you and the country needs you."[60] The president would follow his own advice—to follow doctors' orders.

Howard Bruenn saw Roosevelt frequently (usually three or more times a week) beginning in April 1944 until his death twelve months later. Although the president's signs and symptoms of heart failure improved soon after digitalis was started, it became apparent that he had severe hypertension. Three years earlier Mayo vascular specialist Edgar Allen had written that hypertension "appears to be more common and more deadly than cancer." Acknowledging that the definition of hypertension was debatable, Allen concluded that 120/80 should be considered "the upper limit for normal blood pressure."[61] During the first week of April 1944, Roosevelt's nine blood pressure readings averaged 210/114.[62]

Documenting high blood pressure was relatively easy, but treating it was almost impossible at that time. Edgar Hines, a Mayo physician who was especially interested in the problem, had written in 1941 that there was "no specific treatment for hypertension."[63] Paul Dudley White agreed, noting that many drugs had been tried, "sometimes with slight temporary success, sometimes with toxic effects, sometimes though rarely with prolonged benefit."

The prominent Boston cardiologist stressed that serious hypertension was "frequently followed by congestive failure and death."[64]

Lifestyle changes were the centerpiece of high blood pressure treatment in the 1940s. Edgar Allen recommended that hypertensive patients get nine hours of sleep, nap for sixty to ninety minutes each afternoon, and take frequent vacations. He also advised them to "acquire a calm, philosophic outlook on life and to avoid stresses and strains."[65] But this prescription was problematic if the patient was the president of the United States and commander in chief of millions of military personnel who were fighting on multiple fronts in World War II. Nevertheless, Roosevelt followed recommendations similar to those that Allen outlined in his article.

The war gave White House insiders an excuse for not revealing Roosevelt's exact whereabouts during a month-long vacation in the spring of 1944. He arrived at Hobcaw Barony, Bernard Baruch's 17,500-acre South Carolina estate, on April 9. The following day Steve Early informed the press that the president had left for an undisclosed location in the South where he would "devote himself exclusively to relaxation out-of-doors, in fresh air and sunshine" with the exception of doing work "that is always carried on between the White House and the President regardless of his whereabouts."[66] On April 15 Early sent a telegram to Ross McIntire, who was with the president: "Mrs. Roosevelt asks me to say to you confidentially that she would be 'most grateful' for some word from you about the President, etc. She says she has heard nothing from any one and seems quite anxious for information."[67]

At the end of April, the president told the three representatives of the press who had been allowed to accompany his small party to the secret location in the South: "I am doing very little work. I am resting, sleeping, and absorbing all the sun possible. I am sleeping about twelve hours a day.... They want me to do it for another week or ten days." One of the reporters asked if the president had any trace of bronchitis left. "Very little," he responded. "If I try, I can wheeze."[68] The three reporters remained silent; they were prohibited from sending out any stories until the president returned to Washington.

Roosevelt did not return to Washington for what the *New York Times* described as "the most impressive official funeral service and burial that the capital has seen for years. Many thousands of citizens lined the streets." Seventy-year-old Frank Knox, whom the president appointed secretary of the Navy during the war, had died of a heart attack on April 28, 1944. Roosevelt, the newspaper reported, "was away in the South for his health."[69]

United Press White House correspondent Merriman Smith was one of three reporters staying in a town near Baruch's estate. The men, who rarely saw Roosevelt, were contacted one evening for a specific purpose. "The main reason we were called to Hobcaw that May night," Smith wrote two years later, "was to explain away the President's failure to attend the Knox funeral. The blame was finally placed on McIntire. He, the record said, wanted the President to remain in South Carolina lest his recovery from a bad, coughing winter be interrupted."[70] By this time, Roosevelt had been receiving digitalis for his heart for a month. The president's cardiologist noted that his patient "had no cardiac symptoms, but the blood pressure remained elevated."[71]

Roosevelt Knew He was Sick and Condoned Keeping Secrets

The reporters with the president were told that his problem was bronchitis, but Roosevelt knew that he also had heart disease. When Daisy Suckley reached Baruch's estate early in May, the president handed her two unsent letters. The second one contained very significant, very secret information: "I forgot to tell you that Dr. Bruin [sic] came down, too—He is one of the best heart men—Tho' my own is definitely better—does queer things still—I wish so you were here."[72] Some authors have asserted that Roosevelt did not know he had heart disease, but this letter (first made public a half century later) proves that he did. Now that Daisy was with the president, he shared more details about his medical evaluations with her.

Daisy discussed Roosevelt's health with him and with his cardiologist. She described two May 5 conversations in her diary: "Dr. Bruenn came along & I talked about the P[resident]. He relieved me by saying that the P.'s blood is all right.... From a later talk with the P. the trouble is evidently with the heart—the diastole & systole are not working properly in unison—but there is definite improvement." She then described what happened after Baruch and Bruenn left later that day for Washington: "I had a good talk with the P. about himself—He said he discovered that the doctors had not agreed together about what to tell him, so that he found out that they were not telling *him* the *whole* truth & that he was evidently more sick than they said! It is foolish of them to attempt to put anything over on *him!*"[73]

Roosevelt did not consider it foolish for a national leader to mislead the press under certain circumstances. His advice to Manuel Quezon, the first president of the Philippines, proves the point. In exile during the Japanese occupation of the islands, Quezon was being treated for tuberculosis at the Trudeau Sanitorium in Saranac Lake, New York, when Roosevelt wrote to him in July 1943: "You must certainly stay there...until the Doctors give you a 'clean bill of health.' I think you are right in keeping quiet publicly in regard to your illness."[74] Fifteen months later, Roosevelt praised Quezon's leadership in his statement on American troops landing in the Philippines. He regretted that Quezon had died in August 1944, "on the eve of his country's liberation."[75]

Shortly after Roosevelt returned to the White House from Baruch's estate on May 7, 1944, he wrote to Harry Hopkins. His close friend was recuperating at an Army hospital following a second stomach operation at the Mayo Clinic (his first was in 1937). The letter reveals how health concerns and treatment regimen had reduced the time Roosevelt devoted to his duties:

> My plans—my medical laboratory work not being finished—are to be here about three days a week and to spend the other four days a week at Hyde Park, Shangri-la [later renamed Camp David] or on the Potomac....I had a really grand time at Bernie's—slept twelve hours out of the twenty-four, sat in the sun, never lost my temper, and decided to let the world go hang. The interesting thing is that the world didn't hang. I have a terrible pile in my basket but most of the stuff has answered itself anyway.[76]

Roosevelt's description of his workday reflected his doctors' advice, but it contrasted sharply with the public's perception of a wartime president's responsibilities. Washington-based reporters pointed out in a 1944 *Look* magazine article "The President's Job—Biggest in the World" that he was the commander in chief of 12 million members of the armed forces, in charge of nearly 3 million federal employees, and oversaw a $100 billion budget.[77]

On June 6, 1944, three weeks after Roosevelt described his health-seeking South Carolina vacation to Harry Hopkins, he was sitting behind his desk at the White House, surrounded by about one hundred reporters. Almost all of the questions dealt with the Normandy invasion, launched earlier in the day, but the last question on D-Day targeted the commander in chief: "How are you feeling?" Roosevelt responded: "I'm feeling fine. I'm a little sleepy." The reporters laughed at this quip, which ended the press conference.[78] Taking no chances, Early asked McIntire to meet with reporters two days later to reassure the public about the president's health.

A reporter asked the White House physician on June 8, "Ross, just to get a definitive statement here, what do you think of the president's present health now?" McIntire responded: "His present health is excellent, I can say that unqualifiedly." The reporter then asked, "In all respects?" The doctor declared emphatically: "In all respects. When I say excellent, you can't go much more than that....He is in better physical condition than the average man of his age."[79]

But the journalists persisted. After McIntire mentioned the vacation in South Carolina, one asked, "For the record, Ross, can we have what was wrong with him? He had sinus, bronchitis and the intestinal upset." McIntire interrupted the reporter: "He had his influenza. That was the start of the whole thing. There were complications following influenza.... He had the intestinal upset. Then he picked up this acute cold, which was followed with his sinus infection and his acute bronchitis." What turned out to be the last health-related question referred to "a rumor that there was quite a bit of trouble with his heart, maybe?" Now, McIntire lied: "No. I have been very factual with you. I have given you the exact—" Steve Early stopped the White House physician in mid-sentence, interjecting: "I don't think it is a good thing to start denying rumors. . . . If you do, you just revive them."[80]

"President's Health 'Excellent,' Admiral McIntire Reports" was the headline of a *New York Times* article that summarized the June 8 press conference. The writer referred to Roosevelt's comprehensive evaluation at the Naval Hospital after he returned from Baruch's estate, "where he went to recuperate from a severe attack of bronchitis." Then he summarized the prescription regarding the wartime president's schedule. McIntire "hoped President Roosevelt would continue to observe the new regimen, instituted in recent months, calling for shorter working hours, no business conferences during luncheon and frequent breaks in routine, particularly week-end rests away from the White House." With respect to examinations, the president's physician said, "many physical checks had been made and 'all the checks are well within normal limits.'"[81] Meanwhile, McIntire and Early continued to coordinate a cover-up of Roosevelt's cardiovascular disease. Between March 28, when Howard Bruenn first examined the president, and June 6, D-Day, his blood pressure was recorded more than a hundred times. The average reading, 209/110, was very high by any standard.[82]

Before Roosevelt's month-long doctor-imposed rest at Baruch's estate, Boston surgeon Frank Lahey had examined him with Bruenn, McIntire, and Paullin. Concerned about the potential consequences of McIntire's cover-up of Roosevelt's cardiovascular disease, Lahey wrote a secret memo for his own files:

> I am recording these opinions in the light of having informed Admiral McIntire Saturday afternoon July 8, 1944, that I did not believe that, if Mr. Roosevelt were elected President again, he had the physical capacity to complete a term. I told him that, as a result of activities in his trip to Russia [read Tehran, Iran] he had been in a state which was, if not in heart failure, at least on the verge of it, that this was the result of high blood pressure he has now had for a long time, plus a question of coronary damage. With this in mind it was my opinion that over the four years of another term with its burdens, he would again have heart failure and be unable to complete it. . . . I have told Admiral McIntire that I feel strongly that if he does accept another term, he had a very serious responsibility concerning who is the Vice President. Admiral McIntire agrees with this and has, he states, so informed Mr. Roosevelt.[83]

Lahey's assessment of Roosevelt's life expectancy was consistent with contemporary concepts about the prognosis of heart failure and severe hypertension that Mayo Clinic physicians and others had published.[84]

Roosevelt Keeps Speaking Despite Severe Chest Pain

Roosevelt had a problem that concerned his cardiologist during an August 12 speech in Bremerton, Washington. Thousands of enlisted men stood before him at the Puget Sound Naval Yard, and millions of individuals listened to his speech on the radio.[85] When the president developed severe chest pain during his address, he had to make a decision. If he suddenly stopped speaking, it would suggest that something serious was wrong with him. So the man who had worked hard for two decades to limit public awareness of his polio-related disability kept talking. Roosevelt's secretary Grace Tully, who was with him, considered it "one of the poorest speeches he ever made, both in form and in delivery."[86]

Immediately after the speech, Bruenn examined the president and recorded an electrocardiogram. The heart specialist later described the Bremerton episode as "substernal oppression with radiation to both shoulders," which he interpreted as "coronary insufficiency without evidence of myocardial infarction."[87] Later still, Bruenn explained that he considered this "very disturbing situation...proof positive that he had coronary disease."[88] The printed log of the president's trip, restricted and circulated to very few individuals, contains a clue regarding real-time concerns about the chest pain incident: "Plans for an auto drive about the navy yard after the broadcast were cancelled and the President did not leave the ship."[89]

The president, his physicians, the press, and the public knew that heart disease could kill without warning. In fact, Bruenn had coauthored an article on coronary artery disease a decade earlier, which noted that "the increasing death rate from circulatory disorders has fired the imagination of the laity." The authors reminded readers how often coronary disease "terminates the careers of prominent citizens by sudden death."[90] The president was well aware of this fact. He spoke at the Puget Sound Naval Yard exactly one month after another Roosevelt had died suddenly. Theodore Roosevelt Jr., the son of a former president and a distant cousin of the current one, was among the first to land in Normandy on D-Day. A *New York Times* headline announced five weeks later, "Theodore Roosevelt, 56, Dies on Normandy Battlefield." But the text explained that the brigadier general's July 12 death was "caused by a sudden heart attack" that "took place in camp and not in the full flush of action."[91]

There is no evidence that the president had episodes of chest pain after the Puget Sound incident. In September 1944 Bruenn was with Roosevelt in Quebec City, where he met with Churchill to discuss successes in Europe and challenges in the Pacific. The cardiologist noted that his patient's blood pressure "tended to be higher than usual... but there were no cardiac symptoms.... Phenobarbital was increased from ¼ grain to ½ grain three times a day. Blood pressure ranged from 180/100 to 240/130."[92]

Roosevelt called Daisy when he returned to America, and she wrote in her diary: "He said it was a *good* conference; much was accomplished; he wanted to *sleep* all the time."[93] Phenobarbital, a sedative prescribed as part of the president's regimen for hypertension, contributed to his sleepiness. At a joint press conference with Churchill on September 16, 1944, Roosevelt expressed optimism about the war in Europe. With respect to the possibility of Germany surrendering, he said, "We hope it will come. The quicker the better." Then the Allies could devote full attention to the Far East to bring "the war against Japan to a quick conclusion."[94]

There was no way to predict exactly when the military conflicts in Europe and the Pacific would end, but Roosevelt was involved in a political fight closer to home that was certain to end in less than two months. Daisy Suckley wrote in her diary on September 20, 1944, "The Pres. says he feels there is an excellent chance of his being defeated in the election—that Dewey is making a very good campaign."[95] The nation's newspapers backed Dewey by a four-to-one margin, according to a survey of more than one thousand papers published that month.[96] White House insiders could rationalize that newspaper publishers had traditionally been more supportive of Republicans, but most voters did not think like this. In mid-October, *Life* magazine published an editorial "Why Dewey Deserves the Independent Vote."[97]

The death of a popular political figure always attracted public attention. This was certainly the case when Wendell Willkie "died quietly in his sleep after he had suffered three heart attacks."[98] He was only fifty-two years old when he died on October 8, 1944, a month before the election. Four years earlier, in 1940, more than 22 million Americans had voted for Willkie—who would have been president had he beaten Roosevelt. But 45 percent of the popular vote was not enough to win. Willkie, a decade younger than Roosevelt, had been hospitalized for more than a month after having two heart attacks. The first one occurred in Indiana, where he told a confidant: "Nobody listens to a man with a bad heart... I still have a lot of things I want to say."[99]

Willkie's biographer learned about the former presidential candidate's secret from his press secretary: "It was announced publicly that he was suffering from colitis and needed rest. Walter Winchell, indeed, heard a rumor of a heart attack; but when he telephoned an inquiry, [Lamoyne] Jones lied loyally."[100] Near the end of Willkie's hospitalization for a second heart attack, he developed a streptococcal throat infection. The Associated Press release explained that the strain of this acute febrile illness had affected his heart and that he died as a result of coronary thrombosis.

"A Whispering Campaign Regarding Mr. Roosevelt's Health"

On October 17, 1944, three weeks before the election, a *Chicago Tribune* editorial began, "Boss Hannegan of the Democratic National Committee charges that there is a whispering campaign regarding Mr. Roosevelt's health." The pro-Dewey newspaper proclaimed: "There is no need to whisper. That is one of the principal issues of this campaign.... Mr. Roosevelt is an applicant for a job. The voters to whom he is applying have the duty to satisfy themselves that he is physically capable of discharging it." Claiming that the presidency "broke Wilson and contributed to Harding's death," the editorial writer argued that there was mounting evidence that Roosevelt was not in "physical condition" to meet the demands of the presidency.[101]

The cover of the October 23 issue of *Newsweek* magazine contained a diagonal yellow banner: "Election in Doubt: Trend Is to Dewey." Inside, a new Gallup Poll predicted that Roosevelt would get 243 electoral votes, Dewey would get 228, and 60 votes were a toss-up. In one section, the unidentified *Newsweek* writer explained: "One day after Wendell L. Willkie died, John O'Donnell, anti-Roosevelt columnist for the *New York Daily News*, devoted his entire article to the political importance of the president's health. O'Donnell wrote: 'The life expectancy of Franklin Roosevelt is indeed a definite political handicap for his fourth-term pretensions.'" Under maps showing electoral vote trends in the forty-eight states, the article concluded, "Dewey plainly is stronger today than when he was at the time of his nomination. Roosevelt has lost ground.... The final two weeks of the campaign now appear destined to settle the issue."[102]

On October 23, the same day the *Newsweek* issue appeared, *Time* magazine carried a story "He's Perfectly O.K." Citing recent articles in the "arch-Republican" *New York Sun* and the "rabidly anti-Roosevelt" *New York Daily News*, the *Time* writer explained: "The *Sun* and the *News* were saying out loud what many a citizen has wondered about: is the President too old or tired to live out Term IV? Plainly Franklin Roosevelt's health was a political issue. It was obvious to the White House last week that a report to the U.S. people was needed." The *Time* piece quoted the White House physician: "Nothing wrong organically with him at all. He's perfectly O.K. He does a terrific day's work.... The stories that he is in bad health are understandable enough around election time, but they are not true."[103] But Ross McIntire and Steve Early knew that the stories *were* true.

Both political parties relied on public opinion surveys to help assess their candidates' strengths and weaknesses and to identify issues that concerned voters. Hadley Cantril of the American Institute of Public Opinion and independent public opinion analyst Elmo Roper provided White House insiders with information that could be reassuring or disconcerting. In October Cantril passed on the results of a Republican poll from mid-July;

it revealed that 84 percent of individuals who planned to vote thought Roosevelt was healthy enough to complete a fourth term. Meanwhile, Roper reported that concern about the president's health was causing some likely voters to shift to Dewey.[104]

A Marathon Parade Designed to Dispel Rumors of Bad Health

Steve Early and other campaign operatives wanted to convince voters that the president had stamina, and a big storm provided a perfect opportunity. A headline in the October 21 edition of the *Des Moines Register* was blunt: "F.D.R. Hopes Trip Will End Health Tales." The newspaper's Washington correspondent explained:

> President Roosevelt will reply tonight to what is more than a whispering campaign about his health with a grueling bid for New York State's 47 electoral votes. In the face of a weather forecast of RAIN AND A 50-MILE GALE, he has scheduled a four-hour drive through Brooklyn, Queens, Manhattan, and the Bronx, presumably in an open car.... The state of the president's health has become a real election issue in view of his age and his illness last spring. The usual flood of rumors has resulted, despite repeated statements by Admiral Ross T. McIntire, the president's physician, that except for a bad tooth, he is organically sound.[105]

After the president was paraded before more than a million New Yorkers, *Life* magazine reported: "Candidate Roosevelt came to New York on an October Saturday, just as the big city got caught in the whiplash fringe of the season's second hurricane. The bad weather did not stop the President from driving 51 miles in four-and-a-half hours through a heavy rainstorm in an open car with the top down."[106] Still photographs that had documented the president's weight loss during 1944 seemed to show a man in decline. Now, movie newsreels and pictures of the pre-election parade seemed to show a different person—Roosevelt smiling and waving to crowds in a downpour.

Both Roosevelt and Dewey could produce a parade of celebrities who supported them. Six days before the election, a well-known novelist delivered a fiery five-minute speech in support of the president over the CBS radio network. Sinclair Lewis's message was designed to reinforce the notion that it was risky to replace Roosevelt in wartime. The Minnesota-born author of *Arrowsmith, Elmer Gantry*, and *Main Street* declared:

> Do you know what would be the most fantastic and shocking news that could come to the United States right now? It would be that Winston Churchill had been replaced as Prime Minister of Great Britain, and

replaced by a bright young politician with no great experience in high office, but with lots of driving personal ambition and lots of friends who were hungry for jobs. If, before world peace negotiations, this improbable thing could happen, then we would say, and Russia and China and France would say, that Great Britain had let us down as our ally. And we would be right. And that is what our allies would say if Franklin D. Roosevelt were to be replaced now by that very eloquent young gentleman, Mr. Tommy Dewey.... We want to be represented in the Peace Conference by a man who looks like a President and talks like a President and thinks like a President, and not by a bright young junior partner.[107]

Many individuals, including several in Roosevelt's inner circle, shared a concern that he did not look, talk, or think like he had just a few months earlier. During a radio address the day after Lewis's broadcast, the president complained: "This campaign has been marred by even more than the usual crop of whisperings and rumorings. Some of these get into print, in certain types of newspapers; others are traded about, secretly, in one black market after another." Hoping to put the issue to rest, Roosevelt told his listeners, "The voting record proves that the American people pay little attention to whispering campaigns."[108]

Steve Early Reacts to Rumors Circulating in Rochester

Steve Early knew that some rumors and some news sources were far more significant than others. With the election just days away, he got news from a friend that caused him great concern. Physicians in Rochester had not been involved in Roosevelt's care, but a few of them had been discussing his heart health less than three weeks before the election. The president's press secretary respected the Mayo Clinic and had a personal connection to it. In early October, a Mayo surgeon had operated on his sister at Colonial Hospital in Rochester.[109] But it was Roosevelt's longtime friend Breckinridge Long, who had recently served as assistant secretary of state, who alerted Early to casual conversations in the Minnesota city that might influence voters—and the outcome of the election—if the anti-Roosevelt media reported them.

Breckinridge Long, who lived in Washington, D.C., had been a patient at the Mayo Clinic for several years. Roosevelt had written to him in 1936, "I hope your 'tummy' is well again and that you are ready for one-night-stands and ham and eggs and coffee."[110] Long's abdominal pain persisted, and he went to Rochester where he had an operation for ulcers.[111] His Mayo surgeon Claude Dixon became a friend and confidant. On the eve of the 1940 election, Long described their conversation about a sensitive political issue in his diary: "Tonight I have talked to Dr. Dixon at Mayo's about 'Socialized Medicine' and the reports circulated to our disadvantage that we favor it—which we do not." Long then spoke with Ross McIntire, urging him to have Roosevelt reiterate his opposition to the concept in a pre-election speech.[112]

On July 13, 1944, six days before the Democratic convention opened in Chicago, Long wrote in his diary, "Roosevelt announced yesterday he would accept the Democratic nomination and if elected would serve. My information from Early previously had been to that effect—and further that he wanted to be elected to finish the war—which is quite natural, proper, and, from my point of view, very desirable."[113] Four days after the convention, Long wrote about the vice presidential candidate, a fellow Missourian: "I am glad to help Truman. We have been friends for years."[114] Long then traveled from Chicago to Rochester, where he wrote in his diary on July 25, "Am at the Mayo Clinic undergoing a 'check up' as I have done every year or so since my serious operation in 1936."[115]

Breckinridge Long learned something a dozen days before the 1944 election that he thought had the potential to shift a significant number of votes from Roosevelt to Dewey. On Saturday evening, October 21, 1944, his surgeon-friend Claude Dixon played poker in Rochester with radiologist Byrl Kirklin, three other doctors, the Kahler Corporation's president, and Mayo's chief administrator Harry Harwick.[116] The men surely listened to the live radio broadcast of the president's much anticipated speech to the Foreign Policy Association in New York City. Roosevelt's main theme was what America and the world would be like after the war. But he also described the current situation: "Today, Hitler and the Nazis continue the fight—desperately, inch by inch, and may continue to do so all the way to Berlin. And we have another important engagement in Tokyo. No matter how hard, how long the road we must travel, our forces will fight their way there under the leadership of MacArthur and Nimitz."[117] At some point that evening, the poker players discussed the president's health—specifically his heart health. Claude Dixon, concerned by what he heard, contacted Breckinridge Long.

FBI Agents Interrogate Mayo Clinic Physicians

An FBI memorandum "Circulation of Story Alleging the President Has a Serious Heart Affliction," dated October 29, 1944, describes how federal agents followed the twists and turns of a gossip trail.[118] Claude Dixon's call to Breckinridge Long triggered the emergency investigation that ended with a letter from J. Edgar Hoover (Figure 7.3) to Steve Early. Two FBI agents rushed from St. Paul to Rochester to interrogate radiologist Byrl

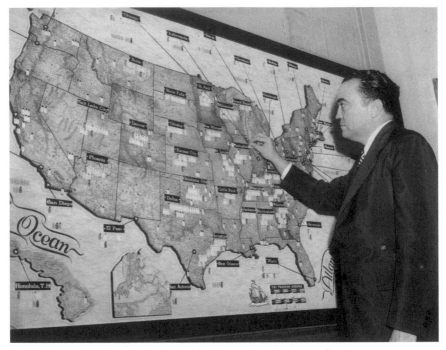

FIGURE 7.3 *J. Edgar Hoover in his office in Washington, D.C., July 1941.*

Original Associated Press (AP) wire photo in the author's possession, used with permission of AP.

Kirklin, who explained that he had eaten lunch at the Kahler Hotel on Saturday, October 21, 1944, with Harry Harwick, Arlie Barnes, and few other Mayo doctors.

The FBI agents reported, "Dr. Barnes had but recently returned from Bethesda, Maryland, where he had attended a meeting of heart specialists. During the luncheon Dr. Barnes stated that the President had a serious heart ailment. Colonel Kirklin heard Dr. Barnes make this comment but stated that Dr. Barnes did not make any further comment and there was no further discussion of the subject at that time." After Hoover's men listed the attendees at the evening poker game, they explained that "Dr. Kirklin quoted Dr. Barnes' previous statement made at the luncheon that the President had a serious heart ailment. No further discussion or comment was made by him or anyone else at this time."[119]

Next, the agents interviewed Barnes, who "admitted making the statement attributed to him by Colonel Kirklin." The Mayo heart specialist explained that while he was in Washington for the National Research Council's Subcommittee on Cardiovascular Disease meeting, his associate Howard Odel had given him a tour of the two-year-old Naval Hospital in nearby Bethesda, Maryland. A member of Barnes's five-man medical section, Odel was stationed at the Naval Hospital during the war. The agents reported: "The two doctors walked around the grounds and...they began discussing Minnesota politics, at which time Dr. Odel made the statement—'The President is a very sick man—heart disease.' Dr. Barnes stated that he asked no questions but that Dr. Odel made the statement as a fact and with no reference to the source of his information. Dr. Barnes stated he had never heard this information from any other source." Armed with this intelligence, a separate FBI team interviewed Odel on October 27.[120]

Howard Odel, who had been a doctor for a dozen years, was used to asking patients very personal questions, but he was unnerved by the FBI agents' interrogation. They described the naval lieutenant as "obviously disturbed and uneasy." Odel denied having made any statements about the president's health. But he acknowledged that the subject had come up at the Naval Hospital after some physicians stationed there had recognized Howard Bruenn, the center's cardiologist, in the *Life* magazine photograph of the president giving his acceptance speech in the train car.[121]

When Hoover's men questioned Odel again the following day, they informed him what Barnes had told their counterparts in Rochester. Tension filled the room as the agents asked Odel more direct questions in an attempt to uncover what the Mayo Clinic doctors had said about Roosevelt's health. They documented the new details:

> Dr. Odel stated to Dr. Barnes that there had been rumors circulating about the President's health and he, Dr. Odel, wondered if the President had heart disease or hypertension. Dr. Odel stated to Dr. Barnes that the President had been at the Bethesda Hospital on two or three occasions for examination and for that reason Dr. Odel had wondered if something was wrong with the President's heart. Dr. Odel advised on interview that while he had no definite recollection as to any further statement made by him to Dr. Barnes, he may have added something to the effect that "I suspect there may be something to it." Dr. Odel stated that he was positive that he had not made a flat statement that the President is a very sick man. He stated that he was certain he had not used the words "very sick man."[122]

The FBI agents reported that Odel "realized his statement to Dr. Barnes had been very imprudent but that he had worked for Dr. Barnes for a period of twelve years and knew of his interest in heart disease because Dr. Barnes is an eminent heart specialist." Odel, hoping to deflect the bright light shining on him, claimed that Roosevelt's health had been a topic of lunchtime conversations at the Naval Hospital and that "at least half of the doctors" stationed there "have been engaged in discussions of this sort." Recognizing his predicament as a physician and naval officer, Odel emphasized that his comments did not represent "any official or authoritative opinion."[123]

Six days before the election, Hoover sent the president's press secretary a copy of the formal FBI memorandum and a reassuring cover letter:

> Dear Steve: I am inclosing [*sic*] herewith a memorandum covering the various interviews which we have conducted of a number of doctors at the Mayo Clinic and at Bethesda, Maryland.... There seems to have been a great deal of gossip and conversation at the Bethesda [Naval] Hospital upon the part of doctors attached there, and the story seems to have originated there and then to have been carried to the Mayo Clinic, where again there seems to have been a lot of loose conversation and talk, all predicated upon the supposition that the President was suffering from some heart ailment by reason of the fact that Doctor Bruenn's picture appeared in the group with the President. If there is anything further you desire me to do in this matter, please let me know and I will be very glad to respond. Sincerely, Edgar.[124]

Early and Roosevelt had relied on Hoover to conduct politically motivated investigations for a decade. The timing and pace of this one reflected the fact that the election was just days away.[125]

Just Before and Just After the 1944 Election

Three days before the election, the *Saturday Evening Post* published a Norman Rockwell cover illustration (Figure 7.4) that portrayed a middle-aged man standing in a voting booth. Looking perplexed, he was holding a newspaper with pictures of Roosevelt and Dewey under a bold headline "WHICH ONE?" An editorial urged voters to elect Dewey, declaring that the "fourth-term campaign is held together by the hope that the people will believe that the President is indispensable as commander in chief, and that he has some formula for perpetual peace too hot for lesser men to handle. This, of, course, is plain nonsense."[126]

Roosevelt was reelected on November 7, 1944, with 53.4 percent of the popular vote. The 3.6 million–vote margin was the smallest of his four elections.[127] Two weeks later, pro-Dewey *Life* magazine published state tallies and argued that "the time-honored statistical game of figure juggling shows that it would not have taken many votes in the right places to swing the election the other way." The writer reminded readers that "a large electoral vote majority can hang on small popular majorities."[128] In his book on the election, historian David Jordan concludes, "It all came together for the President because the country decided it would be unwise to change horses in midstream."[129] Democrats had used this metaphor to bolster support for the wartime president. The few insiders who knew about Roosevelt's hypertensive cardiovascular disease never hinted that they worried he might not survive to get across the stream.

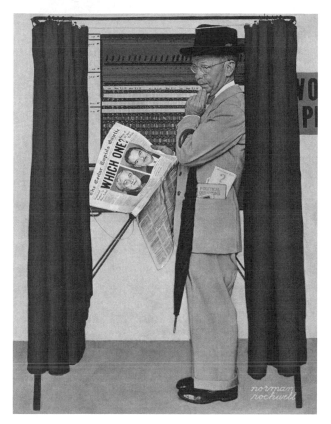

FIGURE 7.4 *Norman Rockwell, "Undecided,"* Saturday Evening Post, *November 4, 1944, cover illustration.*

Reprinted with permission of the Norman Rockwell Family Agency, © 2015 the Norman Rockwell Family Entities and Curtis Licensing.

Three weeks after the election, Roosevelt went to the Little White House in Warm Springs, Georgia, to rest. Bruenn recorded a blood pressure of 260/150 on one occasion during the stay.[130] Daisy Suckley, who was with them, wrote in her diary at the end of November that the president "looks ten years older than last year…Of course I wouldn't confess that to anyone, least of all to him, but he knows it himself."[131] In mid-December she wrote, "I am *hoping* to get a little closer to the doctors, so that they will talk more freely to me. But they put on, or rather, *keep* on, their doctor's manner and tell you nothing. They seem to be concentrating on the Pres.' heart. He himself said it was a 'cardiac' condition."[132] Back at the White House a few days later, Daisy wrote, "I had quite a talk with Anna about her father's health. It is a very difficult problem, & I am entirely convinced that he can *not* keep up the present rate—he will kill himself if he tries, and he won't be so very useful to the world then."[133]

Anna accompanied her father to the Yalta Conference where he, Churchill, and Stalin discussed issues relating to the postwar world. She wrote to her husband on February 4, 1945, the first day of the meeting at the Black Sea resort town:

> Ross [McIntire] and Bruenn are both worried because of the old
> "ticker" trouble—which, of course, no one knows about but those two
> and me.... I have found out through Bruenn (who won't let me tell Ross
> what I know) that this "ticker" situation is far more serious than I ever
> knew. And, the biggest difficulty in handling the situation here is that we
> can, of course, tell no one of the "ticker" trouble. It's truly worrisome—
> and there's not a helluva lot anyone can do about it. (Better tear off and
> destroy this paragraph.)[134]

The paragraph survived, the president's cardiologist was concerned, and the
cover-up continued.

Roosevelt wrote to his longtime friend Supreme Court justice Frank
Murphy on April 9, 1945: "I am down at Warm Springs, 'off the record,' for a
few days and while I want to see you again it may not be for several weeks."[135]
In fact, the president would never again see Murphy or anyone else except the
few individuals (including Daisy Suckley and Howard Bruenn) who were with
him at the Little White House in Georgia. He died of a massive cerebral hemorrhage on the twelfth of April, thirteen months after first being examined
by a cardiologist, five months after winning a close election, and eighty-three
days after beginning his fourth term (Figure 7.5).

The final edition of the *Chicago Tribune* for April 13, 1945, carried a banner
headline "ROOSEVELT IS DEAD!". A brief article, "Here's Ailment Which
Killed the President," explained:

> President Roosevelt died from what doctors call a cerebral hemorrhage,
> which means a sudden extensive bleeding in the brain due to a ruptured
> blood vessel. Nonmedical people recognize a cerebral hemorrhage
> under other names such as a stroke or a stroke of apoplexy. This
> is usually what happens in a case like this: As people grow old their
> arteries lose their elasticity. They become hard, brittle. Usually, with
> advancing age, blood pressure increases. Sometimes arteries in the
> brain grow harder and more brittle than blood vessels in other parts of
> the body. Then some day, usually without warning, a blood vessel in the
> brain gives way. Blood pours thru the brain, paralyzing nerve centers.[136]

Franklin Roosevelt had won the election with the help of Steve Early and others who shaped his public image and suppressed the truth about his health.
He lost his life because there were no effective treatments for severe hypertension, a major contributing factor to cerebral hemorrhage.

Paul Dudley White wrote in his 1944 textbook, "Although heart failure
is the most common of the end results of hypertension, cerebral hemorrhage is also frequent, angina pectoris and coronary thrombosis are next in
order."[137] When Bruenn completed the presidents' death certificate, he listed
cerebral hemorrhage as the immediate cause of death and arteriosclerosis

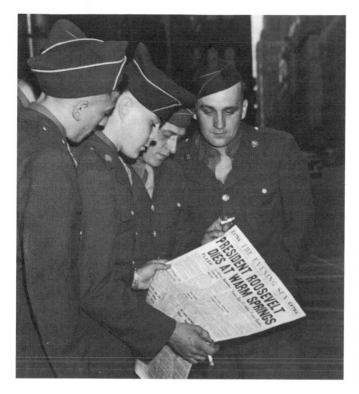

FIGURE 7.5
*Soldiers reading
about Franklin
Roosevelt's death,
April 12, 1945.*
Original wire photo
(without photogra-
pher's name or source
information) in the
author's possession.

as the contributing factor. He did not list any other medical conditions.[138] No autopsy was performed. Whatever other diseases Roosevelt may have had in the closing weeks of his final campaign, they were not Steve Early's concern when he triggered the FBI interrogations of the Mayo Clinic physicians. The president won the election despite his secret cardiovascular disease, but he lost his life to it less than three months into his fourth term.

"Everybody Knew it But the People"

The *Saturday Evening Post* published an editorial "Everybody Knew It but the People" a month after the president died. The writer argued that "the state of Mr. Roosevelt's health was a secret from millions of Americans who voted for the President on the theory that he could reasonably be expected to live out his term of office." Voters who interpreted photographs of the president as showing "signs of serious illness...were continually assured by Admiral Ross McIntire, the President's medical adviser, that his patient was 'in better physical condition than the average man of his age.' "[139]

The *Post* writer concluded that "one purpose of the President's campaign tour through New York during a chilling rain was to dispel apprehensions regarding Mr. Roosevelt's health." Blending conspiracy theory with political reality, he declared, "If the insiders were 'fully aware' of the President's brief life expectancy, they made every effort to discourage the spread of that knowledge. Journalists or politicians who hinted that Mr. Roosevelt was not a well man were rebuked as little better than fifth columnists by the president's associates, who saw their one chance of continued power in the ability of the President to get through one more election."[140] The editorial writer was right. Steve Early had worked overtime to shape news about and images of Roosevelt to improve the odds of his reelection.

Ross McIntire continued to mislead the public after his patient died. Discussing the president's final months, the White House physician wrote in 1946:

> His heart, quite naturally, was our principal concern. Why not? Here was a man of sixty-three, under terrific strain for years, who had been coughing heavily for more than two months in the spring of 1944. Time proved that our fears were groundless, for that stout heart of his never failed.... As for cerebral hemorrhage, it was and is unpredictable. There are some conditions, of course, in which we think we can predict it, such as extremely high blood pressure and advanced general arteriolosclerosis although there is no certainty. President Roosevelt did not have either of these. His blood pressure was not alarming at any time.[141]

Not alarming at any time! Bruenn, who was at the president's side when he died in Georgia, knew the truth. If the cardiologist's diagnoses of severe hypertension and heart failure had been made public before the election, a five-year-old article by Mayo Clinic physicians would have been relevant. They reported that hypertensive patients with the cluster of physical and X-ray findings that Bruenn had documented in his March 1944 examination of the president survived, on average, sixteen months.[142] Franklin Roosevelt would survive less than thirteen months.

In her book *This I Remember*, Eleanor Roosevelt discussed the relationship of her late husband's health to his fourth presidential campaign: "I knew without asking that as long as the war was on it was a foregone conclusion that Franklin, if he was well enough, would run again.... I think that all of us knew that Franklin was far from well, but none of us ever said anything about it—I suppose because we felt that if he believed it was his duty to continue in office, there was nothing for us to do but make it as easy as possible for him."[143] Eleanor Roosevelt's admission that her husband was "far from well" clearly contradicted the reports that McIntire provided to the public during the campaign and what he wrote after the president died.

In 1946 McIntire rationalized the shroud of secrecy that he had helped to erect and maintain: "The health of the chief executive...is his own private business." He claimed that presidents customarily chose an Army or

Navy doctor as their personal physician to provide extra protection against leaks: "These men are officers as well as physicians, and being subject to the iron discipline of the armed services, they can be counted on to keep a close [*sic*] mouth about what they see and hear." McIntire decided which doctors saw Roosevelt as well as when and where:

> Now and then famous consultants were called in, but as a usual thing I relied on our Navy specialists. Not only did I consider them to be as good as the best, but there was the advantage that journeys to the [Bethesda Naval] Medical Center could be made without exciting comment. At no time did I have any quarrel with the co-operation of the Washington correspondents, but a visit of the President to the Mayos or Johns Hopkins, even for a routine checkup, was bound to be played up as big news.[144]

The casual conversations that Mayo cardiologists Arlie Barnes and Howard Odel had in Bethesda and those that followed in Rochester never made the news. If they had, it is quite possible that Thomas Dewey would have won the 1944 election.

The Reinvention of the American Heart Association and the Invention of Cardiac Catheterization

Several medical and scientific research projects initiated during World War II had a major impact on patient care in the postwar era. During the global conflict, the US government pumped massive amounts of money into research on a wide range of projects. The investment led to discoveries, inventions, and innovations that would be incorporated into medical practice.[1] Penicillin is a compelling example of how the war accelerated the development and diffusion of breakthrough therapies. In terms of patients with cardiac disease, this drug could cure some cases of bacterial endocarditis, a heart valve infection that was uniformly fatal before the advent of antibiotics. Penicillin also contributed to a decline in the incidence of acute rheumatic fever, the leading cause of chronic heart valve disease.[2] Cardiac catheterization, a revolutionary diagnostic technique, migrated into practice as an offshoot of wartime studies on traumatic shock.

Science: The Endless Frontier

President Franklin Roosevelt wrote to Vannevar Bush, director of the wartime Office of Scientific Research and Development, on November 17, 1944, ten days after he was reelected. Roosevelt described Bush's office as "a unique experiment of team-work and cooperation in coordinating scientific research and in applying existing scientific knowledge to the solution of the technical problems paramount in war. Its work has been conducted in the utmost secrecy. . . . Some day the full story of its achievements can be told." The president asked Bush to prepare a report on how to maintain the momentum of this wartime experiment in peacetime. Roosevelt explained, "With particular reference to the war of science against disease, what can be done now to organize a program for continuing in the future the work that has been done in medicine and related sciences? The fact that the annual deaths in this country from one or two diseases alone are far in excess of the total number of lives lost by us in battle during this war should make us conscious of the duty we owe future generations."[3]

Roosevelt, eager to review Bush's report, closed his letter with a specific request: "I hope that, after such consultations as you may deem advisable with your associates and others, you can let me have your considered judgment on these matters as soon as convenient—reporting on each when you are ready, rather than waiting for completion of your studies in all."[4] The president would never see the results of the high-priority project. On April 12, 1945, five months after he had written to Bush, Roosevelt lost his top-secret battle with hypertensive cardiovascular disease. Bush submitted his report *Science: The Endless Frontier* to President Harry Truman on July 5, 1945, two months after Germany surrendered and one month before the United States dropped the first atomic bomb on Japan.[5]

Walter Palmer, chief of medicine at Columbia University, chaired the committee that wrote the "war on disease" section of Bush's report. The academic internist boasted about medicine's record during the military conflict and cited therapeutic triumphs, such as penicillin, to justify future federal funding of biomedical research: "When a government wisely invests the people's money in medical research, the people receive huge dividends in the form of better health and longer lives."[6] Individuals who lobbied philanthropic foundations and the federal government for disease-specific research funds after World War II memorized this message and recited it regularly. In his report, Palmer pointed out that cardiovascular disease was responsible for 45 percent of deaths in the United States.

Public Fundraising Campaigns to Support Research and Care

When *Science: The Endless Frontier* was published in the summer of 1945, some leaders of the American Heart Association (AHA) were frustrated by their organization's fragile financial status.[7] A new book on voluntary health organizations had just highlighted the enormous disparity between the annual income of the AHA ($29 thousand) and of the National Foundation for Infantile Paralysis ($8.2 million). The latter organization helped support polio research and treatment for those afflicted by the disease and its consequences.[8]

Franklin Roosevelt, who had been disabled by polio when he was thirty-nine years old, formed the National Foundation in 1938. Comedian and actor Eddie Cantor came up with the "March of Dimes" fundraising concept. He asked listeners of his popular radio program to support the foundation by sending dimes to the White House. Other celebrities also promoted the appeal, which raised more than $250,000 in a few weeks.[9] Individuals concerned about cancer noticed. In 1944 the American Society for the Control of Cancer was transformed into a voluntary health organization and was renamed the American Cancer Society. It launched a fundraising campaign that was soon generating hundreds of thousands of dollars a month.[10]

Boston cardiologist Howard Sprague, secretary of the AHA, and New Haven cardiologist H. M. (Jack) Marvin, chair of the association's Executive Committee, were astonished by how much money the National Foundation for Infantile Paralysis was raising. In 1941 the AHA was coordinating the nation's public health campaign against heart disease through its publications and affiliated clinics. It also held an annual scientific meeting to educate doctors and oversaw the certification of cardiologists. Sprague, ambitious and impatient, submitted a detailed plan that year for expanding the AHA's activities. The Boston cardiologist was frustrated that so little had been accomplished in combating heart disease, but he acknowledged that "the situation of the Association is no more static than is the country itself, and the military emergency overshadows the calmer paths of peace."[11]

The war was only part of the problem; the AHA had always been on the verge of bankruptcy because almost all of its income came from membership dues, which were low. In 1942 Jack Marvin informed the Executive Committee, of which Mayo vascular specialist Edgar Allen was a member, that the association's agenda was "far too limited in its scope and quantity...its limited budget has long been a great handicap."[12] When it came to increasing the AHA's income, the organization's leaders did not have to innovate. They could emulate what the groups concerned with polio and cancer had done in less than five years.

During the 1940s, Mayo physicians Arlie Barnes and Edgar Allen helped transform the 2,400-member AHA from a barely solvent professional society into a big budget voluntary health organization that would award research grants as part of its expanded agenda. Allen was elected to the AHA Executive Committee in 1941, and Barnes joined him on the Board of Directors two years later. In September 1945 Jack Marvin sent a letter to board members, challenging them to take action on the home front now that the war was over: "The public attention has been focused so sharply upon the apparent value of coordinated research, as exemplified by the atomic bomb, the large contributions to cancer research, Senator [Claude] Pepper's many public statements concerning the necessity for federal financing of research, and related matters, that it is beginning to clamor for some action in the field of cardiovascular disease."[13] Marvin wanted the AHA to seize the opportunity.

Arlie Barnes and Edgar Allen were among the seventeen AHA board members who traveled to San Francisco in June 1946 for what would be the most significant meeting in the association's twenty-two-year history. The board made decisions at this gathering that set the stage for a fundraising campaign to broaden the AHA's agenda and increase its impact. Verbatim minutes of the meeting reveal that the Mayo physicians did not speak often, but they contributed to the discussion at critical times. When the board reviewed the proposed $300,000 budget, Barnes complained that there was no allocation for research. He reminded those present that research support was supposed to a key part of the association's expanded mission. After the Mayo cardiologist challenged the board to reaffirm this philosophy, those present agreed to increase the fundraising target to $1 million, with one-third earmarked for research support. This was a very ambitious goal, considering the fact that the association's total income in 1945 was just over $39,000.[14]

Barnes Becomes President of the American Heart Association

The *New York Times* announced on June 7, 1947, "Mayo Clinic Official Named to Head Heart Association."[15] Arlie Barnes used his position as AHA president to promote cardiovascular research as a national priority at a critical time in the history of the association and American cardiology. Along with other AHA leaders, he helped attract the attention of politicians and the public to the problem of cardiovascular disease. Their appeal, which incorporated military metaphors and medical statistics, highlighted the mismatch between disease-specific death rates and the flow of research dollars. Another *New York Times* article described Barnes's advocacy efforts:

> Professor Arlie R. Barnes of the Mayo Foundation for Medical Education and Research, who was elected president of the American Heart Association, urged Congress to take favorable action on the Javits bill which, he said, "was urgently needed to provide the resources to defend the nation against diseases of the heart and circulation which are taking the greatest toll of American lives." More than 587,000 men, women and children, Dr. Barnes said, died of diseases of the heart and blood vessels during 1945. "This figure," he continued, "represents almost twice the number of Americans who lost their lives in battle during World War II. Deaths from these diseases are three times as high as cancer...eleven times as high as tuberculosis, and at least 500 times as high as infantile paralysis....Despite these appalling facts, the campaign against heart disease has been the last to receive public recognition and financial support," he added.[16]

Midway through Barnes's presidential term, the AHA launched a fundraising drive on the "Truth or Consequences" radio show. Ralph Edwards, the popular program's host, explained the "Walking Man Contest" to millions of listeners. Each Saturday night, they would hear the sound of footsteps over the radio, while he provided a clue about whose feet filled the shoes. During the live broadcast, Edwards phoned individuals who had mailed in an entry blank and a donation for the AHA and asked them to guess the walking man's identity. The response was overwhelming. More than 100,000 letters arrived in a single day, and $1.8 million was raised before a Chicago department store clerk guessed Jack Benny, one of America's best-known comedians. The winner, who got a $22,500 prize, had a personal interest in the cause. "My husband died from a heart ailment," she told a reporter.[17] At a Hollywood event celebrating the campaign's success, Edwards explained that Barnes had been "vitally involved in the negotiations between the AHA, NBC, Procter and Gamble and myself" that resulted in the contest.[18]

Arlie Barnes played a significant role in another key aspect of the AHA's transformation into a voluntary health organization: the selection of doctors and scientists who would be invited to join the Founder's Group of a new Scientific Council. The council model established a two-tier membership hierarchy that was designed to extend privileges to certain individuals and to distinguish them from general practitioners. In May 1948 Barnes sent a letter to almost seven hundred physicians and scientists inviting them to become members of the Founder's Group.[19] The list included all 378 physicians who were board certified in cardiovascular disease and 298 medical scientists and physicians who were not board certified but who had established reputations in the field through their research or other activities. Most of Mayo's cardiologists and vascular specialists were invited to join the new Scientific Council, as were nine of its scientists (six physiologists, two biophysicists, and one pathologist). Mayo staff members were also very visible at the AHA's 1948 scientific meeting, where they presented one-sixth of the lectures.[20]

A Blueprint for Building Cardiovascular Research Programs

Between 1946 and 1948, when the AHA was being transformed from a professional society into a voluntary health organization, federal lawmakers and civil servants were busy building an infrastructure to increase the nation's capacity for biomedical research. Rolla Dyer, director of what was then known as the (singular) National Institute of Health (NIH), appointed fellow infectious disease specialist Cassius Van Slyke to lead the new Office of Research Grants in 1946. The NIH director knew that his forty-six-year-old friend was under doctor's orders to limit his workload because he had had a heart attack a few months earlier. Although Dyer assured Van Slyke that the job would not be demanding, it was.[21]

The first sentence of Van Slyke's December 1946 article on new horizons in medical research suggested the scope of his responsibilities: "A large-scale, nationwide, peacetime program of support for scientific research in medical and related fields...is now a functioning reality."[22] Van Slyke described the creation of twenty-one study sections at the NIH that would focus on major categories of research. Study section members had three main responsibilities: to survey the status of research in their fields and identify neglected areas, to stimulate competent individuals to do research, and to review grant applications.

Johns Hopkins cardiologist Cowles Andrus was chosen to chair the newly formed Cardiovascular Study Section in 1946. The following year he asked Mayo physiologist Hiram Essex to conduct a comprehensive national survey of cardiovascular research. Essex, who had just published a review of basic and clinical research on the heart, was enthusiastic. He told Mayo's Board of Governors (Figure 8.1) that his survey would provide a "blueprint of present activities and possible future developments" to help officials decide where to allocate federal funds for cardiovascular research.[23] It is not surprising that the board approved his request to undertake the project. At the time, Arlie Barnes was both chair of the Mayo board and president of the AHA.

Surgeon General Thomas Parran, a longtime admirer of the Mayo Clinic, played a vital role in transforming the NIH into a major resource for intramural and extramural research on cancer and heart disease. He thanked Essex for agreeing to do the survey and welcomed his "advice and counsel in the expanding field of cardiovascular research."[24] When Essex's

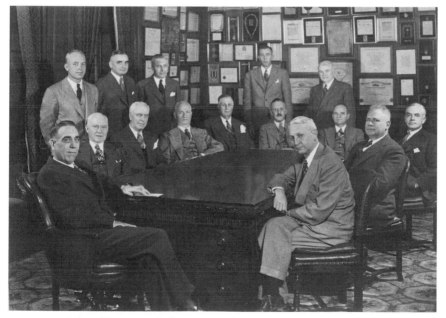

FIGURE 8.1 *Mayo Clinic Board of Governors with cardiologist Arlie Barnes (board chair) seated in the left foreground, ca. 1947.*
Used with permission of Mayo Foundation.

survey was mailed out in March 1948, the amount of money available for cardiovascular research was negligible. The National Heart Institute had not been created, and the AHA had just launched its first fundraising campaign. Although collaboration between academic researchers and the pharmaceutical industry had increased between the two World Wars, the enterprise was still small and there was little emphasis on cardiovascular drugs.[25] Essex sent several copies of the survey to each academic medical center for distribution to divisions that were involved in any type of cardiovascular research. Institutional leaders and individual investigators were asked to answer thirty questions about past, present, and potential research projects. They were also encouraged to brainstorm about how they might use federal funds if they became available.[26]

Debate About and Passage of the National Heart Act

As academic physicians and scientists completed Essex's survey in the spring of 1948, Congressional lawmakers debated the National Heart Act, which was designed to provide support for research relating to diseases of the heart and circulation.[27] There was a precedent. President Roosevelt had signed the National Cancer Institute Act eleven years earlier. Arlie Barnes, as AHA president, testified in support of the heart bill before a Senate subcommittee. Coming from a leading medical center known for providing excellent patient care, generating new knowledge, and producing highly trained specialists, Barnes was a compelling witness.

The Mayo cardiologist emphasized that patients would benefit from a major national investment in biomedical research. This was not a new notion, but attitudes had changed considerably as a result of war-related research that had important implications for patient care. Several concerned citizens now added their voices to the small chorus of academics that lobbied lawmakers, urging them to inject a big bolus of money into the nation's anemic research community. Such an investment, they argued, would result in discoveries and innovations, which, in turn, would improve the diagnosis, treatment, and prevention of heart disease.

Questions about the past, present, and future of cardiovascular research dominated the hearings. Senator Forrest Donnell asked Barnes, "What do the medical schools do now on this heart problem?" The Missouri Republican was mystified "that everything seems to be so far in arrears on the development of the heart study, when the heart is certainly one of the most prominent parts of the body."[28] Barnes responded, "It actually has been very difficult to secure sums of money for research, particularly in this field." He cited the case of the University of Minnesota, where a "considerable amount of research has been carried on ... but it has been done from hand to mouth."[29]

Barnes said that university-based investigators, who depended mainly on small grants from private foundations, did not have enough money to launch even the most promising projects.

Senator Donnell asked AHA board member David Rutstein why medical schools had so little money for cardiovascular research. The Harvard public health professor's response was blunt: "I would say first that medical schools have no funds for research to start off with. In my department, when I try to build up a research program I have got to beg, borrow, or steal to get small amounts. Unfortunately, a great many of us spend a majority of our time trying to find money rather than on investigating scientific projects." Rutstein praised Essex's survey, noting that it would place lawmakers "in a much better position to...evaluate the needs in the field." Personalizing his appeal, Rutstein reminded the committee members of their mortality: "The unfortunate death of Congressman Zimmerman yesterday, I think, is an example that focuses the problem in this sense. You might reasonably ask the question that, if the Congressman had been examined a day earlier, could you have told he was going to have this trouble, and if told, could you have done anything about it."[30] Linking sixty-seven-year-old Missouri Congressman Orville Zimmerman's sudden death from a heart attack to general vulnerability and the lack of effective therapy was part of a strategy to attract attention and money to the problem of cardiovascular disease.

President Truman signed the National Heart Act on June 16, 1948, three days before Arlie Barnes completed his term as AHA president. The association's new research program would complement that of the National Heart Institute, which was created as part of the National Heart Act. Barnes and Allen, as leaders of the AHA, would help decide where the federal money went. They were on a six-man subcommittee of the National Research Council that met in March 1949 to discuss the new National Heart Institute program. During the next fourteen months, the institute distributed $11 million in extramural grants for a "large-scale attack on heart disease." This included $6 million for construction, $3.9 million for research, $650,000 for teaching grants, $215,000 for heart traineeships, and $185,000 for research fellowships.[31] Hiram Essex's survey had identified institutions, investigators, and projects that seemed most likely to benefit from federal support.

Institutional Implications of the National Heart Act

Some ambitious academics, especially those with insider information, moved quickly to help their institutions take advantage of the new funding opportunities. For example, one month after President Truman signed the National Heart Act, New York vascular specialist Irving Wright proposed establishing a "Cardio-Vascular Institute or Division" at New York Hospital, which was affiliated with Cornell University Medical College in Manhattan. In addition to being an influential member of the AHA's Board of Directors, he was on the National Research Council's Subcommittee on Cardiovascular Disease. Wright informed the hospital's chief of medicine, "Large amounts of money are now becoming available for research and training in this field from numerous sources."[32] He argued that their institution should seize the opportunity because it lacked space, equipment, and personnel. And Wright was in a position to influence the flow of funds.

The Mayo Clinic, never a typical academic institution, did not seek government grants. Samuel Haines, vice-chair of the Board of Governors, spoke to the staff in the fall of 1949 about the clinic's strategy for supporting research. He explained that the board had recently reaffirmed a policy of not accepting federal grants, despite being fully aware that "the costs of modern research have increased markedly in recent years." A major concern was the belief that the government would begin to inspect institutions that were awarded grants. But there was more. "Inspection quickly leads to control," Haines claimed, "and control leads to loss of independence. One of the greatest advantages of working in the Mayo Clinic is that the affairs of the institution and of its personnel are self-determined. Any acceptance of funds from the federal government will, to a certain extent, destroy this self-determination."[33]

Haines reassured his audience of physicians and biomedical scientists that the board's decision "does not close the door to future consideration of acceptance of federal funds, but it establishes a definite policy for the present time." Some researchers were disappointed with the decision, but Haines explained that Mayo would continue to support projects that had potential clinical relevance. He also emphasized that "the success of the practice of medicine is dependent, in large part, on the opportunity of studying normal and diseased states by newer methods, and many of these methods which are instituted as research programs soon...become integral parts of the careful examination of many patients."[34] For example, Edgar Allen, Edgar Hines, and Nelson Barker had coauthored a 1946 book on peripheral vascular disease that contained an eighty-page chapter on special methods of investigation, several of which had moved from the experimental laboratory to the bedside. The book also reinforced Mayo's reputation as a world leader in the field.[35]

Edgar Allen, full of ambition, continued his campaign to promote cardiovascular research after the war, when the AHA was being reinvented and the National Heart Institute was being envisioned. In 1947, a dozen years after he had helped form the AHA's Section for the Study of the Peripheral Circulation, the Mayo vascular specialist told members of the association's Executive Committee (of which he was a member), "The heart is a small, although important, part of the cardiovascular system." Allen then presented a resolution that the AHA's president appoint a committee "to consider a more inclusive...name for the organization so that it will indicate the activities of the cardiologists, surgeons, pathologists, physiologists, internists, physicists, and others interested in the broad field of physiology of and diseases of the circulation."[36] Confronting resistance to changing the association's name, Allen shifted his attention to its official journal. He recommended that the *American Heart Journal* be renamed the *American Journal for Circulation* or something similar. No action was taken.

Undeterred, the Mayo vascular specialist carried his message of inclusiveness to the AHA Board of Directors. Their minutes note that "Dr. Allen spoke eloquently of the advantages of union rather than separation" with respect to the relationship of the AHA to other groups whose members were interested in arteriosclerosis, peripheral vascular disease, and hypertension.[37] Allen's plea for cooperation with new organizations, such as the American Foundation for High Blood Pressure, contributed to a decision to incorporate some of them into the AHA's new council structure.[38] His persistence paid off when the AHA dropped the *American Heart Journal* as its official publication in 1949. Jack Marvin, who had become president of the association, emphasized in the first issue of *Circulation* (which was published in January 1950) that the new journal's title was very significant: "We have advanced beyond the limitations of classical 'cardiology' into the overall study of the whole circulation."[39]

Wartime Shock and the Advent of Cardiac Catheterization

The first volume of *Circulation* included articles that reflected current concepts about and contemporary research on a broad range of cardiovascular subjects. One paper by a physiologist addressed the relationship of the peripheral circulation to shock caused by blood loss.[40] Traumatic shock was a life-threatening condition that had attracted a great deal of attention during both World Wars. Harvard physiologist William Townsend Porter, who had studied shock in France during World War I, produced a vivid word-picture of a man near death:

> In traumatic shock, the patient is utterly relaxed, pale as the dead, with eyes like those of a dead fish; he is apparently, but not really, unconscious; his breathing is shallow and frequent, his heart-beat rapid and feeble, and his pulse scarcely to be felt at the wrist. Much of the blood has collected in the great veins, the heart is poorly filled, the driving pressure of the blood in the arteries is less than half the normal—too low for the maintenance of a proper circulation of blood to the brain; the brain cells suffer for lack of food.[41]

Porter explained that traumatic shock was usually fatal unless skilled assistance was available immediately. Even if trained personnel were at hand, treatment attempts were often futile. Other physiologists had studied shock during the World War I, notably Walter Cannon of Harvard, but the subject had attracted little attention during the interwar years.[42]

In a 1935 peacetime review of traumatic shock, Mayo physiologists Frank Mann and Hiram Essex wrote: "At present, the automobile kills and maims each year as many persons as would be injured in a war of considerable dimensions."[43] But this would soon change when the world confronted a war of unprecedented dimensions. Mann was the immediate past president of the American Physiological Society in the summer of 1938, when he sailed to Europe to participate in the International Congress of Physiology in Zurich. More than one thousand individuals attended the meeting, but the mood was somber due to growing regional instability, highlighted by Germany's recent annexation of Austria. Mann informed Mayo Foundation director Donald Balfour: "A feeling of pessimism pervaded the meeting. Many of the scientists reported that their best young men had been taken from them to work on war projects."[44]

By 1940 deaths and serious injuries on European battlefields were soaring. Military surgeons tried to save the lives of soldiers dying from shock by controlling blood loss and restoring intravascular volume with plasma transfusions.[45] Meanwhile, medical scientists were attempting to understand potential mechanisms of shock as a step toward developing more effective treatments. As war spread over the Continent, Alfred Blalock, chief of surgery at Vanderbilt University and an authority on surgical shock, was chosen to head the National Research Council's new Subcommittee on Shock.[46]

Intensive research into the mechanism and treatment of shock during World War II contributed to the development of cardiac catheterization as a diagnostic tool. Blalock was preparing to move from Nashville to Baltimore to become surgeon-in-chief at the Johns Hopkins Hospital in March 1941, when he read an article on cardiac catheterization by André Cournand and Hilmert Ranges of Bellevue Hospital in New York City. Cournand and Ranges opened their paper on catheterization of the right atrium in humans by citing a 1929 article by German surgical resident Werner Forssmann, in which he reported the results of inserting a catheter into a human's heart—his own.[47] Three years later, Johns Hopkins physiologist Arthur Grollman denounced catheterization, declaring it "not only dangerous to the subject but useless so far as cardiac output determinations are concerned."[48] Cournand and Ranges disputed Grollman's claims in their 1941 article, arguing that many animal experiments had demonstrated that the procedure was safe and provided a reliable estimate of cardiac output, a measure of the heart's pumping function.

Physiologists had devised various ways to estimate or measure cardiac output in animals since the nineteenth century, but Cournand and his colleagues sought a more accurate and reproducible method that could be used in humans.[49] Cardiac output, defined as the volume of blood that the heart pumps into the arterial circulation per minute, can be calculated from three variables. Two of them were relatively easy to obtain in humans in 1941: a sample of oxygen-rich blood from the femoral artery, and all of the air expired from the lungs during the brief period of blood sampling. Cournand and his collaborators realized that the third variable—mixed venous blood—could be collected using a cardiac catheter. He inserted a flexible silk catheter (about as thick as a strand of spaghetti and a little more than a yard long) into a vein in the elbow crease and threaded it through the vessel toward the heart. Cournand watched the catheter's progress toward the heart on a fluoroscopic screen positioned over a patient on an X-ray table. Their goal was to place the tip of the catheter in the right atrium, the chamber where venous blood returns to the heart after circulating throughout the body. Once there, he withdrew samples of venous blood for analysis of its oxygen content.[50]

Blalock realized that the Bellevue Hospital team's technique of right atrial catheterization was pertinent to the wartime shock research program. In November 1941 he informed Cournand's collaborator Dickinson Richards that the Army and Navy were "anxious for studies to be carried out on shock in man."[51] Richards responded, "It seems to us that the right auricle [atrium] would be a very interesting place to be in, during shock, with the opportunity thus offered of measuring both pressures and cardiac output, not only once but repeatedly."[52]

Blalock also asked New York University professor Homer Smith for advice. The prominent physiologist replied: "I think one difficulty in the shock situation is that most investigators are busy studying their theory of shock and not studying shock as it actually exists in man." Noting catheterization's potential value as a research tool, Smith declared, "The first results of such a study might well surprise most theorists out of their wits."[53] Eager to proceed, Blalock quickly arranged for the Bellevue Hospital group to get a grant to study shock using cardiac catheterization. Richards recalled, "The United States was by this time at war and further information on the hemodynamics of shock, quantitative measurements of this, and of the effects of treatment, were urgently needed."[54]

The Mayo Clinic Aero Medical Unit

The National Research Council's shock study, which stimulated the development of cardiac catheterization beginning in 1941, focused on injured soldiers who went into shock on the battlefield. Five years later, Mayo would be one of the first institutions in the world to introduce cardiac catheterization as a clinical diagnostic tool. The clinic's early involvement in catheterization was the result of a seemingly unrelated wartime research program that focused on solving problems associated with military pilots flying fast and high. But it was not a coincidence that Mayo was asked to undertake this project. In 1939 a Washington-based newsletter designed to inform the public about developments in science had reported that the Mayo Clinic, "mecca for medical men and the ill, is adding to its tremendous research facilities an aviation medicine laboratory to study problems brought in the train of the air age."[55]

The clinic initially became involved in aviation research in 1937, when Northwest Airlines president Croil Hunter asked Charlie Mayo's son Charles W. (Chuck) Mayo, a surgeon, and Walter Boothby, a pioneer of oxygen therapy, to work with engineers at his company to solve a practical problem. Northwest Airlines, based in St. Paul, Minnesota, had served Rochester for a dozen years, and Hunter wanted Mayo's help in developing a reliable method to deliver oxygen to its pilots so they could fly planes at higher altitudes over the Rocky Mountains. In response, Boothby worked with two other men at Mayo to invent a tight-fitting oxygen mask. Randolph Lovelace II was a surgical fellow and pilot, and Arthur Bulbulian was an expert at creating custom-made latex facial prostheses. The BLB mask, named for its three inventors, delivered oxygen to pilots flying at high altitude and could also be used for patients lying in bed.[56]

Northwest Airlines first tested a prototype BLB mask on July 28, 1938, when Lovelace, six company engineers, and a pilot flew from Minneapolis to Los Angeles via Billings, Montana.[57] The BLB mask received more national publicity in 1940, when President Roosevelt presented the Collier trophy (for major advances in aeronautics) to Boothby, Lovelace, and Bulbulian for their contributions to improving aviation safety.[58]

In the spring of 1941, Mayo's Board of Governors approved a request from the Lockheed Aircraft Corporation to appoint Lovelace as a consulting surgeon for high-altitude aircraft problems.[59] The California-based company was developing high-performance planes for the Royal Air Force after the Battle of Britain and in anticipation of America's entry into the war. It wanted Lovelace's help in developing ways to protect pilots from the physiological stresses that their bodies confronted in new planes that could fly higher and faster, make tighter turns, and pull out of steeper dives. The last maneuver generated such high gravitational forces that a pilot might partially or completely lose consciousness, with potentially catastrophic consequences. The military also turned to Mayo to help solve problems related to high-altitude bailouts.

Physiologist Charles Code played a central role in creating a laboratory at Mayo to study the physiological effects of acceleration and methods to help pilots cope with them. Sickness had shaped Code's career path. He was eleven years old when he contracted polio in 1921. Melvin Henderson, Code's uncle and Mayo's first orthopedic surgeon, was responsible for the Canadian boy's first visit to Rochester for evaluation of lingering leg weakness. This experience and return visits contributed to Code's decisions to go to medical school and then to the Mayo Clinic as a fellow in physiology. After completing his fellowship in 1937, Code spent two years in London, where he worked with several leading British physiologists. He was awarded a PhD in physiology at the University of Minnesota in 1940, after which he returned to Rochester. Soon, Code was devoting much of his time to Mayo's expanding program of aviation medicine research.[60]

The growing role of airpower in warfare became evident during the Battle of Britain, which the Germans launched in the summer of 1940.[61] Late the following year, President Roosevelt delivered one of his most memorable speeches, which began: "Yesterday, December 7, 1941—a date which will live in infamy—the United States of America was suddenly and deliberately attacked by naval and air forces of the Empire of Japan."[62] Three days after the Japanese bombed Pearl Harbor, Mayo's Board of Governors approved a report that Code had written. He encouraged the clinic to construct "a unique machine for the study of the effects of gravity" that Mayo biophysicist Edward Baldes had designed.[63]

Protecting Pilots from High G-Forces: The Human Centrifuge

Code's report included a request for $25,000 to build Baldes's human centrifuge as a tool to study the effects of acceleration and to construct a circular annex to the new Medical Sciences Building, where it would be housed. The acceleration project would be coordinated with a similar program at Wright Field, an Army Air Corps research and testing facility in Dayton, Ohio. Code urged rapid action, emphasizing that the "results obtained may possibly receive immediate application in our armed forces and would be of equal use to our enemies."[64] He listed three staff members who would work on the top-secret acceleration project, along with himself and Baldes. One of them, Howard Burchell, was a cardiologist. Like Code, he was a Canadian medical graduate who had been awarded a PhD in physiology. Burchell had joined the clinic staff in 1940, as a member of Arlie Barnes's cardiology section.[65]

The day after the board approved Code's proposal on December 10, 1941, Germany and Italy declared war on the United States. President Roosevelt got Congressional approval to go to war against the two European nations the same day. The demand for military doctors surged when the United States entered the overseas conflict.[66] Burchell, who was supposed to be a member of Mayo's acceleration group, had become a naturalized citizen

172   *Caring for the Heart*

in 1941 and volunteered for the US Army. His departure contributed to a
decision to hire Earl Wood, a physiologist who would play a critical role in
the acceleration project and the subsequent development of Mayo's cardiac
catheterization program.

Earl Wood had been awarded an MD from the University of Minnesota in
1941, the same year he received a PhD for his work with Maurice Visscher, the
head of physiology. Wood was teaching pharmacology at Harvard Medical
School the following year, when he wrote to Visscher seeking advice about
options for military service. Visscher sent a copy of Wood's letter to Code
in Rochester, adding, "It would be too bad if he were unable to continue
investigative work." The University of Minnesota physiologist thought that
his former student would be more valuable as a researcher "than as a routine
medical officer, considering his lack of experience in practical medicine."[67]
Code responded by informing Visscher that Mayo was planning "a big study
in acceleration" and that he and Baldes were "most anxious to have a man of
Wood's caliber join us as our first assistant." Code closed his letter: "I hope
it will catch Earl's imagination and fire the spark which teaching at Harvard
does not seem to have ignited."[68] It would!

When Wood joined Mayo's Aero Medical Unit in the summer of 1942, a
thirty-four-foot diameter human centrifuge (Figure 8.2) was being installed
in an annex to the Medical Sciences Building. The first of three human cen-
trifuges built in the United States, it incorporated two twenty-ton flywheels

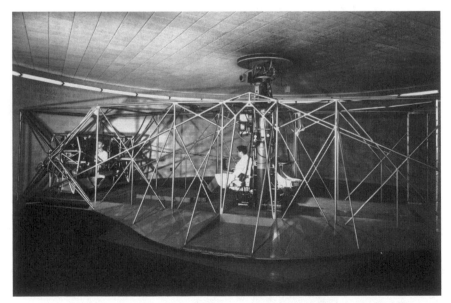

FIGURE 8.2 *Earl Wood in the center of the human centrifuge in Mayo's Medical Sciences
Building, ca. 1944.*

Used with permission of Mayo Foundation.

from a Cincinnati brewery and was powered by a Chrysler automobile engine. A research volunteer sat in a gondola suspended fifteen feet from the center of rotation. Charles Lindbergh, the world's best known aviator, rode in the centrifuge in the fall of 1942, during a ten-day visit to the Mayo Clinic on behalf of the Army Air Corps. Lindbergh developed a severe headache during a spin that generated a force of 5.8 g, and the centrifuge was stopped. He lost consciousness during an experiment in a custom-built low-pressure chamber designed to simulate high-altitude flight. Lucille Cronin, Walter Boothby's longtime laboratory technician, was in the chamber with Lindbergh. She strapped a BLB oxygen mask on him, and he recovered quickly.[69]

The main goal of the accelerator project was to develop special flight suits, known as anti-G suits, to prevent pilots from passing out from high gravitational forces produced by radial acceleration.[70] Wood and his associates studied 300 subjects (including themselves) on the big spinning machine. Code informed the Board of Governors in 1944, "The work on the centrifuge is hazardous. It is definitely a young man's job. Dr. Wood, Dr. Lambert, Roy Engstrom and Dr. Code have voluntarily repeatedly subjected themselves to accelerations which have produced temporary complete blindness and on occasion loss of consciousness. These young men would certainly not be doing this type of work if our country were not engaged in a war and if it were not that they are convinced that they are contributing something towards its prosecution."[71]

In 1944 the Army Air Corps lent Mayo researchers a state-of-the-art dive bomber to test evolving anti-G suit designs under actual flight conditions. Edward Lambert, a physiologist who had joined the program one year earlier, named the Douglas A-24 Dauntless airplane the "G-Whiz." During the final months of the war, combat pilots wore refined versions of the anti-G suit. Yale University physiologist and historian John Fulton claimed in 1948 that pilots who wore these suits "were able to completely outmaneuver the German fighters during the last months of the war and in that way effectively shortened the conflict."[72]

Germany surrendered in May 1945, and Japan was preparing to surrender on August 21, 1945, when Mayo's Laboratory and Research Committee met to discuss the future of the Acceleration Laboratory. Code was a member of the committee, and Wood and Lambert were invited to attend the meeting. The scientists were proud of their practical accomplishments that had supported the Allies' air campaign. Code emphasized that electronics engineers and machinists had played a major role in developing instruments of precision to monitor human subjects as the centrifuge spun them around. These instruments were designed to continuously document a subject's pulse, blood pressure, electrocardiogram, and blood oxygen content. The future of these technologies was secure, but the future of some Mayo scientists who used them was not.[73]

Charles Code and Earl Wood worried that the war's end would lead to the shutdown of their specialized laboratory and to staff cuts. Hoping to avoid this scenario, they asked the Board of Governors to create a formal physiology section at Mayo. Recognizing that Mayo's main mission was patient care, they stressed their willingness to collaborate with clinicians. The physiologists would undertake their main research activities in the Medical Sciences Building, close to where most of the clinic's doctors worked.[74] When the board approved the new section, Code informed Visscher that Wood and Baldes would remain in Rochester, boasting, "I believe that we have a prospect of having the finest physiology division in the world here and at the University under the general auspices of the University of Minnesota."[75] Even before Mayo created a distinct physiology section, Frank Mann had led his institution to prominence in the field. For example, historian Gerald Geison has shown that the Mayo Clinic ranked seventh among all institutional contributors to the *American Journal of Physiology* between 1918 and 1940.[76]

The Advent of Mayo's Cardiac Catheterization Program

As postwar demobilization accelerated early in 1946, Mayo Foundation director Donald Balfour asked Earl Wood about his research priorities. The thirty-four-year-old medical scientist explained that he viewed himself "as a physiologist, not as an aviation physiologist" and that he was quite willing to collaborate with physicians in clinical research.[77] Wood did not know that he would be at the center of Mayo's cardiac catheterization program, which would be launched in December.

Howard Burchell, the cardiologist who would organize the first catheterization in Rochester, had spent four years in the US Army Medical Corps, the last two in Europe. Near the end of the war, he had an experience that would have major implications for patient care at the Mayo Clinic. During a 1945 visit to Hammersmith Hospital in suburban London, Burchell watched Peter Sharpey-Schafer perform a cardiac catheterization. Sharpey-Schafer and John McMichael had done the first catheterization in Britain three years earlier, inspired by Cournand and Range's report of its use as a tool to calculate cardiac output.[78]

Burchell returned to Rochester early in 1946, after completing his military assignment in Europe. In December he arranged Mayo's first cardiac catheterization. The patient was a forty-four-year-old man from North Dakota who had come to the clinic for evaluation of gall bladder disease.[79] When he was a teenager, he had been told there was something wrong with his heart, but he had no symptoms. A physician had heard a heart murmur and detected an enlarged heart in 1941. Since that time, the man had noticed that he became somewhat breathless with exertion. His main problem, however, was upper abdominal pain that had occurred off and on for three years. A local doctor had diagnosed gall bladder disease.

The medical fellow who examined the patient at the Mayo Clinic in mid-November 1946 thought the heart murmur he heard was caused by a ventricular septal defect, a hole between the heart's two main pumping chambers. Burchell examined the man and came to a different conclusion. He thought the murmur was due to an atrial septal defect. This problem, another form of congenital heart disease, results in blood flowing from the left atrium into the right atrium through a hole in the septum between the two chambers. Burchell believed that the diagnosis "would be fairly well confirmed" if cardiac fluoroscopy showed exaggerated pulsation of the pulmonary arteries (reflecting the increased blood flow that resulted from the septal defect). He concluded, "Cardiac condition should *not* make surgical risk prohibitive. Will consider study by auricular [right atrial] catheterization."[80]

The North Dakota patient's preoperative evaluation in Rochester took place one year after cardiologist James Warren and his colleagues at Grady Hospital in Atlanta had published the first article describing how right atrial catheterization could be used to diagnose certain types of congenital heart disease. They concluded that catheterization was "a safe and useful method of differentiating atrial septal defect from other causes of hypertrophy of the right ventricle and prominence of the pulmonary artery."[81] This notion appealed to Burchell, but the patient had come to the Mayo Clinic because of abdominal pain. Shortly before Thanksgiving in 1946, Chuck Mayo removed the man's gall bladder and several gallstones at Saint Marys Hospital (as St. Mary's Hospital had begun to be spelled in the early 1940s).

No one at Mayo had performed a cardiac catheterization, but Burchell knew that anesthesiologist John Pender had extensive experience inserting needles and short flexible tubes into veins for the purpose of administering intravenous drugs and fluids. On December 5, 1946, twelve days after the patient's abdominal operation, Pender inserted a long catheter into a vein in the patient's left arm in an X-ray room at Saint Marys Hospital. Next, the lights were turned off, and the doctors put on red goggles and waited for several minutes so their eyes could adapt to the dark. This was necessary so that they could see the catheter's faint outline on a fluoroscope screen. Radiology resident John Bacon operated the fluoroscope that allowed Burchell to track the thin tube's progress as Pender threaded it through the patient's venous system toward his heart. Finally, blood samples were withdrawn from the inferior vena cava, superior vena cava, and right atrium. Technician Lucille Cronin analyzed the oxygen content of the venous blood samples and arterial blood samples obtained from an artery. Her results confirmed Burchell's diagnosis. The man had been born with an atrial septal defect. But the catheterization had no immediate therapeutic implications because there were no medical or surgical treatments for his problem. He was discharged four days later.[82]

Physiologist Earl Wood was well positioned to develop a cardiac catheterization laboratory in Rochester. On December 5, 1946, the same day he watched John Pender perform the first catheterization at Saint Marys Hospital, Wood wrote to Lewis Dexter, who had begun catheterizing patients at Boston's Peter Bent Brigham Hospital a few months earlier. Wood asked for a reprint of Dexter's recent article on the technique as an aid to the diagnosis of congenital heart disease.[83] Burchell and Wood agreed that future catheterizations in Rochester should be performed in Mayo's Medical Sciences Building, where technologies developed during the war were available to calculate the oxygen content of blood samples and to measure several physiological parameters, such as intracardiac pressures. Wood explained decades later, "We just carried what we had been doing in the war effort into the cardiac catheterization laboratory."[84]

In 1947 Wood performed twenty-two right heart catheterizations (Figure 8.3) with the help of radiologist David Pugh, three physiology fellows, several technicians, and John Pender (who anesthetized children before they underwent the procedure).[85] That year *Life* magazine published "Tube into the Heart," a two-page photo-essay on catheterization that showed a physician making a small incision in a patient's arm in order to insert a "long, thin tube which can be pushed up an arm vein, past the shoulder and into

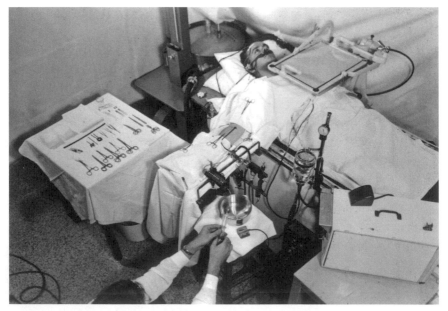

FIGURE 8.3 *Cardiac catheterization (of the right heart) at Mayo, ca. 1951.*
Used with permission of Mayo Foundation.

the heart." The magazine informed readers that doctors at New York's Bellevue Hospital "have perfected this painful-looking but painless operation."[86] The public's interest in medical news increased steadily after World War II, as more voices joined the chorus singing the praises and promise of biomedical research.

Arlie Barnes was simultaneously president of the AHA and chair of the clinic's Board of Governors in November 1947, when he spoke to the Mayo staff about the importance of clinical research. Locally and nationally, aspiring researchers faced problems relating to time, space, and support staff. All these things cost money. Barnes acknowledged that many of Mayo's doctors "desired much more opportunity for clinical investigation." But this would require granting them time away from practice. That was a problem because the clinic was trying to meet growing demands for care in the postwar period. In terms of money, Mayo's research and training programs were supported by income from the practice and investments. The cardiologist reminded his colleagues that the clinic "stands alone as an institution which finances its great research and educational program from its own earnings." Sounding very much like Will Mayo, who had died eight years earlier, Barnes declared that the clinic would "continue to be successful only if its research and educational efforts proceed in closest unity with the practice of medicine.... They all exist in this institution to provide ever increasing improvement in the care of the sick patient."[87]

Worldwide Recognition of Mayo's Catheterization Program

The size and sophistication of Mayo's catheterization program became widely known when the *Proceedings of the Staff Meetings of the Mayo Clinic* (hereafter *Proceedings*) published eight articles on the procedure in the fall of 1948. Fifteen Mayo physicians and scientists contributed to the papers that were presented at a symposium for the staff. Burchell coauthored five articles, reflecting his role in launching the laboratory and his interest in congenital heart disease.[88] The first one, based on sixty catheterizations, discussed the technique's value in diagnosing atrial and ventricular septal defects, patent ductus arteriosus, and pulmonary stenosis. It also announced two technologies that had grown out of the clinic's wartime accelerator program: a photoelectric oximeter to measure blood oxygen content and an electric strain gauge manometer to measure intracardiac and intravascular pressures. Still in the development stage, these technologies provided rapid, almost instantaneous, results during a catheterization.[89] The day the symposium appeared in print, the Board of Governors applauded Wood's laboratory for making "an outstanding contribution... to the development of medical science and the practice of medicine and surgery at Mayo Clinic."[90]

Several pioneers of cardiac catheterization praised the papers that appeared in the *Proceedings* and welcomed the Mayo group into their ranks. A month after the symposium was published, Boston cardiologist Lewis Dexter informed Earl Wood how much he enjoyed the articles and how impressed he was by Mayo's catheterization program.[91] Writing from London, John McMichael commended Wood for "the reports of the excellent work you are now doing."[92] André Cournand asked the Mayo physiologist to send him a copy of the *Proceedings* issue, adding: "I greatly admire the improvement attendant to the instantaneous measurement of oxygen saturation." Cournand wanted to acquire an oximeter for his Bellevue Hospital laboratory.[93] Wood explained that Mayo's engineering section had provided complete specifications and blueprints for the oxygen-measuring instrument to the Waters Conley Company, which planned to market it in the near future.[94] When Cournand published the first book on cardiac catheterization in 1949, six of the twenty-eight references in its bibliography were from the Mayo Clinic.[95]

The photoelectric oximeter and electric strain gauge manometer that attracted the attention of the pioneers of catheterization had been developed for the acceleration project as a result of collaboration between physiologists and biophysicists at Mayo and electronics engineers at the Waters Conley Company. Proximity, personal contacts, and product quality combined to forge a strong relationship between the clinic and the Rochester-based firm. Several years before Glen Waters bought the Conley Company in 1940, its main mission had been to make cameras for Sears and Roebuck. Waters turned it into a company that manufactured phonographs with electronic amplifiers, which required the hiring of electronics engineers. By the end of the war, the company employed ten engineers, several of whom were involved in developing equipment for biophysical and biomedical research.[96]

Richard Jones, Waters Conley's director of engineering, met with Mayo's Laboratory and Research Committee in the fall of 1945 to discuss possibilities for postwar collaboration. Jones provided the perspective of an outsider whose career had been in commercial electronics. The committee minutes reveal his concern that medicine had been slow to adopt or adapt devices and materials already used in various industries. Jones saw many opportunities to apply "electronic instrumentation to medical problems," which had been central to the accelerator project. The committee, chaired by Charles Code, asked the Board of Governors to pay part of Jones's salary so that the electronics engineer could serve as a part-time consultant to the staff.[97]

Edward Baldes went further the following year, informing the board, "During the war we have realized here the necessity and advisability of being able to develop some of our own methods and equipment." Baldes and Mayo's other biophysicists considered Jones the ideal person to coordinate an expansion of the clinic's engineering facilities and staff.[98] It would take time to accomplish this goal, but the board approved the creation of an engineering section in 1948, and Jones was hired to lead it.

When the *Proceedings* published a second symposium on catheterization in 1950, Burchell and Wood said the technique had an established place in helping to diagnose congenital heart defects. They emphasized that a trained team was essential for the safe and successful performance of catheterization in patients, most of whom were children.[99] Wood's laboratory had become a magnet for individuals interested in the technique. Lewis Dexter informed him after a 1951 visit, "I was very much impressed with the type and caliber of the work you are doing.... I learned a lot of new tricks of the trade and came away with a lot of good ideas." The Boston cardiologist was "really impressed with what a smooth-working team you have."[100] Around the time Dexter visited Rochester, Arlie Barnes boasted to Mayo's Board of Governors that Wood's laboratory was "second to none in the country" for the evaluation of patients with congenital heart disease.[101]

Adding Staff and Space to Support Mayo's Research Programs

Earl Wood performed all of the catheterizations in the late 1940s, but most of his time was spent on other activities. The physiologist's main passion was research, and he asked for help with the routine diagnostic procedures as the volume increased. In the spring of 1950, Wood complained to Barnes that "the load of investigational and routine work in the cardiac portion of the Cardio-Respiratory Laboratories cannot be adequately handled by any reasonable degree of effort by a single staff man." He suggested a temporary solution—appointing a senior medical fellow who had more than a year of experience in his laboratory—until a suitable person was recruited for a staff position. "To insure the best possible selection," Wood told Barnes, "it would be most desirable to be able to pick up this man at leisure."[102]

Six months later, Charles Code agreed with another of Wood's suggestions: that they hire a senior technician to set up, supervise, and maintain the apparatus used during a catheterization. As a permanent employee, this person would be more knowledgeable and efficient than the fellows who rotated through the laboratory during their training.[103] Harold J. C. (Jeremy) Swan was hired as a research associate in 1951, with the possibility of a staff position in the future. He had been born in Ireland and trained in medicine and physiology in London, where Henry Barcroft was his main mentor. Code thought the Irishman's interest in pharmacology would complement Wood's emphasis on instrumentation.[104] Swan later recalled being "swept into the new and exciting field of cardiac catheterization" when he arrived in Rochester.[105]

Wartime staff depletion had resolved when Mayo broke ground for a seven-floor addition to the Medical Sciences Building in the spring of 1949.

Charles Code, euphoric about the expansion, boasted that the new facility would "afford a unique opportunity for each of us to work out our professional destinies within a plant more closely approaching the ideal than anything we had believed possible."[106] Mayo's scientists would have more space and staff as they entered the second half of the twentieth century. The Medical Sciences Building's location, just two blocks from the clinic, was ideal. Scientists who worked there were close to scores of proven and potential clinical investigators. When the addition opened in November 1952, it contained a new two-room catheterization laboratory.

The Mayo Clinic invited several national figures to participate in the dedication of the addition to the Medical Sciences Building. They sat in an auditorium named for Frank Mann, whose retirement coincided with the opening of the expanded facility. Vannevar Bush, author of *Science: The Endless Frontier*, gave the keynote address, and James Shannon, associate director in charge of research at the four-year-old National Heart Institute, attended the celebration.[107] The NIH hospital that would be known as the Clinical Center was nearing completion in Bethesda, and Shannon arranged for two medical officers who would help launch its Laboratory of Cardiovascular Hemodynamics to visit Rochester.

Hiram Essex informed his colleagues that Luther Terry and James Callaway were coming "to see the Medical Sciences Building and particularly the circulatory and respiratory laboratories."[108] The visitors were impressed. Callaway told Essex, "Seeing your research facilities will benefit us in many ways. These facilities are surpassed only by the hospitality you and your group extended us."[109] Mayo's physiology section, created at the end of the war, grew dramatically during the next few years. Code's 1952 report to the Board of Governors listed 10 professional staff, 21 fellows, and 43 technical assistants.[110] What had begun as a narrowly focused wartime project had evolved into a world-class catheterization program that would play an increasingly important role in the care of patients with heart disease.

Surgeons Begin Trying to Treat Heart Disease

The origins of cardiac surgery can be traced to the end of nineteenth century, when a few bold surgeons operated in an attempt to save the lives of individuals who had been stabbed or shot in the heart. Most of these trauma victims died within minutes as a result of their wounds, but a few survived for several hours. Some of them developed a condition termed pericardial tamponade, which results from blood leaking into the pericardial sac that surrounds the beating heart. The accumulation of blood causes the pressure inside the pericardial sac to increase to a level that interferes with the vital organ's ability to pump blood. The only hope of survival for such individuals was for a surgeon to remove the blood surrounding the heart and to stop more of the life-sustaining fluid from leaking out of the organ.

In 1896 British surgeon Stephen Paget opened a book chapter on wounds of the heart with a pessimistic prediction: "Surgery of the heart has probably reached the limits set by Nature to all surgery; no new method, and no new discovery, can overcome the natural difficulties that attend a wound of the heart. It is true that 'heart suture' has been vaguely proposed as a possible procedure, and has been done on animals; but I cannot find that it has ever been attempted in practice."[1]

Bold Attempts to Save Lives by Suturing Heart Wounds

That same year German surgeon Ludwig Rehn reported on an experience he had just had and proposed a different vision of the future. He described the case of a twenty-two-year-old man who was dying in a hospital a few hours after having been stabbed in the chest. Rehn performed a procedure that saved the man's life. After making a five and one-half inch incision between the man's fourth and fifth left ribs, he closed a one-half inch hole in the wall of his right ventricle with three silk sutures. The young man recovered from the operation that closed his heart wound. Rehn ended his 1897 report of the patient's story with a plea: "I sincerely hope that this case will not remain a curiosity, but that it will provide a stimulus for further work in the field of cardiac surgery."[2]

Rehn's success inspired other surgeons to attempt the potentially life-saving procedure. In 1902 surgeon Luther Hill of Montgomery, Alabama, performed a similar operation on a thirteen-year-old boy who had been stabbed in a fight. The boy survived. Hill's publication was the first to document a surgical procedure on the heart in the United States. In it, he summarized thirty-eight other attempts to suture heart wounds that had been published since Rehn's report of the surgical breakthrough. European surgeons had done them, and fourteen of their patients survived.[3]

St. Louis surgeon Benjamin Ricketts began his 1904 book on surgery of the heart and lungs on an optimistic note: "Injuries and diseases of the heart have resisted surgery longer than almost any tissues or organs of the human body. They, however, no longer offer such resistance, but find themselves subject to attack on the same surgical principles as other parts of the body." Noting that one-third of fifty-six patients who had undergone suture closure of a hole in the heart caused by a knife or gunshot wound had survived, Ricketts argued that the organ "should no longer be exempt from surgical measures."[4] Where Paget had perceived obstacles, Rehn, Hill, and Ricketts saw opportunities. But performing an emergency operation on the heart of a person dying of a knife or gun wound was not the same as undertaking an elective operation on a patient with chronic heart valve disease or some other cardiac disorder.

Many turn-of-the-century surgeons operated inside the abdomen, but very few of them ever considered operating inside the chest. The main obstacle was the sudden decline in lung function that could result from all but the smallest chest incision. Making a large incision between the ribs to reach the heart allows air to rush into the chest cavity, which causes at least one lung to collapse (a pneumothorax). A collapsed lung cannot perform its normal function of adding oxygen to the blood flowing through it. And contemporary anesthesia techniques could not prevent the potentially life-threatening problem of pneumothorax. The standard anesthetic approach involved dropping ether into a cone placed over the patient's nose and mouth. An anesthetized patient breathed shallowly, but his or her lungs continued to expand so the blood passing through them could absorb oxygen and release carbon dioxide. If a surgeon hoped to open the chest in order to operate on the heart, an anesthetic approach that kept the lungs from collapsing would be necessary.[5]

Will Mayo attended the American Surgical Association meeting in San Francisco in 1905, a few months before the city was devastated by an earthquake and fire. The Minnesota surgeon heard Elliot Rixford discuss what had happened when he removed part of a woman's chest wall in an attempt to reduce the risk of a recurrence of breast cancer. The California doctor described a pneumothorax on one side of her chest, which meant the other (un-collapsed) lung had to maintain respiration: "It was noticed, of course, that the respiration became immediately deeper and more rapid as soon as air entered the pleural cavity, but, aside from the violent flopping of the heart from right to left, terrifying to look at but without noticeable effect on the pulse, there was no special inconvenience to the patient or operator."[6] Despite Rixford's reassurance, very few surgeons were interested in performing a procedure that might produce such a frightening sight with its potential for causing death from asphyxiation.

Samuel Robinson, Mayo Clinic's First Thoracic Surgeon

Samuel Robinson was one of very few individuals in the early twentieth century who attempted to develop techniques to make surgery inside the chest possible. A Harvard Medical School graduate who had extensive experience in experimental physiology, Robinson was well prepared for the task. He had worked with German surgeon Ferdinand Sauerbruch, who had developed a method to prevent pneumothorax when the chest was opened.[7] Robinson had met Sauerbruch at the 1908 International Congress on Tuberculosis in Washington, D.C., where they both presented papers to the surgical session, which Charlie Mayo chaired.

While in America, Sauerbruch visited Rochester and a few other cities to demonstrate how his negative pressure apparatus prevented pneumothorax during operations inside the chest. The German surgeon recalled that the Mayo brothers were particularly interested in his experiments: "They discussed every detail and possibility with me."[8] Robinson was an outpatient surgeon at Massachusetts General Hospital in Boston when he was sent to Germany to study with Sauerbruch in 1909. The following year the two men coauthored an article describing animal experiments that compared techniques to prevent pneumothorax in order to perform lung surgery.[9]

Robinson warned in 1914 that "surgery of the heart is dangerous." He knew that most surgeons would never consider performing an operation to try to sew shut a knife or gunshot wound to the heart; they would "tend to leave such situations in the hands of God, lawyers and police officers."[10] But Robinson, emboldened by the results of his animal experiments, foresaw a future when surgeons no longer feared opening a patient's chest to operate on his or her heart. Robinson's optimism also reflected recent developments that made blood transfusion safer and new anesthesia techniques that reduced the risk of pneumothorax.[11]

During the 1914 meeting of the American Surgical Association, Will and Charlie Mayo heard Robinson present a paper on thoracic surgery at a symposium on the subject. He reviewed recent surgical attempts to treat bronchiectasis, a condition characterized by a chronic cough that produces very large amounts of putrid sputum. Robinson explained that patients with this disabling and incurable disease were often exhausted and emaciated. Although surgery was risky, it might make it possible "to reinstate in society an individual ostracized by the ever-present accumulation of profuse and generally offensive expectoration."[12] Lectures at the chest surgery symposium stimulated the Mayo brothers' interest in the emerging field, and they invited Robinson to Rochester for a job interview. After returning to the East Coast, he informed Will, "I seriously prefer to devote myself to thoracic surgery and its development, provided I can be given the facilities for carrying on its investigation both clinically and experimentally."[13]

During negotiations about salary, laboratory space, and assistants, Will assured the aspiring thoracic surgeon that he was not being recruited "with any idea that there would be any great advantage to us financially, but rather with a view of developing a new field of work."[14] There seemed to be an opportunity to develop the emerging field of thoracic surgery in Rochester. Less than 1 percent of the 10,166 operations performed at St. Mary's Hospital in 1913 involved the chest or chest wall, and only ten involved operating directly on the lung. None involved the heart.[15] Shortly before Christmas 1914, Robinson informed Will of his intention to

> increase the contributions of the clinic to progress in surgery...to impress visiting physicians and surgeons with the fact that thoracic lesions are more thoroughly studied and better treated in Rochester than elsewhere...to build up the slight reputation which I have possibly already acquired in connection with thoracic surgery and to increase the number of consultations thus adding eventually to the income of the clinic...to write and publish the first edition of a volume on thoracic surgery...to carry on animal experimental research....[and] to perfect an ideal intra-tracheal apparatus [for anesthesia] which shall incorporate the best features of those now in use including my own.[16]

The thirty-nine-year-old surgeon from the Northeast was appointed head of a new section of thoracic surgery at the Mayo Clinic in January 1915.

Robinson spoke about the surgical therapy of chest diseases to a group of internists at the annual American Medical Association meeting in 1916. Acknowledging that much had been written about the clinical picture, pathology, and bacteriology of chest diseases, the Mayo surgeon argued that advances in therapy required collaboration: "No region in the body demands the combined efforts of physician and surgeon more than the pleural cavity. The internist occasionally needs the surgeon, and the surgeon never ceases to require the conservative help of the physician. Therefore, kindly regard us thoracic surgeons as your servants rather than as your substitutes, as your consultants rather than your competitors." In addition to promoting cooperation, he championed specialization: "The thoracic cavity is too treacherous a region to become the scene of pastime surgery."[17] Thoracic surgery was not a pastime for Robinson—it was a passion. But World War I and illness changed his life and shifted his career path.

Robinson moved to California in October 1917, after he was appointed chief of surgery at the US Army's Letterman General Hospital. The conflict ended thirteen months later, but it took time for many doctors to resume their prewar activities or to settle into new positions. In 1922 members of the American Association for Thoracic Surgery listened to Robinson's presidential address on the present status and future prospects of thoracic surgery. But someone else read his speech, which opened with an apology for his absence.[18] Sickness had sidelined the surgeon during the war. Shortly after arriving in San Francisco, he developed pneumonia. He moved to Santa Barbara, hoping the Southern California climate would reduce recurrences of bronchitis and pneumonia.

In 1923 Robinson explained that self-preservation had trumped ambition: "In practicing surgery in a small community, I am resigning all hopes of distinction in my profession. Better health is my consolation, however."[19] It is impossible to predict how Robinson might have influenced the development of lung and heart surgery at the Mayo Clinic after World War I if he had not become sick and had returned to Rochester. No other Mayo surgeon would take a real interest in operating on the heart for more than a quarter century after his departure. Edward Churchill, longtime chief of surgery at Massachusetts General Hospital, did speculate about Robinson's decision to leave that institution. He claimed that his hospital "might early have been the creative center for thoracic surgery on this continent" if Robinson had remained in Boston.[20]

The Challenge of Replacing Samuel Robinson

Carl Hedblom, a Harvard medical graduate who had trained with Robinson in Rochester, was appointed head of Mayo's thoracic surgery section in 1919. He helped cardiologist Fredrick Willius treat some patients with pericardial effusion, a condition in which fluid surrounds and may compress the heart, causing shortness of breath and, sometimes, death. In 1922 Hedblom published a report of nine patients who had had pericardial fluid removed by needle aspiration (pericardiocentesis). This was not a new procedure, but Hedblom's article was the first by a Mayo author to describe collaboration between a thoracic surgeon and a cardiologist in Rochester. Hedblom did not write other papers on heart-related surgery. His practice and publications focused on empyema, a collection of pus in the chest cavity caused by infection. This problem was especially common after the influenza epidemic of 1918.[21]

Hedblom was president of the American Association for Thoracic Surgery in 1924, when the group met in Rochester. His address on the evolution of thoracic surgery as a specialty dealt mainly with lung surgery, but he mentioned recent experiments that surgeons Duff Allen and Evarts Graham had done on animals at Washington University in St. Louis. The two men had invented a cardioscope, a metal tube that was designed to be inserted into the heart through an incision in the left atrial appendage. The end that was pushed into the beating, blood-filled heart contained a tiny light bulb covered by a convex lens that allowed the operator to see the mitral valve. Their goal was to develop an operation that might be used to treat certain types of heart valve disease in humans. Hedblom shared their hope that this novel approach would lead to the development of intracardiac surgery as a clinical procedure.[22] His career in Rochester, like Robinson's, was brief. He left the Mayo Clinic in 1924 to become chief of surgery at the University of Wisconsin.

Will Mayo asked thirty-five-year-old Stuart Harrington to succeed Hedblom as head of thoracic surgery. Known for being decisive, Will wasted no time in getting to the point with Harrington, who recalled years later:

Dr. Will Mayo called me to his office about 4:30 on a Friday afternoon in September, 1924, and told me I was head of thoracic surgery at the clinic. I asked him where Dr. Hedblom was, and he said he was leaving the clinic the following week, and I was to take charge of thoracic surgery immediately. As soon as I had recovered from my surprise and could realize the responsibility entailed, both to patients and the clinic, in entering a field of surgery in which I had had no training as well as no special interest, I remonstrated and told Dr. Mayo that I did not think I could accept the appointment but appreciated his confidence in offering me the position.... During our discussion that Friday afternoon, the situation became acute and serious, that is, for me, as at one point he gave me one hour to make my decision.[23]

Will Mayo's sixty-minute deadline stretched to sixty hours after his chauffeur told him it was time to drive to the Mississippi River for a weekend outing on his new 120-foot yacht. On Monday morning, Will embellished the offer. He told Harrington that Hedblom's former first assistant would teach him chest surgery techniques and the clinic would give him time and money to visit hospitals with active thoracic surgery programs.[24] A few days later, Will mentioned Hedblom's sudden departure to dozens of former Mayo trainees, who were in Rochester for their annual alumni meeting: "The Clinic should be prepared to lose its best men. We are glad to see Hedblom go to the University of Wisconsin, where he will be a great asset to the teaching staff."[25]

Harrington spent ten weeks in Europe in 1926, visiting a dozen surgical centers from London to Rome. During this trip, he watched hundreds of operations, but he saw very few chest procedures (and most of them were for treating pulmonary tuberculosis). When Harrington reported his European surgical expedition at a Mayo Clinic staff meeting in 1927, he did not mention seeing any operations involving the heart.[26] This omission is understandable because, as his predecessor Hedblom had said, "Thoracic surgery is largely concerned with infections of the pleural cavity and lung. Diseases of the chest wall, pericardium, and mediastinum are relatively infrequent."[27]

The Rise and Fall of Surgery for Mitral Valve Stenosis

While Stuart Harrington was overseas, Cleveland surgeons Elliott Cutler and Claude Beck were completing a textbook chapter on surgery of the heart and pericardium. The two men had moved recently from Boston's Peter Bent Brigham Hospital, where they had trained under Harvey Cushing, to Cleveland's Lakeside Hospital, where Cutler was now the chief of surgery. Cutler and Beck attributed recent interest in heart surgery to the "modern physiological school of medicine" and to animal experiments that some surgeons had done in an attempt to invent operations that might be performed on humans. "The road to the heart is now open," they boasted, "and a surgical attack in this field may be planned and carried out with some assurance of success."[28] Cushing informed Cutler that he considered their publication "simply A++; a great credit to you and Beck! Nothing so good about the surgery of the heart has ever been put together."[29]

Cutler and Beck declared the surgical road to the heart open in 1927, but almost no one would travel it for two decades. In large part, their optimism was based on two successful attempts to operate on patients with mitral valve stenosis. This disorder, a long-term complication of rheumatic fever, is the result of progressive thickening and fusion of the mitral valve leaflets. As the valve opening continues to shrink, it obstructs the flow of blood from the left atrium to the left ventricle. Patients with mitral stenosis develop progressive dyspnea (shortness of breath) with activity, as well as other symptoms. British cardiologist Carey Coombs had described the final stages of mitral stenosis in his 1924 book on rheumatic heart disease. In addition to disabling dyspnea, such patients develop cyanosis (bluish skin discoloration) due, in part, to low blood oxygen levels: "Usually it takes the form of pinkish-purple coloring of the cheeks, ears, lips, and tip of the nose. When the patient is actually moribund, the face is livid, cyanosis and pallor blending to bring about this result."[30]

Mayo cardiologist Fredrick Willius had shown how serious mitral stenosis was in a 1923 publication that described what happened to 470 patients with the problem who had been seen at the clinic during a six-year period. Mitral stenosis was a disease of young and middle-aged adults: 83 percent of the patients in Willius's series were between twenty-one and fifty years of age. And it was deadly: 37 percent of the patients died an average of sixteen months after having being evaluated at Mayo.[31]

In 1929 Cutler and Beck summarized the published world experience with mitral stenosis surgery. Ten patients had been operated on for the valve problem at six institutions. Despite the fact that 80 percent of the men and women died within a week of surgery, Cutler and Beck argued that "the mortality figures alone should not deter further investigation both clinical and experimental, since they are to be expected in the opening up of any new field for surgical endeavor."[32] Evarts Graham, who had operated on one of the patients with mitral stenosis who died, saw things differently. In 1935 he reflected on the 80 percent mortality rate in the series that Cutler and Beck had reported: "The results speak for themselves.... They clearly indicate that with our present knowledge the operation is at the present time not justified."[33] No one disagreed, and mitral stenosis surgery was abandoned until after World War II.[34]

The Growth of Thoracic Surgery in the 1930s

Thoracic surgery grew significantly during the 1930s, but the surgeons who did chest operations did not operate *inside* the heart. Evarts Graham and two associates published a 1,070-page book on surgical diseases of the chest in 1935, but only one of its twenty-two chapters dealt with operations involving the heart and pericardium.[35] Most of the book was devoted to surgery for various lung diseases. Graham recalled a quarter century later:

> As one who pioneered in the early work in chest surgery before there were transfusions and antibiotics it seems to me remarkable, looking back, that any of our patients survived the operations performed on them.... The high operative mortalities which accompanied our work constituted a vicious circle. The only patients referred to us were those who were in bad condition from chronic infections or from advanced development of their ailments. Our lack of conspicuous success with many of those about to die led in turn to our failure to obtain patients in good enough condition for the operations to justify any reasonable optimism in the surgical treatment of the given diseases. Thus the vicious circle went on.[36]

Despite Graham's grim retrospective assessment, the pace of non-cardiac chest surgery accelerated in the 1930s. In fact, he and his coauthors complained in the preface to their 1935 book that the "difficulty of keeping abreast with the newer developments in this rapidly expanding field has been so great that at times it has seemed to be insurmountable."[37]

The challenge of keeping up with a fast-growing field was addressed at a symposium on thoracic surgery training that was part of the 1936 meeting of the American Association for Thoracic Surgery that was held at the Mayo Clinic. Speaking in Rochester, Graham emphasized that not a single member of the organization was a full-time thoracic surgeon when it had been founded two decades earlier. But things were changing: "Now, there are a few, but as time goes on there will certainly be many."[38] Ethan Butler, a past president of the association, discussed the financial implications of specializing in thoracic surgery: "It is fair at this time to warn the young man who hopes to make thoracic surgery his one and only field of professional endeavor that 75 to 90 percent of all thoracic surgery must be done without hope or expectation of financial remuneration. Those, therefore, who engage in this work to the exclusion of all else must either be subsidized or independently wealthy."[39] Butler's admonition reflected economic conditions during the Depression and the fact that many of the patients that thoracic surgeons helped care for had tuberculosis or other diseases that led to disability and loss of employment.[40]

Mayo surgeon Stuart Harrington, overcoming his initial ambivalence about thoracic surgery, had become a major contributor to the field by the mid-1930s. He published almost fifty articles on the subject between 1925 and 1937, when he became president of the American Association for Thoracic Surgery. None of these papers dealt with the heart, however. On May 9, 1938, Harrington performed a daring cardiac operation at Mayo. The procedure, a partial pericardiectomy, involved peeling off part of a patient's pericardium (the fibrous sac surrounding the heart) that had become thickened and calcified. Partial pericardiectomy was risky and rarely attempted, and this one performed in Rochester was newsworthy. The *New York Times* ran a story in 1938 with the dramatic title: "Feels Heart Beat Again: Melbourne Man Has Stone Casing Cut Away at Mayo Clinic."[41] Harrington's patient, a twenty-seven-year-old Australian with chronic constrictive pericarditis, had deteriorated dramatically in recent months. He was profoundly weak, extremely breathless with almost any activity, and had severe swelling of his abdomen and legs.[42] The surgery was successful, and the man improved.

While the Australian was still hospitalized, Harrington operated on a second patient with constrictive pericarditis. This thirty-eight-year-old man's subjective symptoms and objective signs of heart disease were similar to those of the first patient. Before surgery, doctors used a needle to remove ten quarts of fluid from his massively swollen abdomen. When Harrington opened the man's chest to visualize his heart, he found a markedly thickened pericardium with calcium deposits that were more than one-half inch thick.

The operation was a success, but the patient's recovery was slow. After a month in the hospital, he was discharged without shortness of breath or swelling. Cardiologist Arlie Barnes, during a discussion of constrictive peri-carditis at a staff meeting, said the operation tested a surgeon's courage and skill. Speaking to an audience used to hearing about surgical successes at the Mayo Clinic, he exclaimed, "To see a young man hopelessly crippled by cardiac disease restored to a life of efficiency and happiness, as I believe will occur in this case, is as dramatic as anything one can conceive in medicine."[43] New types of operations for patients with heart disease were on the horizon, and they would be equally dramatic.

New Hope for Some Patients with Congenital Heart Disease

Canadian pathologist Maude Abbott's *Atlas of Congenital Cardiac Disease*, published by the American Heart Association in 1936, drew attention to a rare category of heart disorders that mainly affected children, adolescents, and young adults.[44] Thomas Dry joined Mayo's staff the same year that Abbott's book appeared. Born and trained in South Africa before complet-ing a fellowship in Rochester, Dry was the first cardiologist at the clinic with a special interest in congenital heart disease. In 1937 he published an article on the diagnosis of congenital heart disease in the *American Heart Journal*. It was an uncommon topic: just 4 percent of the articles in the journal that year were devoted to the subject. But Dry claimed that attitudes about congenital heart disease were changing.[45] The real change—one that made headlines—came less than a year later, when a senior surgical resident in Boston performed a new operation that was designed to protect a child from progressive disability and inevitable death.

On August 26, 1938, Robert Gross tightened a braided silk string around a blood vessel inside the left chest of a seven-year-old girl at Boston Children's Hospital. The vessel, the ductus arteriosus, connects the aorta and pulmo-nary artery. Before birth, blood flows through the ductus from the pulmo-nary artery to the aorta, bypassing the fetus's un-inflated, non-functioning lungs. The ductus almost always closes a few days after birth. If it remains patent (open), bloodstream infection, heart failure, and other life-threatening complications may develop.[46] Gross's patient, Lorraine Sweeney, recalled decades later, "I just was very, very weak. I couldn't do anything like other children. They used to go out and play hopscotch and jump rope and all that, and I used to watch them from the window."[47] Gross's procedure went well. Lorraine was able to sit in a chair the day after surgery and to walk around two days later.

Boston cardiologist Paul Dudley White had described Maude Abbott in 1936 as "the most important of the pioneers in establishing congenital heart disease as a living part of clinical medicine."[48] When she died four years later from a cerebral hemorrhage, congenital heart disease had just become a living part of clinical surgery. Abbott's last publication, which appeared in 1940, was a short book chapter on congenital heart defects. Reflecting real-time events, the chapter had two endings. Initially, she wrote that treatment "is necessarily confined to *preventive* and *palliative* measures, for remedial treatment cannot be applied to structural changes in the heart, unless, indeed, by surgical intervention, and this is still in the experimental stage."[49] But the next page told a different story. Surgery for congenital heart disease had just moved from the realm of experiments on animals into attempts to treat humans. Describing Gross's recent operation for patent ductus arteriosus as a brilliant achievement, Abbott declared that "a new era in the treatment of congenital cardiac disease has been inaugurated."[50]

Mayo surgeon Stuart Harrington heard Robert Gross describe his first four operations on patients with a patent ductus arteriosus at the 1939 meeting of the American Surgical Association. During the discussion, Gross's mentor Elliott Cutler congratulated him for plowing "a new furrow in the field of cardiac surgery." He predicted that the success of the ductus operation would stimulate other surgeons to try to develop procedures to treat different cardiac disorders. Cutler championed collaboration and emphasized that innovations depended, in part, on the context: "This type of forward work in surgery represents the things that come from centers where there can be, for the growing young surgeon, all facilities—the laboratory, the intelligent and courageous colleagues in his medical service, and the patients to work upon."[51]

Stuart Harrington remained in Rochester during World War II, and his thoracic surgery practice focused on diseases of the lung and esophagus. By the spring of 1944, however, he had operated on ten children with patent ductus arteriosus and two dozen adults with constrictive pericarditis. He presented his experience with the latter problem at that year's American Surgical Association meeting. Of the patients who had part of their pericardium removed, thirteen improved significantly, two improved moderately, and nine died (six in the hospital and three after discharge). The Mayo surgeon acknowledged that the 25 percent in-hospital mortality rate was high, but he contrasted it with the dismal prognosis of patients without surgery.[52]

One very visible physical sign of severe chronic constrictive pericarditis is cyanosis. This bluish skin tint (usually due to low blood oxygen concentration) is the defining characteristic of a major category of cardiovascular birth defects—cyanotic congenital heart disease. Alfred Blalock, chief of surgery at Johns Hopkins, was among those who heard Harrington speak at the 1944 American Surgical Association meeting in Chicago.[53] When he returned to Baltimore, Blalock was in the final stages of developing an operation designed to improve the survival of children born with a specific type of cyanotic congenital heart disease.

Pediatrician Helen Taussig, director of the Johns Hopkins Children's Cardiac Clinic, had stimulated Blalock's interest in the surgical treatment of cyanotic congenital heart disease. Impressed by Gross's patent ductus operation, she envisioned a procedure to treat severe pulmonary stenosis. The fundamental problem in pulmonary stenosis is reduced blood flow to the lungs, which results in low blood oxygen content, high red blood cell count, and cyanosis. Taussig knew that babies born with this heart defect (often part of a cluster of cardiac abnormalities termed "tetralogy of Fallot") deteriorated after their ductus arteriosus closed naturally after birth. Most infants with the condition died during the first six months, but some survived a few months longer.[54] She speculated that a patient's symptoms might be improved and his or her life might be prolonged if a surgeon created a vascular conduit between the aorta and the pulmonary artery. This would provide a channel for blood to bypass the tight pulmonary valve and circulate through the lungs, where oxygen was exchanged for carbon dioxide.[55]

When Taussig discussed her concept for treating severe pulmonary stenosis with Blalock, she spoke to a surgeon with unusual sophistication in cardiac anatomy and physiology. He also had the advantage of a highly skilled personal research assistant. Vivien Thomas, an African-American who had dropped out of college during the Depression, had worked in Blalock's surgical laboratory at the Vanderbilt Hospital in Nashville. Blalock had brought Thomas with him to Baltimore, where he played a vital role in developing an operation in the animal laboratory that might accomplish Taussig's goal.[56]

The Blalock-Taussig (or blue baby) operation involved attaching the left subclavian artery to the left pulmonary artery to create a vascular channel that carried more blood to the lungs for oxygenation. Performed on blood vessels outside the heart rather than on the organ itself, the operation could transform frail cyanotic children with severely limited exercise capacity into active youngsters. The sudden skin color change—from blue to pink—was obvious to those standing around the operating table.

On November 29, 1944, Blalock operated on sixteen-month-old Eileen Saxon, who weighed just nine pounds and was critically ill as a result of tetralogy of Fallot. In May 1945 the *Journal of the American Medical Association* published Blalock and Taussig's detailed report of Saxon's operation and two others the surgeon had peformed.[57] Baltimore physician Halsey Barker boasted in a 1946 editorial, "Brighter blood for blue babies! Yes, and brighter horizons for the anguished parents of these unfortunate youngsters, the majority of whom succumbed to anoxemia or cerebral thrombosis early in childhood after varying periods of chronic invalidism while the medical profession sat helplessly by.... At the present writing, the conclusion is justified that the operation may be regarded as a God-send to the blue baby."[58]

Life magazine informed the public about "blue baby research" in a 1949 photo-essay that described seven-year-old Michael Schirmer's experience. Before surgery, his "lips and fingernails were always blue, and if he tried to move around too much his whole body turned bluish. He could not even walk across a room without huffing and puffing; he had to be carried up and down stairs and wheeled in a buggy on the street. He had a heart defect that kept his body from getting enough oxygen, and he seemed destined to be a cripple until a premature death." But this would not be Michael's fate. After Blalock operated on him, he was described as healthy.[59]

Surgery for Heart Disease at Mayo and Other Centers

Doctors interested in heart disease recognized the Blalock-Taussig operation as a major breakthrough. Although all forms of cyanotic congenital heart disease were very rare (about 1.4 cases per 1,000 live births), scores of surgeons traveled to Baltimore to watch Blalock operate on patients who had been referred to him from across the continent and from overseas.[60] One early visitor was Stuart Harrington's junior colleague, O. Theron (Jim) Clagett, who would perform Mayo's first Blalock-Taussig procedure. He had joined the staff in 1940, after completing his surgical fellowship at the clinic. Clagett wrote to Blalock in October 1946, saying how much he had enjoyed his recent visit to Baltimore. Then his tone changed: "It is a disappointment to have to tell you that my first attempt at anastomosis for pulmonary stenosis was a failure. The child lived only about four days and died of what was apparently pulmonary congestion."[61]

Blalock, whose mortality rate for his first 110 operations was 23 percent, responded sympathetically: "I hope you will not be disappointed with your fatality in the tetralogy group. This happens to everyone, and I know that you will get a lot of gratifying results. I am very anxious that you should not be discouraged by this single fatality."[62] Clagett wrote back, "I certainly will try not to be disappointed with the loss of my first attempt with tetralogy. There are a couple of others here now that I may have an opportunity to try."[63] Death was a constant companion of the surgical pioneers who hoped to save lives by inventing or performing new operations on patients with serious heart disease.

Mayo cardiologist Thomas Dry opened a symposium on tetralogy of Fallot at a 1947 staff meeting by reciting the traditional fatalistic view of cyanotic congenital heart disease: "Why worry about an anatomic diagnosis when it is impossible to determine the diagnosis accurately, when lesions are frequently multiple and when there is nothing to be done about the condition anyway?"[64] But the invention of the Blalock-Taussig operation had changed all of this. The tetralogy symposium, published in the *Proceedings of the Staff Meetings of the Mayo Clinic* (hereafter *Proceedings*), revealed to the medical world that Mayo had joined the effort to bring new surgical treatments to some patients with congenital heart disease.

In his talk Jim Clagett characterized the Blalock-Taussig operation as a compelling example of so-called physiologic surgery, which referred to operations that were designed to improve the function of organs that cannot be removed. He applauded the Johns Hopkins group's accomplishment: "They saw the problem, studied the physiologic changes that had resulted from abnormal function, developed a theoretic solution based on physiologic principles, proved that their theories were correct in studies on animals and finally applied the technics successfully to the human being."[65] Clagett characterized his own experience with the Blalock-Taussig operation as meager, but he was optimistic about the future of cardiovascular surgery. Citing the invention of operations to treat patients with patent ductus arteriosus, tetralogy of Fallot, and coarctation (narrowing) of the aorta, he predicted that procedures would be developed to treat other types of congenital heart disease.[66]

In July 1947, shortly after the tetralogy symposium, Clagett got a firsthand report on the emerging field of cardiac surgery from Robert Glover, who had completed his surgical training in Rochester six months earlier. Clagett considered Glover one of Mayo's best fellows and was happy that he had won the J. William White Scholarship, which subsidized educational travel. Previous winners had spent time in Europe, but Glover could not follow that path because of the disruption caused by World War II. His American itinerary reflected his decision to devote himself to thoracic surgery, which still dealt almost exclusively with non-cardiac procedures. But Glover's summary of his travels revealed his enthusiasm for the emerging field of heart surgery.

When Glover sent his report to Clagett in the summer of 1947, he was preparing to join thoracic surgeon Charles Bailey's private practice in Philadelphia. The Mayo-trained surgeon soon found himself in the middle of a whirlwind of surgical innovation.[67] Clagett sent a copy of Glover's summary of his eight-city surgical safari to Blalock. He explained in an accompanying letter, "I thought you might be interested in this report since it is an interesting survey of thoracic surgical centers in the United States and particularly because of his reference to the work he saw in Baltimore."[68] Glover, referring to Blalock and Taussig, exclaimed, "Everything at Johns Hopkins Hospital seems to revolve around the work of these two investigators. . . . They have a vast source of material consisting mostly of cyanotic children." This condition was very rare, but the Baltimore institution had become a magnet for children thought to be candidates for the new operation, which Blalock had performed almost four hundred times by the time Glover visited. "In his hands it is beautiful to behold," Glover exclaimed after having watched the Hopkins surgeon operate on eight children with tetralogy of Fallot.[69]

Turning from surgical treatment to preoperative diagnosis, Glover was impressed with pediatric cardiologist Helen Taussig's evaluation of children with congenital heart disease. He found her routine use of fluoroscopy to evaluate a patient's heart and great vessels fascinating because it was not a standard procedure in Rochester. John Parkinson, a leading British cardiologist, had claimed a dozen years earlier that fluoroscopy was "as useful as the electrocardiograph and a necessary complement to it."[70]

Mayo cardiologist Howard Burchell, who had studied with Parkinson and used the X-ray technique in England before World War II, recalled that "fluoroscopy of the heart never flourished at the Mayo Clinic."[71] Mayo's cardiologists did not perform fluoroscopy because the clinic's radiologists controlled all of the X-ray equipment. But the cardiologists and the radiologists who were especially interested in the heart did interact regularly. This arrangement reflected the clinic's tradition of specialization and cooperation, as well as its leaders' resistance to the duplication of technologies.[72]

A Few Surgeons Begin Operating Inside the Heart

Robert Glover spent almost a month in Boston, where he observed Robert Gross perform patent ductus operations. But Gross's procedure, like the Blalock-Taussig operation, involved surgery on vessels outside the heart that were designed to alter the flow of blood through the organ. When he was in Boston, Glover also met Dwight Harken, who was very eager to begin operating *inside* the heart. Harken was a 1936 Harvard Medical School graduate who had done postgraduate training at Boston City Hospital and London's Royal Brompton Hospital, which focused on patients with diseases of the chest.

Harken was working in the surgical research laboratory at Boston City Hospital in 1942, when he submitted a manuscript on experimental intracardiac surgery. In the published article, he predicted that surgery inside the heart had "vast possibilities" once it was "rendered safe for the patient and technically simple." Harken explained that he had "carried out a variety of intracardiac maneuvers on cats and dogs before our laboratory activities were altered by the war."[73] This statement suggested that Harken expected the war to interfere with his goal of developing intracardiac surgery. In fact, the opposite would be true.

On June 10, 1944, four days after D-Day, the first patient was admitted to the US Army's 160th General Hospital, which had been set up in Quonset huts in the English countryside, ninety miles west of London. Harken, who was in charge of the hospital's thoracic surgery unit, decided to tackle a problem that affected 15 percent of the patients admitted to the special section. These soldiers had bullets and other foreign bodies lodged in their chests.[74]

Harken rationalized the risk of removing these battle remnants from in and around the heart by citing complications, such as embolization of them or cardiac rupture, which might occur if they were left alone.

Harken, a very aggressive and supremely self-confident surgeon, removed foreign bodies from 134 men, all of whom survived. In one case, he extracted thirteen objects from inside a patient's blood-filled, beating heart. Another case revealed Harken's tenacity. A twenty-nine-year-old infantryman had been hit by a mortar shell fragment in France in July 1944. In an attempt to remove it, Harken cut a small opening in the soldier's heart on three occasions between August 1944 and February 1945. The first time, he almost retrieved the foreign body from the right ventricle, when it "was pulled from the forceps by the wriggling myocardium" and disappeared. Subsequent X-rays showed that it had fallen back into the right atrium. Harken performed a second operation to retrieve the fragment, but "it escaped again." Finally, during the third operation, he pulled it from the right ventricular cavity "with only moderate difficulty." A photograph of the soldier recovering from the final procedure showed him standing with a healed incision under his left breast.[75] The many daring operations that Harken performed in the Quonset hut hospital disproved once and for all the notion that it was too risky to cut a small hole in the heart's wall in order to operate inside it.

Harken's experiences in England, together with wartime advances in anesthetic techniques and blood transfusion, encouraged him to re-examine the possibility of operating on patients with mitral stenosis, something that his mentor Elliott Cutler had tried and abandoned two decades earlier. Glover, in his report to Clagett, explained that when he met Harken, the Boston surgeon "had just performed his first human attempt at cardiac valvulotomy."[76] This procedure involved cutting away parts of the thickened mitral valve with a small instrument termed a valvulotome.

Although Harken's patient, a twenty-six-year-old man with severe mitral stenosis, died the day after surgery, Glover remained optimistic. Noting that Harken had done many heart procedures in animals, the Mayo-trained surgeon predicted that "within the next few years many developments in this field can be expected from him."[77] Seventeen months later, in November 1948, the *New England Journal of Medicine* published a detailed report by Harken that described two patients on whom he had operated for mitral stenosis. The first one, mentioned by Glover, did not survive. The second patient, a twenty-seven-year-old man, improved dramatically after surgery on June 16, 1948.[78]

On June 10, 1948, six days before Harken operated on his second patient in Boston, Glover had assisted Charles Bailey in performing a successful operation on a woman with mitral stenosis in Philadelphia. Three weeks later, Glover sent Clagett his White Traveling Scholarship report, which he ended with an expression of gratitude: "This opportunity came as the happy climax to a most delightful and profitable period of training under the Mayo Foundation, the results of which I am sure will influence and guide me constantly in my future career."[79] Clagett informed Blalock, "I am sure Dr. Glover is a man that we will be hearing more from."[80] The news would come from Philadelphia, where Glover had just helped Bailey make surgical history.

Robert Glover played a key role in Charles Bailey's first successful mitral stenosis operation in 1948, but the Philadelphia surgeon's passion for the procedure had been inspired by a personal tragedy a quarter century earlier. Bailey recalled his father's struggle with mitral stenosis: "He died when I was only twelve, and when I saw him coughing up blood into a basin as my mother tried to soothe him I just stared at this awful exhibition of how mitral stenosis can terminate a young man's life."[81] Bailey's 1932 Hahnemann Medical College yearbook entry is revealing: "Originality, enthusiasm, individuality.... Hardly had he shaken hands with the circulatory system before an artificial heart and aorta had scrambled forth from his nimble brain. So far no surgeon has been found with sufficient intrepidity to do the transplantation, so Charlie will probably have to do it himself."[82]

Bailey had performed experiments on animals before he first operated on a patient with mitral stenosis in November 1945. The surgeon had hoped to use a tiny knife attached to his finger to open the narrowed valve's fused leaflets, but the man died on the operating table before he got to this point. By the spring of 1948, Bailey had operated on two more patients, but each one died within a week after surgery.[83] His intrepid nature was evident on June 10, 1948, when he performed his fourth and fifth mitral stenosis operations at two Philadelphia hospitals. The first patient died on the operating table at Philadelphia General Hospital, but the second patient, a twenty-four-year-old woman, lived. She was hospitalized on Glover's service at Episcopal Hospital, where the Mayo-trained surgeon assisted Bailey with the operation.[84]

One week after surgery, the woman was well enough to accompany Bailey on a 1,000-mile train trip to Chicago. Bailey introduced her to the audience during his lecture on mitral stenosis surgery at the annual American College of Chest Physicians meeting. Evarts Graham, who had attempted a single mitral valve operation a quarter century earlier, was there. After Bailey finished speaking, the senior thoracic surgeon commented on what he had just seen and heard: "It is thrilling to be here this afternoon and see this patient demonstrated by Dr. Bailey. I congratulate him very much on his success."[85]

Horace Smithy of Charleston, South Carolina, also stood up to discuss Bailey's presentation. Announcing that he had operated on seven patients with mitral stenosis, of whom five had survived, Smithy predicted that more experience with this type of surgery would lead to better results and a lower mortality rate.[86] He was one of the doctors profiled in a November 1948 *Saturday Evening Post* article on recent breakthroughs in cardiac surgery. The subtitle telegraphed a welcome message: "For the Millions Whose

Hearts Have Been Crippled by Disease, There Is New Hope."[87] Most of the patient stories in the article focused on surgery for congenital heart defects, but one discussed Smithy's experience operating on adult patients with mitral stenosis.

Magazine readers learned that Smithy had "slipped a valve knife of his own design into the heart of frail twenty-four-year-old Betty Lee Woolridge of Canton, Ohio, and snipped away part of her thickened mitral valve."[88] Woolridge, Smithy's first patient, had begged him to operate on her because she was incapacitated by severe breathlessness and other symptoms of advanced mitral stenosis: "Couldn't you find some way to even help me? You won't be losing anything. It will be me. I am taking and asking for the chance. . . . Experiment on me, and I will do my part or even more."[89] Smithy operated. Woolridge survived, and her symptoms improved dramatically. The *Saturday Evening Post* writer explained that the thirty-four-year-old South Carolina surgeon had subsequently operated on six other patients. Although two of his seven patients died, the survivors were much improved. A photograph shows Woolridge shaking Smithy's hand as she climbs up the steps to the airplane that would fly her home to Ohio.[90]

Mayo Enters the Emerging Field of Intracardiac Surgery

Mayo thoracic surgeons Stuart Harrington and Jim Clagett did not want to operate inside the heart themselves, but they did want their institution to get involved in this emerging field of endeavor. Cardiologist Arlie Barnes was chair of the Board of Governors in the fall of 1948, when it approved their proposal that Mayo should appoint an ad hoc committee "to study the problems associated with cardiovascular diseases and surgical treatment."[91] The group would include Barnes's protégé Howard Burchell, physiologist Earl Wood, pathologist Jesse Edwards, radiologist David Pugh, and surgeon William Seybold. They were all young men. Burchell, at forty-one, was the oldest. Heart surgery was a new field, and almost all of its pioneers were in their thirties. The Mayo board, committed to developing a first-class program, conceded that the venture would involve "experimental work which will require considerable time and may make it necessary that these men be relieved of some of their routine work." Careful planning and extensive experience in the animal laboratory were considered critical components of a strategy to reduce the risk of performing new cardiac procedures on patients.[92]

John Kirklin was chosen to launch Mayo's intracardiac surgery program. The thirty-one-year-old surgeon had been raised a few blocks from the clinic, where his father Byrl had been head of radiology for several years. He had entered Harvard Medical School in 1938, less than a month after Robert Gross closed Lorraine Sweeney's patent ductus arteriosus at the Harvard-affiliated

Boston Children's Hospital. Gross had a profound impact on Kirklin during his medical school years.[93]

In the summer of 1939, Kirklin went fishing in northern Wisconsin with his father and Arlie Barnes, who were close friends. A half century later, he recalled conversations with the cardiologist: "I would talk to Dr. Barnes about cardiac surgery while waiting for the muskies to strike. He felt an exciting era was ahead when many of the maladies that were unsuccessfully treated would be corrected by surgery."[94] Kirklin graduated at the top of his class at Harvard, where he won the Henry Christian Prize, which was given to the senior medical student "who has displayed diligence and notable scholarship in his studies and offers great promise for the future."[95] This prediction would prove to be true.

Demand for doctors during World War II led to the so-called 9-9-9 plan to accelerate medical training in the United States. Rather than spending one year each as an intern, resident, and senior resident after medical school, a physician in the program devoted nine months to each stage of postgraduate training. After an internship at the University of Pennsylvania, Kirklin returned to Rochester for a nine-month surgical residency at Mayo. He was then sent for a five-week course in neurology and neurosurgery at the University of Pennsylvania before being assigned to O'Reilly General Hospital in Missouri, a 500-bed wartime neurosurgical facility.

When Kirklin resumed his residency in general surgery at Mayo in the fall of 1946, he hoped to get additional training with Robert Gross at Boston Children's Hospital. Clagett was enthusiastic about the plan, and the Mayo board approved a six-month leave of absence to begin in July 1948.[96] Kirklin's future at the clinic seemed secure. When the board approved his leave, they also agreed to make him Clagett's first assistant when he returned to Rochester. The strategy was to groom an individual to lead the Mayo Clinic into the emerging field of heart surgery, but there was no sense of urgency. For two years, Kirklin devoted most of his time to performing routine general and thoracic surgical procedures. He also worked in the experimental laboratory, where he gained experience operating inside the hearts of animals. In October 1950 Mayo's board approved Kirklin's request to take a ten-day trip to Boston, Philadelphia, and Baltimore to observe operations on the heart and aorta.[97]

Cardiac surgery pioneers Dwight Harken, Charles Bailey, Robert Glover, and Alfred Blalock acknowledged in their early publications that success or failure, life or death, depended on more than their own technical skills and an individual patient's condition.[98] One specific individual in the operating room played a critical role—the person who administered anesthesia and checked the patient's vital signs. This is why anesthesiologist John Pender accompanied Kirklin to the East Coast as he prepared to begin operating on patients with mitral stenosis.[99]

Personal contacts ensured that the men from Mayo would be welcome. Kirklin knew Harken from the time he had spent in Boston, and he and Glover had trained together in Rochester. Clagett's friendship with Blalock meant that his junior colleague would not be lost in the swarm of doctors who came to Johns Hopkins to watch heart surgery. Decades later, when Kirklin recalled the period of preparation before he performed his first mitral stenosis operation, he claimed that he had "learned a lot about it, lived and breathed it."[100]

Kirklin performed the first intracardiac operation in Rochester in November 1950, a few days after returning from the East Coast. He used Bailey and Glover's commissurotomy approach for treating mitral stenosis, which involved inserting his index finger into the patient's left atrium through a small incision in the atrial appendage. Kirklin used a tiny knife attached to his finger to separate the fused mitral valve leaflets so blood could flow through them more freely.[101] British surgeon Russell Brock, who had pioneered heart surgery in Europe, wrote that year: "The finger, once within the atrium, rapidly finds the mitral orifice; its shape, the consistency of its edges and of the valve cusps, and the presence or absence of calcification can all be noted; it is almost as if one sees with the finger."[102] Feeling was not the same as seeing—but it had to suffice until methods to temporarily stop the flow of blood through the heart were developed in the early and mid-1950s (which would allow a surgeon to see and work inside the organ).[103]

Surgerical Innovations Stimulate Demand for Catheterization

The advent of surgical techniques to treat some types of congenital heart disease and mitral stenosis stimulated the development of cardiac catheterization as an adjunct to traditional diagnostic techniques, such as physical examination, electrocardiography, and X-ray. There was very little justification for performing the procedure until a patient could be offered surgical treatment for a congenital defect or an acquired valve disorder. Blalock, familiar with cardiac catheterization as a result of the wartime shock study he had coordinated, hired Richard Bing late in 1945 to organize a catheterization laboratory at Johns Hopkins.[104]

Richard Bing, a native of Germany, had been awarded his medical degree in Europe and had received additional training in physiology in New York City, where he had watched André Cournand perform catheterizations at Bellevue Hospital. Blalock stressed the importance of accurate diagnosis because the blue-baby operation was risky and of no value in some types of cyanotic congenital heart disease. In 1946 he reported that 25 of the first 110 patients on whom he had performed the procedure did not survive.[105] After one child died, Blalock's chief resident noted in his diary that the diagnosis was wrong. An autopsy showed that the child had transposition of the great vessels, a very rare type of congenital heart defect that would not be helped by the blue-baby operation.[106] This incident highlighted the limitations of standard diagnostic approaches.

When Robert Glover visited Johns Hopkins in 1947, Earl Wood had just established Mayo's catheterization laboratory. Although Glover had not seen a catheterization in Rochester, he was impressed by the ingenious methods that Bing used in Baltimore to help diagnose congenital heart defects. The postwar inventors of mitral stenosis surgery also recognized the value of catheterization. Boston surgeon Dwight Harken declared in 1948 that performing operations "of such an experimental and hazardous nature in a complex physiologic situation without complete, objective studies is entirely unjustified."[107] Lewis Dexter, who had introduced catheterization in that city three years earlier, recalled that Harken "would have loved for me to have been able to catheterize every patient.... He was a pioneer, and we were running behind him trying to keep up with him."[108] Collaboration among the pioneers of catheterization and heart surgery inspired innovations in both fields.

Mid-Century Optimisim About the Treatment of Heart Disease

The future for cardiac patients looked promising at mid-century. Several things contributed to a sense of optimism. Chief among them was the fact that money to support cardiovascular research and to train investigators was beginning to flow from the National Heart Institute in Bethesda, Maryland, to academic medical centers across the country. The American Heart Association's campaign to raise funds for cardiovascular research was beginning to pay off. In 1950 Arlie Barnes reviewed *You and Your Heart*, a book that four leaders of the association had written for the general public.[109] The volume recorded past progress and future prospects in the treatment of heart disease, a problem that touched almost every American directly or indirectly. At the time, about a third of all deaths in Minnesota, like the rest of the nation, were due to heart disease.[110] Barnes reinforced the book's positive message, explaining that readers who had heart disease "will learn that often their prospects are much better than they expected."[111]

In a 1952 *Reader's Digest* article on heart surgery, a doctor described watching Robert Glover operate on a patient with mitral stenosis in Philadelphia: "A frail wisp of a woman lay on her right side on the operating table. For several years this patient had gone steadily downhill." The woman had become bedridden, but if her surgery was successful "she stood an excellent chance of being restored to good health." Another patient's story reinforced this hopeful message. A thirty-two-year-old woman was so weak before surgery that "she could not climb a flight of stairs; she now does housework, shops, bowls, and dances."[112] The transformation of a young woman who could not climb stairs into one who danced and bowled surely sounded like a miracle.

The *Reader's Digest* story of the woman reanimated by heart surgery paralleled the portrayal of patients who were almost immobilized by rheumatoid arthritis until they were treated with a new drug at the Mayo Clinic beginning in 1948. The focus of the Mayo doctors who first administered an adrenal cortical steroid, which they named cortisone, was on rheumatoid arthritis rather than rheumatic heart disease.[113] Cortisone, like insulin and penicillin, was considered a wonder drug. Its remarkable and rapid effects on the limited joint motion and pain in patients who had been disabled by rheumatoid arthritis attracted a great deal of attention. Shortly after the initial report was published in the *Proceedings*, a *Life* magazine headline proclaimed: "Arthritis: Mayo Clinic Finds a Treatment for Man's Most Crippling Disease." Photographs by Alfred Eisenstaedt showed patients before and after treatment with cortisone. One patient who had been barely able to climb down stairs could "jauntily trot down steps" just eight days after first receiving the drug.[114]

A bright spotlight shone on Rochester in 1950 when rheumatologist Philip Hench and biochemist Edward Kendall shared the Nobel Prize in Physiology or Medicine with a Swiss chemist for their roles in the isolation and therapeutic use of cortisone. That year Surgeon General Leonard Scheele declared, "Medical historians of the future will probably mark the year 1949 as the beginning of a new era in medical research and practice, citing as the precipitating document the report of Hench, Kendall, Slocumb and Polley on the effects of cortisone in the treatment of rheumatoid arthritis."[115] Scheele's celebratory tone reflected his conviction that the discovery of cortisone's therapeutic potential by the Mayo group exemplified the benefits of combining laboratory research and clinical investigation that involved patients when searching for new cures.

Cardiologist Arlie Barnes thought it was possible that cortisone might reduce the risk of patients with acute rheumatic fever developing chronic heart valve disease, such as mitral stenosis. In 1949 he collaborated with Hench and Kendall in a clinical trial of the corticosteroid in three adolescents with acute rheumatic fever. Although the incidence of this serious acute illness was declining, it was still common. And its cardiac consequences could be deadly. The Mayo researchers, impressed by cortisone's apparently beneficial effect on the skeletal muscles and fibrous tissues of patients with rheumatoid arthritis, hoped that it would have a similar effect on the heart muscle and cardiac valves in patients with rheumatic fever.[116]

The three patients they treated with cortisone had typical signs and symptoms of acute rheumatic fever, including an elevated temperature, rapid heart rate, multi-joint arthritis, and cardiac involvement (evidenced by heart murmurs and electrocardiographic abnormalities). Similar to the situation with rheumatoid arthritis, the early results were impressive. Twice daily shots of cortisone resulted in the rapid disappearance of fever, tachycardia, arthritis, and electrocardiographic abnormalities. But the Rochester researchers cautioned that these encouraging effects did not prove that cortisone could prevent chronic injury to the valves or heart muscle.

As clinical investigators in other institutions gained experience with cortisone, there was increasing concern about its obvious side effects and uncertain long-term benefits. These issues were discussed at a three-day symposium on rheumatic fever at the University of Minnesota, which Barnes attended in the fall of 1951.[117] To help sort out cortisone's benefits and risks, the American Heart Association, the Medical Research Council of Great Britain, the National Heart Institute, and other entities launched an international multicenter randomized clinical trial (which was one of the first examples of this research strategy). Although cortisone reduced fever and joint pain, there was no evidence that it cured rheumatic fever or prevented its long-term cardiac complications. Despite disappointment over the drug's apparent lack of benefit in acute rheumatic fever, it was shown to be helpful in other conditions, such as the so-called collagen diseases.[118] Meanwhile, the search for new surgical approaches for patients with serious heart disease intensified.

John Kirklin, who had watched the cortisone story unfold in Rochester, marveled at how rapidly heart surgery was evolving at mid-century. "This field of surgery has fired the imagination of all engaged in it," he exclaimed in 1952. "In many instances a severely handicapped patient can be restored to a healthy, useful existence by means of a properly executed surgical procedure. Although the heartaches of this type of work are occasionally bitter, the rewards can be great."[119] The developing field of cardiac surgery was poised for a sudden growth spurt in the mid-1950s as a result of innovations that would allow surgeons to see and operate inside the heart. Kirklin, who had followed the path of the pioneers of mitral stenosis surgery, would be a world leader in the emerging field of what would be termed open-heart surgery.

Pioneering Open-Heart Surgery at the University of Minnesota and the Mayo Clinic

Operations introduced in the 1940s gave a few children born with heart defects and some adults with acquired mitral valve stenosis a chance to live better and longer lives. But the scope of what came to be called closed-heart surgery was severely limited because there was no way to open the vital organ in order to see and operate inside it. Expanding the boundaries of cardiac surgery would require stopping the flow of life-sustaining blood through the beating heart that pumped it throughout the body. In the early 1950s, about two dozen surgeons in North America and Europe were trying to develop technologies and techniques that would allow them to operate inside the heart. Using very different approaches, teams at the University of Minnesota and the Mayo Clinic proved that what would be termed open-heart surgery could be done with an acceptable mortality rate.

Inventing Ways to See and Operate Inside the Beating Heart

The introduction of open-heart surgery into practice had major implications for the care of patients with heart disease and for the careers of cardiologists and cardiac surgeons.[1] Several names were attached to the technology that allowed surgeons to perform open-heart surgery. The phrase "heart-lung machine" highlighted the two organs involved. And the term "pump-oxygenator" described the two physiological processes that a purpose-built machine temporarily took over for the heart and lungs: pumping blood through the body and the lungs (where carbon dioxide would be exchanged for oxygen). Surgeons, medical scientists, and the media often used the terms "heart-lung machine" and "pump-oxygenator" interchangeably.

Regardless of the term, the principle was the same. A machine served as a temporary substitute for the two vital organs that work in harmony to circulate oxygen-rich blood throughout the body. A pump that substituted for the muscular contraction of the heart was wedded to an apparatus that replaced the respiratory function of the lungs. This technology would maintain the circulation of the blood for upward of thirty minutes, allowing a surgeon to cut open the heart and operate inside it. But there was another challenge. Blood is opaque—it had to be cleared from the heart's chambers so the operator could see the organ's interior structures. This was accomplished by clamping the venae cavae, the two large veins that enter the right atrium and return blood to the heart after it circulates through the body.[2]

Philadelphia surgeon John Gibbon Jr. had begun trying to invent a pump-oxygenator in the mid-1930s. In 1939 he reported using one to take over the functions of the heart and lungs in cats. His method involved a continuous process of withdrawing blood from a peripheral vein, passing it through an oxygenator, and returning the oxygen-rich blood to the animal through a peripheral artery. A few cats survived several months after his apparatus had circulated their blood for as long as twenty-five minutes. Shifting his gaze to humans and the future, Gibbon predicted, "If the flow of blood through the heart and lungs could be safely stopped for 30 minutes, it is conceivable that a new field of cardiac surgery might be developed."[3] Military service during World War II interrupted Gibbon's research, which he resumed in 1946.

The public read about more and more medical breakthroughs at mid-century, when it seemed that researchers were transforming science fiction into nonfiction science on a regular basis. *Life* magazine, a weekly periodical read by millions of Americans, published several medical articles with large and dramatic photographs each year. A story in the May 1950 issue, "Artificial Heart: Mechanical Device Substitutes for Living Organ," highlighted Gibbon's work. The writer described the heart as modern surgery's most important unexplored frontier: "Surgeons have excised lungs, spliced nerves, even probed the brain; but the danger of death from circulatory failure is so great that only rarely is the inner heart exposed. In the near future, however, surgeons may be able to do this routinely with the aid of the world's first mechanical heart and lungs. This robot, a gleaming, stainless steel cabinet as big as a piano, will soon be tested on humans." When it was perfected, a surgeon would be able to "expose and repair damage inside a virtually quiet, bloodless heart."[4] There was no denying that the closed-heart surgery technique to treat mitral stenosis that Dwight Harken, Charles Bailey, and others had developed in the late 1940s helped a specific group of patients. But the prospect of a technology that would allow open-heart surgery was very exciting.

When the *Life* magazine article about John Gibbon's animal research appeared in 1950, Mayo Clinic thoracic surgeon Jim Clagett was on his way to Adelaide, Australia, where he would lecture on recent developments in cardiovascular surgery. After describing operations developed recently for a few types of rare congenital heart defects, he mentioned Gibbon's research.

Clagett, who had introduced the Blalock-Taussig blue-baby procedure at Mayo four years earlier, predicted, "If ever it should be possible to construct a mechanical heart-lung system that temporarily could take over the functions of the heart and lungs, there would be practically no limit to the surgical procedures that could be performed on the heart and great vessels." The Mayo surgeon closed his 1950 talk with an unintentional play on words: "I have not the vision to predict the future but I have the faith to believe that the great days of surgery are ahead." In fact, the future of cardiac surgery would be all about vision—seeing inside the heart.[5] Clagett would never perform open-heart surgery, but his protégé John Kirklin would introduce the procedure at Mayo five years later.

Three influential Mayo surgeons heard Gibbon present an update on his heart-lung machine project at the annual meeting of the American Surgical Association in the spring of 1951. Charlie Mayo's son, Charles W. (Chuck) Mayo, Will Mayo's son-in-law Waltman Walters, and James Priestley were also members of the clinic's Board of Governors.[6] Gibbon described an improved apparatus that had been designed and built by the International Business Machine Corporation (IBM). Much work remained, however, because two-thirds of the dogs he had experimented on died while the technology substituted for their hearts and lungs or shortly afterward. Moreover, these preliminary experiments did not involve operating inside a dog's heart. Gibbon knew that this next step would have to be accomplished safely in animals before anyone attempted to use the apparatus in operations on humans.[7]

The First Attempts to Perform Open-Heart Surgery in Humans

University of Minnesota surgeon Clarence Dennis spoke after Gibbon at the meeting in Washington, D.C. The preliminary program did not include the last five words that appeared in the published version of his talk: "Development of a Pump-oxygenator to Replace the Heart and Lungs; an Apparatus Applicable to Human Patients, *and Application to One Case*."[8] On April 5, 1951, eight days before the meeting, Dennis had used a pump-oxygenator to operate inside the heart of a six-year-old girl who became severely short of breath with any exertion and was "failing rapidly" as a result of a large atrial septal defect. Dennis, whose group at the university had spent four years developing the apparatus, assured his audience that the operation had been "carefully planned and rehearsed in the laboratory during dog perfusions ahead of time."[9]

The heart-lung machine supported the little girl's circulation for forty minutes while Dennis tried to close the hole in the septum between her left and right atria. But problems led to massive blood loss that was followed by heart failure and death on the operating table. Trying to frame this child's death in a positive light, Dennis explained, "The ultimate loss of the patient does not negate the fact that the apparatus proved adequate for the purpose, because it provides promise of a useful tool in further cases, and because much valuable information has been gleaned."[10] Doctors who heard Dennis speak knew that transferring experimental cardiac surgery procedures from the animal laboratory to the operating room was risky. The fact that the original focus of open-heart surgery was on fixing congenital defects—closing abnormal holes between the heart's chambers—meant that almost all of the patients operated on were children.

Surgical pioneers portrayed—and the public perceived—new heart operations as bold attempts to save lives that would inevitably be lost if nothing was done. In a 1952 *Harper's Magazine* article on open-heart surgery, science writer Leonard Engel declared, "The time is close for [a] trial on human patients who have no other chance for survival." He specifically mentioned children with large septal defects, a birth defect for which there was no treatment: "In these cases, any lives saved will be pure gain and the risk involved in employing a new machine is amply justified."[11] It is important to realize that informed consent, as it came to be defined, was an emerging concept in the 1950s. There were no standardized institutional review boards or medical ethics committees when surgeons began operating around and inside the heart.[12]

Open-heart surgery was a complicated undertaking. At the 1951 American Surgical Association meeting, Clarence Dennis emphasized the importance of preoperative planning and teamwork. He outlined the roles of sixteen participants, a record for any operation. In addition to four surgeons, two physician anesthetists, two nurses, and two technicians, six other individuals were involved: four managed the heart-lung-machine, one ran the transfusion apparatus, and another drew blood samples. The University of Minnesota surgeon knew that very few institutions could attempt such a complex procedure. But he predicted that improvements in the technology and in surgical techniques would reduce the number of staff required in the operating room.[13] Johns Hopkins surgeon Alfred Blalock, who had operated on more patients with congenital heart disease than anyone else in the world, stood up after Gibbon and Dennis spoke to applaud their "epoch-making work." He praised Gibbon for his persistence "in a difficult field, which is beginning to bear fruit."[14]

Clarence Dennis worked in a dynamic environment that was energized by Owen Wangensteen, the University of Minnesota's longtime chief of surgery. Wangensteen expected each member of his staff to devote time to experimental surgery and to mentor residents in research. He wanted to encourage surgical innovation and to train surgical trendsetters. Leonard Wilson explains in his book on the history of the University of Minnesota Medical School that Wangensteen would not tolerate trainees who were "mere intellectual parasites, using ideas and methods developed by others."[15] He wanted his residents to be innovators. They worked in a context that stimulated competition, which helps to explain why parallel projects were underway at the university to develop different technologies and techniques for performing open-heart surgery.

John Gibbon performed his first open-heart operation on a human in February 1952. All of the doctors who had evaluated the fifteen-month-old girl with severe congestive heart failure concluded that she had an atrial septal defect. An attempt to confirm this diagnosis with cardiac catheterization was unsuccessful. Using a heart-lung machine built by IBM, Gibbon opened the child's heart and made a disturbing discovery. The preoperative diagnosis was wrong—her atrial septum was intact. She died after surgery, and an autopsy revealed that she had a patent ductus arteriosus (an abnormal vascular connection between the aorta and pulmonary artery) that was not recognized before or during the operation.[16]

Clarence Dennis and John Gibbon's separate case reports describing their first failed attempts to perform open-heart surgery in humans underscored the importance of accurate preoperative diagnosis. Heart surgery pioneers concluded that cardiac catheterization was a powerful tool that complemented the standard diagnostic techniques of physical examination, electrocardiography, chest X-ray, and fluoroscopy. When Gibbon first used his heart-lung machine on a patient in 1952, physiologist Earl Wood ran Mayo's catheterization laboratory. That year, the American Heart Association asked him to serve on a national committee charged with evaluating the risks of catheterization and identifying ways to minimize them. Pooled data from eight leading laboratories demonstrated the procedure's safety in very experienced hands. There were just four deaths in 5,691 catheterizations at these high-volume centers. But the committee stressed that specially trained medical and technical personnel were a major factor in reducing the risk.[17]

Assembling a Mayo Team to Pioneer Open-Heart Surgery

Mayo launched a program to develop a method for performing open-heart surgery in the summer of 1952, when John Kirklin and Earl Wood met with the clinic's Sciences Committee to discuss the "production and experimental use of a mechanical heart in certain types of cardiac surgery."[18] The two men had already discussed the project with Harold J. C. (Jeremy) Swan, a research associate in physiology, and Richard Jones, head of Mayo's Engineering Section. Wood thought there was a 95 percent chance that they would succeed in developing a heart-lung machine within two years if they had the right collaborators. Kirklin wanted David Donald, a skilled veterinary surgeon and physiologist, to be part of the team. They had worked together in the animal laboratory in an effort to invent or improve operations.[19] To jump-start the project, the clinic agreed to send Kirklin, Wood, Swan, Donald, and Jones to institutions where attempts to build a heart-lung machine were underway. Meanwhile, surgeons at the University of Minnesota were competing among themselves to develop techniques to perform open-heart surgery.

F. John Lewis and Mansur Taufic performed the world's first successful open-heart operation on September 2, 1952, at the University of Minnesota Hospital. The patient was a five-year-old girl with an atrial septal defect proven by catheterization. In order to see and work inside the child's heart, the surgeons put loops of braided silk string around the superior and inferior venae cavae and clamped the aorta and pulmonary artery (the so-called great vessels that carry blood to the body and the lungs). This stopped the flow of blood through the heart. Unlike Dennis and Gibbon, Lewis and Taufic did not use a heart-lung machine, so they had to race against time. Normally, the brain suffers irreversible damage if its blood supply is blocked for more than four minutes. Other surgeons had developed the technique of hypothermia to reduce the brain's oxygen demand, which gave them another minute or two to interrupt the circulation. The little girl's body had been cooled to 79 degrees to help protect her brain during the five and a half minutes that no blood reached it or the rest of her body. Lewis opened her right atrium, saw a three-quarter inch hole in the atrial septum, and closed it with silk sutures. Then, the silk strings around the vena cavae were released, and blood flowed through the heart once again. The entire operation lasted fifty-eight minutes, and the child went home eleven days later without a heart murmur, one sign of a successful operation.[20]

Despite this excellent outcome, the inflow-obstruction technique of blocking blood return to the heart had no potential as a routine clinical procedure because it gave a surgeon only five or six minutes to work inside the heart before a lack of oxygen caused brain damage. Lewis's operation was a technical feat, but aspiring cardiac surgeons knew that a heart-lung machine was the only solution to tackling congenital heart defects. No matter how skilled, a surgeon needed more time to correct all but the simplest intracardiac defects.

Ten days after Lewis performed the world's first successful open-heart operation in Minneapolis, Kirklin informed Mayo's chief administrator that if their institution developed a heart-lung machine, it would probably be used about once a month. Despite this projected low number of open-heart procedures, Kirklin argued that "the general prestige gained by the institution in the successful development of such an apparatus would justify the project, let alone the possibility of aiding sick people."[21]

Eight men met at Kirklin's home on October 21, 1952, to discuss the proposed pump-oxygenator project. In addition to the surgeon, the group included cardiologist Howard Burchell, physiologists Earl Wood and Jeremy Swan, biomedical engineer Richard Jones, experimental surgeons David Donald and John Grindlay, and cardiac pathologist Jesse Edwards. The men discussed their goals, what other groups were doing, and which institutions to visit. Members of the Mayo team would visit John Gibbon in Philadelphia, Clarence Dennis in Brooklyn (where he had moved from Minneapolis), and Forest Dewey Dodrill in Detroit. Each of these men had attempted open-heart surgery in humans using machines that they and their collaborators had built and tested on animals.[22]

Competition among the groups trying to develop open-heart surgery was often matched by a willingness to share their knowledge and experience. After Wood visited Dennis, the open-heart surgery pioneer sent him a copy of a progress report that he had prepared for the US Public Health Service, which was funding his research. "If I can be of any further help to you," Dennis declared, "please do not hesitate to call upon me. I am delighted to know of your interest in pursuing this problem. Best of luck to you."[23] The trip to see Gibbon also went well. Wood thanked him for "demonstrating and discussing with us in such a complete fashion the various aspects of the construction and operation of your apparatus. It was indeed impressive." The Mayo physiologist asked the Philadelphia surgeon to help them get the complete engineering specifications for the IBM heart-lung machine he was using.[24]

Gibbon's intervention with IBM on Mayo's behalf was successful. In January 1953 corporate vice president John McPherson informed the clinic's Board of Governors that discussions with the Jefferson Medical College (where Gibbon worked) had gone well. As a result, the company would give Mayo the blueprints for the heart-lung machine and instructions for operating it. The IBM executive thanked the board for its willingness to give credit to the corporation and the medical college "for the pioneer work done in the construction of the machine." He hoped "this original work will be of value in further effort towards the complete solution to this medical problem."[25] Wood, euphoric when the plans arrived, thanked McPherson for his company's willingness to share materials that would be "of inestimable value" in launching open-heart surgery in Rochester.[26]

John Kirklin knew that good surgical results depended on accurate preoperative diagnosis. When the Mayo team was planning to build a pump-oxygenator in February 1953, he thanked Earl Wood for his "marvelous cooperation" and for his first-rate catheterization program: "There is no surgeon in the country dealing with cardiac problems who has the advantage of the superb associates that I have. I know all too well that whatever success we have enjoyed in this field in this institution for the most part is the result of the superb work that you, the medical men, and the other members of the team do."[27] Wood responded in kind: "Your words of praise for the cardiac catheterization setup are very much appreciated. I have very much the same opinion of the surgical side of our team. . . . If a team such as ours cannot be successful in this project, no one can."[28]

Mayo's Board of Governors formally approved "the heart-lung bypass project of Drs. Kirklin, Wood, Donald and Swan" in April 1953 with the understanding that it would cost about $27,000 to build the machine.[29] Two months later, Kirklin sent the board an upbeat report: "This field of surgical endeavor will continue to expand rapidly, particularly when a complete by-pass of the heart and lungs becomes feasible as a repeatable procedure. This time is within the foreseeable future." He hoped the machine that the clinic's engineering group was building (based on the Gibbon-IBM plans) would be ready for use in patients in a year. "If we are able to do this," Kirklin declared, "I am of the definite opinion that we will be in the very center of the stage as far as cardiovascular work in this country is concerned." He knew that a reliable heart-lung machine would be a magnet for patients. Noting that a large number of individuals were already "going to certain centers for cardiac work," he predicted that "many patients in need of medical and surgical treatment for heart disease" would be attracted to Mayo.[30]

The Heart-Lung Machine's Potential is Revealed in Minnesota

John Gibbon performed the first successful open-heart operation using a heart-lung machine on May 6, 1953, in Philadelphia. In an essay on the fiftieth anniversary of this breakthrough, Boston cardiac surgeon Lawrence Cohn wrote, "Curiously, Dr. Gibbon's momentous successful case was not published until one year later in a state medical journal, *Minnesota Medicine*."[31] The original article contains a clue that solves the mystery. Gibbon first reported his path-breaking operation in September 1953 at a symposium on "Recent Advances in Cardiovascular Physiology and Surgery" in Minneapolis. The University of Minnesota and the Minnesota Heart Association cosponsored the three-day event.[32]

The surgical session at the Minneapolis symposium proved that progress was being made in opening the heart in order to operate inside it. Gibbon, one of six participants in the session, reported his experience performing open-heart surgery in four patients using the heart-lung machine that he and IBM had developed. The second patient, an eighteen-year-old female college freshman with an atrial septal defect, was the only survivor. Gibbon attributed the deaths of a fifteen-month-old baby and two five-year-old girls to "human error and not failure of the apparatus."[33]

Gibbon stopped in Rochester on his way home to Philadelphia. Afterward, he told Wood how much he enjoyed visiting Mayo's catheterization laboratory and attending a conference where the management of specific patients was discussed.[34] Many other visitors were impressed by the Mayo Clinic, as they had been for a half century. Alfred Blalock informed Jim Clagett after a 1953 visit to Rochester: "What a grand place you have in the Mayo Clinic. I came back to Baltimore filled with envy. All of you are certainly to be congratulated on the superb job that you are doing."[35] Meanwhile, Kirklin combined his routine clinical work in the operating room with research in the animal laboratory in anticipation of the day he would perform open-heart surgery on a patient.

Kirklin submitted a progress report on the heart-lung machine project to Mayo's Sciences Committee in January 1954. By this time, he had operated inside animal hearts more than seventy times in order to "become intimately familiar with many of the problems inherent in by-passing the heart and lungs." He had also made a list of ten infants and small children that he had seen in consultation who were "doomed to die" without open-heart surgery. The first patients that Kirklin planned to operate on when the heart-lung machine was ready for clinical use would be young children with severe heart failure due to a large ventricular septal defect (a hole between the heart's two main pumping chambers). Repeating his prediction that a large number of patients with congenital heart disease would come to Rochester for surgery once the machine was shown to be safe for surgery on humans, Kirklin boasted, "We have a complete set-up here for the diagnosis, study and treatment of these cases."[36]

As Kirklin prepared his progress report early in 1954, University of Minnesota surgeon C. Walton (Walt) Lillehei was frustrated that his path toward open-heart surgery was being blocked. Owen Wangensteen, the long-time chief of surgery at the university, had told Blalock six years earlier that Lillehei was "a very competent and promising young surgeon" who displayed "a good deal of originality in his attack upon surgical problems in the experimental laboratory.... We will all hear more of him in the years which lie ahead."[37] But Lillehei's promising career had careened off course in 1950, when a lump near his left ear was removed and judged to be lymphosarcoma, a highly malignant tumor. Wangensteen, known for his aggressive surgical attacks on cancer, subsequently performed an eleven-hour operation that required nine pints of blood. The outlook was not good, despite this extensive procedure to remove lymph nodes. The operation left the thirty-two-year-old surgeon very scarred and concerned about whether and when the malignancy might recur. Vincent Gott, one of his residents, believes this situation inspired Lillehei to intensify his efforts to invent operations and make surgical history.[38]

Controlled Cross-Circulation: One Operation—Two Patients

Following months of pain and gradual recovery, Lillehei resumed animal experiments designed to develop a completely new approach to open-heart surgery. In 1953 he was supervising research by surgical residents Morley Cohen and Herbert Warden, who were working on a "controlled cross-circulation" technique. This novel method involved pumping oxygen-rich blood from one dog (the donor) into a second dog (the recipient), whose normal circulation had been blocked temporarily by occluding the venae cavae. The donor dog functioned as a living, breathing, biological oxygenator. This eliminated the need for a mechanical heart-lung machine.[39]

After a series of successful animal experiments, Lillehei was eager to move the technique from the animal laboratory into the operating room. But he faced obstacles. In January 1954 he complained to Wangensteen, "I hesitate to be persistent to the point of being obnoxious; however, sometimes one is driven on by the conviction that he may be right." Lillehei wanted and needed his chief's approval to use the cross-circulation technique for the first time in a human (Figure 10.1).[40]

Gregory Glidden, the prospective patient, was a sickly eleven-month-old child from northern Minnesota who had been born with a large ventricular septal defect. Lillehei, confident that the cross-circulation technique would allow him to close the hole between the heart's two main pumping chambers, told Wangensteen, "His parents are ready, the pediatricians are ready, and we are ready. All that is lacking is your permission." Both surgeons were ambitious and aggressive, but one was in charge. Lillehei pressed his mentor, arguing that the cross-circulation technique was "too good" to be "tied up in the laboratory any longer."[41]

Framing his response in terms of fairness, Wangensteen exclaimed, "Your persistence surprises me." He reminded Lillehei that their colleague John Lewis had used the hypothermia open-heart technique to close atrial septal defects in eleven children, nine of whom had survived. Now, Lewis was working "specifically toward repair of interventricular septal defect." Wangensteen, claiming that "friendly, helpful and sympathetic competition is good," concluded that "the nice thing to do" would be "to let him do the first few cases here."[42] Lewis did operate on two children with ventricular septal defects using his technique, but they both died in the operating room. Lillehei would get his turn.

In mid-March 1954, a week before Lillehei planned to use the cross-circulation technique on little Gregory, he drove to Rochester with the three surgeons who would assist him. They wanted to visit cardiac pathologist Jesse Edwards and to study Mayo's large collection of congenitally deformed hearts. Edwards, a world authority on the subject, had just coauthored

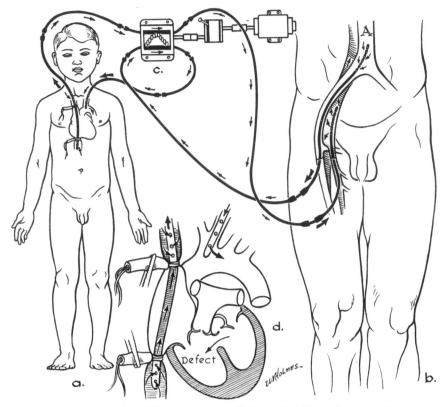

FIGURE 10.1 *C. Walton's Lillehei's technique of "Controlled Cross Circulation" at the University of Minnesota.*

C. W. Lillehei, "Controlled Cross Circulation for Direct-Vision Surgery," *Postgrad. Med.*, 1955, *17*: 389, reprinted with permission of JTE Multimedia.

An Atlas of Anomalies of the Heart and Great Vessels with five Mayo colleagues.[43] He showed the Minneapolis surgeons almost fifty hearts with ventricular septal defects to help them plan Gregory's operation, which was scheduled for March 26.

Back in Minneapolis, Lillehei faced a new obstacle. Cecil Watson, the University of Minnesota's chief of medicine, tried to block the operation at the last minute, declaring it too dangerous. Wangensteen, refusing to yield to his medical counterpart, gave Lillehei permission to proceed. Both chiefs had big egos and a history of defending their territory, but the surgeon won this skirmish.[44] Lillehei, assisted by Richard Varco, operated on March 26, 1954. Lillehei sewed Gregory's ventricular septum shut while Herbert Warden and Morley Cohen attended to his anesthetized father, who functioned as the donor for thirteen minutes while a small pump kept blood flowing between them.[45]

Six days later, Wangensteen boasted to Blalock: "Walt Lillehei has just completed the repair of an interventricular defect using the father as the donor in a cross-circulation operation. It went beautifully." Proud of his protégé, Wangensteen explained: "Together with Morley Cohen, Walt has worked out this technique nicely in the dog laboratory. It looks as though it may come to supplant the complicated pumps which Gibbon and Dennis have been working at—at least for such intra-cardiac procedures which can be completed within a half hour's period of time."[46]

Gregory was doing well when Wangensteen wrote to Blalock, but he developed pneumonia and died eleven days after surgery. Lillehei examined the little boy's heart at autopsy and discovered that the hole in his septum was 90 percent closed. Pressing on, the intrepid surgeon used the cross-circulation technique in seven more patients with ventricular septal defects during the next five weeks. Six of the children (aged five months to five years) survived.[47]

Lillehei's group reported its early experience with cross-circulation at the American Association for Thoracic Surgery meeting in the spring of 1954. John Gibbon stood up after the presentation and told the audience that he was "still convinced that it is preferable to perform operations involving an open cardiotomy by some procedure which does not involve another healthy person."[48] Two lives were at risk with the cross-circulation technique for correcting congenital heart defects: that of the patient and the donor (almost always a parent). But Gibbon had a personal interest in an alternative approach. At the same meeting, he presented his group's experience closing ventricular septal defects in twenty dogs using the heart-lung machine that he and IBM had developed. Eight dogs died, but Gibbon believed that further refinement of surgical techniques and the technology would lead to better results.[49]

Philadelphia was where John Gibbon, Charles Bailey, and Robert Glover practiced surgery. It was also home to the Franklin Institute, which had just opened a popular public exhibit. Bailey had helped pay for constructing a human heart so big that visitors could walk through its chambers as loudspeakers pumped out a rhythmic lub-dub, mimicking the heartbeat. In 1954 *Look* magazine's medical editor Roland Berg published a story titled "New Miracles to Save Your Heart," which included photographs of the Franklin Institute's heart and words that offered hope to thousands of individuals.[50] Familiar with recent breakthroughs in catheterization and cardiac surgery, such as Bailey's closed-heart operations for mitral valve stenosis and Lillehei's cross-circulation technique, Berg explained:

A three-week-old child born with a heart defect that once meant death within weeks; a young mother faced with invalidism because of a heart damaged by a long-forgotten, childhood attack of rheumatic fever; a middle-aged business man sternly warned by his doctor that his last heart attack means giving up business "or else"—these are but a few of countless thousands who have been restored to full and active lives through recent spectacular advances in heart surgery. Disregarding the warnings of surgeons of another era not to tamper with this vital organ, a handful of surgical pioneers have dared the impossible and achieved it.[51]

Look magazine had a circulation of more than 5 million at the time, but just a few surgeons knew the details of the dramatic stories that Berg told.

John Kirklin later recalled that he was "terribly envious" when he heard about Walt Lillehei's first open-heart operation in March 1954. A few days later, he drove to Minneapolis with other members of the Mayo team involved in the pump-oxygenator project to observe a cross-circulation operation. Kirklin's respect for Lillehei "increased exponentially" after he watched him perform the procedure and accompanied him on rounds in the university's Variety Club Heart Hospital where "small children were recovering from these miraculous operations." Back in Rochester, Kirklin had to defend his group's heart-lung project to some colleagues, who considered it a waste of time and money. The surgeon recalled one skeptic's comment: "After all, this young fellow in Minneapolis was successful with a very simple apparatus and did not even require an oxygenator."[52] Despite distractions, Kirklin continued to gain experience operating inside the hearts of animals, and Mayo's Engineering Section worked to perfect a Gibbon-type machine for use in humans.

Mayo's leaders were discussing cost containment when the heart-lung machine project was gaining momentum. Board chair Samuel Haines informed the staff in the spring of 1954 that "things which are not useful should be discontinued."[53] But research was not a specific target. In fact, he emphasized that it was a critical part of the clinic's mission. Shifting his attention to the institution's life blood, Haines said: "We must not forget that most of our patients come from a distance, that they have the expense of traveling to get here, the expense of living away from home, and often the expense of hiring someone to stay at home to take care of the store, the stock, or the children." He argued that it was important that the clinic's charges be "kept as low as is consistent with giving the best care possible."[54]

In Minneapolis, Lillehei forged ahead with his cross-circulation technique. Funding for the project came from several sources, including the Minnesota Heart Association and the National Heart Institute. Meanwhile, Mayo maintained its tradition of funding research internally—even as the National Institutes of Health's total grants to all investigators and institutions skyrocketed from less than $1 million in 1946 to almost $50 million in 1954.[55]

Owen Wangensteen, always eager to get money to support surgical research at the University of Minnesota, was a member of the National Advisory Heart Council. This influential group advised the National Heart Institute's leaders regarding which grant proposals deserved funding. He was present at the council's June 1954 meeting when the cross-circulation technique was discussed. Impressed by what he heard, institute chief James Watt suggested that Lillehei come to their next meeting to show films of how it was done.[56] Three weeks later, Wangensteen wrote to Franklin Yeager, the chief of the National Heart Institute's Grants and Training Branch: "It is a pleasure for me to have the opportunity of affixing my endorsement to this plea for more funds by Doctor Lillehei in support of his research relating to the use of the crossed circulation technique for intracardiac surgery."[57] If Wangensteen wondered whether such advocacy represented a conflict of interest, he kept it to himself. The goal justified the means, and getting to the goal took money.

In September 1954 two thousand doctors from fifty countries attended the Second World Congress of Cardiology in Washington, D.C., where Lillehei spoke at a session on congenital heart disease surgery, chaired by Alfred Blalock. Ten days later, Blalock told the Minnesota surgeon that his presentation was the high point of the meeting.[58] While Lillehei was attracting international attention for his cross-circulation approach to open-heart surgery, Kirklin got some welcome encouragement in Rochester for the heart-lung project. Donald Balfour, a retired surgeon and former head of the Mayo Foundation for Medical Education and Research, visited the animal laboratory. Almost a half century after Balfour had arrived at the clinic, he told Kirklin, "With all my experience here with experimental surgery, I have never seen a project involving so many high-powered details et cetera being worked out with such a marvelous integration." Balfour congratulated him for coordinating the effort and predicted that when the heart-lung machine was perfected for use in patients it would represent "one of the greatest contributions to medicine of all time."[59] Meanwhile, Lillehei seemed to be everywhere, speaking and showing films about the breakthroughs in his operating room.

In November 1954 several Mayo doctors heard Lillehei report his latest clinical experience with the cross-circulation technique at the annual meeting of the Interstate Postgraduate Medical Association in Minneapolis. Chuck Mayo, president-elect of the association and an influential clinic board member, saw him narrate a color film of an operation to close a ventricular septal defect in a two-year-old girl whose mother was the cross-circulation oxygenated-blood donor. Lillehei reported the results of not one but thirty operations: twenty-one to close ventricular septal defects, six to address abnormalities associated with tetralogy of Fallot, and three to correct other forms of congenital heart disease. Eleven patients had died, but all of the parent-donors had survived. Lillehei recognized that better methods for performing open-heart surgery would be developed. Dismissing the "discouragement previously rampant in this field," he predicted that surgery would eventually be developed to correct the vast majority of congenital heart defects.[60]

The public read about Lillehei's cross-circulation technique the same month in a picture-filled *Life* magazine article titled "A Baby's Heart Is Mended: Operation Joins Mother's Bloodstream to Child." The first sentence juxtaposed action and suspended animation: "While surgeons and specialists swarmed around them, two unconscious figures lay stretched out on parallel tables in an operating room of a University of Minnesota hospital." Marsha, a five-month-old with a large ventricular septal defect, was on one table. Her mother, who was "risking her life" to save her child's life, was on another one. The *Life* magazine writer described the complex procedure to a public that had a big appetite for medical breakthroughs. Noting that Lillehei's operation "fulfills an old medical dream of allowing a surgeon to work with a clear view and at leisure inside a living heart," he explained that the "revolutionary technique blocks the heart off from the rest of the body, bypassing blood around it. The patient meanwhile is kept alive by circulating through his body the blood from another human being's bloodstream." The risky procedure that used a mother's lungs to provide oxygen-rich blood was the baby's only chance "to grow up into a healthy, active child."[61]

In November 1954 Lillehei spoke to the National Advisory Heart Council in Bethesda, Maryland. Wangensteen listened as his protégé presented an overview of the cross-circulation technique, showed a film of an operation, and reported his results. National Heart Institute director James Watt applauded Lillehei for this "remarkable achievement."[62] Despite such accolades, no other cardiac surgeons (and there were still very few) used the technique, mainly because operating on one patient's heart could result in two deaths. Harris Shumacker, a former Blalock resident and heart surgery pioneer, had told attendees at the 1954 meeting of the American College of Surgeons that many doctors considered cross-circulation inadvisable because the parent-donor might die.[63]

When Johns Hopkins cardiologist Cowles Andrus heard Lillehei's presentation at the National Advisory Heart Council meeting, he knew that his institution was not in the race to invent open-heart surgery. Charles Bailey had just told Blalock, "Without your inspiration there wouldn't be any real cardiac surgery."[64] But the fifty-five-year-old surgeon-in-chief at Johns Hopkins no longer led the field. After Andrus returned to Baltimore, he shared his impressions of Lillehei's procedure with pediatric cardiologist Helen Taussig. She told Blalock in December 1954, "My group is very anxious for a chance to discuss cross-circulation... with you and Hank [surgeon Henry Bahnson]."[65] Blalock was not interested. His former resident and biographer Mark Ravitch explained, "As open-heart surgery developed and it became obvious that much of the future of cardiac surgery lay in operations with the pump oxy-genator, he made the decision that this was a young man's field, although he was then only fifty-five."[66]

The Mayo Team Prepares For Its First Open-Heart Operation

In January 1955 the Mayo team was preparing to move their customized Gibbon-type heart-lung machine from the animal laboratory into the oper-ating room. Kirklin, pleased with the progress, asked the clinic's Sciences Committee to approve a request to have the Section of Engineering construct a second Mayo-Gibbon machine.

> A second heart-lung by-pass device [would] permit experimental work in animals and operations on clinical patients to proceed as rapidly as possible assuming that the first clinical experience is satisfactory. If the by-pass in man does prove to be practical, there are a number of patients already waiting for such surgery which would occupy the first machine for some time and would not permit the additional experimental studies that are necessary before the by-pass technic can be used for repair of such defects as aortic stenosis, mitral insufficiency and others which cannot as yet be successfully attempted.[67]

Congenital heart disease was the initial focus of open-heart surgery, but Kirklin and other pioneers perceived the potential role of this innovation in treating adults with acquired cardiac problems, such as valve disorders. The Sciences Committee was willing to support his request for a second machine if the early experience in patients was encouraging.

Kirklin sent his annual activity report to the Board of Governors on Valentine's Day 1955. In addition to summarizing his clinical work, the surgeon included a long list of his presentations, publications, and ongo-ing research projects. He predicted that the first human operation using the heart-lung machine at Mayo would be performed within a few months. Admitting that the project was a calculated risk, Kirklin was optimistic that it would be justified by clinical success.[68] Surgeon James Priestley wrote in the margin of the copy that was circulated among board members: "Obviously one of our brightest stars."[69]

Mayo's Section of Publications was expected to manage the media atten-tion that the first open-heart operation was sure to generate. Clinic leaders remembered the frenzy that had followed the report of cortisone's dramatic effect on patients with rheumatoid arthritis seven years earlier, and they wanted to be better prepared this time. The board approved an eighteen-point publicity plan on March 2, 1955. Kirklin, Wood, and their associates were to prepare papers as soon as possible that described the machine and its use in animals. John Gibbon, Jefferson Medical College, and IBM would be thanked for sharing both detailed plans and knowledge with the Rochester group. James Eckman, a PhD member of the Section of Publications, would handle media inquiries. Talking points would include the fact that "the University of Minnesota group has made great contributions, that the cost to the Clinic has been substantial as is the case with so many research projects, and that a substantial amount of donated blood is required." Some information would be not be disclosed, such as the first patient's name, the date of any future procedures, whether the heart-lung machine would be patented, and what the clinic would charge for open-heart operations.[70]

Three days before Kirklin was scheduled to perform Mayo's first open-heart operation, he was participating in the inaugural Henry Ford Hospital International Symposium on Cardiovascular Surgery in Detroit. He heard Lillehei report the results of thirty-nine cross-circulation operations, with a mortality rate of 33 percent.[71] British surgeon Russell Brock, who had been knighted recently by Queen Elizabeth II for his contributions to cardiac surgery, spoke at the black-tie dinner. After citing the contributions of Charles Bailey, John Gibbon, Dwight Harken, and others, Brock said, "To Walton Lillehei we accord the high spot of this meeting; nothing could be more stirring, exciting and significant than his presentation of the work of the Minneapolis team on cross-circulation. Here he has truly shown us that open, definitive intracardiac surgery is here, now, today."[72] As Kirklin listened to Brock, he knew that his team would soon make history in an operating room in Rochester.

The Mayo-Gibbon Heart-Lung Machine is Used in Eight Patients

On March 22, 1955, Kirklin operated on a five-year-old girl with a large ventricular septal defect at Methodist Hospital (the former Colonial Hospital), where Mayo's closed-heart and other thoracic surgery procedures were performed. Mayo's version of the Gibbon machine had been wheeled into the operating room, and Kirklin connected it to his patient. Venous blood flowed into the Mayo-Gibbon machine (Figure 10.2) through flexible plastic tubes that had been inserted into the child's superior and inferior vena cavae. Then a small roller pump pushed the blood into the oxygenator that consisted of fourteen wire mesh screens enclosed in a Lucite case. As a thin film of dark venous blood drained down the screens, it picked up oxygen. The life-sustaining oxygenated blood was then pumped into another flexible plastic tube that Kirklin had inserted into the girl's left subclavian artery. This description oversimplifies a very complex machine that required three individuals to control.[73] The thirty-three-pound patient survived the operation, and the hole in her heart was closed (Figure 10.3).

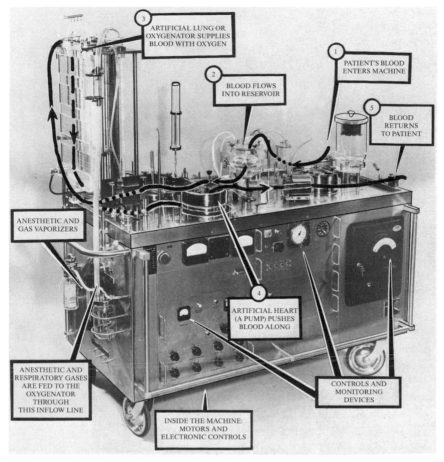

FIGURE 10.2 *Mayo-Gibbon heart-lung machine, ca. 1955.*
Used with permission of Mayo Foundation.

Word of the open-heart operation on the second day of spring in 1955 spread quickly. Science writer Victor Cohn of the *Minneapolis Morning Tribune* called James Eckman's home at 5:40 p.m. the day of surgery. The Mayo spokesperson wrote a memo detailing that evening's telephone trail. It began with a quotation from Cohn: "One of my spies in Rochester has just telephoned me about the first use of a heart-lung circulation machine in an operation on the heart of a human being." Eckman explained that Mayo was not claiming priority and that Gibbon, using the original version of the machine, had performed one successful open-heart operation in 1953. But after three of his first four patients died, he had decided to stop doing open-heart surgery. Nevertheless, Eckman told Cohn that Gibbon knew more than anyone about the development and early use of the machine that Mayo engineers had modified. Pursuing this lead, the Minneapolis reporter

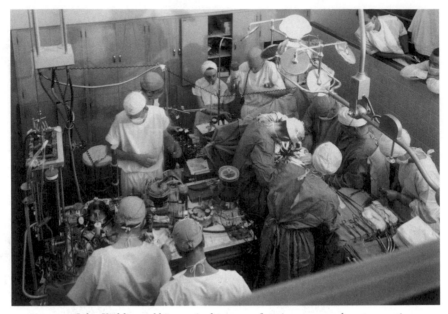

FIGURE 10.3 *John Kirklin and his surgical team performing an open-heart operation,*
ca. 1955.

Used with permission of Mayo Foundation.

phoned the Philadelphia surgeon at home. Gibbon, alerted to the events in
Rochester, called Kirklin at 8:20 p.m. to congratulate him.[74]

The parents of the child who had surgery approved releasing her name,
so the public learned that Mayo's first open-heart operation was performed
on Linda Stout of Bismarck, North Dakota (Figure 10.4).[75] Concerned about
what Cohn might write, Eckman called him at 8:50 p.m. and got him to read
his story's first few paragraphs. The reporter was planning to credit Earl
Wood with heading the project, but Eckman corrected him: "It was explained
to Mr. Cohn that, as in other research projects at the Mayo Clinic, the work
on the development and application of the heart-lung circulation bypass
apparatus actually represented the contributions, in concert, of a number of
investigators each of whose variegated experience and special fields of knowledge were essential and were of particular importance in the success of the
enterprise as a whole."[76]

After speaking with Cohn, Eckman called the editor of the *Rochester
Post-Bulletin* to alert him to the fast-breaking story and to assure him that
the local newspaper would get a detailed background report in the morning.
"First 'Bypass' Operation: Girl Doing Well after Surgery" was the headline
of the *Post-Bulletin* article about the pioneering operation: "A five-year-old
North Dakota girl, who underwent delicate heart surgery here yesterday in
the first human use of a new artificial heart-lung bypass machine developed

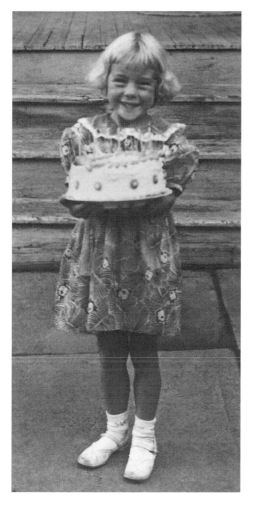

FIGURE 10.4 *Linda Stout, Mayo's first open-heart surgery patient.*
Used with permission of Mayo Foundation.

at the Mayo Clinic, was listed in 'very good' condition today at Methodist Hospital." Readers learned that the child was born with a heart defect "which can cause early death if not corrected by surgery."[77] That evening, an overflow crowd at the biweekly Mayo staff meeting heard two technical talks on the heart-lung machine. Richard Jones, head of the Section of Engineering, discussed the construction of a "Gibbon-type apparatus" at the clinic. Veterinary surgeon David Donald reported the results of its use in ten dogs, nine of which had survived.[78]

British surgeon Russell Brock was visiting the University of Minnesota when news of Mayo's first open-heart operation reached Minneapolis. Richard Varco called Kirklin to ask if their distinguished visitor could come to Rochester to see the patient and watch his next operation. Kirklin recalled: "I had enough on my mind without having a world-famous surgeon sitting in the gallery watching this young guy try to work his way through his second open-heart operation." But Brock's request could not be denied, and he did see Kirklin operate on a seven-year-old child who, like Linda Stout, had a ventricular septal defect.[79] About a month later, Lillehei spoke on the cross-circulation technique at the American Surgical Association annual meeting. Blalock stood up and congratulated him and the university group for their imagination, industry, and courage. After praising the Minneapolis team, the Johns Hopkins surgeon predicted that Gibbon's heart-lung machine would supplant cross-circulation, citing the fact that "Dr. Kirklin, of the Mayo Clinic, has now used it successfully in closing several ventricular septal defects."[80]

After Kirklin performed his eighth open-heart operation, he sent a letter to Earl Wood that provides insight into their relationship and working environment. The surgeon told the physiologist, "I came into this business a complete youngster with no knowledge of cardiovascular problems to speak of and pretty much a surgical neophyte. You and the others in the group took me in and taught me everything I know. I can't forget either that in the earlier days when my experience was limited, I never had the feeling that you people were restless with me because of my inexperience." Kirklin also thanked Wood for his support in the operating room: "You are 100 percent behind me whether I am doing well or am having troubles."[81] And there were troubles.

Like other heart surgery pioneers, Kirklin confronted the gut-wrenching reality of children dying on his operating table. Upset that four of his first eight patients had died, the surgeon opened his own emotion-filled heart, informing Wood:

> The drain on all of the personnel in the operating room, the surgical nurses and everybody, is really pretty heavy. Secondly, by trade I am a surgeon. I enjoy surgical problems. I derive my pleasure from seeing patients getting along well after operation. This bypassing experience with the 50 percent mortality is something new to me. I have never lost so many patients in such a short time. I well understood that the risks were high, etc., etc., etc. but the fact remains that on four occasions there have been four deaths with four families to talk to and four cases that must be explained to my own conscience and to everyone else. It is really very traumatic.[82]

In his letter to Wood, Kirklin outlined a strategy that acknowledged these stresses but would allow the program to proceed in the operating room and the animal laboratory. He told the physiologist that his team would do two bypass operations a week for about a month, followed by a month of animal experiments but no clinical operations. The surgeon did not want the group to "work in the operating room, then rush back to the laboratory to work, and then rush back to the operating room and so on ad infinitum." Returning to the recent series of open-heart operations, Kirklin focused on the children who lived rather than those who died: "We might as well get credit for the four successful cases, the first to be done reproducibly with a mechanical bypass."[83]

Kirklin was the first author of an article in the May 18, 1955, issue of the *Proceedings of the Staff Meetings of the Mayo Clinic* (hereafter *Proceedings*) that reported the results of the first eight open-heart operations on children, who ranged in age from four months to eleven years. Each child was severely symptomatic from congenital heart disease and had a very poor prognosis. The authors emphasized the importance of accurate diagnosis, which involved a review of the patient's medical history and physical findings as well as his or her laboratory, X-ray, electrocardiogram, and catheterization results. Despite the high mortality rate, they concluded that the heart-lung machine functioned well and "established excellent conditions for precise, unhurried intracardiac surgery."[84] The author of a book on the history of heart surgery explains that Robert Frater, who had been a surgical resident at Mayo shortly after the advent of open-heart surgery, thought that each surgeon who pioneered the procedure "carried a small graveyard in his head. It was full of patients he had lost. The graveyards of Kirklin and Lillehei, especially Lillehei, were far bigger and more densely populated. Death comes most to those surgeons who try to be first."[85]

The *Proceedings* reached a large audience because Mayo sent free copies of each issue to approximately 30,000 individuals and 700 medical libraries.[86] Heart surgery pioneer Harris Shumacker later claimed that "the 1955 report of John Kirklin and his colleagues of their first clinical experiences was most important in the history in the development of contemporary cardiac surgery."[87] John Gibbon's longtime goal of inventing a heart-lung machine that would make open-heart surgery possible had been achieved. A series of articles in the *Proceedings* proved that Mayo had entered the race to open the heart. In fact, Kirklin's team was setting the pace.

Aspiring open-heart surgeons welcomed the news that a heart-lung machine had performed well in a series of operations on seriously ill children, although very few centers were prepared to enter the emerging field in 1955. That year, open-heart surgery was done on a regularly scheduled basis in just two institutions in the world: the University of Minnesota and the Mayo Clinic. Surgeons from other states and countries who visited one center often traveled ninety miles to compare what they saw in Lillehei and Kirklin's operating rooms. Donald Ross, who was training with Russell Brock in London at the time, was struck by the contrast:

> I remember going first to Minneapolis to visit Lillehei, and it was like a circus. There was a large gallery in the operating room with about fifty

people. People were rushing in and out. They started about seven or eight in the morning, and Lillehei came in about eleven. The operating room was chaos with pipes and tubes everywhere. The patient did very well, but, I thought, I don't know if I could do this sort of surgery with so much confusion. From Lillehei, I went by bus to the Mayo Clinic to visit Kirklin.... Walking into Kirklin's operating room was like walking into a church; there was no sound, no excitement. We sort of sat in pews watching him as he quietly talked. The door opened, the heart-lung machine was wheeled in and connected to the patient, and he then did the operation. I was dumbfounded that you could do this very complex procedure so quietly with no drama. This was a very important lesson for me. Brock had been my teacher up until then, and he was a very noisy and dramatic operator. Kirklin was cool and calm. I learned a lot from him in this respect.[88]

Cardiac surgeon Norman Shumway, who was Lillehei's resident in the mid-1950s, provides an insider's perspective on the two institutions: "We, at the University of Minnesota, used to joke about the Mayo Clinic. We called it a charm school. There was such a contrast between the atmospheres at the University of Minnesota, which was truly laissez-faire, and at the Mayo Clinic, where everything was carefully regulated. There was little deviation, whether in the dress code of the residents or the methods of doing open-heart surgery."[89]

Older children also formed impressions of the surgeons who would perform heart surgery on them. For example, Mary was nine years old in June 1955, when Kirklin closed a large atrial septal defect using the so-called atrial well technique (which did not require a heart-lung machine). More than a half century later, Mary recalled that he was "Quiet, gentle...I can remember liking him and talking with him and feeling at ease." Her mother recalled being startled by Kirklin's youthful appearance: "But once you talked to him you had all the confidence in the world. He was just great."[90]

Mayo's Heart-Lung Machine Debuts on National Television

The public had an opportunity to see and hear John Kirklin in September 1955, when the "Medical Horizons" television program devoted an entire show to open-heart surgery at the Mayo Clinic. Television was revolutionizing mass communication, and the popular program was broadcast live to about six million viewers each week. The moderator began: "Dr. Kirklin and his associates have agreed to escort us tonight on a rather unique journey, a voyage into the interior of the human heart." The Mayo surgeon explained why some cardiac defects could be treated only by operating inside the heart and how the new heart-lung machine made this possible. Pediatric cardiologist James DuShane discussed the diagnosis and prognosis of various congenital heart defects, and physiologist Earl Wood described how catheterization could help doctors differentiate them. Next, the camera moved into an operating room where anesthesiologist Robert Patrick explained his role. Open-heart surgery pioneers agreed that these risky operations required much more support from anesthesia specialists than closed-heart or non-cardiac procedures.[91]

Finally, the moderator spoke with experimental surgeon David Donald, who had helped refine the Mayo-Gibbon machine and ran it during surgery. The printed script for the television show included a cue at this point. As Donald described why and how blood flowed through the pump-oxygenator, a camera would zoom in on the apparatus and a microphone would pick up the "whooshing sound" it made as it was "flooded with blood." The moderator closed the program: "Well, Doctor Kirklin, my conclusion based on tonight's demonstration is that a skillfully coordinated group effort is required to perform such an operation and that a great variety of abilities are necessary to achieve an advance in medicine." He thanked the five members of the Mayo team "for an exciting and informative look into the 'open' heart and a glimpse of a significant medical horizon."[92]

By the fall of 1955, Wood was encouraged by better patient survival rates after open-heart surgery, despite the fact that many of the children were high risk and had very abnormal preoperative catheterization results. "At present our success with the bypass is unbelievably good," he told former Mayo trainee and aspiring pediatric cardiologist William Weidman.[93] As Kirklin had predicted, the heart-lung machine attracted patients to Rochester. The number of children with congenital heart disease referred to the clinic, which triggered an increase in the volume of diagnostic procedures.[94]

In the spring of 1956, Wood was trying to recruit Irish physiologist John Shepherd to help him and Jeremy Swan in the catheterization laboratory and with research. He informed Shepherd that an average of twenty-six catheterizations and ten open-heart operations were done each month.[95] Along with the clinical practice, the pace of animal research increased. Optimism filled the air on Valentine's Day 1956, when the Engineering Section held a party to celebrate the completion of a second heart-lung machine. A large Valentine-shaped sign in front of the new machine read "Healthy Hearts for All."[96]

The Expansion of Open-Heart Surgery
and Cardiac Catheterization

The advent of open-heart surgery at the Mayo Clinic on the second day of spring in 1955 resulted in a dramatic increase in the number of children with congenital heart disease referred to Rochester for evaluation—from six in January 1954 to forty-one in January 1956.[1] When pediatric cardiologist James DuShane met with the Sciences Committee in February 1956, he mentioned that surgeons at several medical centers were developing heart-lung machines and were performing animal experiments in anticipation of entering the emerging field of open-heart surgery. But DuShane thought it was unlikely "that such procedures will ever be carried out in appreciable numbers at very many institutions."[2]

Two main factors contributed to DuShane's opinion about open-heart surgery's potential for significant growth. When he made his prediction in 1956, open-heart surgery was devoted exclusively to congenital heart defects, which were rare. And the Mayo-Gibbon heart-lung machine, which was used only in Rochester, was very complex. William Stoney, a surgical resident at Vanderbilt University Hospital, visited Mayo in 1956 to watch John Kirklin operate using it. "There were four technicians whose job it was to run the pump," he recalls. "It all worked with precision, and it was very impressive. However, most visiting surgeons were daunted by the complexity and the expense of the Mayo-Gibbon heart-lung machine and concluded that is was beyond their means."[3] It was the size of a horizontal freezer chest, and the commercialized version cost about $20,000, almost as much as a Rolls Royce automobile.[4] In addition to being extremely expensive, the Mayo-Gibbon machine required a lot of fresh blood to fill its tubes and reservoirs. The clinic depended on local donors because eight to ten pints of blood (which had to be the same type as the patient's) had to be drawn the same day as surgery.[5]

When DuShane made his prediction in 1956, more than a dozen groups were racing to construct heart-lung machines that would be less expensive and easier to use than the Mayo-Gibbon apparatus. The University of

Minnesota team, led by C. Walton (Walt) Lillehei, was close to the finish line. Recognizing the shortcomings of his controversial cross-circulation open-heart surgery technique, Lillehei had encouraged Richard DeWall (Figure 11.1), a recent medical graduate working in his research laboratory, to develop a simple pump-oxygenator. Lillehei first used the new apparatus in May 1955 to close a ventricular septal defect in a three-year-old boy. The child died the following day, but five of the next six patients survived. This showed that open-heart surgery, while risky, could save lives that would otherwise be lost due to the consequences of congenital heart disease.

The following January, Lillehei and DeWall were the lead authors of an article that reported the seven-patient series. It announced a technological breakthrough that would greatly accelerate the diffusion of open-heart surgery into practice. They chose a very descriptive title: "Direct Vision Intracardiac Surgery in Man Using a Simple, Disposable Artificial Oxygenator."[6] The words "simple" and "disposable" attracted the attention of aspiring heart surgeons and hospital administrators at a time when other groups were developing their own heart-lung machines. British surgeon Russell Brock claimed in 1957, "There are nearly as many varieties of machine as there are of motor-cars; their basic construction is usually partly dictated by sound mechanical and physiological principles; partly by whim."[7]

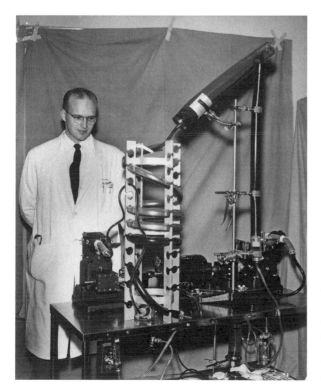

FIGURE 11.1 *Richard DeWall with Lillehei-DeWall helical reservoir bubble oxygenator, ca. 1956.*

Used with permission of the University of Minnesota Archives.

The Cleveland Clinic Enters the Open-Heart Surgery Field

In the fall of 1956, Walt Lillehei declared that "open-heart surgery is a fast moving field at the moment."[8] When the Minneapolis surgeon made this claim, most of the innovation in the budding field was taking place at traditional academic medical centers. But a team at the Cleveland Clinic was eager to join the race. Founded in 1921, this multispecialty group practice in Northern Ohio was modeled after the Mayo Clinic. Three men who had joined the Cleveland Clinic shortly after World War II led its open-heart surgery project. Donald Effler, the group's first thoracic surgeon, was hired in 1948 and developed the clinic's closed-heart surgery program. Mason Sones Jr., one of world's first formally trained pediatric cardiologists, was recruited two years later to launch a cardiac catheterization laboratory to provide diagnostic information that would complement Effler's surgical efforts. Willem Kolff, a Dutch physician and biomedical engineer who had invented an artificial kidney during the war, emigrated to America and joined the Cleveland Clinic's Division of Research in 1950. Five years later, he led the group's effort to build a heart-lung machine [9]

In May 1955, six weeks after John Kirklin performed Mayo's first open-heart operation, Willem Kolff wrote to Earl Wood. He informed the physiologist that he "enjoyed seeing the progress with the artificial heart and lungs" that had been published in the most recent issue of the *Proceedings of the Staff Meetings of the Mayo Clinic*.[10] Hoping to accelerate the Cleveland Clinic's entry into the emerging field, Kolff explained that he "would like to have a plan from which a good mechanic should be able to make one of these Gibbon-type pumps." The Dutchman did not disguise his impatience: "I have asked Dr. Gibbon for it, but he is so slow in responding that I am afraid that I will never get it."[11] Wood, explaining that the Mayo Clinic was not allowed to share the plans, encouraged him to contact the Philadelphia surgeon again. Kolff, based on his experience inventing an artificial kidney, concluded that his group could construct a simpler machine by themselves. And they did.[12]

Donald Effler performed the Cleveland Clinic's first open-heart operation in February 1956, using a pump-oxygenator designed by Kolff. The operation, done to close a large ventricular septal defect in a seventeen-month-old boy, was carefully choreographed. A six-page script written before surgery detailed each person's role and the time that each step should take.[13] Two months later, *Time* magazine published a dramatic description of the operation: "When he was wheeled into the operating theater, the small patient was lost among a task force of fifteen doctors and nurses, led by Surgeon Donald B. Effler. Then, building palisades of clamps, scalpels, retractors, [and] forceps, the surgeons opened the boy's chest." Ultimately, this alarming scene had a happy ending: "Last week, nine weeks after the operation, the youngster was home and hopping." But the *Time* reporter reminded readers that heart surgery was risky—two of Effler's next eight patients died.[14]

Effler's initial death rate was comparable to early experiences elsewhere, but he became concerned when it rose. "My mortality rate was horrendous," he recalled two decades later. "I lost thirty-nine of the first one hundred patients."[15] Effler, Kolff, and Sones, known for their strong personalities, struggled to sort out what might explain the situation. Was Effler's surgical technique the problem? Did Kolff's heart-lung machine function properly? Was Sones's preoperative diagnosis correct? The Cleveland Clinic's official history provides perspective on this situation and reveals Kirklin's role in reassuring Effler and his institution that their open-heart surgery program was sound. After describing the major contributions made by Sones, Kolff, and Effler to the development of cardiology and cardiac surgery at the clinic, the writer explained:

> There were times, however, when these men did not get along. Their effect upon one another became so stressful to them and others around them that the Board of Governors decided that something had to be done and formed a committee to address the issue in 1956. It was headed by William L. Proudfit, M.D., a cardiologist on speaking terms with each of the dissident colleagues. The four men met daily at 8 a.m. and often would talk to each other only through the chairman. Much of the dissension surrounded the death of several high risk patients who were operated on and had been expected to live. At one point, Effler decided to stop operating. However, Dr. John W. Kirklin, then at the Mayo Clinic, said he felt there was nothing wrong with the approach or selection of patients and that the operations should be resumed. His judgment proved correct, and with improved results, bad tempers eased.[16]

William Proudfit, the source of this story, recalled in an interview, "Doctor Kirklin gave the word, the next week we were back to full swing. So that is one way that Mayo Clinic heavily influenced the future of cardiology at Cleveland Clinic."[17]

Kirklin, delighted with his own situation in Rochester, informed Mayo's Board of Governors in 1956, "The environment in which I have been fortunate to have been placed is the most magnificent one in which an individual could be placed. The opportunities for growth and development within it are such that the only limiting factors to accomplishment are the ability, ingenuity and industry of the individuals within it. The materials, assistance and tools for accomplishment and collaboration for research and development are readily available. Surely there must be no institution which offers such magnificent opportunities."[18] Most Mayo staff members had trained at the institution after completing an internship elsewhere, but Kirklin had spent six months at the Boston Children's Hospital, where he had worked with Robert Gross, a pioneer of surgery for congenital heart disease. This experience provided him with perspective that many of his colleagues lacked.[19]

Surgeon Dwight McGoon's Career Path Leads to the Mayo Clinic

Two or three open-heart operations were performed at Mayo each week in 1956. No institution did more, and most did none. Kirklin had trained Henry Ellis Jr., a recent graduate of the clinic's residency program, to use this bold new approach to treat selected patients with very specific types of heart disease. Ellis had assisted the senior surgeon during Mayo's first open-heart procedure performed one year earlier. Initially, it seemed that these two surgeons could manage the open-heart practice. But growing clinical demands and a general surgeon's drowning created an opening for an outsider.[20] Dwight McGoon would become the clinic's third open-heart surgeon and an international leader in the field. Letters that follow provide fascinating personal insights into factors that influenced his career choice and how some outsiders perceived the Mayo Clinic at mid-century. McGoon's many subsequent contributions to surgery also justify this biographical digression.[21]

Dwight McGoon, a Johns Hopkins medical graduate who had spent six years in Alfred Blalock's surgical residency program, was an Air Force surgeon stationed in Germany in 1955 when he began considering future job opportunities. During a trip to the United States to attend his father's funeral in Iowa, McGoon visited Paul Doege, a general surgeon in Marshfield, Wisconsin. Doege wanted to hire another surgeon to help him cope with growing patient demand in his private practice and to perform thoracic and urologic operations.[22] Shortly after McGoon's visit, Doege wrote to Blalock for a recommendation. "The opportunity for a man to work into an enviable position here is great," said the Wisconsin surgeon, "but he must have the prerequisites, namely ability, personality and a determination to reach success through hard work and perseverance."[23] Blalock responded that McGoon was "one of the best residents I have ever had.... He gets along with patients and associates superbly. He is tireless and I know he will be a great success."[24]

Writing from Germany, McGoon told Doege in October 1955, "I am very certain that coming to work with you at Marshfield is a wise choice. It would be no good now, having seen the opportunity there, to think of doing anything else."[25] But a letter crossing the Atlantic at the same time contained news of a tragedy that would alter McGoon's career path and change the history of surgery at the Mayo Clinic. Baltimore surgeon Ridgeway Trimble, who had helped train McGoon at Hopkins, explained that his friend Howard Gray, the head of one of Mayo's surgery sections, had drowned in the Mississippi River. Looking beyond the tragedy,

Trimble saw a potential opportunity for his former pupil: "They may want and need someone of your training who would work up to be in charge of a service at their clinic."[26] McGoon responded, "Your suggestion about the Mayo Clinic is very enticing to me, and I must confess that I had toyed with the idea occasionally myself. However, it seemed to me that they probably had so many men of their own to choose from that there would be little use to explore that possibility.... Of course the medical opportunities there are without equal in many ways."[27]

Trimble contacted James Priestley, a surgeon-friend who was vice chair of Mayo's Board of Governors. Priestley responded that he favored adding some doctors to the staff who had trained elsewhere, but there did not seem to be a place for McGoon because Mayo had three "rather young men" performing thoracic operations.[28] Meanwhile, McGoon was struggling to reconcile his career aspirations with his financial situation. He informed the chief of surgery at the University of Miami:

> It is difficult to see how I could possibly enter academic work at this time. With my present indebtedness, the tremendous cost of living for a family of five, and my complete lack of any reserves...we would have to skimp along for many a year to make ends meet. As opposed to this I have a most attractive opportunity in partnership practice in a central Wisconsin community that offers the assurance of normal living conditions and a busy general and thoracic practice. It is difficult to subjugate my personal desires and ambitions in medicine to so vulgar an influence as money, but when I consider the sacrifices of my wife and family thus far, and consider how little the situation would improve over the years, I must face reality.[29]

One month later, in February 1956, Priestley informed Trimble that his Mayo colleagues had been thinking more about McGoon: "The work in cardiovascular surgery has been very steadily increasing here so that the four members of our surgical staff who work primarily in the chest have been kept busier and busier."[30] Trimble sent McGoon a copy of Priestley's letter, adding, "Since you have already decided to go to Wisconsin, you probably do not want to reopen the whole matter again. Great clinics like the Mayo Clinic have their disadvantages, as well as their advantages. The work load given you is enormous."[31]

McGoon informed Trimble that he was enthusiastic about the possibility of a one-year appointment as a staff assistant.[32] Before Mayo offered McGoon a position, he wrote a letter to Doege, which he described as "the most difficult and miserable task of my career." He reminded Doege of their conversation in Marshfield: "[I] pointed out that my lifetime ambition had been to combine research and teaching with clinical surgery, but that I was forced from an academic atmosphere for financial reasons. Of course, all these ambitions and requirements are met ideally by joining the Mayo Clinic." Aware of the implications of reversing his decision to join the solo surgeon's practice, McGoon pleaded, "I only pray that you will be sympathetic to my standpoint and realize how much this means to me."[33] Doege, who responded that he was "stunned and most unhappy," pressured the thirty-year-old surgeon to join him in Wisconsin.[34]

Doege's wife wrote separately, "We can't believe you would let yourself by-pass such a golden opportunity." Worried about her fifty-eight-year-old husband's physical and financial well-being, she complained, "He works too hard. He just can't get away at all. If he goes for a few days, a big volume is lost. There is no one to take his place."[35] Unwittingly, she was highlighting some advantages of practicing at the Mayo Clinic. They would be summarized four years later in a *Saturday Evening Post* article on the Minnesota group practice: "Fringe benefits help make this a dream shop: no overhead, good retirement income, four to seven weeks vacation; twenty workdays a year, apart from weekends and holidays, to attend medical meetings, largely at clinic expense."[36]

After Mrs. Doege described Mayo as an outstanding institution, she disparaged it: "The established pattern is a complicated one, buried in protocol, red tape, precedence, politics, and all the usual trimmings that go with a mighty institution composed of hundreds of men of various abilities. Personal recognition is subordinated to a kind of institutional routine procedure. We believe they are prone to exploit young men."[37] Whatever challenges McGoon might face in Rochester, he would not be expected to rescue a solo surgeon swamped by the success of his fee-for-service private practice.

Alfred Blalock sent McGoon a three-sentence letter in April 1956: "I had a two hour talk with Jim Clagett of Mayo Clinic about you. The possibilities there seem to be excellent. If you are offered a place I believe you should accept it unless you have gone too far in your other commitments."[38] Two weeks later, Priestley informed McGoon that the board had approved a one-year appointment for him as an assistant to the surgical staff.[39] Blalock told his protégé: "This presents a great opportunity, and I am sure you will make a great success of it. I envy you greatly."[40] Several weeks after McGoon informed Doege of his decision to go to the Mayo Clinic, the Marshfield surgeon's wife wrote: "The only bright spot in our bitter disappointment over your change of mind was your sincere and gracious approach to the matter."[41]

Shortly after McGoon arrived in Rochester in the summer of 1956, he informed Blalock, "All seems to be going well. Fortunately, I am being initiated into the style and manner of Mayo Clinic practice by 'shadowing' Dr. Clagett in nearly all that he does—thus meeting people and learning the ropes through him."[42] Midway through McGoon's year as a staff assistant,

Kirklin told Blalock that his former resident was "a fine surgeon and a fine man, and I am enjoying the association immensely."[43]

McGoon was appointed to the Mayo staff in 1957, just as the focus of open-heart surgery was beginning to shift from congenital heart defects to acquired valve disease. That year, medical journalist Leonard Engel celebrated cardiac surgery's rapid rise in a *Harper's Magazine* article:

> In the space of a decade, surgery of the human heart has graduated from the class of the unusual and unlikely, into an established practice. Operations around, on, and within the heart are being done at a rate of many thousands a year. At half-a-dozen institutions, "open-heart" surgery—with a heart-lung machine keeping the patient alive, while the surgeon works inside the heart—is being done several times a week.... Bringing heart surgery to this point took a lot of doing. There were immense problems to be solved. There were tragic failures and brilliant successes. Above all, there were desperately sick patients pleading for help at any cost, and surgeons with the courage to plunge ahead—frequently over the open opposition of colleagues.[44]

Engel described the heart surgeon as "the Prince of the Operating Room, the man the big-league hospital can't afford to be without" in his 1957 article.[45] How quickly things had changed! Ten years earlier, no hospital in *any* league had a heart surgeon.

Surgeons Develop Operations for Damaged Heart Valves

In a 1958 review of open-heart surgery techniques, Walt Lillehei pointed out that surgeons had entered the last anatomic frontier just a decade earlier with the advent of closed-heart operations. Citing advances in treating patients with leaky heart valves, he emphasized how fast the field was evolving: "Even two years ago such frequently encountered acquired cardiac lesions as mitral regurgitation and aortic insufficiency were beyond the realm of surgical correction. Today, these operations, as well as others not possible a few years ago, are regularly scheduled procedures."[46] The fact that acquired mitral valve and aortic valve diseases were much more common than congenital heart defects encouraged many larger hospitals to establish open-heart surgery programs.

Severe heart valve disease caused disabling symptoms and carried a dismal prognosis. This combination stimulated some surgeons to try to invent operations to treat certain valve disorders in the pre-open-heart surgery era. In 1948 Horace Smithy, Dwight Harken, Charles Bailey, and Russell Brock had operated successfully on patients with mitral valve stenosis.[47] But there were three other kinds of left-sided heart valve disease: aortic stenosis, aortic regurgitation, and mitral regurgitation. The fundamental problem with aortic stenosis, like mitral stenosis, is progressive obstruction of the valve opening, which limits blood flow through the tight valve (Figure 11.2). The causes of aortic and mitral regurgitation vary, but the end result is that some blood leaks backward because the valve does not close completely.

The prognosis for patients with severe aortic stenosis is very poor after they develop symptoms of angina pectoris (chest pain upon exertion), heart failure (usually evidenced by shortness of breath with activity), or syncope (sudden loss of consciousness). About half of the patients who develop these symptoms die within two years. South Carolina surgeon Horace Smithy had a very personal reason for trying to invent an operation for severe aortic stenosis. He had this problem himself and was becoming more and more symptomatic as his valve got progressively tighter. In 1947, he reported a series of experiments on animals that he had done to develop aortic valvulotomy, a procedure to slit open a severely stenotic valve. Smithy told his audience of surgeons: "The need for a safe technical approach to the surgical treatment of chronic valvular disease of the heart has been recognized for many years. Recent developments in cardiac surgery, notably the splendid contributions of Blalock in pulmonic stenosis, have created a stimulus for the reinvestigation of the problem."[48] Soon, Smithy was on his way to Baltimore.

Smithy went to the Johns Hopkins Hospital, hoping to convince Blalock to perform an aortic valvulotomy on him. Once there, the South Carolina surgeon worked in the animal laboratory with surgical resident Denton Cooley and surgical technician Vivien Thomas in an attempt to perfect the valve-opening procedure. The next step was to have Blalock perform the experimental operation on a patient. The senior surgeon agreed, but things did not go well. Blalock and Smithy were scrubbing their hands when Cooley began cutting into the man's chest. Just as he opened the pericardial

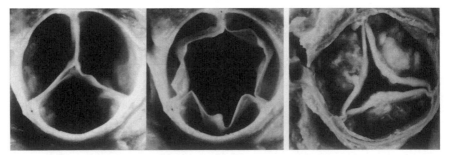

FIGURE 11.2 *Aortic valve: closed, open, and stenotic (obstructed).*

E. R. Giuliani, B. J. Gersh, M. D. McGoon, D. L. Hayes, and H. V. Schaff, eds., *Mayo Clinic Practice of Cardiology* (St. Louis: Mosby, 1996), 1400, figure 32–1; used with permission of Mayo Foundation.

sac, which surrounds the heart, the patient had a cardiac arrest and died. "Smithy was in the operating room," Cooley recalled. "I looked over at him and saw his face fall. He thought that this was the only chance at having a successful operation for himself."[49] Smithy was right. Blalock refused to operate on him. The South Carolina surgeon died in October 1948, a week before a *Saturday Evening Post* article was published that mentioned the pioneering mitral stenosis operation that he had performed on a woman from Ohio.[50]

Robert Glover, who had completed his residency at the Mayo Clinic in 1948, joined Charles Bailey's private practice in Philadelphia, where he would assist the pathbreaking surgeon in the development of valve surgery.[51] Shortly after Bailey operated successfully on a patient with mitral stenosis, he and Glover began developing techniques to treat aortic stenosis. George Lawton, a fifty-three-year-old psychologist, was one of the first patients on whom Bailey operated for this problem. Lawton, who had an aortic valvulotomy in June 1954, wrote a book that described the physical and emotional aspects of his experience. His main symptom was shortness of breath, which had become severe. "Just turning over in bed or getting up and going to the bathroom makes me breathless," Lawton told a friend. "Last night I woke up at three, panting as if I had been in a race."[52] This scary new symptom, termed paroxysmal nocturnal dyspnea, indicated that the man's heart was losing its ability to compensate for his worsening aortic stenosis.

Analyzing his feelings and fears, the psychologist explained, "There is a road toward death that most of us take by rather slow steps. The closing of my aortic valve forced me to follow along this road with ever-increasing speed until in May 1954 my heart and I were really galloping!"[53] Lawton's operation went well, and he was ecstatic after he recuperated from it: "When I first discovered I could walk up *without exhaustion and breathlessness* the inclines and steps that had caused such trouble, my joy and gratitude were really indescribable."[54] Pleased but pragmatic, the psychologist confessed, "Because my operation is so new no one dares predict with certainty what my future will be." But Lawton was more confident about surgery's future: "Heart surgery, whether it gives me a shorter or a longer second chance at life, will be improved greatly each year.... There is hope for heart sufferers."[55] Some patients with symptomatic aortic stenosis surely found this narrative reassuring. Their opinion of the operation would likely have changed if they had read the technical descriptions of it written for surgeons.

John Kirklin performed Mayo's first closed-heart operation for aortic stenosis in November 1953. When he and Henry Ellis reported their experience with aortic valve commissurotomy two years later, they emphasized that aortic stenosis surgery was riskier than mitral stenosis surgery. Their description of the operation reveals some of its very real dangers. Kirklin and Ellis explained that after making a long incision in the chest:

> a purse-string stitch is taken in an avascular portion of the left ventricular myocardium a short distance from the apex. It is important not to tighten this suture too vigorously during manipulations to prevent its tearing through the myocardium. A small stab wound is made in the myocardium, and the guide wire of the Bailey aortic valvulotome is inserted and directed through the aortic valve. The valvulotome is then inserted and guided into position by use of the wire. The valve is forcefully and repeatedly dilated. The instrument is withdrawn, and the opening in the myocardium is closed with interrupted sutures of silk while bleeding from the myocardial incision is controlled by gentle tightening of the purse-string stitch. Although the myocardium is often of poor quality and does not hold sutures well, gentle and accurate placement of stitches allows good hemostasis. Cardiac arrest or ventricular fibrillation may occur following dilatation of the valve. Facilities should be constantly at hand to allow prompt and vigorous therapy should such complications develop.[56]

Although the Mayo surgeons reported that their patients often showed "great improvement" in terms of chest pain and shortness of breath, they warned that the operation's 20 percent mortality rate "demands a sober approach to its use."[57] Kirklin and Ellis's article on aortic commissurotomy appeared in the August 1955 issue of *Surgical Clinics of North America*, less than six months after they had performed their first open-heart operation. When surgeons performed these aortic stenosis operations, they worked blindly inside a patient's beating, blood-filled heart.

Open-Heart Surgery's New Frontier: Diseased Valves

Walt Lillehei at the University of Minnesota was the first surgeon to use a heart-lung machine to operate on patients with aortic stenosis, aortic regurgitation, or mitral regurgitation.[58] In August 1956 he published a case report of the first patient who underwent surgery for aortic stenosis using a pump-oxygenator. Lillehei had operated on the thirty-one-year-old woman in January and reported that three months later she "could climb stairs without difficulty whereas preoperatively this was impossible."[59] Mayo surgeons did not begin to adopt the open-heart approach to treating patients with aortic stenosis until January 1959. Of the first fourteen patients who had open-heart surgery for aortic stenosis in Rochester, one succumbed in the operating room and another died a month later. But half of the survivors described significant improvement in their symptoms. In 1960 Kirklin and cardiologist Harold Mankin described severe aortic stenosis as a very dangerous disease and recommended surgery for patients who were disabled by symptoms associated with it.[60]

Compared with valves that were obstructed, valves that leaked posed problems that were harder for surgeons to solve. Beginning around 1950, a few individuals attempted to devise operations in animals that used artificial materials to substitute for diseased valves that did not close tightly, which allowed some blood to flow backward. These efforts intensified after Georgetown University surgeon Charles Hufnagel implanted the first prosthetic (artificial) valve in a human in 1952. His operation, designed to treat aortic regurgitation, involved inserting an artificial valve in the descending thoracic aorta, just beyond the left subclavian artery. This location was necessary because in the pre-open-heart surgery era it was impossible to remove a patient's damaged valve and replace it with an artificial one. Designed to reduce the leakage of blood back into the left ventricle, the Hufnagel valve consisted of a plastic ball that moved back and forth inside a plastic tube.[61]

In a *Saturday Evening Post* article, a New York City postal worker marveled over how much better he could breathe after having had a Hufnagel valve placed in his aorta: "You'd never think a little plastic gadget no bigger that a man's thumb…could make all that difference."[62] By 1955, Kirklin and Ellis had implanted Hufnagel valves in eight patients, one of whom died in the hospital after surgery. Although the patients who survived had fewer symptoms, none of them returned to normal activity.[63]

Mayo's busy congenital heart disease program overshadowed local efforts to develop artificial valves. Earl Wood informed open-heart surgery pioneer Clarence Dennis in February 1956: "We have been interested in the difficult technical problem of constructing and designing suitable artificial valves."[64] A few months later, Wood mentioned the project to Stanley Sarnoff, chief of the National Heart Institute's Laboratory of Cardiovascular Physiology. Pleased that Sarnoff was interested in refining an artificial valve that Mayo researchers had been trying to develop, he explained:

> Our experimental cardiovascular surgery team is so occupied with other pressing problems involving the heart bypass machine that I am afraid that sufficient time will not be devoted to testing and development of this valve project. This is not due to a lack of interest (which is very keen) but simply that there are just not enough hours in the day to satisfy the very heavy clinical demands for bypass team personnel and still carry out all of the really important investigational aspects of this activity. Your efforts will certainly complement ours, and progress towards the ultimate goal will be expedited.[65]

Dwight McGoon arrived in Rochester a few weeks after Wood corresponded with Sarnoff. Like John Kirklin, his early work in open-heart surgery focused on treatment of patients with congenital heart defects.

Mayo surgeon Henry Ellis was very interested in valve disease, especially mitral regurgitation. In 1958 he and Arthur Bulbulian reported animal experiments with artificial mitral valves. Bulbulian, best known as a co-inventor of the BLB oxygen mask for high altitude flight, had made hundreds of plastic models of pathological conditions (including heart defects) for publications and exhibits.[66] He and Ellis tried to design an artificial valve that was durable and not predisposed to blood clot formation. It would have to open and close with each heartbeat, about 40 million times a year! They used various synthetic materials that were critical for many innovations in cardiac surgery and cardiology. After Ellis implanted valves of various materials and designs in animals, he and Bulbulian concluded that two types were most promising: a Lucite ball valve and a Teflon valve with a floating disk that slid up and down on a central spindle. But continuing problems with clot formation led them to seek other solutions.[67]

At a 1959 surgical meeting in Montreal, Canada, Ellis reported on fifteen patients who had been operated on at Mayo for mitral regurgitation. Surgeons in several centers were working on this problem. A torrent of technical terms in his talk revealed how many methods had migrated from animal laboratories to a few operating rooms, where they were used in patients. Ellis mentioned "hammocks and slings of veins, vein-covered tendon grafts, pericardial grafts, valvular suture, and the intracardiac placement of plastic baffles and obturators."[68] Most of these approaches had been abandoned because they did not work or caused major complications.

Three of the fifteen Mayo patients died in the hospital, and one died suddenly two months after surgery. A majority of the survivors had fewer symptoms, but Ellis warned against the rapid expansion of operations for mitral regurgitation until longer follow-up showed that patients benefited from the procedure. Cleveland Clinic surgeon Donald Effler opened the discussion of Ellis's paper with a comment that amused the Montreal audience: "It is an historic occasion when a discussant can get up and present a series a little larger than the one from the Mayo Clinic (Laughter)."[69] Effler, who had attempted surgery on twenty-seven patients with mitral regurgitation, agreed with Ellis that longer follow-up on patients was critical and cautioned against using the words "cured" or "corrected" in this context.

Dwight McGoon reported a new surgical approach in 1960 that he had used to treat two patients with severe mitral regurgitation caused by ruptured chordae tendineae (thin fibrous cords that connect the valve leaflets to the papillary muscles that protrude from the left ventricle's inner wall). Based on these two cases, he concluded that the leak could be "corrected in certain instances by repair of the leaflets of the valve rather than by mitral annuloplasty or replacement."[70] In a review of mitral valve surgery published in 1965, McGoon coauthored a paper in which he and his colleagues argued that "every effort should be made to restore function by reconstructive methods in patients with mitral ruptured chordae tendineae and cleft or perforated mitral leaflets before the valve is replaced since the long-term results after such reconstructive procedures have been good."[71] These articles appeared before developments in diagnostic technology led to the recognition of mitral valve prolapse, a common cause of regurgitation.[72] Repair would eventually become the preferred method for treating most patients with severe mitral regurgitation due to ruptured chordae and related conditions.[73]

Searching for a Path to Get a Catheter Inside the Left Heart

The introduction of operations for aortic stenosis and mitral regurgitation in the 1950s stimulated a search for better methods to diagnose diseases of the left-sided heart valves. Traditionally, physicians had relied on a combination of physical examination, X-ray, and electrocardiogram findings to help them distinguish various aortic and mitral valve disorders. These techniques had limitations, even in the hands of experienced heart specialists. Making a precise diagnosis did not influence therapy significantly before surgical intervention was possible because there were no drugs that could alter the course of valve disease. Eventually, most patients with severe stenosis or regurgitation developed congestive heart failure, which was very difficult to treat and often led to death. Experimental valve operations offered a few patients some hope, but the risks of these procedures highlighted the importance of accurate preoperative diagnosis.

In the early 1950s, there was no catheterization technique to directly measure pressures inside the left-sided cardiac chambers in humans. So, a few clinical investigators tried to develop an indirect method to assess left atrial pressure. Catheters had already been used to explore the entire right side of the heart in patients by this time. Lewis Dexter's group at Boston's Peter Bent Brigham Hospital had pushed the thin tube the farthest—wedging its tip in small end-branches of the pulmonary artery. Mayo medical resident Daniel Connolly, working in Earl Wood's laboratory, proved that the so-called pulmonary artery wedge pressure (measured by Dexter's technique) was very nearly equal to left atrial pressure measured directly.[74]

Measuring pulmonary artery wedge pressure was a significant advance in the evaluation of patients with mitral stenosis and some other types of heart disease, but the right heart catheterization technique did not provide information about aortic stenosis. The key to assessing the severity of aortic stenosis was measuring the pressure on both sides of the obstructed aortic valve—in the left ventricle and in the aorta. One possible approach was to insert a catheter into a peripheral artery and thread it upstream through the aorta, across the aortic valve, and into the left ventricle. But Dexter's group had issued a stern warning in 1948 against taking this path into the heart. Based on autopsy findings in animals whose hearts had been catheterized by this route, they declared, "Damage found in the chambers of the left side of the heart definitely prohibits the use of arterial cardiac catheterization in man."[75]

Despite this strong admonition, a few investigators tried to develop methods to measure pressures inside the heart's left-sided chambers. Catheterizing the entire right side of the heart was relatively easy. The operator threaded a catheter along an unblocked path from an arm vein through the right heart's chambers and valves and into the pulmonary artery. Advancing a catheter through an artery into the left ventricle (retrograde arterial catheterization) was more difficult because of real and perceived obstacles. For example, arterial spasm could immobilize the thin tube as it was pushed upstream toward the heart.

Cleveland cardiologist Henry Zimmerman, who was not affiliated with the Cleveland Clinic, first reported the technique of retrograde left ventricular catheterization in 1950. The aortic valve was the main impediment to reaching the left ventricle by this route because it opens for just a quarter of a second with each heartbeat. This led Zimmerman to test his technique in patients with severe aortic regurgitation, a condition in which the valve never closes completely. Although he pushed a catheter into the left ventricle in eleven patients, one died suddenly from ventricular fibrillation. Zimmerman speculated that the fatal heart rhythm was caused by the catheter tip entering a coronary artery, thereby interfering with the heart's blood supply. This deadly complication discouraged others from pursuing the retrograde arterial pathway into the left ventricle.[76]

During the early 1950s, Stockholm surgeon Viking Björk, National Heart Institute surgeon Glenn Morrow, and Pittsburgh cardiologist Donald Fisher devised techniques for entering the left heart that did not involve pushing a catheter across the aortic valve.[77] When Mayo cardiologist Howard Burchell chaired the American Heart Association's Research Committee in 1955, he learned about various experimental cardiac procedures before they were reported in journals or at open medical meetings. Burchell, having been responsible for launching Mayo's right-heart catheterization program after World War II, now encouraged Earl Wood to attempt to put a catheter in the left side of the heart.

In 1955 Burchell informed Wood that when he was in Bethesda, Maryland, for a meeting he had seen Glenn Morrow insert a catheter into the left ventricle through a bronchoscope, an instrument used to view the lung's larger air passages. The first step involved pushing a rigid metal tube down a patient's trachea into the left main-stem bronchus inside the lung. Next, Morrow inserted a twenty-inch needle into the tube and advanced it to the point where its tip pierced the walls of the bronchus and left atrium. He then threaded a catheter through the needle into the left atrium, through the mitral valve, and into the left ventricle. Burchell informed Wood, "Allowing for the variation in people's reactions to the bronchoscope, these procedures went very smoothly." But Morrow had accomplished his goal of putting a catheter in the left heart in only two of four patients on whom he performed the procedure.[78]

From the National Heart Institute in Bethesda, Burchell traveled to Pittsburgh, where he watched Donald Fisher use a very different approach to place a catheter in the left heart. First, the cardiologist pushed a six-inch needle through a patient's back. Inserted to the left of the spine, the needle was advanced until its tip punctured the left atrial wall and entered the left atrium. Fisher followed the needle's progress on a fluoroscopic X-ray screen. Next, he threaded a catheter through the needle into the left atrium, through the mitral valve, and into the left ventricle. Then, he pushed the tip through the aortic valve and into the ascending aorta. Having watched Fisher traverse the whole left heart in Pittsburgh, Burchell informed Wood that intracardiac pressures were measured directly and "the patients showed no discomfort whatsoever."[79] Wood responded that he wanted to "push ahead with this project as expeditiously as possible."[80] After discussing the two techniques with some of their Mayo colleagues, Wood and Burchell decided to use Fisher's posterior chest approach. He came to Rochester to demonstrate it to them.

Wood's group reported their experience with Fisher's posterior chest technique for left heart catheterization in twenty-seven patients in 1956. They concluded that the procedure was "practical, carries a reasonably low risk and has much to offer in the accurate diagnosis and study of disease of the mitral and aortic valves." Their article included a picture of a man lying on his stomach with a long needle protruding from his back. The needle was a small part of the technology that Wood used as part of a "rather complicated set of procedures" designed to get the desired information. A caption described a dozen catheters, connectors, tubes, monitors, and measuring devices that were depicted in the photograph.[81] Wood later characterized the Fisher technique as "rather hair-raising," but it did provide unique information that influenced decisions about the care of selected patients.[82]

Howard Burchell presented the first of seven papers at a 1956 Mayo symposium on the diagnostic value of simultaneous catheterization of right heart, the left heart, and the aorta. The main goal of this complex combined procedure was to help decide which patients might benefit from new operations (especially for aortic stenosis and mitral regurgitation). No surgeon wanted to open a patient's chest and heart only to discover that surgery was unnecessary or impossible. Burchell acknowledged that sending a patient to surgery with the wrong diagnosis could be a "humiliating experience for the clinician." It could be deadly for the patient. The seasoned cardiologist cited four common causes of diagnostic mistakes: an inadequate physical examination, the misinterpretation of findings, the overemphasis of single findings (especially laboratory reports), and the failure to discuss difficult cases with colleagues.[83] Kirklin and Ellis, who had been doing open-heart surgery for a year, "heartily welcomed" left-heart catheterization as a tool to improve preoperative diagnosis.[84]

Angiocardiography: An Adjunct to Cardiac Catheterization

Most pioneers of catheterization were physiologists or cardiologists who used the long flexible tubes to measure intracardiac pressures or to collect blood samples in order to calculate its oxygen content. Their goal was to understand cardiac physiology in normal individuals and in patients with heart disease. But a catheter could also be used as a conduit for injecting radiopaque contrast material (hereafter contrast) into blood vessels and the heart to provide anatomical information. Standard X-rays produced a still shadow image of the contrast in a vessel (angiogram) or a cardiac chamber (angiocardiogram). Fluoroscopy made it possible to watch the contrast flow and the chamber outlines move in real time.

Angiocardiography, which involved visualizing the contrast-filled chambers of the heart's chambers, had been invented in the 1930s. It became a clinically relevant technique in the 1940s, following the development of closed-heart surgery.[85] A 1953 American Heart Association report on catheterization and angiocardiography, which Earl Wood coauthored, advised that angiocardiography should be limited to hospitals with "the elaborate equipment and trained personnel essential for maximum yield of information."[86] Johns Hopkins was such an institution because surgery chief Alfred Blalock considered angiocardiography useful in planning operations on patients with congenital heart disease, and radiology chief Russell Morgan was very interested in the technology.

Russell Morgan was perfecting an X-ray image intensifier for fluoroscopy in the early 1950s with the help of biophysicist Ralph Sturm, who had worked with Earl Wood in Mayo's Acceleration Laboratory during World War II. The prototype Johns Hopkins fluoroscopic screen intensifier offered major advantages over commercially available apparatus used to watch moving X-ray images. It produced a picture that was more than 1,000 times brighter than that generated by standard technology. This meant that patients and other individuals near the X-ray source were exposed to less radiation during the procedure.[87]

After Wood saw the image intensifier at Hopkins in 1954, he told Sturm that he was eager to get one installed in his catheterization laboratory. Worried about the $25,000 cost, Wood informed his friend and former colleague that he would try to "convince the authorities" at Mayo that the unit was vital for "the refinement and extension of diagnostic techniques."[88] He was unsuccessful, but in 1955 Mayo did buy a less expensive unit made by Phillips, a Dutch electronics company, that combined a fluoroscopic image intensifier with a 35 mm motion picture camera. Wood thought it would "greatly improve our selective angiography, which has proved to be of considerable value."[89]

Technology for visualizing and recording angiographic images was evolving rapidly in the mid-1950s. Wood became increasingly concerned in 1956 that his nearly new apparatus was not state-of-the-art. Eager to get better equipment, he told two members of the Mayo's Board of Governors that Cleveland Clinic cardiologist Mason Sones was coming to Rochester to lecture on selective cineangiography as a valuable tool for the diagnosis of congenital heart disease. Wood emphasized that Sones had more experience making motion pictures of angiographic images than anyone else in the United States. Confident that viewers would find the visiting cardiologist's films compelling, he pleaded: "I do wish that a representative or representatives of the Research Administrative Committee and the Sciences Committee would make it a point to listen to Dr. Sones' talk and see his motion picture this coming Wednesday."[90]

Five days later, Wood urged the same two board members to support the purchase of a "perfected and proved" Westinghouse Cine-Fluorex unit.[91] Westinghouse promoted their unit in an advertisement as a major advance because it incorporated a motion picture camera that captured "every fleeting [fluoroscopic] image for detailed study of motion."[92] Running out of patience, Wood complained, "We have acute and pressing need for adequate angiocardiographic equipment for use in selective angiography in infants and small children. The Cine-Fluorex equipment will fill this need. It is no exaggeration to say that the methods we are presently using for selective angiography are a disgrace to this institution."[93] The physiologist's frustration was obvious, but he was competing with many others at Mayo who sought institutional support for acquiring new technologies to use in patient care and clinical research.

In 1956 angiocardiography pioneer Charles Dotter declared that radiology was poised "to make really important contributions to cardiovascular medicine." The University of Oregon radiologist explained that "the necessary enthusiasm already exists within our ranks. If encouragement and financial support are forthcoming, the objectives are by no means nebulous."[94] In Rochester, Earl Wood did not find encouragement or financial support for obtaining the state-of-the-art angiocardiography equipment he wanted to install in the catheterization laboratory. Harry Weber, the chief of radiology, worried about the cost of new specialized apparatus. Aware of Wood's concerns and the rapid growth of Mayo's open-heart surgery program, he informed the Board of Governors in 1957 that requests for new equipment for the "mechanically complex procedure of angiocardiography will become more frequent and more insistent before long."[95]

Weber opposed the spread of X-ray technologies among the various outpatient and inpatient facilities in Rochester, where patients were evaluated and managed: "Specialized equipment is very expensive to buy and install; it is also very expensive to maintain and to man, its product is usually expensive to interpret, and most unfortunately it is subject to change without notice." He warned that it was "extravagant and unrealistic to think of installing such equipment in more than one place in the community under Mayo Clinic auspices."[96]

When Earl Wood could not convince Mayo's leaders to equip his laboratory with state-of-the-art angiocardiography apparatus, he redoubled his efforts to develop dye-dilution (or indicator-dilution) techniques, which complemented catheter-based pressure and oxygen content measurements.[97] The dye-dilution method involved injecting a colored dye into a patient's circulation through a catheter tip placed in a blood vessel or cardiac chamber and recording how long it took the substance to reach a sensor in another location. It was used to measure cardiac output and to diagnose some types of congenital heart defects and acquired valve disorders.

Wood's passion for dye-dilution was displayed to Mayo doctors in all medical and surgical specialties in 1957, when he and his colleagues delivered fifteen lectures on the technique at two consecutive biweekly general staff meetings. It is hard to imagine how these physicians and surgeons sat through so many technical talks that had no relevance to their own practices.[98] John Kirklin, who introduced the two-part symposium, confessed that even he found it hard to translate some of the complicated dye-dilution curves into clinically useful information.[99]

Wood's close friend and staunch supporter Howard Burchell closed the dye-dilution symposium by expressing enthusiasm for the technique and praising Mayo medical resident Irwin Fox for helping to develop indocyanine green, an improved dye. Although Burchell admitted that dye-dilution tests could not solve all diagnostic problems, he argued that they could eliminate the need for angiocardiography in some cases.[100] Burchell told the audience at a national meeting that local "interest in the development of dye-dilution techniques... had the result of limiting angiocardiographic experience and collateral investigations" at Mayo.[101] Actually, Burchell's comment about cause and effect reversed the reason for Wood's reliance on dye-dilution techniques. If the physiologist had gotten the angiocardiography apparatus he wanted, he would have been less inspired to develop (and less dependent on) dye-dilution techniques.

Heart Surgery and Catheterization Move to Saint Marys

Mayo's open-heart surgery program moved from Methodist Hospital to Saint Marys Hospital in September 1956. This relocation would have major implications for the future of Earl Wood's world-class catheterization laboratory. At the time, almost all of the patients who underwent catheterization in Rochester were children, and some of them were very sick as a result of advanced congenital heart disease. Kirklin and pediatric cardiologist James DuShane were concerned about moving these children back and forth between Saint Marys, where they were hospitalized, and the Medical Sciences Building, where they were catheterized. The two-mile round trip seemed much longer in winter, when subzero temperatures were common in Minnesota. But proximity was only part of the problem.

Another concern was that Wood collected too much data and repeated too many measurements. Cardiologist Benjamin McCallister, who worked in his laboratory during his training, recalled that a catheterization usually took more than three hours and that Wood "was so meticulous about things that you just measured stuff until your eyes fell out."[102] Some of Mayo's medical and surgical heart specialists expressed concern about the risks associated with prolonging a catheterization to collect data that did not influence the care of an individual patient.

In November 1956, five weeks after the open-heart surgery program moved to Saint Marys Hospital, Wood and his junior associate Jeremy Swan sent a memo to John Kirklin, Henry Ellis, James DuShane, and the heads of Mayo's two cardiology sections. It addressed the thorny issue of balancing routine diagnostic procedures and the catheterization laboratory's academic mission. The memo, drafted mainly by Wood, was written "from the viewpoint of what apparently would be the best interests of the cardiac catheterization laboratory and the institution as a whole."[103] It distinguished two categories of catheterization: those done to "make or complete a diagnosis or make a decision as to therapy or prognosis" and those done "both for diagnostic and for investigative and educational purposes." The section discussing the first category is revealing. After noting that the laboratory was "willing and anxious to carry out all procedures needed for accurate and complete diagnosis," the tone changed:

> Scheduling of purely diagnostic procedures should not be done lightly, however, since they are a very high cost activity from every aspect from

which, after an adequate series of cases of various conditions have been studied there is little chance of extra return on the investment in the form of investigation or education. As you realize, the rather elaborate and unique features of our catheterization laboratory derive their justification for existence on the basis of "extra return" in the form of investigation and education over and above providing the best diagnostic precision possible by these methods. Therefore, cases from which there is little chance of such "extra return" should be scheduled only for *firm* practical diagnostic reasons.[104]

The memo closed with a conciliatory comment, urging the recipients to consider the catheterization laboratory as a cooperative endeavor among Mayo's clinicians, surgeons, and physiologists. But perspective was a problem. Clinicians and surgeons were responsible for the care of individual patients. On the other hand, Wood viewed himself as a scientist who was responsible for furthering knowledge about cardiac function in health and disease.[105]

James Priestley was vice chair of Mayo's Board of Governors when Wood and Swan sent their memo in 1956. In his presidential address delivered to members of the Central Surgical Society two years earlier, Priestley had warned: "If some of us are not careful, scientific thoughts may crowd thoughts of the patient too far into the corner....Well-directed clinical research is essential, but unnecessary laboratory studies are wasteful and not in the best interest of the patient."[106] When Priestley made these points, federal research funding was fueling the growth of many academic medical centers. This, in turn, led to debates about the relative importance of patient care, research, and education.[107] Mayo's main mission had always been patient care. This would not change, even as the institution's capacity for clinical research increased.

After Mayo's Sciences Committee discussed staff responsibilities in the catheterization laboratory in March 1958, its minutes sent a clear message: "The majority of the members of the committee were of the opinion that the best interests of the clinic would not be served in asking members of the Section of Physiology to devote valuable time and effort in the management of diagnostic procedures." They planned a study to determine if the "development of the procedures used in these laboratories for diagnostic purposes has reached a point where it would be logical to have this work performed by persons other than those primarily interested in research."[108] The debate about routine catheterizations was now focusing on where should they be done and by whom.

The Board of Governors agreed in the summer of 1958 that a new laboratory would be constructed at Saint Marys Hospital "in close association with the proposed angiographic center and that these catheterization facilities be planned for ultimate expansion to include all routine clinical catheterizations." The board's choice of the phrase "all routine clinical catheterizations" was very significant. It had decided that the new facility at Saint Marys would be "an independent laboratory entirely under Dr. Swan's jurisdiction as to planning, selection and training of technical personnel, and ultimate operation."[109]

Jeremy Swan would transition into a more clinically relevant role, but his patient care activity would be limited to the catheterization laboratory. In the new hospital-based facility, Swan was expected to "confine his research activities to such investigations as are derived from the clinical work of the laboratory...relinquishing his research interests in other fields of physiology."[110] In his hands, the catheter would be a tool for diagnosis and for clinical research that was relevant to patient care.

In the fall of 1959 Jeremy Swan spent several weeks at Sweden's Karolinska Institute, a world-renowned center for angiocardiography and cardiac surgery.[111] Shortly before the new catheterization laboratory opened at Saint Marys Hospital in March 1960, *Mayovox*, the clinic's newsletter, informed staff that it would be devoted primarily to children. Swan explained that its location and design would permit collaboration between radiologists and cardiologists in using angiocardiography to image the heart.[112] Although Swan had gained extensive experience interpreting angiocardiograms in Stockholm, Mayo's new chief of radiology, Alan Good, insisted that a member of his department's staff rather than Swan dictate the formal test report. Radiologists Owings Kincaid and George Davis, who were already performing aortic angiograms at Saint Marys Hospital, would now help Swan perform angiocardiograms in the new laboratory.[113]

The first catheterization in the laboratory at Saint Marys was done on a Sunday—on a dog. Kincaid recalled that Swan was concerned about subjecting a patient to the new facility and equipment without a trial run on an animal. The two men went to the Medical Sciences Building and anesthetized a dog, which they then carried to the hospital in a suitcase. Swan and Kincaid walked through the lobby and rode a visitor elevator to the sixth floor, where they performed right- and left-heart catheterizations and an angiocardiogram on the animal. Kincaid recalled that "everything worked to perfection." The men retraced their steps, returning the dog to the downtown kennel without attracting any attention.[114] Initially, the laboratory at Saint Marys Hospital was devoted to performing diagnostic tests on patients (mainly children) with congenital heart disease. But this changed in the early 1960s, when the number of adults operated on increased rapidly as a result of the development of artificial heart valves.

The Development and Early Use of Artificial Heart Valves

Acquired heart valve disease was much more common than congenital heart disease, so the invention of artificial heart valves had major implications for tens of thousands of men and women. At the 1960 meeting of the American Association for Thoracic Surgery in Miami Beach, Boston surgeon Dwight Harken (who had pioneered closed-heart surgery for mitral stenosis a dozen years earlier) reported that he had implanted artificial heart valves in five patients with severe aortic regurgitation. Rather than placing the prosthetic valve in the descending thoracic aorta (Hufnagel's approach), he implanted it where it actually belonged—at the junction of the left ventricle and the ascending aorta. Harken cut out the damaged aortic valve and replaced it with an artificial one, composed of a mobile, silicon-covered Lucite ball contained in a stainless steel cage. Only one patient, a thirty-two-year-old woman, left the hospital alive. Harken identified a common theme in the four patients who died: each one had severe left ventricular enlargement and heart failure symptoms. The Boston surgeon concluded that "better valves than the cage-ball valve may well be developed, but the site and technique of insertion described here seem valid."[115]

In September 1960, National Heart Institute director James Watt welcomed 250 individuals to a Chicago conference on artificial heart valves. To underscore the "dizzying pace of progress" in cardiac surgery, he reminded those present that many of them had participated in another institute-sponsored meeting three years earlier. Then, they had gathered "to discuss how to make heart-lung machines work... now they work so well we are practically able to take them for granted."[116] Watt claimed that at least fifty groups in America were trying to develop prosthetic valves. A few prototypes, such as the one Harken had described in Miami Beach four months earlier, were beginning to migrate from laboratories, where they were tested in animals, to operating rooms, where they were implanted in humans.

At the Chicago meeting, the National Heart Institute's cardiac surgery group reported on five of their patients who had undergone mitral valve replacement. The only survivor was a forty-four-year-old woman whose mitral valve had been replaced on March 11, 1960, by Nina Braunwald and Glenn Morrow. Three of their patients had died in the operating room, and another had succumbed fourteen hours after surgery.[117] But that fact that a single patient had survived total mitral valve replacement was perceived as progress at the time.[118]

Henry Ellis, who had performed Mayo's first mitral valve replacement on July 16, 1960, also spoke at this September meeting in Chicago. He reported on this initial operation and three subsequent ones in which he implanted a flexible single leaflet valve that he had helped develop and test in animals. In each clinical case, Ellis used the experimental valve as a last resort, after other surgical approaches failed. Two patients died in the hospital, and the other two survived less than six weeks after discharge.[119] In a 1961 article on Mayo's short-term experience with mitral valve replacement, Ellis and cardiologist John Callahan emphasized that the "proper timing of the introduction into clinical practice of the fruits of laboratory research is always difficult."[120] This was a recurring theme in the risky but rapidly evolving field of open-heart surgery.

University of Oregon surgeon Albert Starr implanted an artificial mitral valve in a thirty-three-year-old woman with severe congestive heart failure in August 1960. Starr's valve, which he had developed with engineer and entrepreneur Lowell Edwards, was modeled, in part, after a cage ball valve that Ellis and Bulbulian had designed in Rochester. The Starr-Edwards valve (Figure 11.3), which opened and closed with each heartbeat, consisted of a Silastic ball that bounced back and forth inside a Lucite (and later a stainless steel) cage attached to a knitted Teflon cloth ring that was sewn in place after the patient's own diseased valve had been cut out. Starr's first patient died suddenly a few hours after surgery, when air trapped inside her heart traveled in the bloodstream to her brain.[121] But the surgeon persisted, and his outcomes improved.

Starr presented the results of his first eight operations using the Starr-Edwards mitral prosthesis in March 1961. His report attracted considerable attention because six patients survived. Up to this point, no patient who had undergone mitral valve replacement had lived more than three months.[122] Encouraged by these results, Henry Ellis implanted the first Starr-Edwards mitral valve at Mayo in April. Starr's successes were highlighted in a 1964 *McCall's* magazine article, "A Miracle for Amanda." It told the story of a twenty-eight-year-old Chinese-American woman who was the second of his patients to survive.[123] Ellis wrote three years later: "Had it not been for the persistence of Starr, successful development

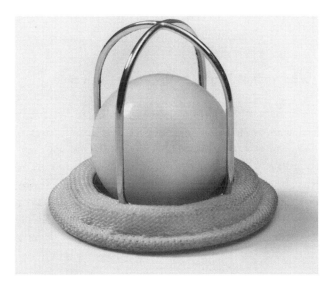

FIGURE 11.3 *Starr Edwards artificial valve.*

Used with permission of Mayo Foundation.

of a prosthetic ball valve suitable for clinical use might have been long delayed."[124] Cardiac surgeon and historian Harris Shumacker considered the Starr-Edwards prosthesis as marking a turning point in valve surgery. It became popular in his opinion because it was easy to implant and it worked very well.[125]

The Starr-Edwards valve was also used in patients with aortic stenosis or regurgitation. Dwight McGoon stunned the surgical world in 1965, when he reported his experience at Mayo with this prosthesis to replace the diseased aortic valves in one hundred sequential patients between February 1963 and December 1964. Each patient left Saint Marys Hospital alive. Noting that several surgeons were now achieving mortality rates in the 4 percent range, he thought it was appropriate to operate on patients before they became severely symptomatic.[126] McGoon, Ellis, and Kirklin began a 1965 article by declaring that surgery for aortic valve disease had changed in less than a decade from being "highly dangerous and uncertain" to being "highly safe and predictable."[127]

Brian Barratt-Boyes of New Zealand, who had trained at Mayo with John Kirklin when the open-heart program was launched, reported implanting a radically different type of prosthetic aortic valve in 1964. The valves had not been made by human hands; they had been removed from the body of a newly deceased human. These human tissue valves, termed homografts, had been removed within fifteen hours of the donor's death, sterilized, and freeze-dried before they were finally prepared for implantation in a patient after his or her own diseased aortic valve had been removed in the operating room.[128] Kirklin implanted the first aortic valve homograft valve in a patient in May 1965, and the early results were encouraging.[129] A quarter century later, Albert Starr reflected on the advent of artificial heart valves and applauded Mayo's surgeons for doing "so much to reduce valve replacement to a standard and predictable operation."[130]

Open-Heart Surgery Expands Dramatically in Just a Decade

When the Mayo Clinic marked the tenth anniversary of its open-heart surgery program in 1965, a heart-lung machine had been used at the institution in 3,897 operations. Noting the advent of artificial heart valves, the author of an article in the clinic's newsletter explained that the number of adults undergoing open-heart surgery was about equal to the number of children. There was a continuous backlog of patients awaiting surgery, despite the fact that Mayo now had four heart-lung machines and seventeen operations were scheduled each week.[131] But open-heart surgery had diffused into practice in the decade since it had debuted as a regularly scheduled procedure in Minneapolis and

Rochester. Doctors who wanted to refer their patients for possible open-heart surgery in the mid-1960s had many choices.

A federally funded survey completed at the end of 1961 (and published four years later) revealed that 303 hospitals in the United States were "fully equipped" for open-heart surgery, closed-heart surgery, cardiac catheterization, and angiocardiography. These findings surprised the authors, who had predicted that about fifty centers provided all four services. Their survey revealed that 8,448 closed-heart operations were performed at 548 hospitals and 8,792 open-heart operations were performed at 290 hospitals in 1961. Because artificial heart valves had just been introduced, it is not surprising that two-thirds of these operations were for congenital heart disease.[132] The survey documented the explosive growth of open-heart surgery, a phenomenon that Mayo pediatric cardiologist James DuShane would not have predicted.

Walt Lillehei published an article in 1966 titled "Should YOUR Hospital Have an Open Heart Surgery Team?" The University of Minnesota surgeon responded, "Yes, if your community can provide a case load of 100 to 150 cases a year and if you can afford the investment in equipment, personnel and training." Linking surgical risk to procedural volumes, Lillehei explained that mortality rates at "experienced centers" had fallen to 2 percent or less in all but the most complex cases. But he warned that mortality above 30 percent was not uncommon in situations where a team performed less than one open-heart operation a month.[133] Lillehei also stressed that accurate preoperative diagnosis was a key component of good patient outcomes. This indisputable fact drove demand for cardiologists who could perform catheterizations and were comfortable advising patients about the new surgical treatment options.

Open-heart surgery had evolved from an experimental procedure in 1955 to a standard treatment technique in less than a dozen years. The field was developing rapidly, and the future looked very promising. Francis Moore, the chief of surgery at Boston's Peter Bent Brigham Hospital, wrote in 1967, "Cardiac surgery has become a distinct branch, growing from the trunk of basic surgical knowledge and technique. Its outward-reaching growth has brought it into new and bright light.... Let us hope that the cardiac branch will never break off its trunk of surgical origin."[134]

Moore was alluding to professional tensions caused by progressive specialization, something that was becoming evident in the relationship between cardiology and internal medicine. The Boston surgeon explained, "Another remarkable dividend of the development of cardiac surgery, bearing on 'surgery in general,' has been the new interface created between the surgeon... and the internist-cardiologist." He noted that the question "What's become of general surgery?" might be rephrased "What's become of internal medicine?" because it, too, was being fragmented among specialists.[135] These tensions became apparent at Mayo in the 1960s, when the clinic's heart specialists confronted increasing competition from academic centers that were growing in size and sophistication as a result of federal research grants.

Beyond Mid-Century

TWO DECADES OF GROWTH AND CHANGE

The two decades after the midpoint of the twentieth century witnessed unprecedented changes in the care of patients with heart disease. This period was also marked by major developments in many areas of science, technology, and culture. For example, in 1950 about 1 million American homes contained a television set and a US air force pilot made the first nonstop transatlantic jet flight. But in 1969 about 125 million Americans watched a live television broadcast of the first men walking on the moon. Meanwhile, in terms of heart care, patients, doctors, nurses, and hospital administrators witnessed the introduction of a host of new diagnostic tests and treatment strategies. Public awareness of the problem of heart disease grew in response to the American Heart Association's fundraising campaigns and media coverage of breakthroughs, on the one hand, and the cardiac-related deaths of celebrities, on the other. The accelerating trend toward medical specialization and subspecialization after World War II had implications for doctors and patients across the nation as well as for the size, structure, and functions of the Mayo Clinic in Rochester.

Mayo Constructs a New Outpatient Building

The front page of a January 1950 issue of *Mayovox*, the clinic's newsletter, showcased an architect's concept drawing of a large new outpatient diagnostic building.[1] Everyone who worked (or received care) in the clinic's 1914 and 1928 buildings knew at mid-century that they were seriously overcrowded. Cardiologist Arlie Barnes, who chaired the Board of Governors, said that space constraints made it impossible for Mayo to "bring its full resources to bear upon what must always be its primary objective...the prompt, efficient care of those patients seeking the medical and surgical services of its staff."[2]

Construction of the ten-story, half-million-square-foot diagnostic building began in the summer of 1950. Like the United Nations Building that was under construction in New York City, it would be an example of the International Style of architecture. When the Mayo building was completed four years later, an *Architectural Forum* article described its light gray exterior as a combination of handsome marble and aluminum (Figure 12.1). Despite this praise, the plain, boxy structure stood in stark contrast to Henry Plummer's carillon-topped limestone and wheat-color brick Art Deco masterpiece across the street.[3] Shifting from the new building's external appearance to its internal functions, the writer explained, "Everything to do with contact between doctors and patients is kept personal, individual, unhurried. But everything to do with the logistics of getting patient, doctor and history into the same place at the same time is clickity-clickity-clickity."[4]

Historian and social reformer Albert Deutsch made a similar point in a 1957 *Consumer Reports* article: "At first glance, the Mayo Clinic has the appearance of a huge medical factory, where patients are processed on a belt-line system, as impersonally as if they were machines in need of repair by skilled mechanics. But a closer view of the system in operation reveals a remarkable network of interpersonal relationships and teamwork under a forbidding front."[5]

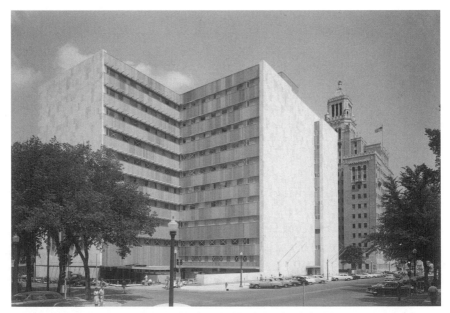

FIGURE 12.1 *New Mayo Clinic building and 1928 (Plummer) building, ca. 1954.*
Used with permission of Mayo Foundation.

Deutsch, a proponent of group practice, compared a patient's experience at the Mayo Clinic with what he or she might encounter in a typical private practice environment. In Rochester, a patient "doesn't have to wait for days to get an appointment with a radiologist...and additional days for the radiologist's report to reach the family doctor. He doesn't have to make an exhausting round of specialists' offices located in different parts of town. He doesn't have to wait for formal conferences or exchanges of correspondence among the medical consultants for a decision on the next step in the treatment of his ailment." In contrast to this scenario, Mayo's "consultants can get into a huddle on the spot."[6] As readers of *Consumer Reports* reflected on their personal travels to see a series of private practitioners, some surely marveled at this description of the Mayo's Clinic's system of highly coordinated specialty care.

Deutsch also detailed the decades-old Mayo system that required all of its internists to function as general diagnosticians, regardless of their medical subspecialty. If a new patient had not been pre-assigned to a specific medical section based on one main health concern, "he is routed to one of the scores of internal medicine specialists who act essentially as general practitioners, or family doctors, following the case through the clinic and coordinating staff work on it." Deutsch dismissed the stereotype of Mayo as being "overspecialized." Noting that almost all staff members were board certified, he explained that "the nearly 100 internal medicine specialists on the staff serve for the most part as general practitioners, giving patients the benefit of their greater training at the important initial examination, and routing them to other specialists as needed."[7]

The author of the 1954 *Architectural Forum* article had made a similar point, explaining that the top three floors of the new diagnostic building were "devoted to general medical sections (analogous to 'family physicians')."[8] The cardiologists, whose combination office-examination rooms were located on the new building's top floor, did not consider themselves family physicians. Tensions surrounding the dual roles of Mayo's hybrid internist-heart specialists increased during the 1960s as a new generation of cardiologists joined the staff. At the same time, medical subspecialization in other fields, such as hematology, was gaining momentum nationally.

Balancing General Medical and Subspecialty Care at Mayo

Mayo's leaders considered the regimented system by which new patients entered the clinic to be a critical component of their institution's long-term success. The Board of Governors distributed a document in 1958 that provides insight into what patients experienced and what the clinic expected of its internal medical specialists, including its cardiologists.

Guiding Principles of the Mayo Clinic Group Practice of Medicine

- Each patient is a private patient and is the responsibility of an individual staff physician who coordinates the diagnostic, surgical and therapeutic measures required for care of the patient.
- The staff physician responsible for a patient is a consultant in internal medicine, unless specific circumstances justify assignment to a physician in a medical or surgical specialty.
- Each consultant in internal medicine, no matter what his special interest, cares for patients with all types of general medical problems.
- On subsequent visits the care of the patient is the responsibility of the same physician who managed his care previously.
- Basic to proper care of the patient are a complete history, obtained through an unhurried interview, and a thorough physical examination, supplemented by properly selected laboratory tests and special studies.
- Consultation with colleagues [having] special knowledge and expertise is freely available and is obtained whenever the patient is likely to benefit from such consultation.
- Medical decisions by members of the staff are based on the patient's medical needs, rather than his ability to pay.[9]

This restatement of a policy that had been in place for two generations was circulated to Mayo's internists when the trend toward subspecialization was accelerating in America.

Mid-century changes in health care delivery created challenges for doctors and patients alike. San Francisco gastroenterologist Dwight Wilbur, who had trained at Mayo in the 1930s, was president of the American College of Physicians in 1959, when he proclaimed, "Internal medicine is the most important, the most rapidly growing, and the least understood specialty in the field of medicine. Laymen in particular, and even members of the medical profession, seem to have little understanding of internists and internal medicine.... The internist has been variously described as the general practitioner and the family physician of the future, the specialist around whom all other specialties will revolve, and the leader in the practice of medicine."[10] Elsewhere, Wilbur described the internist as "a scientifically trained detective" who specialized in the diagnosis and medical treatment of diseases in adults.[11]

Mayo cardiologist Robert Parker, who had joined the Mayo staff in 1937, recalled decades later, "In those early years ... the consultants at the clinic had a strong desire to be internists. In other words we were not cardiologists. We were internists who were specializing in cardiology ... internists with special interests."[12] Parker was describing the partial-specialist model, which is how almost all cardiologists perceived themselves during the middle third of the century. In the 1960s, however, some of Mayo's younger cardiologists became increasingly frustrated because they believed that the clinic's outpatient care model overemphasized general diagnostic work at the expense of subspecialty practice. They were responding to changes in cardiology practice that reflected the introduction of several new technologies and treatment strategies.

America's Increasing Investment in Cardiovascular Research

America's investment in biomedical research after World War II led to many innovations in the care of patients with heart disease, such as cardiac catheterization and open-heart surgery. What had begun as a patchy drizzle of federal research dollars falling on a few academic medical centers turned into a steady rain that drenched many of them. Between 1950 and 1957, total NIH appropriations almost quintupled, from $35 million to $162 million.[13] This unprecedented level of financial support nourished academic centers and promoted the growth of specialties and subspecialties.

Cardiology and cardiac surgery benefited from federal funding more than most other fields because heart disease affected millions of Americans, including celebrities, politicians, and lawmakers. Several prominent political figures had heart attacks in the 1950s, and a few played important roles in getting more federal funds for cardiovascular research.[14] In 1955 Senate Majority Leader Lyndon Johnson had a heart attack while vacationing at a friend's Virginia estate over the Fourth of July weekend. The Texas politician was taken to Bethesda Naval Hospital where Willis Hurst, a thirty-four-year-old cardiologist who had trained with Paul Dudley White in Boston, supervised his care. Lady Bird Johnson wanted Mayo internist James Cain, a longtime family friend and confidant, to see her husband in consultation. He had been involved in Johnson's care at the Mayo Clinic earlier in the year, when the Texas senator was treated for a kidney stone.[15]

James Cain, who subspecialized in gastroenterology, asked Mayo cardiologist Howard Burchell to meet him at the Naval Hospital. Hurst welcomed the senior heart specialist's involvement.[16] Johnson's hospitalization was uneventful. He was recovering at his Texas ranch on September 23, 1955, when President Dwight Eisenhower wrote, "I am delighted to have your encouraging report on your recovery." Literally hours after the Republican president signed the letter warning the Democratic senator not to "try to do too much too quickly," he awoke with severe chest pain.[17]

Eisenhower was at his mother-in-law's home in Denver when he became sick. The White House physician, staying nearby, rushed over to evaluate him. Although the president's pain subsided after a morphine injection, its cause was unclear. Was it indigestion or a heart problem? A dozen hours after the symptoms first appeared, the chief cardiologist at nearby Fitzsimmons Army Hospital made a house call. He recorded an electrocardiogram that revealed an anterior myocardial infarction, which resulted in Eisenhower's hospitalization.[18] This was before the era of coronary care units, so the president was admitted to a private room, where he was placed in an oxygen tent and treated with blood thinners.

One day after Eisenhower was hospitalized, the *Washington Post and Times-Herald* published reassuring words from National Heart Institute director James Watt. He claimed that half a dozen "congressmen who have suffered coronaries in the last few years [are] living normal lives just as if they never had them."[19] But a *Life* magazine article reminded readers of their vulnerability: "The sudden collapse of the President last week focused shocked attention on its cause—coronary thrombosis, the biggest killer in the country." Every year 350,000 Americans died of a heart attack.[20] Understandably, there was debate about whether Eisenhower should run for re-election (Figure 12.2). In January 1956, *U.S. News & World Report* ran a story with a title that implied a consensus among cardiologists: "Heart Specialists Say Ike Could Serve a Second Term."[21] Johnson's recovery was not followed nearly as closely, but he also wanted expert opinions about returning to his life in Washington.

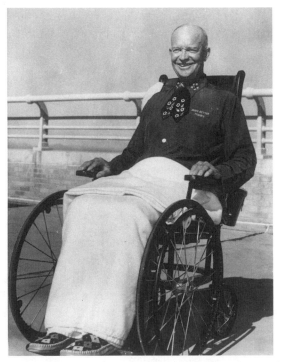

FIGURE 12.2 *President Dwight Eisenhower recovering from his heart attack, with "Much Better Thanks" embroidered on his shirt, November 29, 1955.*

Original Associated Press (AP) wire photo in the author's possession, used with permission of AP.

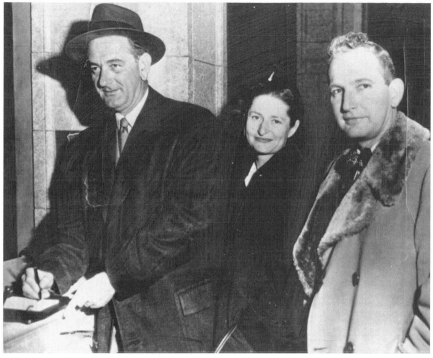

FIGURE 12.3 *Senator Lyndon Johnson, Lady Bird Johnson, and James Cain, MD, in the Mayo Clinic lobby, December 29, 1955.*

Original Associated Press (AP) wire photo in the author's possession, used with permission of AP.

Lyndon Johnson visited the Mayo Clinic shortly after Christmas in 1955 "for a two-day checkup, expected to reveal whether he can resume safely the berth of Senate majority leader after a heart attack earlier this year." The Associated Press circulated this announcement with a wire photo (Figure 12.3) that showed the tall Texan standing beside his wife and James Cain at the clinic's registration window.[22] Johnson did resume his duties in the Senate. Willis Hurst, his longtime cardiologist, recalled decades later, "There is no question about this—Johnson's heart attack stimulated him to increase the funding for cardiovascular research and training."[23] When Howard Burchell participated in Johnson's care in 1955, Mayo did not accept government funds to support any of its research programs. But this was about to change.

Mayo Revises its Policy Regarding External Research Funding

Mayo vascular specialist Edgar Allen became president of the American Heart Association in 1956. Although government grants and private funds were fueling research in several centers, he was frustrated. In his presidential address, he complained about the small amount of money invested in research related to cardiovascular disease:

> The program of medical research represents rebellion against physical deterioration, but the rebellion is still so small that it seems to be hardly more than an insurrection. More scientific minds, more buildings, and more equipment are urgently needed. Almost everyone has had some sorrowful experience with the disease of the heart or blood vessels, or both. Almost everyone we know—a member of his family, a close personal friend, a neighbor or an associate—almost certainly will have or does have heart trouble, or he suffers from the effects of a stroke, of failure of the kidneys to work properly or of poor circulation to the legs. When we consider such all-pervasive facts, we see clearly that there is actually no need to defend a nation-wide, cohesive, planned attack on diseases of the heart and blood vessels.[24]

While Allen was advocating a coordinated national assault on cardiovascular disease, several members of Mayo's Board of Governors were concerned that their institution's tradition of not seeking external research grants threatened its future. Maintaining the status quo—funding research with income from practice and investments—meant that ambitious and aspiring investigators in Rochester would sit on the sidelines as streams of money flowed from Washington to more and more academic centers. Nourished by federal funds, cardiovascular research and training programs were blossoming all across the country. Nearby, the University of Minnesota's cardiac surgery program was in full bloom. In 1956 the National Heart Institute listed 932 active research grants totaling just over $12 million. It was no coincidence that the university received a disproportionate share of the funds—almost one-half million dollars.[25]

Owen Wangensteen, the University of Minnesota's longtime chief of surgery, was an aggressive advocate for his institution's research programs. In 1956 he was a member of the National Advisory Heart Council, the influential group that decided which research grant requests would be funded by the NIH. Wangensteen summarized his congressional testimony in support of cardiac research in a letter to Minnesota Senator Edward Thye. In a letter that began "My dear Ed", the surgeon thanked the senator for his "great and sympathetic interest in this whole matter." Describing a recent visit to Capitol Hill, Wangensteen boasted that he had characterized his department as the home of several "vigorous barrier-breaking surgeons." He had even placed an open-heart surgery article by his protégé Walt Lillehei in the *Congressional Record*.[26] Wangensteen also lobbied American Heart Association leaders for more money. When Edgar Allen was president of the national organization, the Minneapolis surgeon reminded him of a conversation they had had about the need for additional research facilities at the university. Wangensteen explained, "A friendly nod from you in this could perform a miracle for us."[27]

Just before Thanksgiving 1956, the Mayo board made a decision that had profound implications for the institution's future. It unanimously approved a policy permitting Mayo to "apply for and accept grants in support of its programs of medical education and research from appropriate outside sources, both private and public."[28] Board chair Samuel Haines sent a detailed memo explaining the policy change to the clinic's 300 staff doctors and scientists. Each paragraph began with a carefully crafted topic sentence: "Many reasons entered into the Board's decision....The Board has no intention that our entire research program should be supported by grants....The Board is deeply concerned that the new program would be developed circumspectly and properly in all regards." Clear explanations reinforced the notion that Mayo's leaders recognized the significance of this major shift in institutional philosophy.[29]

Haines cited the escalating costs of medical care, research, and education as factors in the board's decision. It was no longer realistic to keep raising fees to maintain Mayo's academic programs at "suitable and proper levels." The board was also impressed by the success of the aggressive postwar public fundraising campaigns of voluntary health organizations, such as the American Heart Association and the American Cancer Society. Noting that many individuals donated money to various disease-specific charities, Haines warned that some patients would resist paying "additional charges of consequence" to help finance medical research in Rochester.[30]

In terms of federal research funding, Mayo got off to a slow start, receiving ten small NIH grants in 1957, totaling just $12,843. The number and size of grants to the institution increased rapidly, however. During the first seven years of the new policy, the institution received $7.4 million in grants: $6.3 million from the NIH and $1.1 million from other public agencies and philanthropic foundations. Even more impressive was the fact that 81 percent of Mayo's 474 grant applications in that period were funded.[31] In 1956, when the clinic's board approved the new policy regarding research grants, its cardiologists were devoting almost all of their time to seeing outpatients. They had little time for research.

Cardiology Structure and Staff at Mayo Between 1950 and 1964

The number of internists at Mayo who focused on heart disease increased significantly between 1950 and 1964. As Tables 12.1 and 12.2 demonstrate, only five of Mayo's sixteen cardiologists in 1964 had been on the staff in 1950.

During this fifteen-year interval, an unprecedented wave of new knowledge, technologies, and procedures stimulated shifts in the scope of their practices. Mayo's comprehensive quarterly listings of staff assignments illustrate how increasing subspecialization influenced the terms associated with (and the content of) the cardiologists' hospital practices in this period. This is reflected in Table 12.3. The most striking change is the appearance and disappearance of the terms "vascular" and "renal" (kidney) in conjunction with "cardio" (heart). In fact, the blending of cardiac, renal, and vascular diseases at Mayo had begun in 1920, when internist Leonard Rowntree arrived in Rochester and the staff was informed that he was "especially interested in cardio-renal-vascular conditions."[32]

Nephrology emerged as a medical subspecialty in the 1950s, mainly as a result of new technologies relevant to the care of patients with serious kidney disease: dialysis to treat acute renal failure and percutaneous needle kidney biopsy as an aid to diagnosis.[33] When Howard Odel was head of a cardiology section in 1953, he recruited James Broadbent (who had just finished a medical fellowship at Mayo) with the expectation that he would care for

TABLE 12.1 Staff Members of Mayo's Two Cardiology Sections, 1950[a]

"Smith Section"	"Barnes Section"
Fredrick Willius (1920)	Arlie Barnes (1925)
H. L. (Roy) Smith (1928)	Howard Odel (1938)
Thomas Dry (1936)	Howard Burchell (1940)
Robert Parker (1937)	Raymond Pruitt (1944)
Charles Scheifley (1946)	Guy Daugherty (1946)
Milton Anderson (1948)	Thomas Parkin (1950)

[a] Adapted from *Quarterly Bulletin...for the Quarter Beginning July 3, 1950*, MCA.

Date the physician joined the staff is in parentheses.

TABLE 12.2 Staff Members of Mayo's Three Cardiology Sections, 1964[a]

"Anderson Section"	"Daugherty Section"	"Brandenburg Section"
Robert Parker (1937)	Howard Burchell (1940)	Robert Brandenburg (1951)
Milton Anderson (1948)	Guy Daugherty (1946)	Daniel Connolly (1955)
John Callahan (1955)	Thomas Parkin (1950)	Emilio Giuliani (1961)
Ralph Smith (1958)	James Broadbent (1953)	Robert Frye (1962)
Robert Schultz (1962)	Harold Mankin (1957)	Stewart Nunn (1963)
		Carlos Harrison (1964)

[a] Adapted from *Quarterly Directory...for the Quarter Beginning July 5, 1964*, MCA.

Date the physician joined the staff is in parentheses.

TABLE 12.3 Mayo-Affiliated Hospital Services That Focused on
Patients with Heart, Kidney, or Vascular Diseases, 1950–1964[a]

Hospital service name	1950	1957	1959	1960	1964
Cardiology	2		2	1	5
Cardiovascular-Renal		3			
Cardiorenal			2	3	
Nephrology					1
Peripheral Vascular	2			2	
Vascular		2	2		3
Total number of services	4	5	6	6	9

[a] Adapted from *Quarterly Bulletin*, July 3, 1950, and *Quarterly Directory*, June 30, 1957;
June 30, 1959; July 3, 1960; and July 5, 1964, MCA. The services were distributed
among three Rochester hospitals: Saint Marys, Methodist, and Worrall.

patients with kidney disease as well as those with heart disease. Two years
later, Broadbent performed the first kidney dialysis procedure and the first
percutaneous renal biopsy at Mayo. Reflecting on that phase of his career
decades later, he emphasized how new technologies influenced the careers of
physicians and the care of patients: "Specialization and careers in subspecialties followed technical developments beginning with cardiac catheterization,
dialysis, renal biopsy, a whole host of things.... There was no master plan.
We simply followed where the developments took us, and the people stepped
forward and said, 'I'll do that.'"[34] In the late 1950s, Broadbent's colleagues
considered him a hybrid heart-kidney specialist, reflecting what he did and
the clinic's cardiorenal tradition.[35]

Mayo's cardiology sections were restructured in the decade around 1960
as a result of the advent of open-heart surgery and the introduction of new
diagnostic techniques and therapeutic procedures pertinent to the care of
patients with heart disease and kidney disorders. In 1959 James Hunt joined
the so-called cardiorenal section after completing his medical fellowship
at Mayo. He was appointed head of a new internal medicine section that
focused on kidney disease four years later. In 1966 *Mayovox*, the clinic's
newsletter, published a primer on the process of subspecialization, using the
development of nephrology to illustrate a major trend in practice at Mayo.
The writer explained that a few years earlier "a substantial number of consultants 'subspecialized' in the whole of cardiovascular-renal disease. More
recently these same consultants have come to concentrate on narrower subspecialty areas—cardiology, peripheral vascular disease, renal disease. The
two-and-a-half-year evolution of the group headed by Dr. Hunt is a current
and important case in point."[36]

Mayo's Cardiologists Develop a Strategic Plan

The shifting boundaries around cardiology practice at Mayo in the early 1960s reflected increasing specialization in medicine, which was one of several interrelated developments occurring at a national level. In 1965 the Association of American Medical Colleges (AAMC) published a report that discussed a dozen intertwined trends affecting health care: accelerating scientific advances; a growing and aging population; increasing individual health expectations; expanding health insurance coverage; unrelenting specialization; growing dependence on technology; increasing institutionalization of care (especially in hospitals); growing teamwork in health care delivery; increasing demand for doctors; a surge in jobs for many other types of health care workers; expanding government involvement in medicine; and rising health care costs.[37] It is notable that the trends described in this fifty-year-old report remain relevant; most of these themes are brought up routinely in current-day discussions of health care in the United States.

The AAMC report was one of several studies of medical practice, training, and research published in the mid-1960s. One major document dealt specifically with cardiovascular disease. President Lyndon Johnson established the Commission on Heart Disease, Cancer and Stroke in 1964, nine years after he had survived a heart attack. Houston cardiovascular surgeon Michael DeBakey chaired the commission, which included Johnson's cardiologist Willis Hurst of Emory University, surgeon Chuck Mayo, and fifteen other doctors and medical scientists. At a White House meeting in April, the president challenged the group: "Unless we do better, two-thirds of all Americans now living will suffer or die from cancer, heart disease or stroke. I expect you to do something about it."[38]

Irving Wright, a New York City vascular specialist and former American Heart Association president, chaired the commission's Subcommittee on Heart Disease. Its 1965 report claimed that tremendous strides had been made during the past fifteen years in the prevention and treatment of the nation's number one cause of death. This was due, in part, to "the wise and intelligent interest and awareness of the U.S. Congressmen who have appropriated increasing amounts of money for medical research."[39] After describing several practical discoveries and developments, the authors recommended that more clinical cardiology fellowships be established to train more heart specialists because these individuals would ultimately carry the fruits of research into patient care.[40] This was one of several issues that Mayo's cardiologists had been considering in the context of national events and a local anniversary.

The Board of Governors chose 1964 as the Mayo Centennial Year to celebrate William W. Mayo's relocation of his medical practice to Rochester in 1864 and the births of his sons Will and Charlie.[41] Beginning in September of that year, many Americans saw the Mayo brothers' pictures in profile on a green five-cent stamp when they sent or received letters (Figure 12.4). This first class stamp found its way into most homes because the government printed 120 million of them at a time when the US population was about 190 million.[42]

In Rochester, the centennial was a time for reflecting on the past, assessing the present, and preparing for the future. *Mayovox* had recently published an article "Long-Term Planning Essential to Insure Future," in which board chair James Priestley urged the staff to look backward because "an organization which forgets its past has no future." As he explained the philosophy of the long-range planning process, the surgeon stressed the interdependence of individuals and their institution.

> A self-critical rather than a self-satisfied attitude; a broad rather than a provincial outlook; search for and ready acceptance of new ideas which appear to have merit; readiness to accept change when this is indicated; a continued eagerness to excel; a constant effort to improve opportunities; a sense of responsibility on the part of each of us for the welfare of each other...full realization that our strength lies in unselfish union, mutual help and cooperation; establishment of long-range goals, by each of us individually, by fields of interest, and for our entire institution.[43]

Priestley's message echoed the words and philosophy of Will Mayo and other former clinic leaders, but he delivered it at a time of increasing unrest in American medicine and society.

When Mayo began celebrating its centennial year, the cardiologists were completing a strategic plan. Coincidentally, the final draft of their

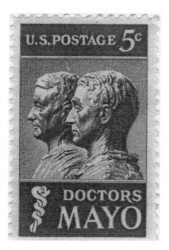

FIGURE 12.4 *The Doctors Mayo first class stamp issued on September 11, 1964.*
In the public domain.

document, "A Prospectus: Adult Cardiology at the Mayo Clinic," was dated January 13, 1964, the same day that Columbia Records released Minnesota-born singer-songwriter Bob Dylan's album *The Times They Are A-Changin'*.[44] Mayo's cardiologists had not heard the song, which reflected the contemporary cultural scene (especially the Civil Rights Movement), but they knew that their specialty was changing rapidly. All sixteen of them signed a letter to the Board of Governors that accompanied their prospectus. This tactic demonstrated unity and a sense of urgency. But their rhetoric was respectful: "We are seeking approval of the concepts in the Prospectus, which we feel would be of assistance to us in recruitment as well as in continued patient care, education, and clinical investigation."[45] They listed six short-term goals:

- The retention and acquisition of adequate professional personnel to maintain excellent patient care.
- The assurance of sufficient concentration of cardiology in practice to insure that a substantial amount of practice time is spent handling cardiologic problems.
- The creation of a sufficient number of hospital services to permit frequent rotation of consultants on the hospital services (approximately one month out of each quarter would be optimal).
- Time and space opportunity for clinical investigation and research for those desiring it.
- Improved liaison with laboratory scientists who are pursuing investigation and research in cardiology.
- The furtherance of improved educational opportunities for consultants and Mayo Clinic fellows and special trainees in clinical cardiology.[46]

The cardiologists viewed the provision of high-quality patient care as their primary role, but they were also concerned about the academic aspects of their practice. Mayo had been an international leader in developing cardiac catheterization and open-heart surgery, but the heart specialists now thought that their institution had fallen behind: "The great stimulus for investigation and research which was present a decade or two ago with the development of cardiac catheterization and operative cardiac surgery has reached a noticeable plateau," they wrote in 1964.[47]

Academic physicians and scientists have long considered the number of articles published in peer-reviewed journals to be a critical measure of research productivity. In 1963 Mayo's sixteen cardiologists published a total of just twenty-five papers. They attributed this low output to "the great press of work involved in patient care."[48] Most full-time faculty members at traditional academic medical centers were granted protected time for research, but this was uncommon at Mayo. In 1962 just twelve of the clinic's twenty-one internal medicine section heads reported that any of their staff members were granted time away from practice for research.[49]

Each Mayo cardiologist fell along a spectrum of enthusiasm with respect to interest in doing research and willingness to support others who did (or hoped to do) it. As a group, however, they identified issues that could influence individual attitudes and actions. For example, they recommended granting clinicians "some time off from routine duties" if the appropriate committees approved "a well-conceived, properly planned project."[50] But the main challenge was having enough cardiologists available to manage the large volume of patients, many of whom were assigned to their sections for general (non-cardiac) diagnostic workups. In 1964, for example, the six physicians in Robert Brandenburg's cardiology section saw more than 6,500 patients in the outpatient practice, in addition to their inpatient and other responsibilities.[51]

As the cardiologists developed their strategic plan, the balance between patient care, research, and education was being debated not only at the Mayo Clinic but at many academic institutions. George Thorn, physician-in-chief of Boston's Peter Bent Brigham Hospital, had explained in a 1963 speech that the number of full-time faculty members at traditional academic medical centers "began to increase geometrically when research funds became available in relatively generous proportions" after World War II. The Harvard endocrinologist reminded his audience of "the often quoted criticism that departments of medicine are more concerned with research effort than with patient care."[52] No one could claim that this was the case at the Mayo Clinic. The author of a 1965 *Business Week* article "Mayo's Magic: The Human Touch" observed, "Critics have charged that the clinic is too patient-oriented at the expense of research.... On the other hand, the chief of another medical center says, 'Who is to say if critics cloistered in university research have not gone too far in removing themselves from patients? Who is to say Mayo is not right?' "[53]

More Specialization and a Cardiology Fellowship Program

Very few Americans received care at academic medical centers, and most patients were unconcerned about how physicians in those institutions divided their time between clinical and research activities. In many contexts, however, the accelerating trend toward subspecialization did affect the care that men and women received. Magazine and newspaper articles, motion pictures, and television programs informed the public about a shift toward more specialized care in the 1950s and celebrated a series of medical and surgical breakthroughs.[54] Albert Deutsch declared in his 1957 *Consumer Reports* article on the Mayo Clinic, "The day when the bearded man with the little black bag could comfortably retain in his head most of the essential medical knowledge of his time—and use it—has long since passed. Today there are no less than 36 recognized medical specialties and subspecialties...the Age of Specialism is definitely established."[55]

In 1959 a *Life* magazine writer discussed the dynamics of specialization: "Many doctors have reasoned that only by focusing all their energy and attention on the details of a certain condition or organ can they hope to keep up with technology. Although this narrow focus does tend to make some of them forget that patients are whole human beings, specialists are essential at today's high level of medicine. Patients may not like being sent to unfamiliar specialists or paying their fees, but it improves their chances of being cured."[56] Mayo's cardiologists, acknowledging these trends, concluded that the type of training they had received (and that their institution still offered) was no longer sufficient for physicians aspiring to be heart specialists.

Mayo's pioneering three-year medical fellowship model was fifty years old in 1963, when physiologist Victor Johnson, director of the Mayo Foundation for Medical Education and Research, drafted a memorandum, "Proposed Training Program in Advanced Cardiology." The plan that he summarized had been described to him by Robert Parker, James Broadbent, and Daniel Connolly, who represented the clinic's three cardiology sections. When the concept of a formal cardiology fellowship was first discussed in Rochester, several academic medical centers had already established such programs.[57] The one-year program proposed at Mayo would consist of four quarters divided among outpatient cardiology, hospital-based cardiology, the catheterization laboratory, and pediatric cardiology.

Traditionally, hospital administrators viewed interns, residents, and fellows primarily as workers rather than advanced learners. Victor Johnson, alluding to the balance between service and education, concluded that the cardiologists' proposal appeared "to be loaded a little more in favor of what a fellow will receive as compared to what he will give." But he was confident that it would be "an excellent program for prospective cardiology staff members."[58] Section head Milton Anderson made the same point in his annual report to the board. He also predicted that the fellowship program would stimulate the staff to become more involved in research because it could "be done in a supervisory way with the trainees serving in the capacity of a proxy."[59] This model was standard in research-oriented institutions. Mayo's formal one-year cardiology fellowship training program was launched on July 1, 1963. Robert Corne, the first fellow, had completed medical school and an internship in his native Canada before spending three years as a medical resident in Rochester.[60]

Specialty training was changing rapidly in the mid-1960s. The cardiologists' 1964 prospectus included a proposal to establish a two-year fellowship that would provide "more intensive training" for doctors who planned to "practice primarily in the field of cardiology."[61] Each fellow would spend nine months in adult cardiology, three months in pediatric cardiology, six months in the catheterization and electrocardiographic laboratories, and six months in research related to cardiac pathology, physiology, or pharmacology. In September 1964, section head Milton Anderson sent a memo to representatives of the other two cardiology sections, explaining that he was eager to proceed with planning this two-year fellowship. Rather than focusing on training cardiologists for private practice, he stressed the importance of producing "cardiology specialists" with sufficient research experience to qualify them for "positions of teaching and investigation" in medical schools.[62] In fact, Mayo-trained physicians, surgeons, and scientists had long been attracted (and attractive) to academic institutions. A 1961 report had shown that 40 percent of approximately 3,000 former Mayo trainees held academic appointments in 73 medical schools in 36 states.[63]

Mayo launched a two-year cardiology fellowship program in January 1966. Paul O'Donovan, the first fellow, was a native of Ireland, where he had graduated from medical school and completed an internship. Prior to beginning his cardiology fellowship, O'Donovan had completed a second internship in Massachusetts and a three-year medical residency in Rochester. The new training model was successful and soon became the standard at Mayo and other academic medical centers.

Mayo's Medical Residency Program is Put on Probation

The Mayo Clinic's enviable reputation and its record of producing thousands of specialists over one-half century did not shield it from rules and regulations governing medical training that were implemented in the 1960s.[64] The American Medical Association had established the Citizens Commission on Graduate Medical Education in 1963 to evaluate the training of interns and residents. The commission's lengthy report, published three years later, rejected the status quo and demanded action. A single sentence revealed its expectations: "Graduate medical education needs an organization that can and will turn its spotlight into many nooks and crannies, that will seriously consider serious problems, and that will exert strong leadership in bringing about improvements already known to be desirable and other improvements that will later be recognized."[65] In fact, another national body was already in a position to accomplish some of those goals, and one of its actions had a major impact on the Mayo Clinic.

The Residency Review Committee for Internal Medicine, made up of representatives of the American Board of Internal Medicine, the American College of Physicians, and the American Medical Association Council on Medical Education and Hospitals, was responsible for accrediting internal medicine training programs in the United States.[66] After representatives of the committee visited Rochester in December 1965, they raised concerns that resulted in Mayo's internal medicine residency program being placed on probation the following summer. During the year surrounding the Mayo site visit, the committee placed 10 percent of 311 internal medicine residency programs on probation and withdrew approval for another 10 percent.[67] Mayo took the probation very seriously. Loss of accreditation would cripple its ability to recruit potential medical residents, the main source of future staff members.

The Residency Review Committee for Internal Medicine was concerned that Mayo's medical residents spent too much time in the outpatient practice. Residents in almost every other training program devoted essentially all of their time to caring for hospitalized patients. A related issue was the work that a Mayo medical resident actually did when he or she was assigned to the outpatient practice. Basically, these trainees performed five general diagnostic evaluations each day with one-to-one supervision by a staff physician.

A *Look* Magazine Editor Describes His Mayo Experience in 1964

A senior editor at *Look* magazine, who detailed his experience as a patient at the Mayo Clinic in 1964, described the institution's approach to training medical residents. Jack Star sat in one of the 225 chairs in the tenth floor waiting room. Soon, he was taken to one of the floor's 96 combination office-examination rooms that were shared by almost four dozen staff physicians. Next, he met "a bouncy man of middle age" who was "a specialist in internal medicine." David Carr, a pulmonary subspecialist whose main interest was lung cancer, would function as Star's "personal physician" during his evaluation in Rochester. Douglas Gracey, a first-year medical resident, would take a history and perform a physical examination. After Gracey finished, he called Carr, who returned to examine the magazine editor and formulate a plan for his further evaluation.[68]

Star's blood pressure averaged 150/100, and Carr decided to order a comprehensive hypertension workup. Effective antihypertensive drugs had been introduced during the past decade, and this coincided with increased emphasis on trying to identify a specific cause for a patient's high blood pressure. These developments had led to the establishment in 1958 of a Hypertension Clinic that was staffed by members of Mayo's two vascular medicine sections.[69] As part of Star's hypertension evaluation, he underwent tests of his kidneys and adrenal glands. After they were completed, he returned to see Carr, who was coordinating his visit. Next, Alexander Schirger, one of the vascular specialists who focused on hypertension, joined the two men and gave the editor-patient a series of recommendations: "Get enough rest, don't get overtired, don't smoke, have your blood pressure checked once a month by your family doctor—he can prescribe medication if it remains high. The blood vessels in your eyes show some narrowing so you should have your eyes checked once a year, along with the rest of you."[70]

Pleased with the results of his thorough evaluation, the *Look* editor ended his story: "I shake the doctors' hands and take the elevator down to the lobby. There, I pay my bill, which by now totals $450. 'It's all those tests that run them up,' the clerk explains. 'I know what you mean,' I say as I gratefully walk out into the cool Minnesota country air."[71] Star's experience as an outpatient was typical for the Mayo Clinic, but it was not what members of the Residency Review Committee for Internal Medicine expected from a medical training program. The committee concluded that Mayo residents performed too many routine outpatient examinations and were not involved in the final decision-making process.[72]

In terms of a medical resident's inpatient experience, the committee faulted Mayo in 1966 for not having a system for the "graded increase of responsibility for conduct of the patient's course while in the hospital."[73] This concern reflected opinions held by many leading academic physicians. For example, James Warren, a cardiologist who chaired Ohio State University's Department of Medicine, argued in 1966 that good training programs must give residents increasing responsibility as they gained experience. He also expressed concern about training programs that relied on private patients. Warren warned that under those circumstances "the young physician is apt to be given very little responsibility and the staff physicians literally take over," with the result that the residents occupy an "almost clerk-like role."[74] In fact, this seemed to describe the situation at the Mayo Clinic and its affiliated hospitals, where all individuals were considered private patients. Staff physicians were actively involved in the care of each one, whether they were outpatients or inpatients.

Mayo's Hospitals Focus on Patient Care, Not Medical Teaching

Johns Hopkins Medical School dean Thomas Turner had expressed an opinion in 1963 that many of his peers in academic medical centers shared. He argued that an "asset of the greatest importance in the teaching hospital is the presence of a certain number of so-called service cases which become the principal responsibility of the senior resident staff. The availability of such patients is essential to post-doctoral education."[75] Turner claimed that "the primary purpose of a teaching hospital is to serve the teaching needs of the medical school, that is, the preparation of young men for careers in medicine."[76]

Unlike Johns Hopkins and other traditional academic institutions, Mayo did not have a medical school in 1966, when its medical residency program was put on probation. And the primary purpose of its affiliated hospitals was to provide care to patients. Turner, aware of the national context, acknowledged that "the trend in the economics of medical care will inevitably lead to fewer service cases in the future…much of the teaching of the doctor of the future will of necessity be around the diagnosis and treatment of private patients."[77] Johns Hopkins had two parallel medical residency programs: one focused on so-called service cases (patients without insurance) and the other on private patients.[78] This distinction did not exist at Mayo, where all individuals were treated as private patients.

Mayo moved quickly and deliberately to address the concerns that the Residency Review Committee for Internal Medicine had raised in order to justify placing the clinic's internal medicine training program on probation. For example, the Board of Governors changed local trainee terminology to conform to national standards—the term "resident" would replace "fellow" (except in the case of advanced post-residency positions). Individual trainees would be categorized as a resident, senior resident, or chief resident to reflect the fact that they would be given greater independence as they progressed through the program. A senior resident, who was usually in his or her third postgraduate year, would assume "primary responsibility for patient care, diagnostic or therapeutic, or both, under direct supervision of a permanent faculty member." The chief resident would have "full responsibility for patient care, diagnostic or therapeutic, or both, under direction of a permanent faculty member."[79] Vascular specialist John Spittell, who was put in charge of the medical residency program, would coordinate several significant structural and philosophical changes.[80]

Charles Code, who became director of the Mayo Foundation for Medical Education and Research during the 1966 probation episode, explained six years later, "The crisis afforded the opportunity to introduce change. The principle was simple; shift the responsibility for selection of residents, for development and maintenance of programs, from the paternalistic-central control of the past to the periphery—to the departments where the training was done. We called it the peripheralization of responsibility and control. We had the talent, the brains, the knowledge and the skill to develop as fine programs as there were in the world."[81] Code boasted that the changes had returned Mayo to the forefront of national and international postgraduate training programs.

Mayo Creates a Department of Internal Medicine

One of the most significant changes that resulted from the probation incident was the creation of a Department of Internal Medicine in 1967.[82] This development highlights a fundamental difference between the Mayo Clinic and traditional academic medical centers that were framed around a medical school. The conventional departmental structure originated in the nineteenth century.[83] Rosemary Stevens explains in her history of American hospitals: "Even small hospitals were expected to have at least divisions of medicine and surgery in the 1950s.... Department chairmen in the largest teaching hospitals were becoming controlling czars of substantial domains."[84] But Mayo's structure was very different before its training programs came under intense scrutiny in the mid-1960s. On the basis of several interviews, the author of a 1960 magazine article on the Mayo Clinic concluded that "there are no 'chiefs' in the medical school sense, only section heads with purely administrative duties. Every staff man has equal status in handling patients. No one has the prerogatives of a university chief, but no one is under a chief's thumb either."[85]

Internist and gastroenterologist Richard Reitemeier, the first chair of Mayo's Department of Internal Medicine, recalled, "Prior to the time that the department was organized [in 1967], there was a very highly structured arrangement of sections, each with its own individual autonomy.... These reminded me a little bit of fiefdoms in the Middle Ages."[86] In fact, Reitemeier's original title, "Chairman of Sections of Internal Medicine," respected this institutional tradition. When he was selected to head the clinic's twenty-three internal medicine sections, Mayo was moving from a horizontal to a pyramidal administrative structure.

John Kirklin had been selected to be "Chairman of Sections of General Surgery" in 1964, and Robert Brandenburg was chosen to be "Chairman of Sections of Cardiology" the following year.[87] When the board considered whom to choose to chair general surgery, cardiology, and internal medicine, it stated explicitly that "the appointee will not be selected on the basis of seniority."[88] This major shift in philosophy acknowledged the need to select leaders based on their perceived potential to help their colleagues negotiate the increasingly complex and competitive spheres of medical practice, research, and postgraduate training.

Mayo Cardiologists Want to See Patients With Heart Disease

National trends toward more subspecialization in training and practice led some Mayo cardiologists to challenge another long-standing institutional tradition. Shortly after Robert Brandenburg became chair of the three cardiology sections in 1965, he complained to the board about the number of general diagnostic evaluations that he and his colleagues were expected to perform. Concerned that the ratio of patients with cardiovascular disease to those with other medical problems was "still not high enough for ideal training and experience in our subspecialty," Brandenburg proposed a radical solution: "If the percentage of cardiology problems cannot be increased by better selection at the admissions area and through physician calls and correspondence, and I believe this is possible, then I believe consideration of our functioning as a strict subspecialty section (that is, like neurology) will be warranted." This suggestion struck a nerve.[89]

Board chair Emmerson Ward, an internist-rheumatologist, wrote in the margin of Brandenburg's report, "I do not think this is feasible, and if the Board of Governors agrees we should tell Bob so, otherwise some undesirable undercurrent may get started."[90] Ward was concerned about setting a precedent that would disrupt the half-century-old Mayo model of care whereby all internists (regardless of their subspecialty interest) were expected to perform a large number of general diagnostic evaluations. If the cardiology sections were excused from this duty, other medical sections might make the same argument in an attempt to focus their outpatient practices on patients whose main problem fell within their chosen subspecialty field. One potential solution was to add physicians to the staff who would function exclusively as general internists rather than as hybrid general internist-medical subspecialists.[91]

There was a precedent at the Mayo Clinic for having a group of physicians function as general internists, but these doctors cared for local patients, who represented a very small portion of the practice. The board had addressed the issue of how to provide general medical care to Rochester residents in 1947, when it established a new medical section that was charged with caring for local patients.[92] By this time, virtually all independent physicians who had practiced in the city during the early decades of the twentieth century had relocated, retired, or died. And Rochester was unattractive to doctors seeking to build private practices because its hospitals limited admitting privileges to physicians and surgeons who were on the staff of the Mayo Clinic. These dynamics led clinic leaders to support the formation of two autonomous entities in the city in 1953: the Olmsted Medical Group and the Olmsted Community Hospital.[93] The Olmsted group practice included eleven doctors four years later, but the vast majority of Rochester residents continued to seek care at Mayo.

In 1959 Mayo's leaders debated whether the general medical section that had been formed to provide care to local patients should be expanded or broken up. The board-appointed committee that studied the issue produced majority and minority reports. This unusual outcome reflected deep philosophical differences about how to provide general medical care to Rochester residents in the face of increasing subspecialization.[94] Committee members interviewed almost every internist under fifty years of age in the clinic's nineteen internal medicine sections. More than two-thirds of these physicians did not want to assume more responsibility for local patients. In fact, many of the younger internists were grateful for the general medical section's existence because it freed them up "to some extent...to pursue and further their subspecialty interest."[95] Ultimately, the board voted to maintain the general medical section and to supplement it with additional internists committed to providing care to the local population.[96] This strategy did not address the coordination of care for the vast majority of patients who came to the Mayo Clinic, however.

Robert Brandenburg brought up the issue of balancing cardiology and general medicine responsibilities again in 1968. He cited "the paradoxical situation of our colleagues occasionally complaining of difficulty getting cardiac consultations when at the time of the request, the cardiologist is occupied by a patient with a gastrointestinal disorder, headache problem, or other non-cardiac problem."[97] Milton Anderson, who chaired one of the cardiology sections, agreed. The following year he informed the board that several members of his section had expressed "considerable displeasure" with the percentage of time they were required to function as a "general practitioner." Anderson explained that the younger members were especially eager to see a "greater concentration of cardiology patients to maintain expertise and to develop the experience to be intellectually productive in their field."[98] Mayo's heart specialists were also expected to care for patients hospitalized for non-cardiac problems. In the late 1960s, for example, cardiology fellows assigned to hospital rotations were informed that "like other hospital services, the cardiology services receive on rotation their quota of patients with such problems as back pain, prostatic obstruction and metastatic carcinomas."[99]

In 1969 almost all of the cardiologists signed a letter to the board that summarized their concerns about the scope of their practice:

> It is our conviction that the future growth of excellence in the practice, investigative and educational aspects of this particular subspecialty demands an extensive cardiology practice as distinct from a general internal medicine practice. Because of this we strongly support Doctor Brandenburg's proposal for re-organization of the sections and believe that any plan which in substance does not afford the in-depth practice as proposed would necessarily be inadequate for the development of superior clinical cardiology at the Mayo Clinic. Without superior clinical cardiology, education and research must also suffer.[100]

In fact, Brandenburg had not proposed any radical changes. His main request was to shift the balance between general medicine and cardiology in the outpatient practice. If the proposal was accepted, a cardiologist would be expected to see general medical patients in the clinic two months rather than three months each year. The board approved the proposal "in principle" but took no action.[101] Brandenburg kept up the pressure. In a 1970 letter to the chair of medicine, he cited "the wave of unrest and general unhappiness which now seems to affect many members of the Department of Medicine." Acknowledging that many factors contributed to this situation, the cardiologist explained:

Solutions, in part, to these difficulties must rely on identification by members of each area of specific goals which are attainable in their areas of endeavor. It must also, I believe, involve the opportunity of achieving excellence in a specific area. The "general patient" is the problem which in part prevents attainment of excellence and yet clearly is necessary for our economic well being. As I indicated earlier I believe major new approaches to the problem of care of the "general patient" must be made in the Department of Internal Medicine.[102]

Brandenburg knew there were no simple solutions, but he continued to advocate for shifting the evaluation of patients who presented to the clinic with non-cardiac problems to individuals who considered themselves general internists.[103]

In response to the needs of local patients and the growing reluctance of Mayo's medical subspecialists to function as primary care physicians, the board established the Division of Rochester Internal Medicine as part of the Department of Internal Medicine in 1970. The members of this newly named division drafted a document "Delivery of Health Care by Internists" that outlined a range of issues and potential solutions. This same year, Mayo established a policy that physicians practicing in southeastern Minnesota could refer patients "for consultation in any of twelve subspecialties in internal medicine without the necessity of a general examination at the clinic." Developed by the Department of Internal Medicine, this plan addressed concerns that Mayo internists, regional physicians, and patients had raised. It was presented as a way to "expedite care for certain recognized problems, to decrease time spent at the clinic, and to avoid added cost of a general examination when this is unnecessary."[104]

Mayo's Vascular Specialists and Board Certification

The accelerating national trend toward subspecialization in internal medicine stimulated greater interest in board certification. A 1972 survey of doctors who had graduated from medical school in the early 1960s revealed that "the vast majority of United States graduates consider specialty-board certification an important prerequisite for independent practice.... [It] is in effect becoming a de facto requirement for practice." The authors who summarized the national survey results listed several factors that encouraged doctors to seek board certification, such as income potential, perceived status, academic advancement, and hospital admitting privileges. They predicted that "the pressure for all physicians to obtain specialty certification will increase in the future as academic medical centers expand their involvement in health care delivery [and] as third-party payers increasingly recognize specialty certification in determining fee schedules."[105] Mayo had instituted a policy in 1969 that required all staff members to be certified "or in the process of meeting the requirements for certification" by the appropriate specialty and subspecialty boards. If a doctor was not certified within five years after becoming board eligible, his or her role at the clinic would be reviewed by their section and the Board of Governors.[106]

Mayo's vascular specialists faced a dilemma as specialty and subspecialty board certification gained momentum in the late 1960s. Their institution had been a world leader in vascular medicine for more than a generation when the fourth edition of the Mayo-authored book *Peripheral Vascular Diseases* was published in 1972. In their introduction to the 797-page volume, the co-editors cited problems with their field and suggested a remedy: "There is inadequate coverage of peripheral vascular disorders in medical school and during postgraduate training.... Because of this lack of interest in this specialized field and since larger and larger numbers of patients suffer from disorders found in this specialty, one could make a plea for better recognition of peripheral vascular disease as a specific subspecialty of cardiovascular disease."[107] But they realized that their only hope of gaining the status of certified subspecialists was to take the examination in cardiovascular disease that was administered by the American Board of Internal Medicine.

The international prominence of Mayo's vascular medicine program helps to explain why there were thirteen physicians in the clinic's two vascular sections in 1968, compared to twenty physicians in its three cardiology sections.[108] No institution in America had more vascular medical specialists on its staff. That year, the members of Mayo's vascular sections, headed by John Spittell and John Fairbairn, "devoted considerable time and effort" to discussing a merger with the cardiology sections in order to form a unified cardiovascular section. Their main incentive was to forge a formal link to "a recognized sub-specialty of medicine." In a report to the board, Spittell expressed his colleagues' concern about their field's future. They wanted to be sure that Mayo maintained a "dedicated and expert group of specialists in peripheral vascular disease and hypertension."[109]

John Fairbairn told the board in 1969 that his vascular colleagues supported the plan to appoint Brandenburg as chair of the five sections. Sharing Spittell's concern about their subspecialty's future, Fairburn emphasized that "neither Dr. Brandenburg nor our sections want the talents of the vascular sections...abolished or diminished by this amalgamation. Indeed, it is imperative that these talents be recognized as *unique* to this institution and the country and that they should be enhanced rather than diminished."[110] In 1969 the board approved uniting the cardiologists and vascular specialists in a "Division of Cardiovascular Diseases and Internal Medicine" that Brandenburg would lead. It took time for the members of the three cardiology and two vascular sections to adjust to the new administrative model, but a consensus emerged that it had advantages in terms of their activities in patient care, research, and education.[111]

Philanthropy as a Means of Ensuring Mayo's Future

Mayo's leaders made many decisions during the 1960s in an attempt to address local issues, such as the medical residency probation incident and the reluctance of a growing number of medical subspecialists to function as primary care physicians for Rochester patients. Other decisions reflected broader concerns, such as the increasing size and sophistication of academic medical centers that had benefited from federal research grants and corporate and individual philanthropy. By the early 1960s, the Board of Governors had concluded that their institution needed more resources in order to maintain its momentum in patient care and to enhance its educational and research programs.

Chuck Mayo, the son and nephew of the clinic's founders, appointed a committee in 1962 to reevaluate the Mayo Association, an entity that had evolved from the Mayo Properties Association, which Will and Charlie Mayo had created forty-three years earlier. The committee, chaired by San Francisco internist Dwight Wilbur, included Warren Burger, a former St. Paul lawyer who was one of the judges with the US Court of Appeals in Washington, D.C. The Wilbur committee report included a recommendation that members of the Mayo Association's governing body (which was distinct from the Board of Governors) be designated trustees and that it include more public members.[112] As a result of the Wilbur committee report, the Mayo Association was renamed the Mayo Foundation, which would play a significant role in attracting philanthropic support.

In 1968, a dozen years after the Mayo Clinic's Board of Governors approved applying for federal research grants, the Mayo Foundation Board of Trustees authorized a new program to encourage private gifts to support the institution's tripartite mission. Former President Lyndon Johnson, the newest public trustee, said shortly after leaving the White House in January 1969 that he considered it "an honor to be called upon to serve one of the nation's great medical institutions." The former president explained that accepting a position on Mayo's Board of Trustees meant that he would have an opportunity to continue his "interest in raising the quality of health care and medical research for the benefit of every American."[113] When Johnson joined the board, Mayo was poised to launch a new initiative to strengthen its academic programs that supported patient care.

The 1969 booklet *Trusteeship of Health* announced Mayo's development campaign. The publication, which outlined the institution's achievements, current status, and ambitions, began with an explanation: "It may seem superfluous to describe the medical complex at Rochester, Minnesota, collectively best known as Mayo Clinic. Few enterprises in the field of medicine are as familiar by name as this. Yet, as is often the case with 'household terms,' the story is more interesting and more involved than most people know. The life, the work, and the future of the Mayo institutions are of importance to medicine, to health care, and to people everywhere."[114] Mayo Clinic may have been a household term, but the institution's leaders and their outside advisors agreed that targeted fundraising was an important ingredient for ensuring a successful future.

Cultural changes and new patterns of payment for medical services, especially the launch of Medicare in 1966 and the continued growth of private health insurance, contributed to Mayo's decision to seek philanthropic support: "Social ethics and medical standards do not permit in these times the generally much higher fees which years ago were commonly charged to wealthy patients. Nowadays, fees have become standardized and applicable to all alike."[115] The strategy was not to launch "a conventional, short-term, public fund-raising drive." Instead, Mayo would "present its hopes and plans in a quiet way" to a range of institutions and individuals, such as philanthropic foundations, corporations, and former trainees.[116]

Philanthropic support would also help to bring Mayo's complementary programs of practice, research, and education into proper balance: "There is agreement now that research must grow at Mayo to twice its present scope to bring it to optimum proportions for continued delivery of the finest possible patient care." The institution's main mission of patient care had always influenced the type of research done in Rochester, and this would not change: "Researches particularly suited to Mayo are those close to the bedside, close to sickness—disease-oriented investigative programs, programs related to organ systems (e.g. nervous system, cardiovascular system), programs studying living, healthy or diseased cells and their tiny parts, and reactions at the molecular level in health and disease."[117]

The *Trusteeship of Health* booklet also explained that the Board of Trustees had decided that the institution should establish a medical school because "a medical school will broaden and deepen Mayo educational programs, provide a further source of scholars for the residency program, add to the productive and stimulating atmosphere at Mayo, and fulfill a growing desire at Mayo to help in producing doctors needed for the care of the sick of our state and nation."[118] Initially, the concept of launching a medical school in Rochester was controversial because Mayo's educational programs had always focused on advanced postgraduate training. Physiologist Charles Code raised the issue in a 1966 speech to the medical staff. Having recently been appointed director of the Mayo Foundation for Medical Education and Research, he described a recent review of the institution's academic mission:

If in our study we find that a medical school will aid us in maintaining our position in medical practice, education and research, if it would aid us in developing improved programs for the care of the sick, improved programs for the education of scholarly physicians and research workers, and if it would forward our goals in research—then we should have it. We are not interested in a medical school for its own sake. If it can be a handmaiden, an adjunct, an important asset to the main thrust of our institution, then, if someone else will pay for it, we should have one![119]

Code made these remarks in the context of a major national movement to build new medical schools to help address a serious and growing shortage of physicians. Several pieces of federal legislation in the mid-1960s were drafted to encourage the expansion of the supply of doctors, nurses, and other health care personnel.[120]

The Mayo trustees set an ambitious goal—raising the institution's endowment to more than $100 million: "Though a large sum, it is by no means startlingly so, when it is recalled that there are at least 22 American foundations with larger assets, not to mention the fact that at least 18 American colleges and universities have larger endowments."[121] The *Trusteeship of Health* booklet included other big numbers to emphasize Mayo's size and impact. More than 2.8 million new patients had registered at the clinic in the previous six decades. In 1968 just over 200,000 new patients were seen and 28,000 operations were performed at the clinic's two affiliated hospitals, which contained almost 1,600 beds. Mayo employed about 500 full-time physicians and scientists, 700 residents, and 2,600 allied health and other personnel. The cardiologists and cardiac surgeons were a small part of a massive enterprise, but their twin specialties were changing rapidly and were poised for growth in the face of new technologies that promised to transform the care of patients with heart disease.[122]

Technologies Transform Heart Care and Stimulate Subspecialization

Creating Coronary Care Units and Empowering Nurses

Clark Gable finished filming *The Misfits* with Marilyn Monroe on November 4, 1960, four days before John Kennedy was elected president. But the fifty-nine-year-old actor did not have a chance to celebrate the movie's completion or cast his vote. Gable was admitted to Hollywood Presbyterian Hospital with a heart attack on November 6. Former President Dwight Eisenhower, who had spent a month in bed after an acute myocardial infarction five years earlier, wrote to the actor the day after his admission: "I learned from the paper this morning that you have suffered a mild coronary thrombosis. I trust that your recovery will be rapid and complete."[1] Gable's recovery went well until the tenth day, when he died suddenly in his hospital room. The actor was not connected to a heart monitor, and no one was aware that he had a cardiac arrest, an abrupt life-ending event usually caused by ventricular fibrillation (an exceptionally rapid heart rhythm that causes the left ventricle to quiver rather than contract and pump blood).[2]

Gable's sudden death was big news because he was a celebrity, but Americans were reminded regularly that coronary artery disease could kill without warning. A 1963 *Look* magazine article described heart disease as the "most critical medical and public health problem facing the nation." And no one was immune: "Good teachers, prominent businessmen, scientists, artists and other useful citizens...[are] cut down in their prime."[3] The consequences of coronary disease were staggering. A US Public Health Service official reported in 1964 that it killed one American adult "every minute of every day" and that about 1.5 million men and women had a heart attack annually.[4] Johns Hopkins University's public relations director Lynn Poole claimed that year: "A high percentage of American men are terrified of a heart attack, of the possibility of being alive one minute and dead the next." Having survived three myocardial infarctions, he spoke from experience.[5]

In the summer of 1965, *Life* magazine reported that Adlai Stevenson, the Illinois senator who had lost the presidency to Dwight Eisenhower twice in the previous decade, was walking on a London street when "with no warning, he fell to the sidewalk." A friend "gave artificial respiration, but it could not help. Adlai Stevenson was dead, at 65, of a heart attack."[6] A recent study from the Mayo Clinic had confirmed the impression that sudden death was usually caused by coronary artery disease. About one-half of the men and women who died suddenly as a result of an acute myocardial infarction never reached a hospital.[7] Although it was impossible to predict whether, where, or when an apparently healthy person might have a cardiac arrest, a few doctors thought of a way to improve the odds of survival of one group of individuals—hospitalized patients who were recovering from a heart attack. The idea was to provide these men and women with a safety net created from a combination of specially trained personnel, new resuscitation techniques, and state-of-the-art electronic technologies.

The key components of the coronary care unit (CCU) concept, first outlined in 1961, included placing patients at risk of sudden death as a result of an acute myocardial infarction in a special hospital space that was equipped with oscilloscopes for continuous electrocardiographic monitoring and staffed by nurses who had been trained to recognize life-threatening heart rhythms and to help perform cardiopulmonary resuscitation (CPR). The CCU concept, which was implemented at hundreds of American hospitals in the mid-1960s, would transform the care of patients, the careers of cardiologists, and the boundaries of nursing practice by the end of the decade.[8]

The Origins of the Intensive Care Unit

The CCU was an extension of the intensive care unit (ICU) model that had been introduced in the 1950s, which, in turn, was a direct descendant of the recovery room concept developed during World War II. Mayo anesthesiologist John Lundy pioneered this approach in Rochester, where a Postanesthesia Observation Room opened on March 17, 1942.[9] The observation room at Saint Marys Hospital (as St. Mary's Hospital began to be spelled around this time) was designed for postoperative patients awakening after general anesthesia. Prior to this innovation, these individuals were taken directly from the operating room back to their hospital room. A nurse assigned to the floor had to postpone her routine duties so she could observe the patient until the effects of anesthesia had worn off. In 1943 Mayo's anesthesiologists emphasized that the recovery room provided a dedicated staff and all the equipment necessary to care for patients recovering from general anesthesia. They argued that it was efficient and appealed to patients, nurses, doctors, and administrators.[10]

Two Chicago anesthesiologists described the unit at Saint Marys in 1949 as "a new innovation in hospital construction and management."[11] Five years later, an anesthesiologist, a surgeon, and a hospital administrator (from another Chicago institution) linked the recovery room and ICU concepts in an article subtitled "The Intensive Therapy Unit Is a Further Development of the Recovery Room to the End of Providing Maximum Care for Medical as Well as Surgical Patients." They outlined the key components of an ICU, explaining that "the patient at a most critical time is surrounded by physical equipment of all types ready for immediate use by trained personnel." Although the focus would remain on postoperative patients throughout the 1950s, these authors acknowledged a "natural tendency for other medical specialties to desire such intensive care for their patients."[12] Historian Rosemary Stevens, noting the "public fascination with both the efficacy and drama of specialized, high-technology medicine," explains that "the most pervasive image of hospital technology in the 1950s was the hospital intensive care unit."[13]

The advent of open-heart surgery at the University of Minnesota and the Mayo Clinic produced a new type of postoperative patient. Marjorie Traufic, a nursing instructor at the university, described this situation in 1956. She had a unique perspective because she was helping to care for some of the first open-heart surgery patients and was married to a doctor who had helped pioneer the procedure. "It is an exciting time for the surgical nurse," Traufic proclaimed, "for she is assuming a most important role as one of a team whose objective is saving lives which once were considered lost." The nurse's job in this unique context was very challenging because "she must be a mechanic at the bedside," able to use and maintain the elaborate equipment that was now part of postoperative care.[14]

Earl Wood Proposes Postoperative Monitoring to Save Lives

John Kirklin and other members of Mayo's open-heart surgery team reported the results of the first forty operations performed with the Mayo-Gibbon heart-lung machine in July 1956. Twenty-four of the patients were alive three months after surgery. Most of those who did not survive had died in the early postoperative period. The authors emphasized that many of the patients (most of whom were children) who had open-heart surgery were critically ill before the procedure.[15] Hoping to reduce the mortality rate, physiologist Earl Wood, who performed the preoperative catheterizations and monitored physiological parameters during surgery, proposed a project. In July 1956, the same month their article appeared, he asked Kirklin for permission to do studies to evaluate postoperative complications, which he considered "the greatest problem in the bypass

game." Wood argued that the "disturbingly high incidence of postoperative mortality could be greatly reduced if we had more knowledge of what
was going on."[16]

Wood wanted to monitor arterial and venous pressures and the electrocardiogram continuously and to calculate cardiac output periodically. Although
this would require leaving catheters and other monitoring devices in place
after a patient left the operating room, he thought it could be accomplished
"with little discomfort to the patient or interference with the usual postoperative care."[17] Wood envisioned keeping patients in a "postoperative recovery
room" for up to four days to record data that "might prove of value as additional guide-posts" in their care. The physiologist knew what he wanted, but
he respected the surgeon's role: "You are boss on the bypass project and the
above is for your consideration." Pediatric cardiologist James DuShane wrote
in the margin of a copy of the proposal: "I favor this *very* much...[and] think
a postoperative room or ward absolutely essential for this. Believe it worth
any effort."[18]

When Earl Wood recommended monitoring postoperative open-heart
surgery patients in the summer of 1956, Mayo's Board of Governors had
just approved moving John Kirklin's surgical service from Methodist
Hospital to Saint Marys Hospital when an addition to the latter opened
in the fall. Initially, the Franciscan sisters who operated the hospital had
planned to create an ICU for selected neurology and postoperative neurosurgical patients who required frequent checks of their mental status, vital
signs, and reflexes. Acknowledging the unique needs of patients recovering from open-heart surgery, the sisters agreed to postpone opening a
neurological unit and to use the space for a Postoperative Cardiovascular
Unit.

Mayo's open-heart surgery program formally moved to Saint Marys
Hospital on September 30, 1956, and the first patient who had open-heart
surgery there was admitted to the new unit two days later.[19] It was the
world's first ICU designed to care exclusively for patients recovering from
open-heart surgery. Sister Maristella (later Sister Elizabeth Gillis) was in her
mid-twenties when she was appointed supervisor of the new Postoperative
Cardiovascular Unit. "Our nurses were outstanding," she recalled, "but none
of us knew anything about caring for cardiac surgery patients. I went up to
the University of Minnesota for one day and observed surgery. Another day
I went to Methodist Hospital where Dr. Kirklin first performed open-heart
surgery, and that was it." Earl Wood's proposal for comprehensive pressure
and pulse monitoring was not implemented. "There were no machines to tell
us how a patient was doing," the sister explained. "It was all observation, and
we had to be acutely observant. We were learning all the time, and so were
the doctors."[20]

Sister Mary Brigh and the ICU at Saint Marys Hospital

Patient experiences, some of them catastrophic, encouraged the creation of intensive care units. The head nurse of the new neurology-neurosurgery ICU, which opened in 1958, and Sister Mary Brigh, the administrator of Saint Marys Hospital, wrote that year, "After having assisted with serious emergencies on general wards where nursing personnel scattered to several areas for specialized equipment when an emergency occurred, one is deeply impressed by the ease with which the unit enables the nurse to meet a sudden serious patient need." Turning to the objects and the observers of care, they reported that "patients and relatives testify to the confidence and feeling of security they experience, knowing that everyone in the unit is familiar with and personally concerned with their care."[21]

St. Louis University's Department of Hospital Administration invited Sister Mary Brigh to speak on intensive care in 1959. She claimed in her lecture that the ICU concept had led to many "discussions, displays, articles and arguments" and that administrators had "rated it all the way from the most revolutionary advance hospitals have made in the past decade to a device of the devil."[22] The sister-nurse, who had earned an MBA in hospital administration from the University of Chicago and was on the Catholic Hospital Association's Board of Directors, noted that intensive care was one of five parts of a new progressive patient care model promoted by Faye Abdellah, a nursing educator in the US Public Health Service. Sister Mary Brigh said the main stimulus for developing ICUs was the advent of "operations and treatments that ten years ago seemed as remote as outer space." Suddenly, however, outer space seemed less remote. She spoke shortly after the Soviet Union had launched Sputnik, the world's first satellite.[23]

In her 1959 speech in St. Louis, Sister Mary Brigh outlined the key components of the ICU concept: "It concentrates in one area the patients needing expert care, the personnel best qualified to give that care, and the special equipment needed to give it, in a manner that no ordinary hospital unit has or can duplicate. If any of the components is missing or diluted, you do not have an intensive care unit." Gazing into the future, she predicted that the ICU would be taken for granted in six years, just as the recovery room was when she spoke.[24] In another 1959 talk, she addressed the care model as it pertained to cardiac surgery:

Much time and effort of highly trained personnel and much costly equipment and supplies are used during...open-heart surgery, yet it may be all in vain unless the care given after surgery can maintain the patient at a level where recovery is possible. The difference between the immediate observation and treatment of a serious symptom and its observation and treatment ten minutes later may be the difference between success and failure, life and death. In no section of the hospital is the line drawn more clearly than in the intensive care unit.[25]

The ICU movement gained momentum in the late 1950s as more doctors, nurses, and administrators acknowledged the care model's benefits. "Special Unit Saves Lives, Nurses and Money" was the title of a 1957 article by a surgeon and an administrator at a Hanover, New Hampshire, hospital. The seven-word title spoke volumes about the potential impact of an ICU.[26]

Using Electronic Technologies to Combat Cardiac Arrest

Mary Fordham, a nurse born and trained in England, had succeeded Sister Maristella as supervisor of the Postoperative Cardiovascular Unit shortly after it opened in 1956. Six years later, she published *Cardiovascular Surgical Nursing*. Written before Fordham left Rochester in 1960, the book described the layout, equipment, and functions of the postoperative unit at Saint Marys Hospital. One photograph showed a mobile emergency cabinet that contained cardiac drugs and surgical instruments for acute complications, such as a collapsed lung. Another photograph depicted a cart with an oscilloscope electrocardiogram monitor and an artificial pacemaker for stimulating a stopped heart to beat. Fordham did not mention another electronic treatment technology—the defibrillator.[27]

Patients recovering from open-heart surgery were very different from those recuperating from an acute myocardial infarction. Although heart attack patients could have a cardiac arrest as a result of asystole if the heart stopped beating, they were more likely to die suddenly as a result of ventricular fibrillation. This was the most feared heart rhythm disorder because it could occur without warning and was invariably fatal. Scottish physiologist John MacWilliam had painted a vivid picture of ventricular fibrillation decades earlier: "The ventricles are thrown into a tumultuous state of quick, irregular, twitching action; at the same time there is a great fall of blood pressure…. The cardiac pump is thrown out of gear, and the last of its vital energy is dissipated in a violent and prolonged turmoil of fruitless activity in the ventricular walls."[28] Although ventricular fibrillation during the administration of anesthesia or during a surgical procedure was very rare, it was in this context that a treatment strategy was introduced that would eventually be refined for use in patients who had a cardiac arrest somewhere other than in an operating room.

Years of research on using an electric shock to convert ventricular fibrillation to a regular heart rhythm had come to fruition in 1947, when Cleveland surgeon Claude Beck reported the first successful human defibrillation. He was operating on the sternum of a fourteen-year-old boy who had pectus excavatum (funnel chest deformity). "During closure of the wound in the chest, the pulse suddenly stopped and the blood pressure sounds could not be heard. The patient was apparently dead."[29] Beck's aggressive resuscitation technique included immediately cutting open the teenager's chest and squeezing his fibrillating heart by hand in order to pump blood through his anesthetized body. The surgeon then placed metal electrodes on the heart's quivering surface and sent a jolt of electricity through it. A regular rhythm returned, and the boy survived. Beck reported the case and promoted his aggressive resuscitation technique to surgeons who might confront cardiac arrest in the operating room.[30]

Research had shown that a brain deprived of oxygen for more than four minutes suffered severe and irreversible damage. But resuscitating an anesthetized patient required that someone in the operating room recognize that his or her heart had stopped beating. The traditional approach relied on the anesthetist periodically feeling the patient's pulse. A cardiac anesthesia pioneer explained, "First the diagnosis is made by recognition of the absence of carotid artery pulsations by the anesthetist. The surgeon is told that the patient is dead." Survival depended on vigilance and immediate action.[31]

During the 1950s, oscilloscopes began appearing in operating rooms to monitor the heart rhythms of unconscious patients. Two California cardiologists insisted that "there is no time to think when cardiac arrest strikes... all operating personnel must have been indoctrinated and all equipment prepared beforehand so that immediate action can be taken with the speed of a reflex action and the precision of a fire drill."[32]

Resuscitating Individuals Who Have Had a Heart Attack

In 1956 Claude Beck proposed extending his emergency operating room resuscitation technique (which required cutting open a patient's chest) to men or women who had a cardiac arrest while they were in a hospital recovering from a heart attack. Patients with coronary artery disease who developed a sudden life-threatening arrhythmia (heart rhythm disorder) could be saved if "supplies and personnel trained in resuscitation methods are available as soon as the patient dies." The surgeon told a story to prove his point: "A physician dressed in his street clothes died from a heart attack while leaving the hospital. He was successfully resuscitated. This one experience indicates that resuscitation from fatal heart attack is not impossible and might be applied to those who die in the hospital and perhaps also to those who die outside the hospital."[33]

Moving Beck's open-chest cardiac massage technique out of operating room and into the real world was impractical. When a person had a cardiac arrest outside a hospital, there was almost no chance that a doctor would be present, let alone a surgeon armed with a scalpel and willing to slash a chest open in order to massage the heart. Boston cardiologist Lewis Dexter declared in 1958, "Not being a surgeon, and not being an anesthesiologist, I am not going to open these chests. I wouldn't even think of doing it."[34]

Cardiac arrests, although very rare in patients undergoing surgery, are the most common cause of unexpected death in the general population. Sudden death was a recognized complication of acute myocardial infarction in the 1950s, but there was no consensus about the need to hospitalize patients when they had a heart attack. At a 1955 symposium on atherosclerosis at the University of Minnesota, New York cardiologist Henry Russek argued against routine hospitalization:

> For many patients, being jostled in an ambulance or admitting office, then subjected to the psychic trauma of a hospital room and bed and of being placed in an oxygen tent, often when oxygen is entirely unnecessary, and being repeatedly punctured for prothrombin and coagulation times, hardly constitutes optimum management during this early critical period. In most instances, any form of treatment deemed necessary can be initiated in the patient's own home and removal to hospital can be accomplished if indicated, when this critical period has passed.[35]

But Russek seemed to contradict himself with respect to the "critical period" because he pointed out that most deaths after an acute myocardial infarction occurred during the first forty-eight hours as a "result of ventricular fibrillation, cardiac asystole, shock, or congestive heart failure."[36] These life-threatening complications could not be treated in a patient's home.

In response to Russek's remarks at this 1955 symposium, Mayo cardiologist Howard Burchell explained that most patients in the Rochester area were hospitalized when they had an acute myocardial infarction. The main reason was to draw blood daily to adjust the dose of an oral anticoagulant (Dicumarol or Coumadin), which many doctors administered routinely to patients after a heart attack. Burchell, who was interested in heart rhythm disorders, discussed sudden death from a theoretical perspective at the Minneapolis meeting: "Assuming that this might be caused by ventricular fibrillation, then this is an avenue of investigation that must be further encouraged."[37] In contrast to Burchell, who recommended research, Boston cardiologist Paul Zoll called for action. He had been working with a Massachusetts electronics company to commercialize a defibrillator that sent a life-saving shock through the chest wall. This technology, which did not require cutting open a patient's chest to shock the surface of the heart, helped set the stage for a new approach to resuscitation that, in turn, was critical for the development of the CCU.[38]

In 1960 Johns Hopkins researchers published an article titled "Closed-Chest Cardiac Massage" that described an alternative to Claude Beck's open-chest technique. Because their approach did not involve a surgeon wielding a scalpel, they declared that "anyone, anywhere, can now initiate cardiac resuscitative procedures." The Hopkins team had combined external chest compressions with artificial respiration in five patients, four of whom had suffered sudden cardiovascular collapse in an operating room. Each one recovered after a few minutes of closed-chest CPR.[39]

The fifth patient's story was different. A forty-five-year-old man, who had come to the Johns Hopkins Hospital emergency room with "excruciating chest pain radiating down his arms," collapsed while taking off his clothes in preparation for an examination. Doctors started CPR immediately and documented ventricular fibrillation with an electrocardiogram. They continued chest compressions and artificial respiration for the twenty minutes it took to bring the hospital's only defibrillator to the dramatic scene. Two electric shocks restored a normal heart rhythm, and the man survived sudden death to begin "the usual course of treatment for myocardial infarction."[40] There is no mention of admission to a CCU because the care model had not been proposed in 1960. When the Hopkins group described its experience with CPR the following year, Beck proclaimed, "This contribution speaks for itself. Death has been reversed without opening the chest."[41]

Imagining and Implementing the Coronary Care Unit Concept

Mayo cardiologist Robert Parker was an early advocate of extending the ICU model to selected patients with acute heart disease. In December 1960 Sister Mary Brigh informed the members of the Joint Conference Committee that he had asked "about the possibility of setting up an Intensive Care Unit for medical patients, particularly cardiology patients," at Saint Marys Hospital.[42] The committee, which included three other Franciscan sisters and four Mayo Clinic doctors, met regularly to facilitate communication between the independent but interdependent institutions. Minutes summarized Sister Mary Brigh's concerns about Parker's proposal:

> Such a project had been discussed by the hospital as a future project. It is best, however, when the request comes from the Medical Staff as it gives added assurance of their assistance and cooperation in setting up and using such a unit. Several problems would need to be worked out in order that such a unit could be set up. Staffing the unit with a sufficient number of registered nurses on all shifts presents additional staffing problems. Many of these patients seem to require longer periods of

care than surgical patients and therefore there would be danger of the unit becoming a chronic care unit and less well supervised by Medical Consultants.... Much more careful and detailed planning will need to be done before such a unit can be opened.[43]

As Saint Marys Hospital's chief administrator, Sister Mary Brigh was responsible for helping the large institution adapt to a rapidly changing medical milieu. In 1960 "Quiet Hospital Zone" signs still surrounded buildings with corridors and spaces that were becoming busier and noisier as more complex technologies, tests, and treatments were introduced. A volatile mixture of medical, technological, and cultural forces was revolutionizing the actions and attitudes of doctors, nurses, and administrators.[44]

During a 1962 speech in South Dakota on emerging hospital problems, Sister Mary Brigh expressed concern about growing government involvement in health care, increasing regulation by the Joint Commission on Accreditation of Hospitals, declining nursing school enrollments, and increasing costs. America was entering what would be called the Electronic Age when she complained, "The salesman can point to amazing savings but when you try to find them reflected in the expense account at the end of the month they are usually invisible. Then you comfort yourself that at least you have given better care and perhaps you are correct. In at least some cases, you have done nothing more than keep up with the Joneses." Referring to new technologies that disturbed a hospital's tranquil atmosphere, she quipped, "All that beeps is not better."[45] In fact, most hospitals had little if any equipment that beeped in 1962. None of Sister Mary Brigh's listeners could have imagined the cacophony that would surround patients in ICUs of the future, following the introduction of a multitude of noise-making monitoring and treatment technologies.[46]

The first intensive care unit in America designed specifically to monitor and treat patients with acute myocardial infarction opened at Bethany Hospital in Kansas City, Kansas, on May 20, 1962. One year earlier, the John A. Hartford Foundation had awarded a grant to the hospital to implement and evaluate the innovation under the direction of cardiologist Hughes Day. The foundation's minutes summarize the decision to support the project and describe how ICUs and CCUs differed:

> Intensive care units in most hospitals are designed to provide continuous qualified general nursing for the critically ill medical and surgical patients. Bethany Hospital proposes to implement an intensive care program which is oriented especially to the care of the acute coronary patient, who comprises the majority of the critically ill medical group, and to demonstrate that many of these patients can be saved and

rehabilitated by specially trained personnel and by the use of electronic monitoring and treatment facilities.[47]

The 200-bed hospital's "Intensive Coronary Care Area" consisted of four private rooms adjacent to a seven-bed medical and surgical ICU.[48]

Los Angeles cardiologist Morris Wilburne published the first description of the CCU concept in 1961 as a brief abstract in the journal *Circulation*.[49] Two years later, he and surgeon Josh Fields published a detailed article on the CCU. Reminding readers that "sudden death due to cardiac arrest in patients convalescing from acute myocardial infarction is an ever-present threat," they challenged the status quo. Arguing that implementation of the CCU model could transform the "early stages of death [into] a two-way threshold," they complained that "the present practice of random assignment of patients with acute coronary disease to various locations in the hospital is, therapeutically, an antiquated procedure."[50]

Three months after Wilburne and Field's article appeared in print, two Mayo Clinic physicians cited it in a manuscript they submitted to the *American Heart Journal*. Published in 1964, Ralph Spiekerman and Malcolm Lindsay's article "Re-evaluation of Therapy of Acute Myocardial Infarction" was the first paper about the CCU model written by Mayo physicians. Neither author was a member of one of the clinic's cardiology sections. Spiekerman, who had recently completed his medical residency, was in the section responsible for providing care to Rochester residents. In that role, he cared for patients hospitalized with heart attacks and followed them after they were discharged. Mayo did not have a cardiology fellowship program at the time, and Spiekerman's internal medicine training (which included cardiology rotations), research interest in coronary artery disease, and publications were sufficient to classify him as a cardiologist in most contexts. He invited medical resident Malcolm Lindsay Jr. to coauthor the article.[51]

Spiekerman and Lindsay summarized the main components of the CCU model that Wilburne and Fields, British cardiologist Desmond Julian, and Hughes Day had described during the previous two and one-half years:

Ideal therapy for acute myocardial infarction must include constant nursing supervision plus the use of electronic instruments necessary for the detection and management of acute coronary failure [cardiac arrest]. We envisage the development of an intensive-care ward, similar in principle to the postcardiac surgery ward, to meet these needs.... The intensive-care ward would be staffed by specially trained nurses and physicians who are intimately familiar with each step of resuscitation and external cardiac massage and with the cardiac monitor, pacemaker, and defibrillator. Ideally, there should be continuous electrocardiographic monitoring of the cardiac rhythm.[52]

This Mayo article was among the first to promote the establishment of CCUs. When it appeared, there were fewer than a dozen units devoted exclusively to the care of patients with acute myocardial infarction in the United States.

Saint Marys Hospital opened a twelve-bed medical intensive care unit (MICU) on December 7, 1964. It was designed for critically ill non-surgical patients, including those with cardiac problems, such as an acute myocardial infarction or severe congestive heart failure.[53] Deciding which patients to place in the 1,000-bed hospital's new MICU presented a challenge. Staff were informed that the decision to admit a specific individual was made jointly by the "physician in charge of the patient" and the "nurse in charge of the unit."[54]

In 1965 Sister Mary Brigh wrote an essay on the MICU to accompany her application for fellowship in the American College of Hospital Administrators. In it, she described the construction, organization, and utilization of her hospital's unit in Rochester. Forty patients had been admitted during the first month it was open, sixteen of them with a diagnosis of heart attack. Interviews of doctors, nurses, patients, and relatives revealed "general satisfaction with the unit." Two patients who had been hospitalized previously for a myocardial infarction "noted how much more secure they felt in the unit." Costs, a concern shared by patients and hospital administrators, were considered acceptable. A charge of $20 per day for intensive care was added to the charge of $22 for a standard double room. Sister Mary Brigh emphasized that this supplement was less than the charge of $54 per day for a private duty nurse to provide around-the-clock care in a regular room.[55] Cardiology section head Robert Brandenburg told Mayo's Board of Governors in 1965 that the MICU resulted in "more expert care of seriously ill cardiac patients" due to a combination of advanced nursing practices and new technologies designed to detect and treat life-threatening arrhythmias.[56]

Diffusion of the CCU Model and the Empowerment of Nurses

The CCU movement (and heart care in general) got a big boost from new legislation and increased federal funding in the mid-1960s. In 1964 several hundred doctors attended the Second National Conference on Cardiovascular Diseases in Washington, D.C. Mayo cardiologists Howard Burchell and Robert Brandenburg, cardiac surgeon John Kirklin, and vascular specialist John Spittell were members of the conference's Central Advisory Committee. Congressman John Fogarty, who welcomed the participants, had a personal interest in the subject, having survived a heart attack a decade earlier. After reminding his audience that "heart disease continues to head the list of killers," the Rhode Island Democrat predicted that more than "one million of our relatives, friends, neighbors, and fellow citizens in these United States" would die as a result of it that year.[57]

Fogarty was a key member of a very effective health lobby that included doctors, scientists, lawmakers, and citizen activists. Alabama Senator Lister Hill, NIH director James Shannon, and two wealthy women, Mary Lasker and Florence Mahoney, were the other main participants. The author of a 1967 *Atlantic Monthly* article "The Health Syndicate: Washington's Noble Conspirators" described one of their chief strategies: "Reminding the lawmakers of their mortality has been consistently effective in raising the ante for health research.... Fogarty, Hill, Shannon, and Lasker performed each year as a highly polished quartet."[58] When the article appeared, one member of the quartet had just left the stage—forever. Fogarty was just fifty-three years old in January 1967, when he died of a heart attack while sitting at his desk on Capitol Hill.[59]

Los Angeles cardiologist Eliot Corday became president of the American College of Cardiology in 1965, and he took advantage of his position to champion the CCU movement. Interested in cardiac arrhythmias and well connected in Washington, Corday created and chaired the college's Special Committee for Liaison with Congress, the Surgeon General, and the National Institutes of Health. This audacious title reflected the California cardiologist's ambition and agenda.[60] His term as president of the college coincided with Lyndon Johnson's signing of the Heart Disease, Cancer, and Stroke Amendments of 1965 (the Regional Medical Programs Act), which accelerated the creation of CCUs. It authorized grants to assist in the establishment of regional cooperative arrangements among medical schools, research institutions, and hospitals for research, for training, and for demonstrations of innovations in patient care in the fields of heart disease, cancer, and stroke. The act was also designed to help physicians and hospitals make new approaches to the diagnosis and treatment of these diseases available to patients in a timely fashion.[61]

Corday also created the American College of Cardiology's Bethesda Conferences, theme-based meetings that brought together a small number of heart specialists who were experts on specific subjects with government representatives and others to discuss a particular topic and to produce a report. He invited CCU pioneer Hughes Day to chair a Bethesda Conference on the care model and sent him a list of a dozen doctors and four nurses he wanted to participate. Twenty-five individuals attended the December 1965 meeting that was designed to "describe the expanded role of the nurse in the Coronary Care Unit and to identify the special training needed to prepare her for the responsibilities she will have as a key member of the unit staff."[62]

The widespread establishment of CCUs in the late 1960s contributed to a very significant shift in the traditional relationship between doctors and nurses.[63] Physicians recognized the life-saving potential of the technologies clustered in CCUs, which Corday characterized as "an electronic sales-man's paradise."[64] Initially, a significant number of doctors were reluctant to let nurses control the unit's most powerful technology—the defibrillator. Support for granting specially trained nurses authority to defibrillate patients grew during the second half of the decade. Proponents argued that this approach would result in more survivors of sudden death because it would reduce the delay between recognizing a life-ending arrhythmia and delivering a life-saving shock. The notion of nurses using defibrillators also gained popularity in practice because it represented an alternative to having a doctor less than five minutes away from vulnerable patients at all times. There simply were not enough physicians to provide instantaneous round-the-clock coverage, especially at community hospitals without interns or residents.[65]

Mary Fordham, who had been the supervisor of the Postoperative Cardiovascular Unit at Saint Marys Hospital in the late 1950s, played a significant role in promoting the notion that nurses should be granted greater autonomy in caring for patients in CCUs. In January 1965 she started working as head nurse of one of the world's first CCUs, a four-bed unit at the New York Hospital-Cornell Medical Center. Fordham already knew a lot about caring for unstable patients with serious heart disease from her experiences at Mayo.[66] She recalled the dynamics of defibrillation in the Manhattan hospital's CCU, where members of her staff were responsible for watching the oscilloscope heart monitors. When a patient's heart went into ventricular fibrillation, one of her staff would have to find a doctor to discharge the defibrillator. Fordham explained that she became frustrated because it took "much too long for that patient to be resuscitated by running outside [the unit] to get a doctor, whereas we felt that if there was a nurse, someone at the bedside who could immediately defibrillate...we could probably save that patient."[67]

Cardiologist Thomas Killip, who founded and directed New York Hospital's CCU, shared Fordham's concern, and the institution established a policy that permitted specially trained nurses to defibrillate patients. He later recalled that Fordham "realized, far more than we did, what nurses were capable of."[68] Killip's protégé Stephen Scheidt, who began working in his unit in 1968, cited the "vigorous championing of increased responsibility for nurses" as one of their CCU's most important contributions.[69] Still, it took time for individuals and institutions to accept and implement these revolutionary concepts and practices.

Mayo general internist Ralph Spiekerman and cardiologists John Callahan, James Broadbent, and Emilio Giuliani coauthored a 1967 article on the organization of the MICU at Saint Marys Hospital.[70] Sister Henry (later Sister Charlotte Dusbabek), the unit's first head nurse (Figure 13.1), contributed to a second paper that summarized the treatment of 1,000 patients admitted between December 7, 1964, and June 11, 1966. Two-thirds of these patients

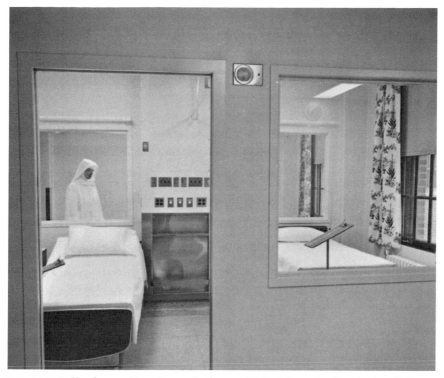

FIGURE 13.1 *Head nurse Sister Henry in the new Medical Intensive Care Unit at Saint Marys Hospital, Rochester, Minnesota, December 1964.*
Used with permission of Mayo Foundation.

were admitted with a cardiovascular diagnosis, and one-fifth of them were considered to have had an acute myocardial infarction. Resuscitation was attempted in fifty-eight patients, and twenty-two of them survived without clinical evidence of serious brain damage from lack of oxygen. The authors concluded that the unit "fulfilled the expectations of the planners and has operated to the satisfaction of patients, nurses, and physicians." Nurses had used the defibrillator rarely, but in view of "the growing tendency in other such units, plans are being formalized to have certain nurses authorized to proceed with defibrillation without waiting for a physician."[71]

Saint Marys Hospital approved a policy in 1968 authorizing specially trained nurses to use a defibrillator if a doctor was not immediately available to deliver the potentially life-saving shock to a patient who had had a cardiac arrest.[72] That year, Sister Henry spoke on the expanding role of nurses in coronary care to members of the Illinois Heart Association. Emphasizing that "electronic gadgetry is not enough," the Saint Marys Hospital head nurse addressed the life-saving role of specially selected and trained personnel. She outlined the ideal CCU nurse's traits: willingness to care for critically ill patients eight hours a day, interest in self-improvement, performance under pressure, initiative, ability to adapt to change, emotional maturity, and mechanical aptitude. Shifting her gaze from nurses to the men and women lying quietly in CCU beds, Sister Henry warned, "It is very easy for the nurse to lose sight of the patient in the midst of monitors, loose electrodes, false alarms, real alarms, 60-cycle interference, etc." When they cared for vulnerable patients, CCU nurses were expected to exhibit compassion amidst the technology: "In the strange electronic atmosphere of the unit, the professional nurse must strive to retain her ability to have face-to-face communication with the patient because she is his link with the human, warm, personal world.... We cannot stress enough the concept of viewing the patient as a person with a disease."[73]

In 1967 Chicago cardiologist Oglesby Paul coauthored an article that described how a CCU's atmosphere affected patients: "The design of the unit should provide for maximal patient tranquility and privacy without sacrificing the principles of constant surveillance and the proximity of help.... We would warn against including the coronary care unit in the general intensive care area where unsettling signs and sounds and general hubbub from postoperative, traumatic and other acute medical cases cannot be eliminated."[74]

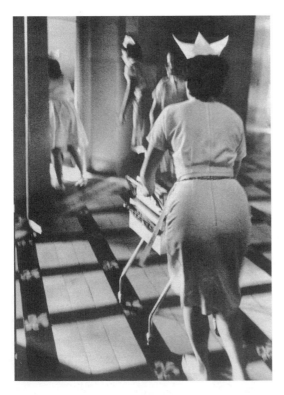

FIGURE 13.2 *Charles Harbutt, "Hurrying Nurses" during a cardiac arrest.*

Life, February 28, 1964, 52B [*sic*], used with permission of Charles Harbutt.

Oglesby Paul's article did not address one common scenario. When a patient had a cardiac arrest, the CCU environment would change from calm to chaos in seconds. Nurses and doctors raced to the dying patient's bedside to initiate CPR and deliver a life-saving shock if the arrest was due to ventricular fibrillation. The scene was even more chaotic if a patient had a cardiac arrest in a regular room rather than a CCU because staff members ran much further—up and down halls and stairwells, passing other patients and visitors who could tell that something was terribly wrong or that someone was dying (Figure 13.2).

Creating Special Teams to Resuscitate Hospitalized Patients

Some of the pioneers of CPR promoted the concept of creating special teams to transport life-saving techniques and technologies to patients scattered around a hospital. It was a pragmatic approach to a serious problem. During the first five years that closed-chest CPR was employed at the Johns Hopkins Hospital (1958–1963), it was used in an attempt to save the lives of 301 patients who had a total of 340 cardiac arrests. These patients had cardiac arrests "on the hospital wards, in private rooms, in the emergency department, in the cardiac catheterization laboratories, in the x-ray department, and even in the hospital elevators."[75]

Kansas City cardiologist and CCU pioneer Hughes Day published the first comprehensive description of a cardiac arrest team in 1962. His hospital's "Code Blue Emergency" team of specially trained staff responded immediately to an arrest. One person raced to the scene with a "crash cart" full of emergency medicines and life-saving electronic equipment.[76] During the 1960s, patients and visitors began hearing phrases (which often included the word "code") over hospital public address systems that were the equivalent of a pistol shot signaling the start of a race at a track meet. But this was a race to save someone's life.

Life magazine published a photo-essay on the role of the cardiac arrest team in 1964 that included several dramatic action-filled pictures of one patient's successful resuscitation:

> Somewhere in the hospital someone's heart stops. Or he stops breathing. A nurse calls in an alarm. An urgent voice comes on the public address system: "Attention please! Attention please! Code 99!" That means a man is dying. It tells doctors to come on the double. Nurses run for a cart already loaded with equipment. In seconds a remarkable new kind of medical team is at the patient's bedside, a team which may literally bring him back from the dead.... This emergency had a severe heart attack. Suddenly his heart stops pumping. The first two people who

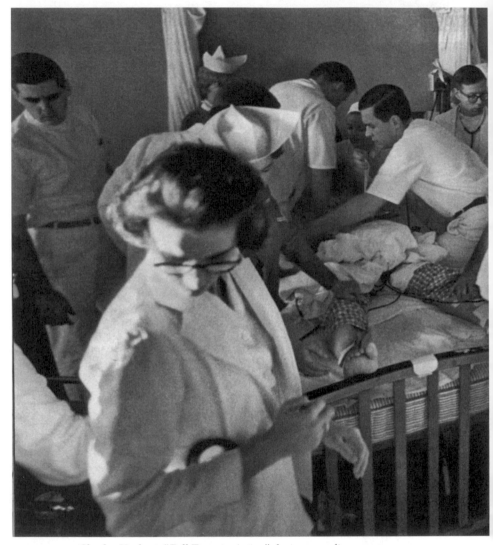

FIGURE 13.3 *Charles Harbutt, "Full Team in Action" during a cardiac arrest.*
Life, February 28, 1964, 56–57, used with permission of Charles Harbutt.

arrive at his bedside do the two most urgent jobs: they get air into the
patient's lungs and blood into his brain. One of them puts his mouth
directly down on the patient's mouth and blows in air, hard, until his
chest expands.... The other person starts massaging the heart. He
places the heels of his hands on the breastbone and leans. He depresses
the bone up to two inches and squeezes the heart against the spine until
the blood inside it spurts into the arteries.[77]

One photograph (Figure 13.3) showed more than a dozen doctors and nurses
filling this patient's room during the resuscitation! Another one reproduced

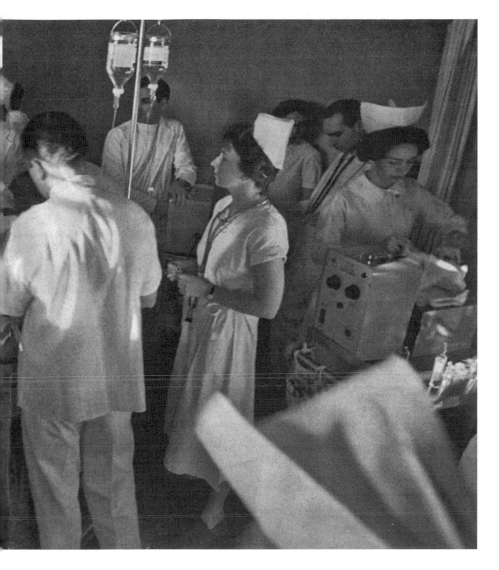

his electrocardiogram, which revealed ventricular fibrillation. The text explained that a defibrillator shocked the dying man's heart "back into action with a 550-volt jolt of electricity." But there was lingering uncertainty: "It is fifteen minutes since the code was called and the immediate emergency is over. The patient is alive, perhaps for years, perhaps for another day."[78]

In many hospitals, anesthesiologists played a major role in establishing and coordinating a cardiac arrest team. They were experienced in helping to manage catastrophes in operating rooms and were experts in artificial ventilation. Mayo anesthesiologist Paul Didier met with the clinic's Executive Committee

in May 1965 to encourage the creation of emergency resuscitation teams at
Saint Marys Hospital and Methodist Hospital. Concerned that these programs
would require special personnel, equipment, training, and a communication
strategy, Mayo's leaders appointed a committee "to study this matter in depth
and to make definitive recommendations for the development and operation
of an emergency resuscitation team."[79] Didier chaired the group that included
cardiologists John Callahan and Harold Mankin, cardiac surgeon Robert
Wallace, and two other doctors. In November 1965 he urged the Executive
Committee to approve implementation of an "inpatient emergency resuscitation system" as soon as possible.[80] Its launch was delayed as various individuals
and committees considered a range of logistical, legal, and ethical issues.[81]

In the fall of 1966, Howard Burchell described the MICU at Saint Marys
Hospital as "a place where we are learning a great deal more about people with
coronary disease and sudden death." Noting that "there are patients who die
suddenly in all parts of the hospital," the Mayo cardiologist expressed frustration that his institution had not established a cardiac arrest team: "Repeatedly
I have emphasized to our administration that there are problems in the periphery of the unit and plans must be made to handle these.... One must have a
means of getting to the patient in various parts of the hospital in a hurry...as
yet, we have not solved the problem to our satisfaction."[82] Unlike most community hospitals, Mayo and its two affiliated hospitals were large bureaucratic
institutions. Committees, however well intentioned, sometimes functioned as
webs—snaring innovators and stopping (or at least slowing down) the processes of decision-making and program implementation.

After months of planning and training nurses to perform CPR, Mayo
launched the "Code 45" program at its two hospitals on July 5, 1967. The team
charged with responding to the overhead emergency announcement included
a nurse, an anesthesiologist or nurse anesthetist, a cardiology trainee, and a
member of the pharmacy staff.[83] During the first six months of operation, the
Code 45 system was activated 105 times at Saint Marys Hospital. Ninety-six of
the patients died immediately or within two months (which they spent in the
hospital). Of the nine survivors, four had been discharged, and five were still
hospitalized.[84] These dismal survival statistics lent support to the concept of
clustering patients considered most vulnerable to a cardiac arrest in a CCU,
where specially trained staff and life-saving technologies were close at hand.

A Rochester Physiologist Becomes a Los Angeles Cardiologist

Eliot Corday was president of the American College of Cardiology in 1966,
when he wrote an editorial on how the launch of Medicare and the Heart
Disease, Cancer, and Stroke Amendments of 1965 would affect cardiology. He argued that federal agencies would not give money to "medical

institutions merely because they are there."[85] If a hospital's leaders could not demonstrate that they were committed to implementing programs and technologies designed to improve the diagnosis and treatment of heart disease, there was little chance that their institutions would attract new federal funds. After reviewing the situation at his own Los Angeles institution, Corday recruited Jeremy Swan from the Mayo Clinic to help him. In July 1965 the Irish-American physiologist became the first full-time director of cardiology at Cedars of Lebanon Hospital, which had recently merged with Mount Sinai Hospital to form Cedars-Sinai Medical Center.

Serendipity played a significant role in Swan's sudden career shift. Corday had spent two weeks overseas with him in the spring of 1964, when they lectured in Bulgaria, Greece, and Romania. They were members of a five-person delegation sent abroad as part of the International Circuit Courses educational program that was co-sponsored by the American College of Cardiology and the US State Department. Swan, listed as a professor of physiology at the Mayo Clinic, spoke on cardiac catheterization, his area of expertise.[86] One year later, the Rochester *Post-Bulletin* reported that "a noted Mayo Clinic cardiologist and director of Saint Marys Hospital catheterization laboratory" was resigning to become "chief of cardiology at the new Cedars-Sinai Medical Center in Los Angeles... on the outskirts of Beverly Hills."[87]

Swan's colleagues were stunned by his sudden transformation from a cardiac physiologist who performed catheterizations into a clinical cardiologist.[88] Swan's decision to leave Mayo in the summer of 1965 reflected his perception of the professional and social advantages associated with the new position at Cedars-Sinai. He would be the first full-time director of a cardiology program with significant academic potential in a large city with many cultural attractions. Decades later, Swan told a former Mayo colleague, "[I] came to the personal conclusion that my goal was more that of a physician than a physiologist.... My training as a clinical cardiologist was limited, yet I believed I had gained sufficient insight into clinical practice to be successful. This was not possible in the well-structured Mayo practice, and I decided to seek opportunities elsewhere."[89]

Corday propelled Swan to the front ranks of the CCU movement by inviting him to be one of sixteen physicians who participated in the American College of Cardiology conference devoted to the emerging care model in December 1965. Several of those doctors were CCU pioneers, but Swan was not. Cedars of Lebanon Hospital, where his office was located, would open its unit one month after the conference.

Swan's role in Rochester had been confined to the catheterization laboratory, where the focus was on congenital heart disorders and to a lesser extent acquired valve disease. He recalled years later, "The practice at Cedars-Sinai at that time was that of a community hospital not, as Mayo, a referral center. So, congenital heart disease, my area of expertise, didn't exist for practical purposes... [and] valvular heart disease was not all that common."[90]

Swan explained that his "appreciation of cardiovascular disease changed dramatically" at Cedars-Sinai, where coronary heart disease was "endemic with its associated dysrhythmias, heart failure, unstable angina, and acute myocardial infarction. Of necessity, my...clinical and research goals had to change."[91] His expertise in catheterization facilitated his new institution's entry into a federally funded research program to study heart attacks that was launched a year after he arrived in Los Angeles.[92]

When Robert Grant became director of the National Heart Institute in March 1966, he published an article that began with a warning: "Coronary heart disease is far and away the leading killer among the variety of disorders which are collectively termed cardiovascular-renal disease, snuffing out the lives of more than half a million Americans each year."[93] A few months later, Grant announced an institute-funded extramural research program designed to identify more effective heart attack treatment strategies. One initiative would fund the construction and operation of Myocardial Infarction Research Units (known as MIRUs) at selected institutions beginning in 1967.[94]

Grant would never visit any of the units; he died suddenly less than six months after taking charge of the National Heart Institute. Eugene Braunwald, who worked with the fifty-year-old cardiologist at the NIH, wrote in an obituary: "Ironically, one of his major efforts at the time of his untimely death was the organization of a nation-wide effort on the disease that claimed his own life—acute myocardial infarction."[95] But sudden death was common among doctors. The issue of the *Journal of the American Medical Association* published the day Grant died included the obituaries of forty-nine physicians. Fifteen of those between the ages of forty-four and sixty-five had died of coronary disease.[96]

The National Heart Institute funded nine Myocardial Infarction Research Units, including one at Cedars-Sinai, where Swan led a team of ambitious young clinical investigators. Mayo did not have such a unit, but Paul O'Donovan (who had been born and trained in Ireland before completing his cardiology fellowship at Mayo) launched a catheter-based study of patients who developed shock after a heart attack in 1968. Shock is characterized by a constellation of abnormalities, including very low blood pressure, cold and clammy skin, low urine output, and confusion. Cardiogenic shock as a complication of extensive heart muscle damage due to acute myocardial infarction was almost always fatal. The initial focus of the CCU movement was on reversing sudden death due to cardiac arrest. By the late 1960s, however, it was apparent that about 90 percent of patients who succumbed in a CCU after a heart attack died as a result of severe left ventricular failure and shock.[97]

Cardiology section chief Milton Anderson addressed the problem of shock in his 1968 report to Mayo's Board of Governors: "It is hoped that through study of such patients by hemodynamic means treatment can be made more adequate and mortality statistics will improve."[98] In 1970 Jeremy

Swan coauthored an article describing a new technology that helped accomplish this goal. The so-called Swan-Ganz catheter became a fixture in CCUs because it could be inserted into a vein and pushed into the right heart at the bedside. It allowed continuous monitoring of intracardiac pressures, simplified cardiac output measurement, and provided information that could be used to guide treatment with intravenous drugs or fluids.[99]

Cardiologists Take Control as the CCU Movement Matures

As more complex technologies and treatments were introduced into the CCU, questions arose regarding who was qualified to care for patients with heart attacks. The Inter-Society Commission for Heart Disease Resources, established by the American Heart Association, published a position paper on the optimal care of patients with acute myocardial infarction in 1971. In the section on CCU staffing, the Study Group on Coronary Heart Disease stated that the director of the unit should be a "physician well trained in cardiovascular medicine."[100] This statement was published at a time when a very small percentage of doctors who considered themselves heart specialists had completed a formal cardiology fellowship.

There was growing recognition that not every self-styled heart specialist was comfortable with (or capable of) caring for patients in a CCU, with its expanding array of electronic equipment, catheter-based technologies, and powerful intravenous drugs. The editors of an 820-page book on coronary care outlined the challenge in 1972: "Although just ten years have elapsed since this new plan of care was first proposed as a possible means of reducing the awesome mortality from acute myocardial infarction, thousands of articles have already been published about every aspect of the program."[101]

In Rochester, more than a dozen Mayo cardiologists took turns staffing the CCUs at Saint Mary Hospital and Methodist Hospital in 1969. Robert Brandenburg, chief of cardiology at the time, recalled how the arrangement affected care: "This ended up being entirely too many people having the service too infrequently, causing much distress and discomfort to the CCU [nursing] personnel because everyone had a slightly different idea about the management of coronary care problems." The cardiologists concluded that a limited number of consultants should be assigned to staff the unit, specifically those who had a special interest in this demanding area of hospital practice.[102]

Paul O'Donovan was appointed director of a new Intensive Cardiac Care Service that was established in 1970. He met with MICU head nurse Sister Henry (Sister Charlotte Dusbabek) and other nursing representatives in July to develop policies relating to the care of patients with acute heart problems at Saint Marys Hospital. One message was clear: "*All* cardiac patients admitted to [the MICU] will become the responsibility of the Intensive Cardiac Care Service for the duration of their stay in [the unit] and the adjacent monitored beds."[103] The creation of this special CCU service had implications for the careers of some Mayo general internists who had cared for local patients in the unit.

Ralph Spiekerman, who had coauthored the first Mayo article that described the CCU model in 1964, recalled that he "used to enjoy taking care of coronary patients." He and his colleagues in the general medicine section responsible for the care of patients from Rochester had "real mixed feelings when it became known to us that we would have to give that up to the cardiologists, which I knew was the right thing to do but was not something I really wanted to do."[104] This phenomenon played out at large hospitals across the country. By 1972, a policy was in place at New York Hospital that transferred responsibility for the care of patients admitted to the CCU from his or her personal attending physician to a small team of full-time cardiologists led by Thomas Killip. This strategy exemplified the impact that new technologies might have in terms of defining the scope of a doctor's practice in some contexts.

The CCU movement fueled the demand for formally trained cardiologists. Between 1960 and 1972, the number of cardiology fellowship programs in the United States quadrupled from 72 to 280, and the number of cardiology fellows skyrocketed from 142 to 1,260.[105] After these fellows completed their training, they carried cardiology's new knowledge, technologies, and techniques to community hospitals across the country.

The Mayo Clinic played a significant role in an educational program launched in 1969 that was designed to improve the care of patients hospitalized with heart attacks in Minnesota. A state survey had revealed that traditional nurse training programs provided very little education about coronary heart disease and that there were not enough nurses to staff the CCUs that were being planned. It also found that "medical directors were not generally available for supervision of coronary care units and there was some reluctance on the part of physicians to assume this responsibility."[106]

Mayo Helps Train Minnesota Nurses to Work in a CCU

Paul O'Donovan led a project to train nurses to work in CCUs, which was funded by the Minnesota Heart Association and the Northlands Regional Medical Program. Between 1969 and 1972, more than two hundred nurses from around the state completed the four-week program in Rochester that was designed "to prepare the nurse for her role as a highly skilled member of the coronary care team."[107] Nurse Judith Thierman directed the course, which used a full-size, fully equipped, two-bed mock-up CCU created at Methodist Hospital. Demand for these specially trained nurses was strong because the number of Minnesota hospitals with CCUs or portable heart monitors increased from eighteen to more than one hundred between 1967 and 1972.

In a 1974 review of CCUs, Mayo cardiologist John Callahan explained that the terms "ICU" and "CCU" were used "somewhat loosely" because local circumstances influenced how the special spaces were utilized: "At one end of the scale is the unit in which all critically ill patients are placed, including postsurgical patients, post-trauma patients, medical patients and so forth. At the other end is the strict cardiac unit, limited to patients with myocardial infarction or suspected infarction."[108] Turning from patients to the individuals who cared for them, Callahan explained: "The intensive-care nurse is not a patchwork person composed partly of electrical engineer, partly of physician and partly of nurse. She is a new person with expanded capabilities, special training and increased responsibility." Describing the traditional physician-nurse relationship as "one of almost military authority, feudal allegiance and unquestioned omniscience," the Mayo cardiologist emphasized how the idea of the CCU had challenged and changed the status quo:

> The intensive-care nurse is able to read electrocardiograms, use complex respiratory-assist equipment and conduct cardiopulmonary resuscitation, including defibrillating countershock—in short, record observations and make decisions which had been the exclusive domain of the physician. When a physician finds that his nurse can "read" dysrhythmias on the moving beam of the oscilloscope screen more rapidly and more accurately than he can, some kind of adjustment in relationship has to begin. The most reasonable reaction would be a feeling of gratitude that the patient-care team has been so wondrously enlarged and enriched. We hope that this reaction soon will be universal.[109]

Callahan coauthored this review with Robert Bahn, a pathologist who chaired Mayo's Computer Committee. This paring of authors reflected the introduction of computer technology into a sixteen-bed dedicated CCU that opened at Saint Marys Hospital early in 1974.

Using Computers to Monitor Patients and to Collect Data

The groundwork for using computers at Mayo to help monitor, record, and study the heart's function had been laid more than a dozen years earlier. In February 1959, sixteen months after the Soviet Union had launched Sputnik, the clinic's newsletter announced that Mayo's huge human centrifuge, which had been dormant for a dozen years, was "being tuned up for a new series of investigations to be carried out at the request of the United States Air Force." The writer predicted that the research was "expected to have immediate application to presently available and proposed high speed aircraft. It has potential application to rocket and space flight."[110] The so-called Space Race, with its emphasis on technology and human physiology, had implications for patients on the ground in Rochester.

Earl Wood, who directed the centrifuge project, later explained that the Air Force and NASA funded the acquisition of state-of-the-art technology that converted analog data recorded during acceleration studies into a digital format that could be analyzed by an IBM 650 computer at the company's Rochester facility: "This development was the initial major basis for IBM and NIH support of analog and digital research computer facilities in our laboratory. This in turn expedited automated electrocardiographic and intensive care monitoring and analysis in clinical laboratories."[111] These dynamics were reminiscent of events in Rochester after World War II, when Wood played a major role in adapting technologies that had been developed as part of the wartime accelerator project for use in the cardiac catheterization laboratory.

Mayo introduced computer technology to monitor hospitalized patients with heart disease in 1968, when an IBM 1800 computer was installed at Saint Marys Hospital. It was used to record and store up to eight physiologic parameters (such as blood pressure and cardiac output) in individuals recovering from open-heart surgery. Financed by the clinic, the hospital, and IBM, this computer project meant that "all of the cardiac surgeons and a large number of cardiologists have direct experience with the performance of the computer as it relates to the care of patients."[112]

University of Utah physiologist Homer Warner was an American pioneer of biomedical computing. His interest in the field had developed when he worked with Earl Wood and Jeremy Swan in Mayo's catheterization laboratory in the early 1950s. In the middle of that decade, Warner launched the catheterization program at the Latter-day Saints Hospital in Salt Lake City. In 1968 he described how he had introduced computers into patient care in his hospital's catheterization laboratory, operating room, and postoperative ICU during the past decade. Warner explained that nurses and doctors felt that they were busier as a result of the computerized monitoring of heart rate, blood pressure, cardiac output, and other physiologic parameters because "they now know much more about their patient and are forced to make many more decisions than before when they were, to a greater extent, in the dark about what was going on physiologically."[113]

The desire to obtain objective, real-time data to help manage sick patients, such as those recovering from cardiac surgery or a heart attack, stimulated the development and diffusion of computer-based monitoring technologies at Mayo. They were already in place in the postoperative cardiac surgery unit at Saint Marys Hospital when a decision was made to send newly trained Mayo cardiologist Barry Rutherford to Salt Lake City to spend a year with Warner. When he returned to Rochester in July 1971, Rutherford succeeded O'Donovan as CCU director. He would coordinate the implementation of a state-of-the-art computer monitoring system in the new dedicated CCU (separate from the MICU) that opened at Saint Marys Hospital in 1974. That year, eight cardiologists were identified as members of an expanded "coronary care group" that assumed responsibility for caring for patients in the CCUs at Saint Marys Hospital and Methodist Hospital.[114]

Carlos Harrison was appointed director of the CCU in 1976, when Rutherford left Mayo to join a cardiology practice in Kansas City, Missouri. Two years later, the clinic's newsletter published a story about Harrison and the role of computers in the care of patients with heart disease who were hospitalized at Saint Marys. It began by stressing the impact of computers: "This is the age of the computer. From balancing our checkbooks to guiding rockets to the moon, computers have proved their usefulness in scores of ways in our society." Explaining that the introduction of computers into patient care had lagged behind other applications of the technology, the writer boasted, "Saint Marys Hospital provides a dramatic exception to the rule." Citing the computerized monitoring systems that had been installed in the hospital's CCU, catheterization laboratory, and cardiac surgery postoperative unit, the article claimed that "computers participate in patient care to a greater degree than perhaps anywhere else in the world." The technology in place in these three areas at Saint Marys was "helping doctors make more informed decisions and relieving nurses of some routine repetitive tasks so they can give patients more personal attention."[115]

It took several months for the doctors and nurses in Rochester to conclude that the constant monitoring of heart rhythm, blood pressure, fluid administration, and other things offered advantages over traditional pre-computer care in the CCU. Improvements in the computer programs and monitoring equipment influenced the attitudes of the physicians and nurses who worked there. Cardiologist Byron Olney noted that these changes resulted in a system that "is a very useful adjunct to the care of my patients." CCU head nurse Jean Lee agreed: "I finally am seeing that the computer is doing something for us once in a while, rather than us just feeding it data all the time.... Having been around under the old system, I can say it saves a lot of wear and tear on patients. We don't have to be bothering them every minute." But Olney pointed out that computers could come between a patient and his or her caregivers: "You can become so enamored of the technology that you forget about the patient. You punch buttons and look at displays and forget to talk to the patient."[116] This was a computer-era version of a concern that doctors had raised for decades as more laboratory tests and technologies were introduced that seemed to compete with rather than complement the traditional diagnostic methods of interviewing and examining a patient.[117]

The Mobile CCU: Transporting Technology to a Patient

CCUs saved lives because they provided a safety net for patients who suffered a cardiac arrest while being monitored continuously. But several factors influenced whether a patient with a heart attack might be admitted to such a facility. One important obstacle related to the fact that many individuals did not seek medical attention when symptoms consistent with an acute myocardial infarction first appeared. A 1972 *Newsweek* article "Heart Attack: Curbing the Killer" explained that more than one-half of men and women with symptoms consistent with the diagnosis "never reach a hospital, with its life-saving technology."[118]

Almost every reader had some experience with this phenomenon, having had a relative, a friend, or an acquaintance die suddenly. The sudden death of a public figure, something that happened regularly, was a reminder of how someone could be well one minute and dead the next. For example, the *Newsweek* article noted that forty-seven-year-old baseball legend Gil Hodges had died a few days earlier while playing golf. And no one could have known that his former Brooklyn Dodgers teammate fifty-three-year-old Jackie Robinson would have a cardiac arrest at his home a few months later. Although both sports celebrities had survived earlier heart attacks, their deaths came without warning.[119]

The 1972 *Newsweek* article described an innovative approach designed to save lives that had first been employed five years earlier in Belfast, Ireland: "Since every minute after a heart attack counts, hospitals now use mobile CCUs to bring the life-saving benefits of cardiac monitoring and resuscitation to the patient stricken at home."[120] *Newsweek* reported how a mobile CCU had transported one of America's most prominent citizens to the University of Virginia Medical Center in April 1972. Former president Lyndon Johnson, who had survived a heart attack seventeen years earlier, was at his daughter's home in Charlottesville, Virginia, when he developed severe chest pain. Charles Robb, his son-in-law and a law student at the university, called cardiologist Richard Crampton. He rushed to the Robbs's home at the same time a special team raced there in the hospital's one-year-old mobile CCU.[121]

The former president, pessimistic about his chances for full recovery, spent less than a week at the hospital before insisting that he be flown to Brooke Army Center in San Antonio, Texas. Johnson was released from the Texas hospital to recuperate at his ranch, but he continued to have frequent episodes of chest pain. On January 22, 1973, he telephoned his Secret Service agents for immediate help. They arrived at his bedroom in minutes, but Johnson was unconscious. CPR was unsuccessful, and the sixty-four-year-old former president was declared dead on his way to the hospital.[122]

Lyndon Johnson was a member of Mayo's Board of Trustees at the time of his death, and the clinic's newsletter celebrated his service to the institution in February 1973. It quoted comments that the former president had made in Rochester two years earlier: "Here, under the umbrella of a single institution, we have an opportunity to strike a blow against heart disease, against cancer.... Whatever time I have left, I want to spend it trying to contribute to the great undertaking that Mayo's skilled talents have pledged themselves to."[123]

Ironically, the same page of *Mayovox* that mourned the former president contained an article that began, "EMERGENCY! The patient has just four minutes to live." The article announced the imminent launch of an electrocardiogram telemetry system that would connect trained personnel in special Gold Cross ambulances with the CCU at Saint Marys Hospital. Anesthesiologist Roger White and CCU director Paul O'Donovan were collaborating in the development of a "Prehospital Life-Support System" that would be inaugurated in the Rochester area.[124]

White was inspired to start the program after visiting Miami, Florida, where the telemetry approach had been pioneered in 1967. One hurdle that White faced related to the Federal Communications Commission (FCC), which had to allocate unused ultrahigh frequency bands to carry the data and voice communications. He explained in 1973: "We had the help of our Congressmen—Albert Quie, Hubert Humphrey and Walter Mondale—in petitioning the FCC to get dedicated channels."[125]

The Rochester-based initiative had national implications because it resulted in the FCC granting dedicated frequencies across the country for the transmission of emergency cardiac data. The strategy to save lives in Rochester involved attaching a portable electrocardiogram to a patient in an ambulance and transmitting the signal to Saint Marys Hospital, where it would be displayed on an oscilloscope screen and could be printed on paper. The CCU resident evaluated the rhythm and radioed instructions to the ambulance crew that was with the patient. If instructed to do so, these specially trained men and women could use an onboard defibrillator. Mayo funded the program that White predicted would save the lives of about 10 percent of the patients who had a cardiac arrest in a Gold Cross ambulance each year.

The Mayo-sponsored "advanced pre-hospital life support system" was launched on June 8, 1973. During its first eighteen months of operation, three of seventeen patients who had a cardiac arrest were resuscitated "at the scene." Roger White and Paul O'Donovan attributed the low survival rate of patients who had out-of-hospital cardiac arrests to inadequate (or no) CPR prior to the arrival of an ambulance crew with the knowledge and equipment to resuscitate a patient. The other big problem related to the time delay between the onset of symptoms and the decision to seek medical attention. White and O'Donovan were hopeful that an aggressive campaign to educate the public about the warning signs of a heart attack would help to reduce this delay and save lives.[126]

The decade of the 1960s witnessed a sea change in the management of patients with acute myocardial infarction. It began with some men and women with heart attacks dying suddenly in hospital beds. Their hearts were not monitored, and cardiac arrest teams did not exist. By the end of the decade, the CCU model had spread to a majority of American hospitals and was beginning to spread out of these institutions by way of ambulances that carried a crew trained to use life-saving technologies and techniques.

A "Biology-Watcher" Warns About Halfway Technologies

In the midst of a chorus of enthusiasm about CCUs, one dissonant voice arose in 1971. Lewis Thomas, a prominent medical scientist and administrator, published an essay "Notes of a Biology-Watcher: The Technology of Medicine" in the *New England Journal of Medicine*. Based on the title, many readers assumed it would be a typical celebratory piece. But Thomas set them straight in the first paragraph: "Technology assessment has become a routine exercise for scientific enterprises on which the country is obliged to spend vast sums for its needs. Brainy committees are continually evaluating the effectiveness and cost of doing various things in space, defense, energy, transportation and the like.... Somehow medicine, for all of the 60-odd billion dollars that it is said to cost the nation, has not yet come in for much of this analytical treatment."[127]

Thomas coined the phrase "halfway technology" to describe things that are done to "compensate for the incapacitating effects of certain diseases whose course one is unable to do very much about." He singled out the CCU as an example:

> An extremely complex and costly technology for the management of coronary heart disease has evolved, involving specialized ambulances and hospital units, all kinds of electronic gadgetry, and whole platoons of new professional personnel, to deal with the end results of coronary thrombosis.... It is a characteristic of this kind of [halfway] technology that it costs an enormous amount of money and requires a continuing expansion of hospital facilities. There is no end to the need for new, highly trained people to run the enterprise. And there is really no way out of this, at the present state of knowledge. If the installation of specialized coronary care units can result in the extension of life for only a few patients with coronary disease...it seems to me an inevitable fact of life that as many of these as can be will be put together, and as much money as can be found will be spent. I do not see that anyone has much choice in this.[128]

Thomas argued that the only way to escape halfway technologies, such as the CCU, was through research.

In a very real sense, he was lobbying for his community of academic biomedical scientists: "If I were a policy-maker, interested in saving money for health care over the long haul, I would...give high priority to a lot more basic research in biologic science." The media contributed to the public's infatuation with halfway technologies, in Thomas's opinion. Newspaper and television reports tended to present each innovation or procedure as "a breakthrough and therapeutic triumph, instead of the makeshift that it really is."[129] His message resonated with some of his contemporaries, but it was drowned out by the cheers for new diagnostic and therapeutic technologies and techniques to deal with heart disease and other conditions that could not be cured in the sense that an antibiotic could eliminate an infection.[130]

{ 14 }

Coronary Angiography
THE CLEVELAND CLINIC LEADS THE WAY

Coronary care units, first established in the early 1960s, focused on patients with an acute myocardial infarction because they were at risk for having a cardiac arrest, the most dramatic and deadly complication of coronary artery disease. By the end of the decade, tens of thousands of Americans had been admitted to these specialized units. But millions of men and women were living with angina pectoris, a chronic symptom of coronary disease that is characterized by chest discomfort associated with activity. Angina is usually caused by blockages in one or more coronary arteries, which results in a reduction in the amount of oxygen-rich blood available to nourish the contracting heart muscle.[1]

In the 1950s, a patient who informed a physician that he or she had chest pain brought on by exertion was assumed to have coronary artery disease. The diagnosis was more certain if they had a history of a heart attack or if their electrocardiogram showed the classic pattern of a prior myocardial infarction. But in the absence of these two things, it was almost impossible to say with certainty that a patient with exertional chest discomfort did or did not have coronary blockages. A new diagnostic test, coronary angiography, would change all of this in the 1960s.

Coronary angiography is a catheterization procedure that makes the coronary arteries visible by taking X-ray pictures of the heart just when a radiopaque contrast medium (hereafter contrast) flows through those blood vessels. The result is a series of images that show the three main coronary arteries and their progressively smaller branches. If narrowed segments are present in these main arteries or their larger branches, a coronary angiogram reveals the location and severity of the blockages. The X-ray test produces a composite picture that is analogous to a road map. Although this would seem to be very valuable information in terms of taking care of some patients with chest pain, it took more than a decade for the pioneers of coronary angiography to convince many physicians that the test's benefits outweighed its risks.[2]

The story of how coronary angiography became a common clinical tool to help doctors make treatment decisions in individual patients with angina focuses on the Cleveland Clinic. And some very interesting parts of it have never been published. Cardiologist Mason Sones Jr., who joined the Ohio group practice in 1950 to establish a catheterization laboratory, was largely responsible for developing coronary angiography.[3] He also played a central role in catapulting the Cleveland Clinic to the forefront of the diagnosis and surgical treatment of coronary heart disease during the 1960s and early 1970s.

Several things contributed to Sones's success in developing coronary angiography, including his obsession with perfecting angiography as a diagnostic tool, colleagues who shared his interests, internal and external funding, and access to patients. Coronary angiography would set the stage for the invention of operations performed directly on the coronary arteries and catheter-based procedures performed inside them. This cluster of treatment procedures would have a profound effect on the care of millions of patients with coronary heart disease, and it would greatly stimulate the growth of cardiology and cardiac surgery as specialties.

Angiography: Mapping Blood Vessels as a Guide to Therapy

The history of coronary angiography can be traced to 1907, when German physicians Friedrich Jamin and Hermann Merkel published the first X-ray images of human coronary arteries filled with contrast. These images were sold as a boxed set of actual photographic prints of angiograms that had been mounted side-by-side on thick cards, designed to be looked at with a handheld stereoscope viewer. Jamin and Merkel's stereoscopic pictures of the coronary arteries were stunning, but they had been made by injecting contrast into the blood vessels of hearts that had been removed from deceased persons.[4] More than four decades would pass before a few researchers began publishing X-ray pictures of the coronary arteries in living humans. During that interval, doctors in several countries developed techniques to produce angiograms of other blood vessels in patients.

Mayo internist Leonard Rowntree coauthored a 1923 article with specialists in urology and radiology that contributed to the advent of angiography as a clinical tool. But the Rochester researchers had not set out to visualize blood vessels. They wanted to develop a technique to take X-ray pictures of a patient's urinary system without performing ureteral catheterization—a painful procedure that involved pushing a thin flexible catheter into the urethra, through the bladder, and up a ureter. The Mayo researchers' alternative method involved injecting sodium iodide (a contrast agent) into a vein and taking sequential X-rays of the urinary tract as a patient's kidneys excreted the substance. In their article, they described an incidental discovery and its implications:

> Much is offered by this method in the study of the vascular system. Under the fluoroscope, the cephalic vein has the appearance of a steel wire, from the point of injection of the iodide at the elbow to the juncture of the cephalic vein with the subclavian. This has been noted following the use of 10 and 20 percent solutions of sodium iodide. In all probability, with variations in the technique, important results will be obtained with regard to the venous returns and the peripheral arterial circulations.[5]

This observation, an example of serendipity, inspired St. Louis surgeon Barney Brooks to use sodium iodide to produce X-ray pictures of the peripheral arteries in humans. Seven months after the Mayo article was published, he injected contrast into a woman's femoral artery to visualize the blood supply to her leg. An X-ray proved that her circulation was adequate despite weak pulses and skin changes that seemed to indicate reduced blood supply. Brooks boasted in 1924 that angiography was the first method for objectively assessing how blood vessel disease affected the circulation to the extremities.[6]

In 1928 Mayo vascular specialist George Brown and orthopedic surgeon Melvin Henderson coauthored an article on peripheral vascular disease. Acknowledging the confusion that surrounded the diagnosis of arterial disorders, they advocated angiography as a method to assess the condition of a patient's peripheral blood vessels in challenging clinical situations. The resulting images would provide unique visual information that could help a surgeon decide whether a patient might be harmed rather than helped by an amputation.[7]

Four years later, Mayo vascular specialist Edgar Allen and radiologist John Camp reported the results of peripheral angiography in twenty-five patients. An injection of contrast into a brachial (arm) or femoral (leg) artery had helped to define the type and severity of vascular disease in patients and to identify collateral (small connecting) vessels.[8] In 1934, during a lecture at the annual American Medical Association meeting, Allen and Camp predicted that the technique would soon be used to visualize most of the arteries in humans. During the discussion period, New York vascular specialist Irving Wright congratulated them: "Although other men have done this work abroad, they have been the men in this country who have interested us and inspired us to attempt this technique."[9]

World War II led to an unprecedented number of blood vessel injuries, and military surgeons treated them with a range of new approaches that were later used in civilian practice.[10] After the war, the scope of vascular surgery expanded rapidly due, in large part, to the introduction of antibiotics, anticoagulants, and synthetic materials that could be fashioned into flexible tubes to replace large blood vessels. By 1953, Mayo surgeon John Kirklin was among those operating on aneurysms of the aorta (a localized dilated segment of the body's biggest vessel). Like other surgeons, he recognized that angiography played a vital role in planning these major vascular procedures.[11] Mayo orthopedic surgeons Joseph Janes and John Ivins, who also did vascular surgery, performed peripheral angiograms in the early 1950s. But radiologists Owings Kincaid and George Davis assumed this responsibility as the scope and volume of angiograms increased in Rochester in the middle of the decade.[12]

Challenges in the Diagnosis and Treatment of Angina Pectoris

Experience had shown by mid-century that it was safe to flood a patient's aorta and peripheral arteries with contrast to produce X-ray pictures of those vessels. But there was reluctance to apply angiography to the coronary arteries because they carried oxygen-rich blood to the body's most vital organ. For example, Cincinnati cardiologist Harold Kotte warned in 1950, "The danger of introducing a foreign, oxygen-free [contrast] medium into a coronary circulation already seriously compromised by arteriosclerosis is probably great, and anginal pain, dangerous arrhythmias or sudden death are to be feared."[13] During the 1950s, a few researchers sought a safe way to make X-ray pictures of the coronary arteries by injecting contrast into the ascending aorta. Although some of the contrast would flow into the coronary arteries, it rarely produced complete pictures of them. The individuals who were trying to develop coronary angiography in this era were motivated by the belief that it could provide unique information that would help a physician care for a patient. This general phenomenon was not new. The desire to use objective data to help identify and sort out the potential causes of a patient's subjective symptoms had stimulated the development of countless laboratory and X-ray tests since the nineteenth century.[14]

In his 1956 book *Diseases of the Heart*, New York cardiologist Charles Friedberg listed several medications that physicians prescribed to patients thought to have angina. There was no consensus about which ones were beneficial except for nitroglycerin, a nineteenth-century remedy first used by homeopathic practitioners. Friedberg noted that sedatives, such as Phenobarbital, were among the most widely prescribed drugs for angina. He claimed that many physicians encouraged their patients to drink an ounce of alcohol to relieve an acute attack of angina.[15] But Friedberg explained that the main treatment strategy was to have patients avoid activities that predictably caused the distressing symptom:

> Patients with angina pectoris rapidly learn by themselves to avoid those forms of bodily exertion which are the commonest immediate causes of pain. Usually it is necessary to reduce the distance and

especially the speed of walking. To avoid being conspicuous, many patients stop repeatedly in front of stores and pretend they are window shopping. Often the patient may avoid pain by changing his manner of transportation so as to reduce the walking distance to his train or subway. He may have to change his route if it involves walking uphill. Running for buses or trains must be prohibited. The patient must learn to allow sufficient time so that hurrying is unnecessary.... Walking in cold weather, especially against the wind, should be avoided when possible. If feasible, the coldest month or months of the year should be spent in a warm climate.[16]

Several of Friedberg's recommendations, which reflected the fact that he practiced in New York City, were irrelevant for many patients—especially those whose lives involved physical labor.

When Mayo cardiologist Howard Burchell spoke at a symposium held at Manhattan's Waldorf-Astoria Hotel in January 1957, he did not emphasize the plight of a farmer or a laborer who had angina. Like Friedberg, he focused on patients with white-collar jobs. In discussing the benefits of taking nitroglycerin just before an activity that predictably brought on an attack of angina, Burchell explained: "Nitroglycerin has been of great advantage to patients, not to entice them into foolish feats of strength or endurance but to allow certain scheduled common-sense activities, such as walking from parking lot to office against a cool wind, to be done without anxiety or pain."[17]

The serious shortcomings of drug treatments for angina stimulated a few surgeons to try to develop operations that might improve the heart's blood supply. Mayo surgeon John Kirklin published an editorial on operations for coronary heart disease in 1955. He listed several procedures, none of which involved operating directly on the coronary arteries:

Attempts have been made to stimulate the ingrowth of myriads of extremely small vessels by the production of pericardial adhesions or of adhesions between the heart and such organs or tissues as the pectoral muscle, the omentum or isolated loops of intestine. The implantation of the internal mammary artery into the ischemic myocardium recently has been proposed as a more direct approach to the problem of bringing arterial blood into the cardiac muscle.

Summarizing the situation, Kirklin stitched together three key questions: "Do these procedures truly increase the blood supply to the myocardium and by virtue of this increased blood supply relieve the pain of angina pectoris and prolong life?"[18] Like almost all heart specialists, Kirklin considered the evidence inconclusive.

In September 1955, one month after the publication of Kirklin's editorial, almost 500 physicians, surgeons, and scientists attended a symposium on arteriosclerosis at the University of Minnesota. University surgeon C. Walton (Walt) Lillehei (who, like Kirklin, had become world famous for pioneering open-heart surgery) spoke at the meeting after a presentation on thromboendarterectomy. This tongue-twisting term referred to a new operative technique that was designed to peel out the diseased inner lining of an obstructed peripheral artery and sew the outer layers back together in order to reconstruct an open vessel and to restore blood flow.[19] Lillehei was eager to apply endarterectomy to the coronary arteries, but he hoped to develop another procedure that involved operating directly on the vessels.

Based on animal experiments, Lillehei had concluded that it was possible to create an end-to-end anastomosis (connection) between an internal mammary artery (which runs down the inner chest wall) and a coronary artery (which runs over the surface of the heart). He described the biggest obstacle to the application of this technique to patients, and he suggested a solution. A surgeon needed to know precisely where a coronary artery was blocked, and Lillehei predicted that improved angiographic methods could provide this critical information.[20]

Mason Sones Invents "Selective" Coronary Angiography

Cleveland Clinic cardiologist Mason Sones Jr. was responsible for a breakthrough in coronary angiography that would provide the information that Walt Lillehei considered indispensable in order to operate directly on a diseased coronary artery. In the summer of 1956, Sones submitted a research grant application to the National Institutes of Health (NIH) for a project titled "Contrast Visualization of the Coronary Circulation." The application form and other unpublished documents dispel some myths and correct some recollections about Sones's invention of what would be called selective coronary angiography. The Cleveland Clinic cardiologist's goal was to use a combination of new X-ray technology and standard motion picture equipment in order to improve the quality and clinical usefulness of coronary angiograms.

The few researchers who were trying to image the coronary arteries in the mid-1950s took a series of still-frame X-ray pictures of the heart during the few seconds that contrast flowed through those small vessels that supplied it with blood. The contrast that flowed into and through the left and right coronary arteries had been injected into the proximal aorta (just above the aortic valve). But this approach had limitations, as Sones explained in his grant application: "Single X-ray exposures, or exposures made at rates presently obtainable with conventional angiocardiographic equipment, frequently fail to demonstrate areas of the coronary circulation because of the heart's motion or because of the failure of all branches of the coronary tree to fill at precisely the same time after any single injection of contrast medium. High speed motion picture photography during contrast visualization significantly reduces the possibility of such technical failure."[21] The $17,500 NIH grant that Sones applied for would help pay for a new eleven-inch image intensifier and a 35 mm motion picture camera.

Sones explained in his grant application that his Cleveland Clinic colleagues in radiology, biophysics, surgical research, and cardiac surgery supported the project. His co-investigators included radiologist Robert Hughes, biomedical engineer Willem Kolff, and cardiac surgeon Donald Effler. Sones also cited ongoing research at the Ohio clinic regarding "the development of effective surgical techniques to bridge or bypass segmental occlusions in the coronary circulation, by the use of frozen dried arterial grafts, or by direct arterial anastomosis with the internal mammary arteries during induced cardiac arrest and maintenance of the circulation with a pump-oxygenator."[22]

Sones indicated that the subjects would be patients who had symptoms consistent with coronary heart disease. He would compare their angiograms with those from patients with congenital heart defects or acquired heart valve disease who did not have symptoms or signs of coronary disease. The research grant application did not mention informed consent. This concept and the processes to address it were the subject of discussion at the time, but no formal standards had been developed.[23] Sones emphasized the project's potential clinical implications. The advanced technology he hoped to use should make it possible to "visualize the precise location of points of arterial occlusion or segmental narrowing." In turn, this information would facilitate "the development of surgical techniques for the direct re-establishment of coronary artery flow."[24] Sones's grant application, just eight pages long, proves that he had a clear goal in sight. And he would attain it with the support of his institution and his colleagues.

A University of Minnesota Surgeon Communicates With Sones

Owen Wangensteen, the longtime head of surgery at the University of Minnesota and Walt Lillehei's mentor, had inside knowledge about Sones's coronary angiography project. He was a member of the National Advisory Heart Council, which was charged with reviewing his research grant application. At the time, Wangensteen was supervising research on coronary artery surgery that his resident Alan Thal was doing. Wangensteen encouraged Thal to write to Sones in November 1956 in order to learn about the coronary angiography research at the Cleveland Clinic. Sones responded:

> At the present time, our experience has been limited exclusively to study of laboratory animals and incidental opacification of the coronary arteries in patients studied by selective cardioangiography with varying

types of congenital heart disease. From a philosophical standpoint, we have rather anticipated that direct surgical attacks on the coronary arteries would probably be one of the last things accomplished in the field of cardiovascular surgery, with congenital and acquired heart lesions constituting the evolutionary basis for a possible later approach. With the advent of elective cardiac arrest [during open-heart surgery], the hurdle of ventricular arrhythmias during manipulation of the coronary vasculature became a thing of the past, and it immediately appeared feasible to entertain the idea of coronary artery surgery with the object of specific re-vascularization by the use of grafts or internal mammary [artery to] coronary [artery] anastomoses. It was also quite apparent that we had no really acceptable method for specifically determining the precise location and magnitude of segmental occlusions or points of narrowing and no really precise method of evaluating the status of the disease.[25]

Sones told Thal that he was welcome to visit the Cleveland Clinic. But he warned the surgical resident that he "might be disappointed in finding no tremendous concentrated full-time effort in this direction" because the work was undertaken "at odd times when we have been able to snatch short periods from an extremely busy clinical schedule."[26] Thal thanked Sones for his letter and explained that the Minnesota group was also conducting experiments in animals to visualize and operate on the coronary arteries.[27]

Sones received word about his grant application in a letter that National Heart Institute director James Watt sent on December 26, 1956. It contained news that was surely better than any Christmas present the cardiologist might have received. Sones's proposal had been approved, and his project would be funded.[28] The special equipment was installed in 1957, and the following year the *Cleveland Clinic Newsletter* boasted that the high-speed motion picture and X-ray apparatus in Sones's laboratory "opened the door for a whole new series of techniques for precisely assessing illnesses like congenital heart defects, valve lesions, and coronary artery disease."[29]

Sones Documents the Breakthrough Coronary Angiogram

Mason Sones had a big scare the day before Halloween 1958. During what began as a routine procedure, the tip of his catheter came very close to entering what was considered to be forbidden territory—the ostium (opening) of a coronary artery. The Cleveland Clinic cardiologist was very concerned when contrast injected close to the ostium flooded his patient's right coronary. He recounted this particular procedure in talks and articles. Other individuals, including his colleagues, also described the events. But the definitive account, based on previously unpublished material, is presented here for the first time.

As was his practice, Sones dictated a detailed procedure note shortly after he completed the case on October 30, 1958. His patient was a twenty-six-year-old man from West Virginia with valve disease who had been referred to the Cleveland Clinic for a cardiac catheterization and possible surgery.[30] After making an incision in the man's brachial artery, Sones inserted a catheter and threaded it up the vessel to the point where the tip was in the ascending aorta just above the aortic valve. He followed its progress on a fluoroscope screen and prepared to record the contrast injection on 35 mm motion picture film. After Sones threaded the catheter tip through the aortic valve into the left ventricle, an automated pressure syringe injected 50 cc of contrast into the chamber. His note details what happened next:

> The second injection of 50 cc. of 90% Hypaque was made directly into the ascending aorta above the aortic valve annulus. During this injection, which was...accomplished quite slowly, it was seen that the catheter tip lay nearly in the orifice of the right coronary artery and the pressure injection was made too slowly to really fill the root of the aorta so that almost all the contrast media passed into the right coronary artery, perfusing it heavily. The injection was made under too low a pressure to effectively perfuse the left coronary artery or the entire aortic root. This resulted in extremely heavy opacification of the right coronary artery selectively. Immediately after the injection was completed the patient developed a bradycardia which in a period of 4 seconds progressed to asystole which persisted for 5 seconds. There was prompt return to a slow sinus rhythm which during the next 10 seconds returned to a rate of 64 beats per minute. At no time during the injection did any ventricular premature beats occur. With this second injection the patient developed moderate diaphoresis and a sense of faintness which persisted for about 3 minutes.[31]

Sensing the significance of the situation, Sones wrote: "This is the first instance in which we have seen extremely heavy opacification of a single coronary vessel with contrast media." Because his patient "tolerated the procedure very well," Sones's fear that filling a coronary artery with so much contrast would cause a life-threatening ventricular arrhythmia gave way to a feeling of "considerable satisfaction regarding the further diagnostic evolution of this technique."[32] This is a compelling example of serendipity contributing to a major medical breakthrough.

Emboldened by his experience, Sones had a company in Syracuse, New York, produce custom-made, tapered-tip catheters that were designed to inject contrast directly *into* the left and right coronary arteries. He first used the special catheters in April 1959. Sones's technique would be termed "selective coronary angiography" because it involved injecting contrast directly into the vessels. In October 1959 Sones showed a movie of the technique during a

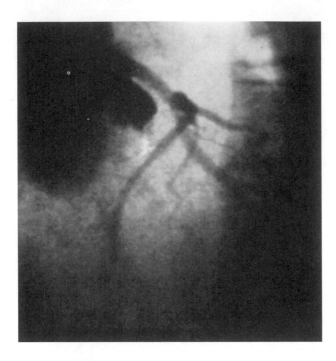

FIGURE 14.1

A semi-selective coronary angiogram. Image of left coronary artery made when Mason Sones Jr. injected contrast into the left anterior sinus of Valsalva.

B. L. Gordon, ed., *Clinical Cardiopulmonary Physiology*, 2nd ed. (New York: Grune & Stratton, 1960), 141, figure 10-6, reprinted with permission, Cleveland Clinic ©2013.

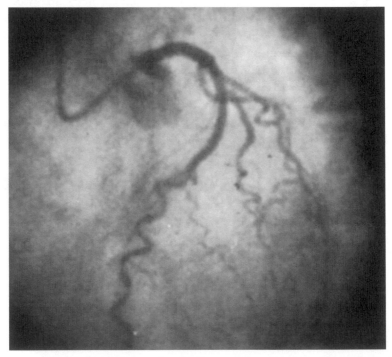

FIGURE 14.2 *First published image of a selective coronary angiogram. Mason Sones Jr. had just injected contrast directly into the left coronary artery.*

B. L. Gordon, ed., *Clinical Cardiopulmonary Physiology*, 2nd ed. (New York: Grune & Stratton, 1960), 142, figure 12, reprinted with permission, Cleveland Clinic ©2013.

lecture at the American Heart Association meeting. His very first publication on selective coronary angiography, which appeared in a 1960 textbook on cardiopulmonary physiology, has been overlooked. Sones's book chapter is historically significant because it contains his description, supplemented by pictures, of the evolution of coronary angiography from a non-selective (central aortic injection) to a semi-selective (sinus of Valsalva injection) to a truly selective (intracoronary injection) technique (see Figures 14.1 and 14.2).[33]

The Cleveland Clinic Sees Coronary Disease as an Opportunity

Just before Valentine's Day 1960, a headline in the *Cleveland Press* proclaimed, "Clinic Team Scores Breakthrough in Heart Diagnosis." Earl Shirey, a cardiologist who worked closely with Sones in the catheterization laboratory, had shown movies of coronary angiograms "to an overflow audience of general practitioners at a clinic seminar." The newspaper reporter boasted that "a historic breakthrough in understanding of coronary artery disease, the great killer, has been made at the Cleveland Clinic." Unlike some supposed breakthroughs trumpeted by innovators, institutions, or the media, this one appeared to have real relevance to patient care. Impressed by the procedure's potential, the writer explained that "the cardiologist knows at once whether there is blockage in the coronary, and if so, where." In some instances, the test revealed that a patient who was thought to have had a heart attack had no coronary disease at all. If that were the case, "a young executive of 40 could take on the offered promotion and avoid a restricted life with a false coronary." The newspaper article's final sentence echoed a statement that Sones had made four years earlier in his NIH grant application: "This technique is expected to open new frontiers in coronary surgery."[34]

In March 1960 Cowles Andrus, the former chief of cardiology at Johns Hopkins, gave a small but very influential audience an opportunity to see what Sones had accomplished. At a meeting of the National Advisory Heart Council in Bethesda, Maryland, he showed a movie that Sones had made of a series of selective coronary angiograms. Mayo cardiologist Howard Burchell, a member of the council, was present and heard Andrus remind the audience "of the intensity with which research in the field of coronary disease has been pushed" during the dozen years the council had been in existence. "Finally," Andrus exclaimed, "there has been a very striking advance in the visualization of the coronary vascular system by angiography. This is the consequence of a fortunate collaboration of electronic engineers, radiologists, chemists, physiologists, and clinicians." The Johns Hopkins heart specialist acknowledged that "angiography has been made possible by a certain amount of daring."[35]

Mason Sones was a daring and very strong-willed individual who had become obsessed with perfecting and performing coronary angiography. He got support from his surgical colleague Donald Effler, who was unwilling to simply watch the future of heart surgery unfold—he wanted to help shape it. In November 1960 Effler informed Fay LeFevre, a vascular medicine specialist who chaired the Cleveland Clinic's Board of Governors, that their institution had a strategic advantage as a result of Sones's technique of coronary angiography: "Cleveland Clinic has the best possible set up for the surgical treatment in selected patients with coronary artery disease."[36]

LeFevre responded that he had read Effler's proposal for operating on patients with coronary heart disease with great interest and thought the project should have top priority. Displaying institutional pride and entrepreneurial spirit, the Ohio vascular specialist declared: "We should move ahead as rapidly as possible with this procedure as we are in a better position that anyone else in the country to carry it out."[37]

The implications of developing complementary programs of catheter diagnosis and surgical treatment of coronary heart disease impressed Richard Gottron, the Cleveland Clinic's business manager. In the spring of 1961, he asked Sones to "dream a little" in preparing a ten-year plan for the administration.[38] Three months later, Gottron reflected on the cardiologist's ambitious agenda: "Viewed in its entirety, Dr. Sones' requirements are of such a magnitude as regards space, manpower, and money as to deter even his most enthusiastic supporters." But the financial analyst saw opportunities: "Dr. Sones' success in the field of cardioangiography leads us to believe that a substantial further development of this field has important potentials for the Cleveland Clinic Foundation. New techniques in heart surgery, vein and artery surgery, and neurosurgery could be developed as a result of Dr. Sones' efforts. All of this could serve not only to enhance the professional standing of the Cleveland Clinic, but could also lead to important economic advantages."[39] Gottron's predictions could not have been more correct.

Syracuse cardiologist Goffredo Gensini, an early adopter of Sones's technique, put the procedure in perspective in 1961, when he and two coauthors predicted that "the introduction and widespread application of coronary angiography may very well take the precious information now only available in a postmortem report and place it in the hands of the cardiologist, the radiologist and the surgeon."[40] The hope was that putting this information in the hands of a living patient's physicians would influence treatment so that an autopsy was irrelevant. Accurate diagnosis was the first step to appropriate therapy.

This same year that Gensini encouraged the adoption of coronary angiography as a diagnostic tool, two internists provided practical advice about how to determine the likely cause of an individual patient's symptoms: "Sutton's Law needs to be kept in mind by the diagnostician." After advising physicians to proceed "immediately to the diagnostic test most likely to provide a diagnosis," they described the origin of the phrase: "When Willie Sutton, a hold-up man, was being interviewed by newsmen he was asked why he always robbed banks. Sutton, with some surprise, replied, 'Why, that's where the money is.' "[41]

Sones applied Sutton's Law in Cleveland every time he performed a coronary angiogram to prove whether or not a patient had coronary disease. But his main motivation was not money; it was passion for his procedure. In fact, this was how Sutton explained his career of crime. Claiming that some enterprising reporter had invented the quotation attributed to him, Sutton confessed, "Why did I rob banks? Because I enjoyed it. I loved it. I was more alive when I was inside a bank, robbing it, than at any other time in my life."[42] Sones, who certainly loved doing coronary angiograms, provided his colleagues with maps of the heart's arteries that helped guide their decisions about a patient's care.

Mason Sones, Donald Effler, Fay LeFevre, and Richard Gottron shared a vision of the future: coronary disease would become the centerpiece of the Cleveland Clinic's cardiology and cardiac surgery programs. They were being pragmatic. Johns Hopkins health economist Herbert Klarman estimated that the total economic costs attributable to cardiovascular diseases in the United States in 1962 were $30.7 billion. Although many assumptions went into this estimate, no one could deny that coronary artery disease accounted for much of the cost.[43] The Cleveland Clinic group would focus on coronary disease, which was very common. Meanwhile, the Mayo Clinic group continued to devote much of its energy to congenital heart defects, which were rare.

Mason Sones and Earl Shirey, his colleague in the catheterization laboratory, published a concise review of selective coronary angiography in the July 1962 issue of *Modern Concepts of Cardiovascular Disease*. Published by the American Heart Association, this monthly bulletin was sent free to almost 100,000 physicians. By the time the Cleveland Clinic cardiologists' brief article appeared, they had performed selective coronary angiograms in 1,020 patients. The fact that only three patients had died as a result of the procedure proved that the dire predictions about what would happen if contrast was injected directly into a coronary artery were unwarranted. But Sones and Shirey cited other problems: "Inept performance, inadequate instrumentation, and overimaginative or undiscerning interpretation provide the means of opening a Pandora's box of misinformation which may plague the physician, harm his patients, and retard the evolution of a better understanding of human coronary artery disease."[44]

The Cleveland Clinic cardiologists emphasized how the test could help practitioners and their patients:

> The largest group of patients which may be studied with benefit are those in whom the diagnosis of coronary artery disease is suspected, but ill-defined, or questioned because of atypical clinical features.... Normal coronary arteriograms have been demonstrated in a number of such patients following years of well-intentioned treatment with vasodilators, sedatives, or anticoagulant drugs. In some, the combination of pain, unresolved hopelessness, and personality maladjustment, compounded by poor medical management, led to narcotic addiction. In others, pericardial poudrage, internal mammary artery ligation, or the

production of myxedema with radioactive iodine, have been needlessly performed.[45]

Despite Sones's obvious passion for coronary angiography and the publicity it received, very few institutions introduced the technique in the early 1960s. Most physicians did not see any need to refer a patient for the invasive catheter procedure when there was no accepted surgical treatment for coronary heart disease.

In 1962 sociologist Everett Rogers published his classic five-category system for describing how individuals respond to innovations. Sones belonged to the first category—innovators. The remaining categories were early adopters, early majority, late majority, and laggards.[46] Several factors may encourage or stifle innovation. In most situations, innovators require more than personal passion to succeed. If they work in an institutional context, they depend on the support of individuals who are empowered to provide time and other resources necessary to move a project or a program forward. It is also important to acknowledge the importance of personal relationships and the ability of innovators and potential early adopters to persuade individuals and committees that a specific proposal is worthy of investment.

Early Adopters of the Sones Technique at Johns Hopkins

A cardiac surgeon, a radiologist, and two cardiologists at the Johns Hopkins Hospital were early adopters of Sones's technique of selective coronary angiography. David Sabiston recalled that when he was the chief surgical resident at the Baltimore institution, Alfred Blalock offered him a full-time staff position with the understanding that he would try to develop methods to improve the blood supply to the heart.[47] In 1960 Sabiston and radiologist Erich Lang began using selective coronary angiography to help decide if a patient was a candidate for a coronary endarterectomy.[48]

Later that year, two cardiologists at Hopkins began performing coronary angiograms. Richard Ross, who had just succeeded Cowles Andrus as chief of cardiology, and Gottlieb Friesinger, a cardiology fellow, visited the Cleveland Clinic to observe Sones and Shirey perform the procedure.[49] Cardiology and cardiac surgery research was thriving at the Baltimore institution as a result of grants from the National Heart Institute and the American Heart Association that helped support an ambitious group of young clinical investigators. Ross, Friesinger, and cardiologist Michael Criley also had access to a new catheterization laboratory. Funded by the London-based Wellcome Trust, it was equipped with state-of-the-art angiography equipment.[50]

Sabiston and Blalock reported their experience with coronary endarterectomy in six patients in 1961. They explained the rationale for the procedure by drawing an analogy between symptoms caused by peripheral vascular disease involving the legs and symptoms attributed to coronary artery disease. Patients with significant blockages of the femoral artery in the leg often have claudication, a severe pain in the calf muscle that comes on with walking and is relieved by rest. The pain is due to ischemia, which results from inadequate blood supply to the contracting muscle.

The Hopkins surgeons explained, "In the recent past it has been shown that direct removal of obstructing lesions in such cases often produces relief of symptoms. It is perhaps logical to assume that the removal of similar lesions from the coronary arteries might be a rational method of therapy for patients with angina pectoris."[51] Based on their experience with coronary thromboendarterectomy in six patients who had severe angina, Sabiston and Blalock thought the operation had potential. Nevertheless, they concluded that "additional cases and an extended period of observation will be necessary before definite conclusions may be drawn regarding the ultimate role and efficacy of this procedure."[52]

Cleveland Clinic Surgeon Donald Effler Becomes Impatient

Donald Effler performed the first operation for coronary disease at the Cleveland Clinic in January 1962. He did a coronary endarterectomy on a forty-five-year-old man with severe angina who had a 90 percent narrowing of his left main coronary artery. Effler covered the opening in the vessel with a small patch taken from a vein in the man's leg. When he reported his experience with four patients at the annual meeting of the American Association for Thoracic Surgery in April 1963, Effler expressed frustration during the discussion period. After listening to Oxford University surgeon Philip Allison's comments about surgery for coronary heart disease, Effler grumbled, "I can't remember when so much has been said by people who know so little about the most important subject that is the future of cardiovascular surgery."[53] The following month, a *Time* magazine article provided insight into the Ohio surgeon's personality: "'To be great,' says the Cleveland Clinic's Dr. Donald B. Effler, 'a surgeon must have a fierce determination to be the leader in his field. He must have a driving ego, a hunger beyond money. He must have a passion for perfectionism. He is like the actor who wants his name in lights.'"[54]

At the American Surgical Association's 1965 meeting, Effler complained: "The treatment of coronary occlusive disease by the direct approach, either excision or bypass of the occluding lesion, is not popular. Only about *200 patients have survived such procedures*—a paltry figure when one considers that the number of persons with coronary artery disease in this country alone must be counted in the millions." Revealing his impatience, Effler exclaimed: "We have got a real chore cut out for us. If we can get more clinical surgeons like the Kirklin group [at the Mayo Clinic], who get excellent results in pediatric surgery, to employ their talents in this field of acquired vascular disease, namely coronary atherosclerosis, it will not be too soon."[55]

Turning to Mason Sones's technique of coronary angiography, the Cleveland Clinic surgeon took aim at medical heart specialists: "The last break-through that is mandatory—and this will be the hardest nut of all to crack—is to bring our cardiologists out of the *deep sleep*." Speaking to an audience of surgeons, Effler argued that angiography was indispensable for evaluating individual patients and for advancing the operative attack on coronary disease: "But to get our cardiology friends—and I have very few of them left, I might add—to consider this progressive step and to stop wallowing in the glory that came with the development of the electrocardiogram...will be something that we may not live to see."[56] When Effler made these caustic comments in the spring of 1965, Sones and his associates at the Cleveland Clinic had performed more than four thousand selective coronary angiograms. No one at the Mayo Clinic had performed the procedure, but that was about to change.

Mayo's Cautious Approach to Surgery for Coronary Disease

Several factors contributed to the lag between the time when Howard Burchell had a front-row seat for the special screening of Mason Sones's selective coronary angiography motion picture at the National Advisory Heart Council meeting in 1960 and when Mayo cardiologist Benjamin McCallister first performed the procedure in Rochester in 1965. Despite the five-year gap, Mayo entered the field at a time when it would best fit into sociologist Everett Rogers's early majority category.

In 1960 Mayo's medical and surgical heart specialists, like most of their peers in other institutions, were unconvinced that any of the operations that very few surgeons performed for coronary heart disease were beneficial. This attitude is exemplified by a speech that Mayo cardiologist Robert Parker delivered to a group of insurance agents in 1958. His audience was surely mystified by the technical terms that Parker used to describe eight different indirect surgical procedures on patients thought to have angina pectoris. None of the procedures involved operating on the coronary arteries themselves: "Implantation of a systemic artery into the myocardium, ligation of the coronary sinus, creation of a shunt between the aorta and coronary sinus, pericardial implantation of pulmonary, pleural, or other tissues, chemical removal of epicardium with phenol, the insertion of abrasive material in the pericardial sac and, finally, coronary endarterectomy and also bilateral ligation of the internal mammary arteries."[57]

Parker explained that none of these procedures had been performed on patients in Rochester and that he had never referred a patient to a surgeon who did any of them. Why not? Because there was no proof that any of the operations increased blood flow to the heart muscle or improved its pumping function. In 1958, the same year that Parker spoke, Mayo surgeons John Kirklin and Dwight McGoon published a review of open-heart surgery. They devoted ten pages to operations for congenital heart defects and three pages to operations for valve disease. But Kirklin and McGoon wrote fewer than one hundred words about surgery for coronary heart disease, explaining, "Only for completeness should it be mentioned that investigative work is underway in many institutions oriented toward the direct relief of occlusion of the coronary artery under conditions of extra-corporeal circulation." Although the Mayo surgeons considered this research very preliminary, they were optimistic that "certain carefully selected patients with localized coronary artery occlusion someday may be amenable to reparative operations by these techniques."[58]

In order to gain firsthand information from surgeons who performed and promoted the two most promising procedures, Mayo's Board of Governors approved a two-week trip for surgeon Henry Ellis and cardiologist Milton Anderson to visit Baltimore, Philadelphia, Cleveland, and Montreal in 1958.[59] David Sabiston in Baltimore and Charles Bailey in Philadelphia were performing coronary endarterectomy. Claude Beck at Western Reserve University in Cleveland was performing an indirect operation that he claimed led to the development of anastomoses (tiny connecting channels) that carried blood to the coronary arteries.[60] Montreal surgeon Arthur Vineberg had developed an operation that involved dissecting the left internal mammary artery away from the inner chest wall and implanting its bleeding end into a tunnel that he had made in the heart muscle (Figure 14.3). Based on animal experiments, Vineberg claimed that the implanted artery developed anastomoses to branches of the left coronary artery, thereby improving the heart's own blood supply.[61]

Mayo's heart surgeons were aware of other experiments that had been conducted closer to home, in Minneapolis. When University of Minnesota surgical resident Alan Thal had corresponded with Mason Sones in 1956, he mentioned ongoing animal research that involved attaching the end of an internal mammary artery directly to a coronary artery.[62] Mayo surgical resident Norman Baker and surgical research director John Grindlay reported similar animal experiments in 1959. Just as the Minneapolis group had done, they performed aortic angiograms (non-selective coronary angiograms) to assess the results several weeks after they had created an anastomosis.

Baker and Grindlay concluded that it was "possible to locate segmental occlusive disease by means of coronary arteriography." Citing the publications on non-selective coronary angiography from the University of Minnesota and the Cleveland Clinic that predated Sones's selective technique, they explained that this X-ray procedure "has been done experimentally and of late clinically with excellent results." Although the Baker and Grindlay found that one-half of the grafts were occluded in the four animals that survived, they predicted

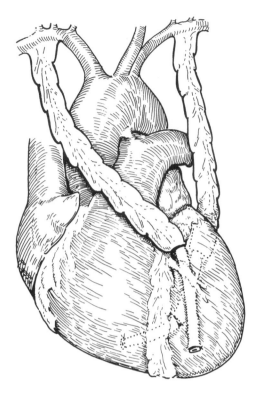

FIGURE 14.3 *Vineberg internal mammary artery implant operation (with two arteries inserted into tunnels made in the left ventricle).*

R. Favaloro, *Surgical Treatment of Coronary Arteriosclerosis* (Baltimore, MD: Williams & Wilkins, 1970), 80, figure 6.26, reprinted with permission of Wolters Kluwer Health/ Lippincott Williams & Wilkins.

that "in selected cases, with the aid of coronary arteriography, occlusive disease of the coronary vessels may be benefited by a direct surgical procedure, as is occlusive disease situated elsewhere."[63]

In 1961, two years after Baker and Grindlay expressed optimism about the potential of coronary angiography and its implications for operating directly on the coronary arteries, another group of Mayo researchers came to the opposite conclusion. Medical resident Joseph Eusterman presented the results of research at the annual American Heart Association meeting that he had undertaken with internist Richard Achor, radiologist Owings Kincaid, and pathologist Arnold Brown. They had combined pathological and radiological techniques to evaluate whether angiography produced an accurate picture of coronary artery disease.

The Mayo researchers had removed the hearts from fifty patients who had died of various causes. Next, they injected the coronary arteries with contrast and X-rayed the isolated organs. Finally, they sectioned the arteries and studied them under a microscope. Based on what they considered to be "rather poor agreement of arteriographic and anatomic findings," Eusterman, Achor, Kincaid, and Brown warned that coronary angiography "either for selection of patients to undergo direct coronary operations or for evaluation of coronary disease for diagnostic, therapeutic, or prognostic purposes should be accepted conservatively and hesitantly." They concluded that "too much dependence on the reliability of coronary arteriograms for the exact evaluation of coronary disease seems unwarranted at this time."[64]

Angiography pioneer Charles Dotter and pathologist Nelson Niles of the University of Oregon delivered a very different message at this same 1961 meeting in Miami Beach. In contrast to the Mayo authors' lack of enthusiasm for coronary angiography, they argued that it would be "essential to any surgical attack likely to succeed."[65] Elsewhere, Dotter had chastised clinicians for being complacent about coronary disease: "In the face of the staggering annual loss of over a half-million American lives, it is disconcerting to note that the current and widely accepted treatment for arteriosclerotic heart disease amounts to little more than supportive nonintervention."[66] This criticism reflected contemporary medical practice and general skepticism about the operations for coronary heart disease, which very few surgeons promoted.

Early in 1961, when Mason Sones was actively promoting selective coronary angiography, Mayo's chief of radiology Allen Good was expressing concern about the implications of expanding general (non-coronary) angiography in Rochester. He warned the clinic's Board of Governors that staffing his department was becoming more difficult because of departures of staff members and the fact that radiology was changing so rapidly. Mayo's X-ray specialists, like its heart specialists, confronted challenges as new technologies and techniques were transforming their fields at an unprecedented rate.

Because some imaging procedures, such as angiocardiography, were "complicated and sometimes hazardous," Good explained that it had become necessary for the radiologists to develop special interests and to divide their energy between the day-to-day "bread and butter" radiology (such as interpreting routine chest X-rays) and a particular subspecialty. But progressive subspecialization posed its own problems. For example, it reduced a radiologist's ability to choose when he or she might want to go on vacation or attend a professional meeting. And all of this increased "the difficulty already encountered in finding time to pursue research."[67] Good concluded his report to the board:

> In considering the future, it seems likely that further additions to the permanent staff will be necessary. It also seems likely that additional expensive and complicated radiographic equipment with limited usefulness will be required to carry out the newer examinations and those which will be developed in the future. All of this leads to the conclusion that expense will increase faster than income and that the Section of Diagnostic Roentgenology will not produce the same proportion of the revenue of the Mayo Clinic as it has in the past. In spite of this gloomy prediction, it seems obvious that, if the Mayo Clinic is to maintain its position as a leader in Medicine, it will be

essential for the Section of Diagnostic Roentgenology to remain abreast of the times, to apply new techniques as they develop and to continue to render the best possible and most expeditious service to the patient and consulting physician.[68]

When members of Mayo's board were reading Good's report in 1961, the Cleveland Clinic was committing significant resources to coronary angiography.

Mason Sones, the human dynamo that powered the Cleveland Clinic's aggressive coronary angiography program, worked in a multispecialty group practice that was modeled after the Mayo Clinic. But there were several differences. For example, Sones, like his institution's other heart specialists, was not expected to perform general medical diagnostic examinations.[69] Mayo's cardiologists had to share this responsibility with the clinic's other medical subspecialists. When Howard Burchell was recruiting Robert Frye in 1959, he explained to Mayo officials that he had informed the Johns Hopkins resident that there would be "a fair percentage of work in general diagnosis and in internal medicine" in addition to cardiology-related activities.[70]

The Mayo Clinic had no individual comparable to Mason Sones, who functioned as a hybrid cardiologist-physiologist-angiographer and spent most of his time in the catheterization laboratory. Physiologist Earl Wood, who had directed Mayo's catheterization laboratory since its inception shortly after World War II, had collected reams of research data for potential publication. Sones did not. Wood had lobbied for better angiography equipment in the mid-1950s, but he did not get it. Sones, on the other hand, had access to state-of-the-art imaging technology and did not have to rely on a radiologist to help him perform or interpret the X-ray studies that complemented his hemodynamic catheterizations.

Mayo's catheterization program was in a state of flux at a critical period in the development of coronary angiography. When it was reorganized in March 1960, Wood remained in charge of the original catheterization laboratory in the Medical Sciences Building, where adult patients would continue to be studied. Cardiac physiologist Jeremy Swan was put in charge of a new laboratory at Saint Marys Hospital, where children would undergo catheterization. By 1962, however, several of the cardiologists had become frustrated with Wood's focus on research. As the number of patients referred to Rochester for evaluation of valve disease increased, some Mayo cardiologists began directing adult patients to Swan, whose catheterizations were more clinically oriented and less time-consuming than Wood's.

The Board of Governors acknowledged these concerns in 1963, when it made a decision that marked the end of an era in Mayo's catheterization program. Going forward, Swan's catheterization laboratory at Saint Marys Hospital would assume responsibility for diagnostic procedures on adults as well as children. Wood's laboratory in the Medical Sciences Building would be "maintained for special investigations…made by special arrangements between the consultants concerned." This strategy acknowledged the loyalty that some cardiologists, especially Howard Burchell, felt toward Wood and the world-class cardiac catheterization program he had launched fifteen years earlier.[71]

Experiences at Johns Hopkins Influence Attitudes at Mayo

Richard Ross, chief of cardiology at Johns Hopkins, contributed to a symposium on coronary angiography that was published in 1963. He described three stages that a new diagnostic test passed through before its role in practice could be determined: "During the first stage, the test is used by its developers on a limited group of patients. During the second stage, the test is applied widely as clinical investigators explore possible new applications. Coronary arteriography is in this second stage at present and has not yet passed into stage three, where the indications, applications, and contraindications are clearly defined."[72] Ross cited a recent lecture by Canadian heart surgeon Wilfred Bigelow to illustrate one role for angiography. It had been used to prove that the Vineberg mammary implant operation could result in the formation of tiny anastomoses between the implanted artery and a patient's coronary arteries. Sones had shown this by injecting contrast into the mammary arteries of a few patients on whom Bigelow had performed the Vineberg procedure.

Bigelow, in his published report, cautioned against the widespread adoption of the Vineberg operation: "Even in the most carefully selected group of patients represented here, the results are good but not dramatic." But he was impressed by the postoperative angiograms that Sones had performed. The Canadian surgeon declared, "The remarkable feature is the radiologic confirmation that an open and bleeding [internal mammary] artery implanted into the heart will remain patent and apparently provide a source of blood supply to the heart."[73]

Impressed by Bigelow's report, Ross argued that coronary angiography "should be an essential part of the evaluation of any such revascularization procedure" because it provided unique visual evidence.[74] Although enthusiasm for the diagnostic procedure remained low, there were pockets of support. For example, a 1961 editorial writer in the *British Medical Journal* had declared that Sones "deserves great credit as a pioneer in this field and as the first to put coronary angiography on a practical and worth-while basis."[75]

By 1963 John Kirklin had concluded that Mayo should enter the evolving field of surgery for coronary heart disease, despite the controversies that continued to swirl around it. But starting a surgical program for coronary disease would require that someone perform selective coronary angiograms. Kirklin asked Robert Frye, who had joined the cardiology staff one year earlier, to accompany him to Johns Hopkins, where they would meet with surgeon

David Sabiston, who had operated on a few patients for coronary disease. They would also see the facilities for coronary angiography and meet with the individuals who performed it. Frye was a logical choice for launching coronary angiography at Mayo. He had recently completed a medical residency at Hopkins and had done right heart catheterizations (but not angiograms) during the two years he had worked in Eugene Braunwald's cardiology section at the National Heart Institute.[76]

Kirklin and Frye returned to Rochester convinced that it was reasonable to initiate a clinical trial of the Vineberg mammary implant procedure with pre- and postoperative coronary angiograms to assess the results. The program was in the planning stage when Frye suddenly left the Mayo Clinic in the summer of 1964 to join the Menlo Park Clinic in California. Disappointed with that experience, he returned to Rochester in the fall. Shortly thereafter, the Board of Governors approved a plan whereby Frye would spend a month working in Jeremy Swan's laboratory at Saint Marys Hospital to supplement his prior catheterization experience. The board also approved a plan whereby Frye and Benjamin McCallister, who had nearly completed his training at Mayo, would spend half of their time (on an alternating basis) performing adult catheterizations in Swan's laboratory beginning in 1965.[77] This represented a significant shift in philosophy and policy at the clinic. During the time that Frye and McCallister were assigned to the catheterization laboratory, they would not participate in traditional patient care activities.

In February 1965 Mayo sent McCallister and Franz Hallermann, a radiologist who had recently joined the staff and who performed aortograms, to the Cleveland Clinic to learn about the equipment and techniques used to do coronary arteriograms.[78] McCallister, who visited Sones on another occasion to observe the procedure, began doing coronary arteriograms at Saint Marys Hospital later that year. Frye recalled that he never had any formal training in the procedure beyond watching Sones perform them: "Ben and I kind of learned as we went along.... We just started doing it."[79]

Jeremy Swan's surprise announcement that he was leaving Rochester in July 1965 to become chief of cardiology at Cedars-Sinai Medical Center in Los Angeles led to a restructuring of Mayo's catheterization and cardiology programs. The Board of Governors appointed cardiologist Robert Brandenburg, surgeon John Kirklin, and pediatric cardiologist James DuShane to an ad hoc committee charged with making "recommendations not only for the future staffing of the cardiac catheterization laboratory, but also for an over-all plan for the development of cardiology generally within the institution."[80]

In anticipation of Swan's departure, the board appointed Donald Ritter, a pediatric cardiologist who had joined the staff two years earlier, and Shahbudin Rahimtoola, a research assistant in physiology who had received cardiology and catheterization training in England, as co-directors of the catheterization laboratory until a permanent director was chosen. Owings

Kincaid and George Davis were already well established as cardiac radiologists and angiographers. Although they would continue to assist the cardiologists with angiocardiograms, Kincaid and Davis would not perform coronary angiograms.[81] Mayo's programs for the diagnosis and surgical treatment of congenital heart disease and acquired valve disorders continued to thrive. But now, five years after Sones published his first description of selective coronary angiography, the technique would be available in Rochester to evaluate some patients with known or suspected coronary heart disease.

The Cleveland Clinic's Coronary Heart Disease Program Grows

Donald Effler and Mason Sones presented the Cleveland Clinic's early experience with the Vineberg operation at the annual meeting of the American Association for Thoracic Surgery in March 1965. Sones explained that angiograms done in patients nine to twelve months after surgery proved that blood flowed through two-thirds of the implanted mammary arteries.[82] During the discussion period, Toronto surgeon Wilfred Bigelow declared, "With typical American decisiveness and enterprise, Dr. Effler and Dr. Sones and their associates have moved into the field of revascularizing the heart with obviously attractive and excellent results, as you would expect." Bigelow saluted Sones for providing a yardstick to measure success and predicted that his angiographic technique was "going to change the complexion of surgery for coronary artery disease." Closing the discussion, Sones estimated that 25 million Americans had symptomatic coronary disease and challenged surgeons to "get at it" and develop better operations to bring more blood to the heart muscles of more patients with angina.[83]

In the spring of 1965, shortly after Sones spoke to surgeons in New Orleans, his colleague William Proudfit addressed an audience close to Rochester. The Cleveland Clinic cardiologist was participating in a symposium on coronary heart disease sponsored by the Iowa State Medical Society. Proudfit explained that Sones and Shirey had done more than 4,000 angiograms and that Effler and his surgical colleagues had performed almost 200 Vineberg procedures with a 4 percent mortality rate. Proudfit, like Canadian surgeon Wilfred Bigelow, was impressed that angiograms done several months after a Vineberg operation showed that a majority of the arteries that had been implanted into the heart muscle were open and that some blood flowed through them and into tiny branches of a coronary artery.[84]

Turning from pictures to patients, Proudfit told the Iowa practitioners, "Surgical therapy is not a cure, but the risk nowadays is low in suitable patients, and symptomatic improvement and probably increased life expectancy result." The Cleveland Clinic cardiologist cautioned, however, that "more general employment of surgical procedures must await widespread use of selective coronary cine-arteriography for the necessary preoperative and postoperative evaluations of the patient's circulatory status."[85]

Despite the ongoing efforts of cardiologists, surgeons, and radiologists at a few referral centers to promote selective coronary angiography, the procedure remained controversial and was not widely available in 1965. The following year, an editorial writer in the London-based *Lancet* protested that it "seems at present to offer little that cannot be more easily obtained by much simpler methods, such as good history-taking and electrocardiography."[86] Effler attacked the anonymous author, insisting that interest in coronary angiography was increasing every day and predicting that facilities for performing it would "multiply many times over within the next year or two."[87]

The public continued to read about the Cleveland Clinic's aggressive approach to coronary disease. For example, the *Wall Street Journal* published a front-page article, "Healing the Heart," in 1966 that described the Vineberg operation and credited Sones with using angiography to prove its effectiveness. "Backed by such evidence," the writer explained, "a small but growing number of surgical centers are beginning to use the artery implant operation." He quoted Effler, who acknowledged that "all patients with coronary heart disease aren't candidates for surgery and no one operation is applicable to all candidates." Based on the prevalence of coronary disease, however, it appeared that "several hundred thousand persons might benefit from the operations." The writer closed by noting, "These operations on clogged arteries, however, are being performed on only a small number of angina sufferers at present and are being attempted by only a few surgeons, chiefly in Cleveland, Miami and Houston."[88] This publicity surely pleased Cleveland Clinic's business manager Richard Gottron, who had predicted five years earlier that Sones's breakthrough would enhance the institution's image and income.

Most medical and surgical heart specialists remained unconvinced about the two operations (endarterectomy and internal mammary implantation), despite the boost they received from coronary angiography. David Sabiston had begun operating on patients with angina at Johns Hopkins in the late 1950s. Shortly after he became chief of surgery at Duke University Medical Center in 1966, Sabiston reviewed the role of surgery in coronary heart disease, concluding:

> Coronary endarterectomy and internal mammary implantation would appear at this time to remain in an investigational state. The results of both techniques require further evaluation and careful preoperative and postoperative study, including selective arteriography. While progress clearly is being made, additional research remains to be done in this important field. The accumulation of more objective data in centers which possess complete facilities necessary for thorough preoperative evaluation and critical postoperative assessment is a mandatory obligation which remains for the future to fulfill.[89]

When Sabiston wrote this, the Cleveland Clinic had far more experience with coronary angiography than any institution in the world. This was evident from a two-year National Heart Institute–sponsored study of complication rates associated with catheterization and angiocardiography that ended on October 31, 1965. The Mayo Clinic had a tradition of developing new catheterization techniques, so it had been chosen to participate, along with the Cleveland Clinic, Duke University Medical Center, the Johns Hopkins Hospital, the Peter Bent Brigham Hospital, and eleven other centers.[90] One of two-year study's most striking findings was that 81 percent of the 3,312 coronary angiograms had been done at the Cleveland Clinic. The remaining 642 procedures were spread (unevenly) among the other centers involved in the survey.[91] When the study ended in the fall of 1965, Benjamin McCallister and Robert Frye had just begun performing coronary angiograms at Saint Marys Hospital in Rochester.

With Jeremy Swan's departure in the summer of 1966 and the introduction of coronary angiography at more institutions, Mayo adopted a new staff model in the catheterization laboratory. Physiologists had run the facility for two decades, but that changed when cardiologist Robert Frye became a full-time laboratory-based diagnostician. Robert Brandenburg informed the board early in 1967: "For the first time in the history of the laboratory it has been solely under the supervision of clinicians, and it has been the opinion of all of us that it has never functioned more effectively."[92] Mayo had also just entered the slow-growing field of coronary heart disease surgery.

Robert Wallace performed Mayo's first Vineberg mammary implant operation in 1966 at Saint Marys Hospital. He had come to Rochester three years earlier as a special fellow in cardiovascular surgery. This experience supplemented his earlier training in New York City and Houston, Texas, where he had spent a year working with leading cardiovascular surgeons Denton Cooley and Michael DeBakey. Kirklin arranged for Wallace to spend a week at the Cleveland Clinic with Effler and Sones to learn when and how to perform the Vineberg operation.[93] The number of coronary angiograms performed in Rochester grew very slowly, as did the number of Vineberg operations. In 1968, for example, McCallister and Frye performed 115 coronary angiograms. By that time, Sones and his associates were performing more than ten times that many studies each year.[94]

Two weeks before Christmas 1968, René Favaloro, one of Donald Effler's junior surgical associates, submitted a manuscript to a journal that described a new operation for patients with angina. The procedure, which came to be known as coronary artery bypass graft surgery (CABG), would solidify the Cleveland Clinic's reputation as the world's leading center for the diagnosis and surgical treatment of coronary artery disease. It would also stimulate the diffusion and rapid growth of coronary angiography.[95]

Coronary Artery Bypass Surgery Stimulates the Growth of Angiography

In January 1968 the *New England Journal of Medicine* published a review of cardiovascular surgery by Dwight McGoon in its Medical Progress section. The Mayo surgeon devoted just two paragraphs of his eleven-page paper to coronary artery disease, despite acknowledging that it was far more common than any other heart problem. At the time, most medical and surgical heart specialists remained skeptical about the value of the indirect operations that a few surgeons had developed for the treatment of patients with known or suspected coronary heart disease. "Like alchemists of old," McGoon declared, "surgeons have devised and applied method after method, first with fanfare and then with dwindling enthusiasm."[1]

Attitudes about surgery for coronary heart disease were gradually changing as a result of the more widespread use of Cleveland Clinic cardiologist Mason Sones's technique of selective coronary angiography. McGoon acknowledged that angiograms done after the Vineberg (internal mammary artery implant) operation had shown that blood continued to flow through the vessel that had been inserted into the heart muscle and that some of this blood reached the coronary circulation through tiny anastomoses (connecting vessels) that had formed in the months following surgery. Nevertheless, the Mayo surgeon concluded that "only a long and carefully controlled comparison of patients with coronary disease who have received an arterial implant or any other regimen of treatment with those who have not will allow establishment of the [Vineberg] method as anything more than investigative."[2]

The Cleveland Clinic Champions the Vineberg Operation

Dwight McGoon was cautiously optimistic about the Vineberg operation, but Cleveland Clinic surgeon Donald Effler was wildly enthusiastic about it. In November 1968, ten months after McGoon's review appeared, Effler published an editorial "A New Era of Surgery for Ischemic Heart Disease." He shared McGoon's skepticism about the smorgasbord of surgical procedures that a few surgeons had designed and done in the 1950s: "These procedures, each traumatic in its own way, were alleged to bring new blood to the ischemic myocardium or to redistribute the diminishing supply.... The era of pioneer surgery for the treatment of coronary arterial disease ended with general disillusionment, and the attitude was that medical treatment, despite its obvious inadequacies, was preferable to what the surgeon had to offer."[3]

But Effler emphasized that new era of surgery for coronary disease had begun in the early 1960s after his colleague Mason Sones had invented selective coronary angiography. This novel X-ray procedure "permitted accurate demonstration of coronary arterial disease and defined the precise needs of the individual patient." During the decade, Cleveland Clinic's medical and surgical heart specialists aggressively promoted coronary angiography *and* the Vineberg operation. When Effler's editorial appeared in 1968, the Ohio group had performed more than 12,000 coronary angiograms and more than 2,000 Vineberg procedures.[4]

The surgical treatment of coronary heart disease was about to undergo a sea change when McGoon and Effler's articles appeared. Soon, a technique that involved operating directly on the coronary arteries would first supplement and eventually replace the indirect Vineberg procedure. In August 1969 Cleveland Clinic surgeon René Favaloro published an article, "Saphenous Vein Graft in the Surgical Treatment of Coronary Artery Disease: Operative Technique."[5] This operation would come to be called coronary artery bypass graft surgery and would commonly be referred to as CABG (an acronym pronounced "cabbage"), or simply bypass surgery.

The operation that Favaloro described involved removing a segment of saphenous vein from a patient's leg and suturing one end of it into the aorta, just above the aortic valve, and its other end into a coronary artery beyond an area of blockage (Figures 15.1 and 15.2). This vein graft, which functioned as a conduit around the obstruction, carried oxygen-rich blood from the aorta to an area of heart muscle that would normally have been nourished by the narrowed coronary artery. Unlike the Vineberg operation, coronary bypass surgery produced immediate results. The injection of radiopaque contrast into a vein graft during a postoperative angiogram proved that blood flowed through it right away. Bypass surgery seemed to be a logical strategy for treating a blocked coronary artery. And doctors could use a simple plumbing analogy to explain the procedure to patients.

In April 1969, four months before Favaloro's article was published, Donald Effler had presented the Cleveland Clinic's experience with saphenous vein graft surgery at the annual meeting of the American Association for Thoracic

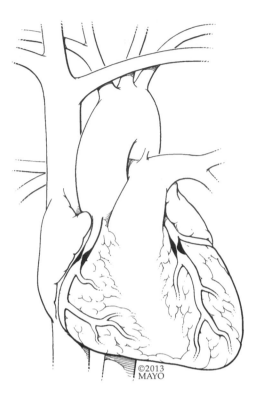

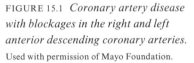

FIGURE 15.1 *Coronary artery disease
with blockages in the right and left
anterior descending coronary arteries.*
Used with permission of Mayo Foundation.

Surgery.[6] At the same meeting, Dudley Johnson of Milwaukee described a
more aggressive surgical approach that involved bypassing two blocked
arteries rather than just one. During the discussion period, San Francisco
heart surgeon William Kerth declared, "It seems as though the indications
for direct coronary artery surgery have gone from an estimated 4 percent,
several years ago, to perhaps 80 or 90 percent of patients at this time."[7] If
Kerth's prediction came true, bypass surgery would have profound implications for the management of patients, the careers of surgeons, and the cost of
health care.

Kirklin Leaves Mayo as Cardiac Surgery Enters a New Era

John Kirklin was also on the program of the 1969 meeting of the American
Association for Thoracic Surgery, but he was no longer at the Mayo Clinic.
His unexpected departure three years earlier to become chief of surgery at the
University of Alabama Medical Center in Birmingham had stunned the staff
in Rochester and the surgical world. It would also affect Mayo's ability to
compete with the Cleveland Clinic and Houston's Texas Heart Institute, centers that took the lead in performing and promoting coronary bypass surgery.

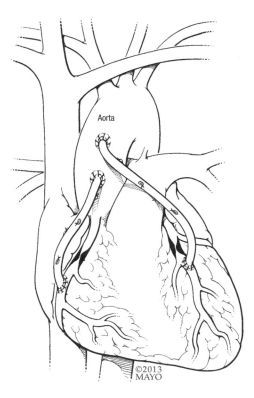

FIGURE 15.2 *Coronary artery bypass graft (CABG) surgery with two vein grafts carrying blood from the aorta into the coronary arteries beyond blockages.*

Used with permission of Mayo Foundation.

Kirklin had shared a secret with his protégé Dwight McGoon in 1966: "It is an extremely difficult thing for me to...tell you that I will be leaving the Mayo Clinic as of the first of September. I wanted you to know this prior to the official announcement because of my great esteem for your work."[8]

In addition to Kirklin's central role in Mayo's cardiac surgery program, he was the chair of general surgery and a member of the Board of Governors. As soon as Kirklin announced his plans, the board appointed McGoon as head of cardiac surgery. McGoon told the board one year later that the senior surgeon's "sudden departure" caused a serious problem because the clinical load was "already excessive." It also had an effect on the academic aspects of Mayo's cardiac surgery program. McGoon explained, "We feel acutely his absence in many spheres."[9]

On the first anniversary of his departure, Kirklin compared his new and old contexts in a letter to McGoon: "I have responsibilities which are as great, and I work as hard, but I have more freedom in accomplishing my goals *perhaps....* I do feel quite free now, within the limits of these responsibilities." Turning from where he was to where he had been, Kirklin admitted, "At times, since coming here, I've been *heartsick* that I ever left Rochester. It is very difficult at age 50 to move oneself & one's family. Yet it is at the same time exciting and stimulating. The enormous *security* of the Mayo Clinic is hard to leave, and I suppose at times I consider myself a fool to have wandered away from it into the outside world." Comfortable confiding in his former colleague, Kirklin confessed, "It's hard to say whether my leaving Rochester could actually have been prevented. Somehow, I felt the last 5 years or so that I was there that I probably would someday leave. Why I decided against leaving on several different occasions, and did leave this time, I don't know."[10]

Kirklin's departure in 1966 was very disruptive to Mayo's heart surgery program. But earlier resignations had also attracted the attention of outsiders who had been impressed by the overall stability of the clinic's staff. Cardiologist Raymond Pruitt had left Mayo in 1959 to become chair of the medical department at Baylor College of Medicine in Houston. The following year, cardiac pathologist Jesse Edwards moved to St. Paul to become laboratory director at a large community hospital that did not have a heart surgery program.

Donald Effler, who had spoken with Edwards about his decision, told the chair of the Cleveland Clinic's Board of Governors that the world famous pathologist's departure "puzzled many of his professional friends and admirers." Effler explained, "I believe the reasons can be digested briefly into the following: (a) inadequate remuneration, (b) reduction in personal incentive and (c) a reactionary and inflexible policy on the part of the Board of Governors." Effler had also chatted with Pruitt, who had expressed frustration about Mayo's travel policy, "which he found quite restrictive and, again, not conducive to personal incentive."[11] Arguing that Edwards and Pruitt were "not malcontents, but the highest type of professional colleagues," the Cleveland Clinic surgeon concluded:

> There is no question in my mind that the efforts of our Board of Governors and Trustees over the past ten years are being rewarded by attitudes that stimulate the individual rather than force him to conform or else. In the past we have had a natural tendency to look toward Rochester for precedent and help before arriving at decisions. In view of the current trends, I would question the need for this in the future. For myself, I am convinced that we are going in the right direction and it would be difficult to find a better team. Whereas my views in the past have been critical, and in some respects still are, I for one am grateful for what the institution has [accomplished] and will accomplish.[12]

Effler's letter illustrates how institutional philosophies and policies have the power to influence important career decisions. The attitudes and actions of leaders and committees certainly affect the atmosphere of an organization and the satisfaction of its staff.

When Kirklin left Rochester with little warning in the late summer of 1966, the clinic's cardiac surgery program stuttered. Mayo would not be well positioned to enter the field of surgery for coronary heart disease, which was about to shift from indirect procedures to the bypass operation. This situation was due, in part, to the clinic's international reputation as a center for congenital heart disease management and the demands that this placed on its staff.

Following Kirklin's departure, McGoon's practice became more focused on patients with congenital heart defects. University of Pittsburgh surgeon Mark Ravitch, who like McGoon had trained with Alfred Blalock at Johns Hopkins, described his friend: "Quiet, modest, a masterful technician achieving results in the 'standard' operations of cardiac surgery ranking with the world's best, presenting in some areas of complicated congenital anomalies a dazzling and almost unique experience which has led to his being termed 'Mr. Surgery-of-the-Impossible' in congenital heart disease."[13] The large number of pediatric cardiologists on the Mayo staff in 1970 reflected the significance and geographic reach of the clinic's complementary medical and surgical congenital heart disease programs. This is exemplified by the fact that there were five board certified pediatric cardiologists in Rochester, a city of 50,000, compared to six each in Boston and Minneapolis and two in Baltimore.[14]

Mayo's congenital heart disease practice was supported by a robust program of animal research that received a big boost during the 1960s from Giancarlo Rastelli. The recent Italian medical graduate, who had come to Rochester in 1960, performed hundreds of animal experiments in an attempt to improve or invent operations for complex congenital heart defects. Although Rastelli spent almost all of his time in the surgical research laboratory, he eventually functioned as an assistant in the operating room, where he helped Mayo's surgeons introduce some of his innovations into practice. By the time Rastelli died of Hodgkin lymphoma in 1970 at the age of thirty-six, he had coauthored almost fifty papers, mainly on congenital heart disease.[15]

Lingering Uncertainty About Surgery for Coronary Disease

The Mayo Clinic, like most cardiac referral centers, moved cautiously into the unsettled field of coronary heart disease surgery in the 1960s—before the introduction of bypass surgery. Robert Wallace, who had arrived in Rochester as a senior resident in 1963, recalled that Kirklin encouraged him to visit the Cleveland Clinic in order to learn how to perform the Vineberg operation and to determine when it might be indicated. Wallace did the first Vineberg procedure at Mayo in 1966.[16]

In the late 1960s, Wallace collaborated with cardiologists Benjamin McCallister and Robert Frye and radiologist Franz Hallermann in a clinical research project designed to assess whether the Vineberg operation actually improved the heart's pumping function. Their study of two dozen patients showed that the internal mammary artery implants provided some blood flow through tiny collaterals to the coronary arteries in fourteen subjects. But there was objective evidence of improved left ventricular function in just two patients. By the time their paper was published in 1970, Favaloro had already reported his bypass surgery technique. Familiar with the Cleveland Clinic surgeon's work, the Mayo authors acknowledged that it was possible that this new direct revascularization procedure might provide more adequate blood supply to the heart muscle, which, in turn, might improve left ventricular function.[17]

The introduction of coronary artery bypass surgery did not lead to the sudden abandonment of the Vineberg operation. Cleveland Clinic surgeons had performed almost 2,000 Vineberg procedures when Effler claimed in a 1968 article in *Minnesota Medicine* that "true revascularization of ischemic myocardium can be provided by a properly executed internal mammary implant procedure. Proof of this has been established repeatedly by postoperative internal mammary arteriography."[18] Skeptics—and there were many—considered the words "proof" and "repeatedly" problematic.

Henry Zimmerman, a catheterization pioneer who was chief of cardiology at St. Vincent Charity Hospital in Cleveland, charged in a 1969 editorial that "the surgical management of coronary disease is in a state of almost total chaos." Although he did not mention the Cleveland Clinic by name, most readers of the *American Heart Journal* knew that he was referring to it when he ridiculed an unnamed group for showing one patient's angiogram "hundreds of times" to demonstrate blood flowing from an implanted mammary artery through tiny collaterals into a coronary. "For every one case like this," Zimmerman declared, "there are hundreds of other cases which show only a small tuft of few vessels arising from the internal mammary artery."[19] Effler chastised the cardiologist across town for his "thinly veiled jibes at the Cleveland Clinic." He told Zimmerman that "revascularization surgery is accelerating steadily as more and more qualified people participate in this surgical endeavor. Your diatribe may appeal to others who think as you do, but in no way will it change the direction of revascularization surgery."[20]

Henry Zimmerman pounced again when Favaloro published his first paper on coronary artery bypass surgery in 1969. In an editorial titled "And Now—Vein Grafts," Zimmerman reminded readers that "numerous surgical procedures have been devised to provide 'so-called' revascularization of the myocardium." Each one had been "introduced with much fanfare, including the blowing of bugles and beating of drums," but there was no proof that any of them prolonged life or improved cardiac function. Characterizing bypass surgery as "the latest rage," Zimmerman dismissed the notion that it was a "cure-all" for problems associated with a localized partial or complete obstruction of a coronary artery. The cardiologist demanded evidence: "Only a very critical objective evaluation carried out on a well-planned study will give the final answer. In the meantime, the cardiac surgeons will have another field day doing procedures by the hundreds, basing their proof on the premise that the 'patient who has been revascularized feels better.'"[21]

Dwight McGoon wrote a response to Zimmerman's stinging editorial. Although the Mayo surgeon objected to the cardiologist's cynical tone, he agreed that an objective assessment of the results of bypass surgery was needed. Accustomed to collaboration, McGoon predicted, "By a co-operative effort of cardiologists, surgeons, physiologists, radiologists, and others to develop and apply a critical objective evaluation, a method of treating patients whose lives are abbreviated in their prime by coronary arteriosclerosis *will* be developed, and all can share in the 'field day' of administering that treatment to *thousands* of patients."[22] McGoon considered evidence much more compelling than testimonials from surgeons whose passion for a procedure might cloud their objectivity.

Cardiac surgeon Gordon Danielson had joined the Mayo staff in 1967. Trained at the University of Pennsylvania and the Karolinska Institute in Stockholm, he had been chief of cardiac surgery at the University of Kentucky in Lexington before moving to Rochester. Danielson performed his (and Mayo's) first coronary bypass operation on June 24, 1968. During the next three years, he performed the procedure on ninety-one patients, more than two-thirds of whom received two or more vein grafts to diseased coronary arteries.[23] McGoon was pleased that Danielson adapted quickly to Mayo's culture, but he was still concerned about his group's workload. Shortly after the new surgeon arrived, McGoon told the Board of Governors that the "extremely demanding" field of cardiac surgery was "made still more difficult by the fact that the present surgical staff cannot comfortably handle the volume of patients coming to the Mayo Clinic requiring this type of care."[24]

Mayo's heart surgeons were very busy, but physician workforce was just part of the problem at the time when the Cleveland Clinic group was pioneering coronary bypass surgery. Nurses were also in short supply. When McGoon wanted to schedule twenty-six open-heart procedures each week beginning in the summer of 1968, Mayo Clinic and Saint Marys Hospital's Joint Conference Committee, chaired by Sister Mary Brigh, warned, "With the present shortage of nursing staff, it may not be possible to staff the operating rooms at all times for this heavy surgical load."[25] Mayo surgeons performed 772 open-heart operations in 1970. Although this was fewer than McGoon had hoped for, it was far more than almost any other institution in the nation. A 1969 survey of 6,600 hospitals in the United States revealed that only thirty-eight institutions were doing more than 200 open-heart operations a year.[26]

Turf Battles Over Who Should Perform Coronary Angiography

The growing acceptance of bypass surgery stimulated demand for coronary angiography, the diagnostic tool that was indispensable for determining whether a patient might be a candidate for the operation. As angiography gathered momentum outside Cleveland in the late 1960s, disputes arose in some contexts about who should perform the procedure. One of the earliest turf battles between cardiologists and radiologists took place in Rochester. Mayo had sent cardiologist Benjamin McCallister and radiologist Franz Hallermann to the Cleveland Clinic to observe Sones perform coronary angiography in February 1965. These ambitious men were in their mid-thirties when they joined the Mayo staff that summer. By the end of the decade, relations between them had become severely strained as a result of Hallermann pushing to perform coronary angiograms and McCallister pushing back.[27]

McCallister made his position clear in a 1970 article: "It is essential that the coronary arteriographic study be under the direction of a physician familiar with cardiovascular hemodynamics and not be considered a radiologic procedure separated from the diagnostic cardiac laboratory." The cardiologist outlined the indications for coronary angiography, which included "selection of patients for medical or surgical therapy, postoperative evaluation of surgical results, diagnostic explanation of chest pain, investigation of electrocardiographic abnormalities, clarification of ill-defined heart disease, and evaluation of the coronary circulation in patients with valvular heart disease."[28] Most of these activities were in the realm of clinical patient care—something that was an integral part of cardiology (but not radiology) practice.

When McCallister's article on coronary angiography appeared, he was no longer at the Mayo Clinic. In 1969 he had moved to Kansas City, Missouri, where he joined cardiologist James Crockett's private practice. Hallermann moved to Corpus Christi, Texas, the same year. McCallister later recalled, "It was a very difficult time. We were trying to develop coronary angiography and ran into tremendous conflicts with the radiologists because it was a turf battle."[29] In this context, Mayo's leaders decided that cardiologists rather than radiologists would perform the procedure in Rochester. John Hodgson, who had become head of radiology at Mayo in 1966, later recalled that the volume of traditional diagnostic X-ray studies was increasing steadily in the 1960s and "new services [were] being added all the time." Addressing technology and turf, he explained that "new methods of imaging and the competition for these newer methods with other subspecialty divisions within the clinic and elsewhere were constantly being attended to."[30]

Mayo physiologist John Shepherd, who had performed cardiac catheter-izations in Earl Wood's laboratory, informed the Board of Governors after meeting with Hodgson in 1970 that "cardiovascular radiology is still his bête noire."[31] Hodgson told the board a few weeks later, "One of the chronically recurring problems the department has faced for many, many years is the staffing of the cardiovascular area. With the exception of George Davis, no one in the department has been interested in making a career out of car-diovascular radiology. As a matter of fact, Dr. [Owings] Kincaid, who has spent many years in this special area, requested to be relieved of any further duties in this area." Hodgson explained in his report to the board that Davis was willing to devote his full time to cardiovascular radiology but noted that "he is getting older and coronary arteriography should probably be done by younger individuals." Davis was fifty-seven years old, and Mayo had a policy of mandatory retirement at the age of sixty-five.[32]

Radiologists Perform Coronary Angiograms in Some Contexts

In order to understand the turf battle over coronary angiography in Rochester, it is necessary to appreciate the prominent role that radiologists played in developing and performing the procedure in some institutions. In general, those radiologists had been performing peripheral angiograms, aor-tograms, and angiocardiograms when selective coronary angiography was introduced outside Cleveland in the early 1960s. This situation is exemplified by the University of Minnesota, where the prominent role of radiologists in cardiac and coronary angiography was due, in part, to a conflict over patient care that involved heart surgeon C. Walton (Walt) Lillehei and chief of medi-cine Cecil Watson.

Walt Lillehei, a strong-willed surgical innovator, bristled whenever a per-son or a policy blocked his path. In 1958 he protested arbitrary limits that Cecil Watson had imposed on the preoperative evaluation of his patients. After the two men met with Owen Wangensteen, the chief of surgery, Lillehei complained to his mentor: "It must be apparent to you after our meeting with Dr. Watson the other day that Medicine is bankrupt mentally." The two surgeons had nothing in common with the internist-administrator, whose background was in biochemistry. Lillehei argued that "the backbone of modern cardiological evaluation of patients consists of the classical physical and auscultatory findings buttressed by left heart catheterization, dye dilu-tion curves, and selective angiocardiography where indicated." The ambi-tious surgical pioneer was furious that "the last three forms of study are specifically prohibited on the Medical Service by Dr. Watson's edict." As a result, Lillehei saw no point in admitting his preoperative patients to a medi-cal service.[33]

Lillehei told Wangensteen in 1958, "We are well into the beginning of a new era in the treatment and management of cardiac disease. Heart disease is a surgical condition. This is perhaps a bitter pill for some of the older 'diehard' clinicians to swallow but nonetheless it is true." He attributed the "deplorable state of affairs in adult cardiology" at the university to the fact that "Dr. Watson has discouraged the development of young men interested in cardiology in his own department." Lillehei explained that the cardiac surgeons had taken matters into their own hands: "We are developing, of necessity, a fairly satisfactory program of diagnostic services on our own service."[34] This program included having radiologist Kurt Amplatz do angiograms for the surgeons. An innovator and educator, he would train several radiologists at the University of Minnesota to perform coronary angiography. Explaining his active role in coronary angiography, Amplatz later recalled that Lillehei "did not send anything to the cardiologists."[35]

Wangensteen watched his protégé Lillehei invent or improve several cardiac operations and mentor many heart surgeons during the late 1950s and early 1960s. When Wangensteen approached retirement in 1967, he warned the medical school's dean that Lillehei would probably leave the University of Minnesota if he was not selected to succeed him as chief of surgery. When an outsider was chosen for the position, Lillehei moved to New York City to become chief of surgery at the New York Hospital-Cornell Medical Center.[36] This move had implications for coronary angiography at the prestigious Manhattan institution because Lillehei took Harry Baltaxe, an Amplatz-trained vascular radiologist, with him. When Baltaxe arrived at New York Hospital, he faced no competition in terms of performing coronary angiograms.

Thomas Killip, who was chief of cardiology at New York Hospital when Lillehei and Baltaxe arrived, explained that Daniel Lukas, the cardiologist who directed the cardiac catheterization laboratory, "was very skeptical of coronary arteriography." As a result, Baltaxe and his protégé David Levin "developed a monopoly" on the procedure until the early 1970s, when cardiologist Susan Kline began to perform coronary angiograms in the catheterization laboratory.[37] In 1973 Baltaxe, Amplatz, and Levin coauthored the first English-language book on selective coronary angiography. Although they acknowledged cardiologist Mason Sones's seminal contributions, they stressed that radiologists had pioneered many angiographic techniques and had developed special catheters for injecting contrast into the coronary arteries.[38]

Another turf war over coronary angiography took place in Boston. It began after radiologist Herbert Abrams, an acknowledged angiography expert, moved from Stanford University in Palo Alto, California, to the Peter Bent Brigham Hospital in Boston in 1967. Brigham cardiologist Richard Gorlin, a catheterization pioneer who also did coronary angiograms, recalled that Abrams's arrival as the new chief of radiology "created an immediate conflict as to who exerted control over the procedure."[39]

The turf war escalated when cardiologist Eugene Braunwald became head of medicine at the Boston hospital in 1972. Three years later, tensions increased further when Abrams recruited David Levin from New York Hospital to be co-director of cardiovascular radiology. The official history of radiology at the Brigham explains that Levin "found himself immediately in a struggle between his chief [Abrams] and Eugene Braunwald, the chief of medicine, over the performance of cardiac imaging studies. Both sides were well equipped with their own catheter laboratory, their own fellows, and their own qualified angiographers. Of course, the cardiologists had patients, and the radiologists had to rely upon referrals."[40]

Levin and Abrams proclaimed in 1977 that coronary angiography "is first and foremost a radiological procedure; it should be performed by radiologists!" Recognizing that their rhetoric did not reflect reality, they acknowledged that radiologists "play a minor role in or have been excluded from clinical coronary angiography at important cardiac centers."[41] The same year, Levin and Abrams reported survey results revealing that radiologists did all of the coronary angiograms in just 3 percent of 299 hospitals in the United States. These two men had passion for performing the procedure, but most radiologists did not. Just one of 426 so-called refresher courses offered at the 1975 and 1976 annual meetings of America's two major radiological societies was devoted to coronary angiography.[42]

Cardiologists Gain Control of Coronary Angiography

Cardiologists gained control of coronary angiography when it became an indispensable (and profitable) clinical tool during the 1970s. New York radiologist Harry Baltaxe predicted in 1971 that the diffusion of bypass surgery would cause the number of coronary angiograms to "skyrocket to the point [that] there will be an acute shortage of physicians capable of performing the procedure."[43] He was right, but there was already a shortage of radiologists, and very few of them wanted (or had the opportunity) to become angiographers. Radiologists and cardiologists had very different career goals and traveled down separate paths to reach them. Radiologists were image-oriented diagnosticians who did not provide direct patient care. Cardiologists were internists with additional training that focused on the clinical evaluation and management of patients with a wide range of heart problems. Importantly, cardiologists were trained to manage unstable cardiac patients.

Although surveys showed that coronary angiography was generally a safe procedure, catastrophic complications could occur. Cardiac arrest was the most dramatic one. In rare instances, a coronary angiogram could cause a heart attack. This, in turn, could trigger acute pulmonary edema, a frightening condition characterized by a patient gasping for air as his or her lungs filled up with fluid. Cardiologists were trained to treat such life-threatening problems; radiologists were not.[44] Gradually, the few dozen radiologists who did coronary angiography were marginalized in most institutions. Radiologists did continue to perform angiograms that did not involve injecting contrast into the coronary arteries.

Demand for cardiologists who could perform coronary angiography grew dramatically in the 1970s as the number of coronary bypass operations surged. Mayo vascular specialist John Spittell told the Board of Governors in 1971 that some of the clinic's cardiology fellows were frustrated by the lack of opportunity to learn how to perform coronary angiography. These aspiring heart specialists were convinced that they needed "this experience to be competitive with most other young well-trained cardiologists in private practice."[45] That year, Cleveland Clinic surgeon Donald Effler wrote, "Sones's catheter pried open the lid of a veritable treasure chest and brought forth the present era of revascularization surgery."[46] The twin technologies of coronary angiography and bypass surgery were fueled by reimbursement to hospitals and doctors as a result of the launch of Medicare in 1966 (Figure 15.3), and the fact that three-quarters of Americans had some form of private health insurance by that time.[47]

Increased income potential encouraged some heart specialists and hospitals to adopt new technologies to diagnose and treat coronary disease, but new knowledge also contributed to a major shift in the management of patients. Ohio State University cardiologist James Warren declared in 1973, "We are passing through a major revolution in our thinking about coronary artery disease." The former American Heart Association president described research that had yielded new insights into coronary disease and its complications, including angina pectoris, acute myocardial infarction, heart failure, and sudden death. Warren also mentioned dramatic new treatment strategies, such as coronary care units and bypass surgery.[48]

Approximately 800 coronary angiograms were done at Mayo in 1971, a tenfold increase in just four years. This surge reflected the fact that the clinic's cardiologists had gained respect for the diagnostic test and that Gordon Danielson had begun performing coronary bypass surgery two years earlier.[49] After Benjamin McCallister left Mayo in the fall of 1969, Robert Frye was assigned to the catheterization laboratory on a full-time basis. This meant that he did not see outpatients in the clinic or have responsibility for an inpatient cardiology service. Beginning in 1970, cardiologist Gerald Gau, who had just joined the staff, was assigned to help him. Gau had learned to perform coronary angiography at London's Hammersmith Hospital, where

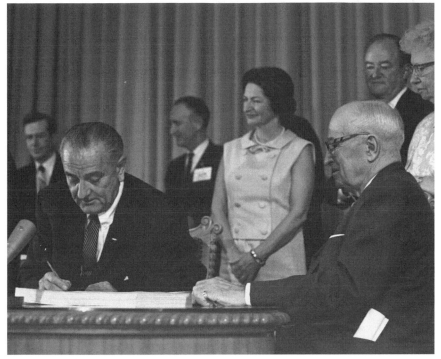

FIGURE 15.3 *President Lyndon Johnson signing the Medicare Bill with Harry Truman looking on, July 30, 1965.*

LBJ Presidential Library, Austin, Texas, in the public domain.

he had spent two years as a cardiology trainee after completing his medical residency at Mayo.[50]

Controversies Surrounding Coronary Artery Bypass Surgery

Unlike the Vineberg operation, coronary bypass surgery immediately re-established blood flow to heart muscle normally nourished by an artery that had become blocked. Post-procedural angiograms documented this, and most patients who underwent the operation reported improvement in their angina. The short-term subjective results were impressive, but some doctors raised questions about the long-term impact of bypass surgery in terms of preventing heart attacks and prolonging life. Randomized clinical trials had begun to gain momentum during the 1960s as a strategy to evaluate the effectiveness of new therapies, and several cardiologists called for such trials to assess coronary bypass surgery's indications and long-term effects.[51] These concerns were reflected in editorials published in medical journals in the early 1970s with titles such as "Surgical Treatment of Coronary Artery Disease: Too

Fast, Too Soon?" and "Direct Coronary Revascularization: A Plea Not to Let the Genie Escape from the Bottle."[52]

The general public read articles that made it seem that the genie was already out of the bottle and that bypass surgery could grant a welcome wish to a patient who had severe angina. For example, a 1971 *Life* magazine article was titled "Lifeline for a Man with a Dying Heart: New Surgery Saves Doomed Coronary Victims." It told the story of Jack Cronin, a forty-two-year-old man who had recovered from his first heart attack thirteen months earlier. The father of two young girls had a second heart attack while driving his car. Cronin made it to a coronary care unit where he was treated with morphine. As he recovered, it seemed that "life from now on would be a trek on eggshells." But there was an option. Reporter Rick Gore described recent developments in patient care, explaining that "one operation in particular, called bypass grafting, has saved some two thousand lives and enabled close to 90% of those undergoing it to return to normal existence, totally freed from debilitating pain."[53] Although the *Life* article noted that the operation was less than three years old, it implied that the benefits lasted indefinitely. Actually, only time would tell how an individual patient would fare.

Some members of the medical profession and other interested observers wanted more than success stories about individual patients and testimonials from surgeons who profited from the procedure. In 1971 the National Advisory Heart and Lung Council appointed a four-man Subcommittee on Coronary Artery Surgery.[54] John Kirklin, now at the University of Alabama in Birmingham, chaired the group, which included a cardiologist and two cardio-pulmonary physiologists. The council accepted its six recommendations regarding bypass surgery. One of them was especially blunt:

> That the National Heart and Lung Institute and its Council recognize the highly controversial and emotional nature of this subject; recognize that only by taking *no* position some other perhaps less-knowledgeable branch of the Government *will* soon, and perhaps improperly, label surgical procedures for coronary artery disease as "experimental" (and thus non-fundable by private or government insurance programs) or "therapeutic" (and thus fundable, albeit at great cost, as presently done).[55]

The council members knew that a lot of money was at stake. Medicare, signed into law by President Johnson in 1965 and implemented the following year, meant that the government faced enormous expenditures if bypass surgery grew unchecked. On the other hand, most patients would not be able to afford the operation if their insurance did not pay most of the costs associated with it.

Lyndon Johnson's concern about his health contributed to his decision not to run for re-election in 1968. He explained three years later, "My heart attack of 1955 seemed well behind me, but I was conscious that it was part of the background of my life—just as I was conscious of my family's history of stroke and heart disease.... I frankly did not believe in 1968 that I could survive another four years of the long hours and unremitting tensions I had just gone through." These tensions included the Vietnam War, racial conflicts, urban unrest, an inflationary economy, protests on college campuses and the streets, and a growing generation gap.[56]

Shortly after leaving the White House in 1969, Johnson became a member of the Mayo Foundation Board of Trustees. The following year he spoke at Industry Day, an event that brought more than sixty executives to Rochester. The clinic's newsletter explained that the meeting's main purpose was "to invite corporations to give financial support to an expansion of Mayo medical research and education."[57] Johnson outlined three opportunities, one of which was to extend "Mayo's long and productive efforts in the field of arteriosclerosis, the chief cause of both heart disease and stroke, and the main public health problem facing this nation." The former president also revealed a personal decision: "I've been offered positions on some of the boards in the country and I've not accepted those assignments because I felt this way—whatever time I have left, I want to spend it trying to contribute to the great undertaking that Mayo's skilled talents have pledged themselves to."[58] After Johnson had a second heart attack in 1972, Houston surgeon Michael DeBakey concluded that he was not a candidate for coronary bypass surgery. The former president died suddenly at his Texas ranch the following year.[59]

When Lyndon Johnson died in 1973, the role of coronary bypass surgery was still being actively debated. Theodore Cooper, the director of the National Heart and Lung Institute (who had trained as a cardiac surgeon), advocated a clinical trial to help clarify the operation's place in patient care. Describing the devastating impact that coronary disease had on patients and American society, he explained that it had accounted for 22 million doctor visits in 1971. It was also the principal diagnosis on most hospital discharge summaries and the largest single cause of days spent in a hospital.[60]

Cooper appointed Dwight McGoon and nine other doctors to the Ad Hoc Policy Advisory Board on Coronary Artery Surgery in 1972. The board, estimating that 20,000 coronary bypass operations had been performed the previous year, concluded that there was "a critical need for objective data on the long and short term effects of coronary artery surgery" in terms of mortality and quality of life. It recommended "collaborative randomized studies comparing surgical to medical management in carefully defined subsets of patients with ischemic heart disease."[61]

The author of a 1973 editorial on bypass surgery in the *Lancet* placed the problem in perspective:

> The pioneer work at the Cleveland Clinic has led to many thousands of such operations in the United States, and the snowball is still increasing in size and momentum. The implications and potential repercussions are immense. If the operation is shown to be effective, then there will be demands for rapid expansion in heart investigation and surgical services; if no scientifically reputable appraisal of the results is made, then we are at risk of making many serious errors of judgment, both for the individual and in general policies.[62]

Describing bypass surgery as a remarkable achievement from a mechanical point of view, the writer thought it was "understandable that many major cardiac centres have gone straight ahead in organizing a production line for thousands of such operations."[63] When this editorial appeared in the highly regarded London medical journal, the Cleveland Clinic's production line was already running at top speed.

The Cleveland Clinic Sets the Pace in Coronary Bypass Surgery

In 1973 Mason Sones, Earl Shirey, and their associates at the Cleveland Clinic were doing twenty coronary angiograms a day, and five surgeons were performing fifty open-heart operations a week, most of them coronary bypass procedures. *Cleveland Magazine* published a cover story that year with a very long, attention-grabbing title: "Effler and Sones and the Boys at Cleveland Clinic Have Taken the You-Bet-Your-Life Out of Heart Surgery, So Don't Wait Around to Get Zapped by a Heart Attack, Head It Off at the Coronary Artery." Senior editor John Mearns, who had spent two weeks watching patients being evaluated and treated at the clinic, detailed the case of Norman Rice, a forty-nine-year-old man who had developed angina at rest and was "on the verge of a heart attack." Mearns recounted a telephone conversation that Sones had had with Rice's private physician: "Well, Goddammit, we can only do twenty of these things a day, and that's more than anybody else can do, and we've got 300 people on line right now.... But O.K., get him right over here and we'll check him out. He's the kind we like to get hold of."[64]

This crusty quotation from Sones did not surprise anyone who knew him. For example, his longtime Cleveland Clinic colleague Irvine Page characterized him as "eccentric, blunt, and sometimes rude."[65] Mearns described Sones preparing to do an angiogram on Rice, whom he considered to be "a perfect candidate for a heart attack" because he was an overweight middle-aged man who smoked two packs of cigarettes a day. "But Sones is about to make a road map of his heart, and would tell you with great confidence and conviction, 'This guy ain't going to have *his* heart attack.' "[66]

The *Cleveland Magazine* editor also described meeting Effler: "With his longish, graying hair, his aviator glasses, the conviction with which he talks, one could easily subtract the white coat, add a business suit and see him as the president of an electronics company talking about research, sales and employment policy." Turning to the economics of heart surgery, Mearns explained, "Nobody at the clinic wants to talk about personal incomes, but if one listens long enough one can hear that the clinic's billings for Effler's professional services are something more than ten times his salary. The salary doesn't reach six figures, but the billings reportedly go over seven." One unnamed insider did discuss profit: "As long as we plow it back into the clinic, Uncle Sam doesn't touch it, and we have enough say about how the money is spent around here that we get to do the things we really want to do." The profits would help fund a 330-bed addition to the Cleveland Clinic Hospital and would allow Sones to move "out of his basement catacombs to a new laboratory which will be able to handle 70 patients a day, instead of the present 20. Effler will move to a new surgical suite and be able to handle 1,250 more patients a year."[67]

The *Cleveland Magazine* article opened and closed with Norman Rice, who went home ten days after undergoing an operation that included a coronary artery bypass graft and a Vineberg internal mammary implant. "He may draw some attention in the locker room; the scar will always be there, looking as if the doctors had installed a zipper down the middle of his chest. But Norman Rice never did have the heart attack that was all ready to happen to him. You could say he's lucky."[68] This confident conclusion reflected the opinions of Effler, Sones, and several of their Cleveland Clinic colleagues. Other heart specialists were not so sure.

Advocating for a Clinical Trial of Coronary Bypass Surgery

Richard Sautter, a cardiac surgeon at Wisconsin's Marshfield Clinic, argued in 1974 that a prospective, randomized clinical trial of coronary bypass surgery was necessary to prove whether or not the operation really prevented heart attacks or prolonged lives. Shifting from outcomes to incomes, Sautter said that the bypass operation "has been the salvation of many cardiologists and cardiac surgeons and preserved many heart surgery programs." Putting these "vast economic considerations" aside, he urged all cardiac surgeons to support such a trial "in order to provide more rational and, therefore, better care for our patients."[69]

Responding to Sautter, Effler rejected the notion that coronary bypass surgery "rests on a shaky foundation which can only be firmed up by a randomized prospective study" and boasted that "the Cleveland Clinic team

plans to escalate the volume of revascularization surgery."[70] When these dueling letters to the editor were published in 1974, the Marshfield Clinic and the
Mayo Clinic were among fifteen sites that had been chosen to participate in
the National Heart and Lung Institute–sponsored Coronary Artery Surgery
Study (CASS). Launched in 1973, CASS was a prospective, randomized trial
designed to compare the results of medical and surgical treatment in patients
with coronary artery disease that had been documented by angiography.[71]

Several surgeons resisted clinical trials of bypass surgery, but Effler was
the most vocal early critic of the approach. He cited the Cleveland Clinic's
enormous experience with surgery for coronary heart disease as proof that
the bypass operation was effective. Physician-historian David Jones, in his
analysis of controversies surrounding the surgical treatment of coronary
disease, concludes, "Members of the Cleveland Clinic team had been particularly outspoken in their opposition to the need for trials."[72] For example,
shortly after Dwight McGoon and the other members of the National Heart
and Lung Institute's Ad Hoc Policy Advisory Board on Coronary Artery
Surgery proposed a major clinical trial in 1972, Mason Sones griped, "I hope
we do not let the Federal government, through the insistence of the National
Heart and Lung Institute, con us into a prospective randomized study in
institutions which now 'enjoy' a 2–3% surgical mortality rate in an attempt to
tell us whether we can do a good job prospectively."[73]

The number of coronary bypass surgery programs and procedures performed in America grew quickly during the 1970s. For example, a study of
cardiac surgery trends in the city and state of New York between 1970 and
1977 revealed a striking sevenfold increase in the number of operations for
coronary disease.[74] Boston cardiologist Eugene Braunwald estimated that
approximately 70,000 bypass operations would be performed in America in
1977 at a total cost of nearly $1 billion. Concerned that "this rapidly growing enterprise is developing a momentum and a constituency of its own," he
explained:

> Because of the magnitude and seriousness of the problem of coronary
> artery disease and the frequent dramatic symptomatic improvement
> resulting from CABG, this procedure has received a great deal of
> attention in both the lay and professional press. As a consequence, it
> is now very much in the public (and even political) eye. Patients, their
> families and, in some cases, their primary physicians are applying
> pressure on cardiologists to carry out coronary arteriography and on
> cardiac surgeons to perform these operations even in patients without
> severe angina; these pressures are not always resisted vigorously.[75]

Braunwald considered the government's funding of the CASS trial to be a wise
investment because "the outcome will affect such a large number of patients
and such a substantial fraction of medical resources."[76] In 1979 Stanford

University surgeon Norman Shumway observed that coronary bypass surgery was the most common operation performed in most medical centers and claimed that "only the Comstock Lode has contributed more riches to so few in so brief a period of time."[77]

The Cleveland Clinic's medical and surgical heart specialists continued to resist clinical trials of bypass surgery. In 1975 Floyd Loop was selected to succeed Effler as chief of cardiac surgery, and William Sheldon was appointed to head a newly created Department of Cardiology. Three years later, the two men coauthored an editorial that began with the observation that coronary artery surgery was under fire. After conceding that clinical trials had "enormous value," Loop and Sheldon summarized problems associated with using them to evaluate bypass surgery. Their concerns included issues surrounding the selection of patients, physician bias, conflicting results from participating hospitals, high crossover rate from medical to surgical treatment, and "poor quality of surgery found in many participating hospitals." These problems could "introduce inaccuracies into the study, leading to erroneous conclusions that further confuse the physician."[78] Another factor that influenced physicians' attitudes about treating patients with coronary disease was introduction of the beta-adrenergic blocking drug propranolol into practice at the beginning of the decade. Research had shown that it reduced the heart's demand for oxygen, which meant that some patients experienced fewer episodes of angina.[79]

Although controversy continued to swirl around operations for coronary disease, physicians and the public considered open-heart surgery to be a medical miracle. In 1974 San Francisco physiologist Julius Comroe and Philadelphia anesthesiologist Robert Dripps described their survey that asked physicians and medical scientists to list the most important clinical advances in cardiovascular and pulmonary medicine since World War II. Open-heart surgery was at the top of almost every respondent's list. They explained that the general public considered it to be "the pinnacle of surgery, comparable to the conquest of Mt. Everest."[80]

Growing Acceptance of Coronary Bypass Surgery

In 1973 Mayo's team of cardiac surgeons, anesthesiologists, and heart-lung machine technicians who worked together in the operating room gathered for dinner. The celebration was organized to honor the technicians on the occasion of the 10,000th open-heart operation performed at the institution since John Kirklin had closed Linda Stout's ventricular septal defect eighteen years earlier.[81] Mayo was a world leader in the total number of open-heart operations in the mid-1970s, but it lagged behind the Cleveland Clinic and a few other institutions in the adoption of coronary bypass surgery.

Cardiac surgeon Robert Wallace was Mayo's chief of surgery when he told the Board of Governors that the number of thoracic and cardiovascular surgical procedures had declined in 1977 compared to the previous year. "The reasons for this are not readily apparent," Wallace admitted, "but one wonders if the reputation that we have acquired for long waiting times, both for evaluation and surgery, are not now proving detrimental. Our approach to coronary artery surgery has been somewhat conservative as compared to other institutions; however, with increasing experience I feel that surgery for coronary artery disease will be the mainstay of treatment for those patients with far advanced disease and anticipate further growth in this area."[82]

On September 16, 1977, the Cleveland Clinic hosted an international symposium "The First Decade of Bypass Graft Surgery for Coronary Artery Disease." Cardiology chief William Sheldon, who had suggested the event, boasted to the chair of the clinic's Board of Governors, "Few contributions in the history of medicine have had the impact upon the medical community as has bypass graft surgery."[83] None of the sixty cardiac surgeons and cardiologists who spoke at the celebration in Cleveland could have imagined the significance of a catheter-based procedure that was first done that very same day on the other side of the planet. German cardiologist Andreas Grüntzig performed the world's first percutaneous transluminal coronary angioplasty (PTCA) on a patient in Zurich, Switzerland. The procedure, which is discussed in Chapter 16, was developed as an alternative to bypass surgery. It would revolutionize the treatment of men and women with coronary artery disease during the 1980s.[84]

In 1980 Mayo cardiologist Robert Frye chaired a thirteen-member panel that listened to and summarized almost two dozen talks presented at a National Heart, Lung, and Blood Institute–sponsored consensus conference on coronary bypass surgery. The presentations included reports on CASS and two other prospective, multi-institutional clinical trials of bypass surgery. The panel concluded that the operation resulted in "an improvement in the quality of life, a decrease in myocardial ischemia, and an increase in survival...in selected subsets of patients."[85]

Medical reporter Gina Kolata informed readers of the journal *Science*: "The consensus, reached after two days of animated discussions among the meeting participants, was conservative. Although the panel declared bypass surgery a 'major advance,' it did not claim miracles for the treatment.... It concluded that the operation can improve blood flow to the heart, can improve the quality of life, and can, in some patients, prolong life. But it stopped short of concluding that the great number of bypass operations performed each year is fully justified."[86]

Cleveland Clinic cardiac surgeons Delos (Toby) Cosgrove and Floyd Loop and cardiologist William Sheldon coauthored a paper for the 1980 National Heart, Lung, and Blood Institute conference that reported their institution's twelve-year experience with bypass surgery.[87] Their heart program was riding a wave of positive publicity at the time. During an ABC television network special on coronary bypass surgery in 1983, the announcer proclaimed that "the Cleveland Clinic is proof that practice makes perfect. It is a mecca for bypass surgery."[88] High surgical volumes and teamwork contributed to low operative mortality, which, in turn, attracted more patients.

By this time, the Vineberg operation had disappeared from the repertoire of surgeons at Cleveland Clinic, the institution that had given the mammary artery implant procedure its biggest boost in the 1960s. Effler, who had coauthored several articles praising the procedure, described a phenomenon that pertained to this situation. He had once told surgeons, "Scientific papers can be like old love letters in that the content written in all sincerity may be embarrassing when read years later."[89]

The Cleveland Clinic Chooses Cardiac Surgeons as its Leaders

Floyd Loop and Toby Cosgrove would not only become prominent figures in cardiac surgery, they would eventually lead the Cleveland Clinic. Loop was chosen as chair of the Board of Governors in 1989, and Cosgrove succeeded him fifteen years later. In part, their selection reflected the Cleveland Clinic's determination to grow its reputation as an international center for cardiac surgery. Cosgrove's career path had been shaped by a summer experience at the Mayo Clinic in 1965, when he was a medical student at the University of Virginia. He spent two months in Rochester as one of fifty-three "medical students in residence." This was seven years before Mayo opened a medical school. Cosgrove recalled his Mayo experience as "a very exciting exposure to surgery" and as "one of the most formative things" in his early career. After watching John Kirklin operate and visit patients in the hospital, Cosgrove concluded that he was "an absolute beacon of intellectual energy and physical energy."[90]

Toby Cosgrove, who would do most of his surgical training in Boston, recalled thinking that "the difference between the organization of the Mayo Clinic and the organization and the practice of medicine at Harvard was just like night and day." His Rochester experience influenced a critical career decision: "I wanted to go to a place like the Mayo Clinic where I would have that huge experience and have that wonderful opportunity." After completing his surgical training in 1972, Cosgrove interviewed at the Cleveland Clinic. "I remembered the experience at the Mayo Clinic...[and] I saw the same thing." The combination of high-volume cardiac surgery and a very efficient system of patient care impressed him: "The exposure to John Kirklin. The exposure to the system was just pivotal in what I thought about how medicine ought to be practiced."[91]

Loop and Cosgrove would coauthor more than forty papers on cardiac surgery by 1985. That year, Loop explained in an editorial on CASS that the number of coronary bypass surgery procedures performed in America had reached a plateau: "The current moderation has not come about solely as a result of adverse publicity surrounding clinical trials. Medical treatment has undergone a major transformation in the 1980s with the advent of new drugs, a greater appreciation of risk-factor intervention...and overall, more efficacious medical therapy." Loop admitted that CASS "has dampened enthusiasm for operating on all patients with severe coronary arterial narrowing, irrespective of symptoms." Praising the sixty-six publications that had resulted from that federally funded clinical trial, he concluded, "The stream of useful information that is being obtained justifies the 24 million dollar cost of the CASS project, which provides the best perspective on coronary artery surgery to date."[92]

Robert Frye was the first of five Mayo authors of a 1987 review of randomized trials of coronary bypass surgery. After summarizing several trials, they concluded:

This approach, with all of its problems and limitations, still provides one of the more important methods that should distinguish medicine, namely, the application of the scientific method to an analysis of how we treat patients. It is one method of achieving objectivity in the "laboratory" of clinical practice. We have attempted to point out the limitations of randomized clinical trials; all physicians who make judgments based on such trials should have a clear understanding of their limitations, including adequacy of study design, considerations of sample size, and applicability to other patients. While the trials of CAB[G] have aroused considerable debate and discussion, it is important not only to focus on the results that are in conflict, but also to acknowledge those points where there is consistency in results reported.[93]

Frye coauthored a chapter on coronary angiography with cardiologists Hugh Smith and Guy Reeder that appeared in the 1987 textbook *Cardiology: Fundamentals and Practice*. In their contribution to the Mayo-authored textbook, Reeder, Smith, and Frye emphasized that "a thorough understanding of coronary arteriography is essential in today's practice of cardiology." They concluded that the technique had "revolutionized the diagnosis and management of coronary artery disease" during the past two decades.[94] That is what Mason Sones and Donald Effler had predicted, and they were right.

Transforming Cardiac Catheters
into Treatment Tools

Beginning in the mid-1960s, a few inventive radiologists and cardiologists transformed intravascular catheters from diagnostic to treatment tools. University of Oregon radiologists Charles Dotter and Melvin Judkins helped launch this transition when they described a catheter-based technique for opening blocked leg arteries in 1964. *Life* magazine reported that Dotter had saved a seventy-five-year-old man from having his leg amputated "by applying a bit of know-how straight out of the plumber's manual." By pushing progressively larger stiff Teflon catheters through a narrowed artery, the radiologist created a new channel to supply the man's leg with "life-giving blood."[1] Dotter and Judkins predicted that what they termed "transluminal recanalization" might eventually be used to treat other localized blood vessel blockages, including "severe proximal narrowing of the coronary artery."[2] This goal would be achieved in Europe during the next decade.

The European Origins of Catheter-Based Coronary Treatments

In 1971 West German radiologist Eberhard Zeitler taught cardiologist Andreas Grüntzig (who had left East Germany fourteen years earlier) how to perform the so-called Dotter procedure to treat narrowed leg arteries. In 1975 Grüntzig began a series of animal experiments in an attempt to develop a new catheter-based technology to treat some patients with angina by opening a narrowed coronary artery. To accomplish his goal, Grüntzig constructed a catheter with an inflatable balloon near its tip that could be threaded into a coronary artery over a flexible guide wire. Once the balloon was positioned in the narrowed arterial segment, it was inflated to expand the vessel so more blood would flow through it. Grüntzig was optimistic that his tiny sausage-shaped inflatable balloon could transform a traditional diagnostic coronary catheter into a therapeutic device. The technique would be termed percutaneous transluminal coronary angioplasty (PTCA) or simply angioplasty.[3] The mechanism of angioplasty as it was understood in 1980, is depicted in Figure 16.1.

Coronary artery bypass graft surgery (CABG) was a decade old when Grüntzig performed the world's first PTCA on a thirty-seven-year-old man with severe angina at the University Hospital in Zurich, Switzerland, on September 16, 1977. He reported his experience with the procedure in five patients in a letter to the editor of the *Lancet* that was published in February 1978.[4] Grüntzig spoke at a symposium on coronary heart disease in Frankfurt, Germany, that same month. Describing the results of the procedure in eight patients, he explained that angioplasty "is comparatively simple in the hands of an experienced angiographer and has the advantage of providing instantaneous revascularization without open-heart surgery." He concluded that the procedure "might be a new breakthrough in the direct relief of ischemic heart pain in selected patients."[5]

Mayo cardiologist Carlos Harrison, who was in the audience, was very impressed by Grüntzig's presentation. When he returned to Rochester, Harrison urged junior staff member Ronald Vlietstra to visit the German cardiologist, who was then working at the University of Zurich.[6] In April 1978 Vlietstra spent two days with Grüntzig, who had done fifteen PTCAs by this time. Although he did not witness an actual angioplasty, the Mayo cardiologist was mesmerized by the coronary angiograms that Grüntzig made before and after the intracoronary balloon-dilatation procedures. The brief letter

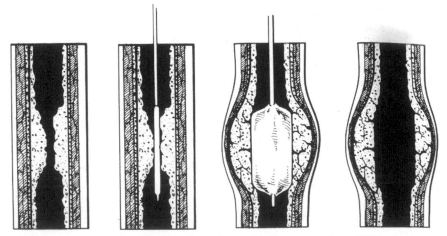

FIGURE 16.1 *Presumed mechanism of transluminal balloon angioplasty, 1980.*

W. R. Castaneda-Zuniga, A. Formanek, M. Tadavarthy, Z. Vlodaver, J. E. Edwards, C. Zollikofer, et al., "The Mechanism of Balloon Angioplasty," *Radiology*, 1980, *135*: 570, figure 11; reprinted with permission of the Radiological Society of North America.

in the *Lancet* had included three still photographs, but the motion pictures had much greater visual impact. Vlietstra recalls thinking that he had "seen a miracle."[7]

Angioplasty crossed the Atlantic Ocean in March 1978, when Richard Myler in San Francisco and Simon Stertzer in New York performed the first PTCAs outside Zurich and Frankfurt.[8] In July the American public read about one of Stertzer's patients in a *Time* magazine article "Blowup in the Arteries." Robert, a forty-seven-year-old chauffeur, had been admitted to Lenox Hill Hospital in Manhattan after being "stricken with suffocating spasmodic chest pains of severe angina." Stertzer performed an angiogram that revealed that his patient was a candidate for coronary bypass surgery. "But with Robert's approval, Lenox Hill doctors decided to forego surgery and try a new and highly experimental alternative: a procedure with a tongue-twisting name of 'percutaneous transluminal coronary angioplasty.'"[9]

Stertzer completed the PTCA in less than an hour, and a post-procedure angiogram proved that he had opened the chauffeur's clogged coronary artery with Grüntzig's balloon catheter. "Two days later, his angina gone, Robert left the hospital and returned to work," according to *Time* magazine. Angioplasty had substituted for bypass surgery for this individual patient, and the article reported that PTCA might be feasible in up to 15 percent of patients who were candidates for CABG "at about one-tenth the $15,000 average cost of a bypass." Stertzer, shown holding a balloon catheter, acknowledged that angioplasty was still experimental, but he was optimistic: "If 80 percent of the arteries are open after a year, we're into a revolution in cardiology."[10]

Grüntzig was eager to show others what PTCA could accomplish and how to do it. In August 1978 he hosted his first live demonstration course in Zurich, where twenty-eight individuals watched him perform angioplasties on seven patients. PTCA was still experimental at this point, but Ronald Vlietstra was anxious to pioneer the procedure at Mayo. He would begin, as Grüntzig had, by working in leg arteries, a vascular territory that was more forgiving than the coronaries, which supplied blood to the heart muscle. In November he presented a proposal to Mayo's Cardiovascular Practice Committee: "Evaluation of Percutaneous Transluminal Balloon-Catheter Dilatation Technique for Treatment of Peripheral Atherosclerotic Occlusive Disease." The committee approved the protocol, but it raised the larger issue of how new technologies were incorporated into practice. The members suggested forming an ad hoc committee "for the purpose of reviewing clinical developments, such as the balloon-catheter dilatation technique...which do not appear to fall exclusively within either a research or clinical practice realm."[11]

Planning and Preparing to Perform PTCA in Rochester

Ronald Vlietstra met with the Cardiovascular Practice Committee in March 1979 to submit a formal proposal to introduce PTCA as a clinical procedure at Mayo. He was accompanied by co-investigator Geoffrey Hartzler, who had joined the staff two years earlier, following completion of a cardiology fellowship in Rochester.[12] Catheterization laboratory director Hugh Smith, whose name appeared first on the proposal, was a member of the committee. The three cardiologists explained that about 100 PTCAs had been performed at a few medical centers in Germany, Switzerland, and the United States in the nineteen months since Grüntzig treated his first patient. Two-thirds of the individuals who had undergone angioplasty "experienced significant, and so far, sustained clinical benefit as manifested by less angina, improved treadmill exercise tolerance, less exercise perfusion defects on isotope scans, and improvement in coronary lumen size at angiography one to six months later." Their references to treadmill exercise tests and radioisotope imaging of the heart reflected a trend toward using more objective means to document the results of treatments for coronary artery disease.[13]

In their proposal, Smith, Vlietstra, and Hartzler summarized their strategy to prepare to perform PTCA and outlined the criteria for selecting potential patients. First, they would test the equipment and technique on animals in Mayo's experimental surgery laboratory. At least one of them would visit Grüntzig in Zurich or Myler in San Francisco to watch a procedure. Two of Mayo's senior clinical cardiologists would review and approve the selection of each patient. More teamwork would come into play if an acute complication, such as sudden complete occlusion of a coronary artery, occurred during an angioplasty. Each PTCA "would be scheduled in close cooperation with one of the cardiac surgeons so that, if problems arise, prompt saphenous vein bypass grafting [CABG] could be performed."[14] The key components of the new treatment technology were already in Rochester. Grüntzig had arranged for a Zurich firm to send Vlietstra a set of balloon catheters, guiding catheters, and guide wires. Mayo's engineering department had built a compressed air pump for rapid inflation and deflation of the angioplasty balloons.[15]

In March 1979, the same month the Mayo cardiologists submitted their protocol to an internal committee, the National Heart, Lung, and Blood Institute (NHLBI) published a one-page position paper on PTCA in the journal *Circulation*. The institute also announced that it would host a workshop on angioplasty in June. Citing Grüntzig's experience with thirty patients, the authors of the position paper predicted, "On the basis of this early reported experience, it appears that PTCA has limited promise as a therapeutic technique for a small number of categories of patients with obstructive coronary disease."[16] Conscious of coronary bypass surgery's explosive growth during the previous decade, they concluded, "The complexities and cost of conducting cardiovascular research and providing the best care to the patients with cardiac disease demand that the evaluation of any new or potentially promising technique, such as PTCA, be conducted in a rational, scientific manner."[17] But this idealistic approach did not reflect the realities of the medical marketplace.

Two Philadelphia cardiologists complained in February 1979 that news media were playing too great a role in shaping public opinion about PTCA. Referring to recent articles on the procedure in *Time* magazine and the *New York Times*, as well as television coverage on the *CBS Evening News*, they explained, "Last summer the popular news media, ever eager for a 'breakthrough,' gave a good bit of space and time to a new approach to the treatment of coronary heart disease.... News promotion of coronary angioplasty has even extended to encouraging patients with angina to consult their physicians about a less risky, less costly alternative to saphenous vein bypass, free of the discomforts of coronary surgery."[18]

These physicians were frustrated that such publicity preceded objective scientific reports on PTCA. Earlier in the decade, others had raised similar concerns about the rapid, unregulated diffusion of coronary bypass surgery. The Philadelphia heart specialists called for "controlled studies, statistical analysis, objective assessment of coronary reperfusion, and long-term follow-up" to assess the relative merits of PTCA, CABG, and drug therapy in the treatment of patients with angina.[19] They issued this challenge when angioplasty was performed at fewer than a dozen hospitals in the United States.

About 275 angioplasties had been attempted at nineteen centers in Europe and North America by June 1979, when Grüntzig co-chaired the NHLBI-sponsored PTCA workshop. The early results were encouraging. Cleveland Clinic cardiologist Mason Sones, who had invented selective coronary angiography two decades earlier, expressed his "profound admiration of the magnificent efforts" of Grüntzig and his associates for developing PTCA. But Sones cautioned that the "casual angiographer" should not attempt angioplasty, which required a "very high level of technical skill and tenacity." He argued that it should be done by "individuals with great experience, excellent judgment, and a proven capacity to respond immediately and decisively to the stresses which are certain to be encountered."[20] Sixty years old when he spoke, Sones would not perform angioplasty. Almost everywhere, younger cardiologists would introduce the technique. Vlietstra and Hartzler, who attended the NHLBI workshop, were in their early thirties.

Geoffrey Hartzler Performs Mayo's First Angioplasty

When Vlietstra and Hartzler returned to Rochester, they redoubled their efforts to launch PTCA at Mayo. In a revised and expanded protocol, which they submitted in October 1979, they noted an increase in the number of angioplasties at the few centers where it was done and emphasized that the early results were encouraging.[21] By this time, PTCA pioneers Martin Kaltenbach from Frankfurt and Richard Myler from San Francisco had visited Rochester to discuss the procedure with Vlietstra and Hartzler, who had gained experience performing it in animals. One section of their revised proposal to begin performing PTCA stood out. It was titled "Case Report." Hartzler had seen a patient who seemed to be an ideal candidate for the procedure, and he had acted. Vlietstra, who had expected to perform Mayo's first angioplasty, was out of town. He recalled, "Geoff apparently was keen to be the one to do the first case, and he went ahead without saying a word to me ahead of time. The next day he came up to Toronto, to the same meeting, and casually broke the news to me."[22] Vlietstra was frustrated, but there was nothing he could do—the first PTCA at Mayo had already been done.

On October 9, 1979, Geoffrey Hartzler, assisted by Hugh Smith, performed Mayo's first angioplasty on a sixty-year-old-man from Iowa. Four days earlier, Hartzler had recorded the onset and progression of Harvey Grummitt's angina:

> The patient was in good health until the morning of August 6, when on his usual six-block walk to work he experienced progressive chest pain commencing at about the third block. The pain increased with a tightening and "strangling" quality until he reached work, then gradually lessened over the subsequent 15 minute period as he rested. . . . Since that time he has had daily episodes of angina pectoris with radiation to his neck and left arm. Typically the discomfort comes with emotion and anxiety, minimal physical activity as climbing one flight of stairs, and following meals.[23]

Three weeks after the middle-aged man began having angina, he saw an internist in Waterloo. The physician supervised a treadmill exercise test that triggered chest pain and electrocardiographic abnormalities consistent with inadequate blood supply to his heart. As a precaution, the doctor admitted Grummitt to his hospital's coronary care unit and ordered scheduled doses of two standard anti-anginal drugs (Isordil and propranolol), in addition to sublingual nitroglycerin as needed.

Despite this medical regimen, Grummitt continued to have daily attacks of angina. A Waterloo cardiologist who had completed his training at the Cleveland Clinic two years earlier performed an angiogram that revealed an 85 percent narrowing of the patient's proximal left anterior descending coronary artery.[24] This coronary artery had acquired the reputation of being a "widow-maker" because sudden total occlusion of it could cause a massive heart attack and cardiac arrest.

Harvey Grummitt's persistent angina and worrisome angiogram led his cardiologist to refer him to the Mayo Clinic, where he saw Hartzler. A repeat treadmill exercise test on October 8 caused angina and disconcerting electro-cardiographic changes, despite the fact that he was now receiving the anti-platelet drugs aspirin and Persantine, in addition to the three anti-anginal medications prescribed in Iowa.

Hartzler, eager to perform a PTCA to open the narrowed artery, docu-mented his plan of attack, which included admitting the man to Saint Marys Hospital and having cardiac surgeon Francisco Puga review his case. Puga, who had recently joined the staff, saw the patient promptly and wrote in his record, "Reviewed. As per Dr. Hartzler. Single tight LAD lesion. Class III angina unrelieved by medical Rx. Agree [it] is reasonable to proceed with [P]TCA. Proceed with immediate coronary revascularization if unsuccessful or if complications. Discussed fully." Two medical residents also interviewed and examined Grummitt. Their notes state that he was scheduled for "coro-nary artery balloon dilatation" in the morning. Hartzler wrote, "All appears ready for attempted transluminal angioplasty tomorrow. Patient understands that this is a new therapeutic procedure & that operation may be required."[25]

Hartzler started the procedure at 7:38 a.m. on October 9, 1979 (Figure 16.2). The jargon-filled report created at the end of the case detailed the birth of Mayo's angioplasty program. It also described technologies used to assess the procedure's progress and its immediate effects on blood flow through the cor-onary artery, which was thought to be causing the patient's symptoms:

> Transluminal coronary angioplasty was performed using a Grüntzig #9 French guiding catheter and #4 French dilating catheter with a 20 mm. length, 3.7 mm. diameter balloon. Initially, the balloon would not pass the mid left anterior descending lesion and was inflated proximal to the obstructed area five times. Subsequent to passage of the lesion, the balloon was inflated twice with increase in distal left anterior descending pressure from 33 to 74 mm Hg. Simultaneous coronary sinus blood flow measurements by reverse thermodilution recorded a 19% increase in total coronary flow coincident with expansion of the lesion. Subsequent angiography suggested a marked decrease in obstruction at the site of previous 95% narrowing.[26]

Harvey Grummitt was discharged two days after his angioplasty. Hartzler documented his patient's progress during a return visit: "Outstanding result since angioplasty 13 days ago. Returned to work 6 days ago. Feels 'wonderful. Working like a horse.' Recently put in 20 hour day draining a water tower.... No angina or other symptoms [of] heart disease." A repeat treadmill exercise test was normal, and a coronary angiogram revealed a residual 20 percent ste-nosis (blockage) at the site of the angioplasty. The following month Hartzler wrote to his patient, "By now I hope that you have recovered from all the

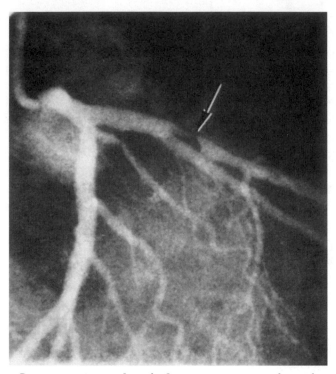

FIGURE 16.2 *Coronary angiogram from the first percutaneous transluminal coronary angioplasty (PTCA) at Mayo, 1979. The arrow points to blockage before balloon dilatation.*

G. O. Hartzler, H. C. Smith, R. E. Vlietstra, D. A. Oberle, and D. A. Strelow, "Coronary Blood Flow Responses during Successful Percutaneous Transluminal Coronary Angioplasty," *Mayo Clin. Proc.*, 1980, 55: 46, figure 1; used with permission of Mayo Foundation.

'invasive' things that we did to you during your recent visits to Rochester." Pivoting from past procedures to lifestyle changes, Hartzler added, "I also hope you are continuing to not smoke, losing a little bit of weight, and working somewhat less than 20 hours per day!"[27]

Three weeks after Hartzler performed Mayo's first PTCA, the Cardiovascular Practice Committee approved a detailed protocol that identified him and three other cardiologists as the investigators. David Holmes, who had recently joined the staff, was listed, in addition to Ronald Vlietstra and catheterization laboratory director Hugh Smith.[28] There were three dozen cardiologists on Mayo's staff, but these four physicians were the only ones who performed coronary angiograms. This arrangement reflected the clinic's tradition of subspecialization and a conviction that concentrated procedural experience contributed to better outcomes. Hartzler was lead author of the report of Mayo's first PTCA, which was published in the *Mayo Clinic Proceedings* in January 1980, three months after it was performed.[29]

Andreas Grüntzig Grows Restless and Looks to America

On the other side of the Atlantic, Grüntzig had grown restless. In January 1980 he hosted his third live demonstration course in Zurich, which Vlietstra, Smith, and Holmes attended. On a train afterward, Grüntzig sat beside Emory University cardiologist Spencer King, who had performed several thousand coronary angiograms. As they traveled through the Swiss countryside, Grüntzig told the ambitious Atlanta heart specialist that he was considering job opportunities in the United States. "He mentioned Harvard and Stanford as potential options," King recalled, "but seemed to prefer the offer he had received from the Cleveland Clinic because of its worldwide reputation in bypass surgery."[30]

Mason Sones, who had praised Grüntzig's presentation at the 1979 PTCA conference, encouraged his colleague William Sheldon, the chief of cardiology, to try to recruit him.[31] The German cardiologist had already visited the Cleveland Clinic twice by the time Sheldon asked its Board of Governors to hire him. Sheldon explained that Grüntzig had an international reputation as the developer of a "method to dilate segmental stenotic lesions in coronary arteries with a balloon catheter. This technique has attracted considerable interest, and we have been interested in exploring its feasibility in our patient population." Hoping to lengthen his institution's lead in the race to diagnose and treat coronary disease, Sheldon declared, "Doctor Grüntzig's presence and his new therapeutic modality will result in additional patient referrals."[32]

In January 1980 the Cleveland Clinic's board approved Grüntzig's appointment as a clinical fellow, beginning in July.[33] But the plan was derailed after the German cardiologist spoke with Spencer King of Emory in Switzerland. The Cleveland Clinic, a large multispecialty group practice modeled after the Mayo Clinic, was not affiliated with a university. King later recalled his conversation with Grüntzig: "He said he would like to be a 'Professor.' Coming from the European tradition, this title of 'Professor' seemed to be particularly important for him.... I advised him that since, at the time, the Cleveland Clinic had no medical school, the title of professor would not be possible.... I suggested that he visit me in Atlanta and consider the possibilities at Emory."[34] J. Willis Hurst, Emory's chief of medicine and one of the world's leading cardiologists, played a critical role in the recruitment effort. He helped the German cardiologist over several hurdles, such as getting a visa and a Georgia medical license.

Grüntzig's last demonstration course in Europe in August 1980 attracted 212 participants. The charismatic German pioneer of angioplasty arrived in Atlanta two months later. Grüntzig's move to America accelerated the diffusion of PTCA into practice. It was perceived as a powerful treatment tool that was capable of enhancing the care of patients, advancing the careers of cardiologists, and boosting the reputations of hospitals. King recalled, "Hundreds of patients from all around the world came to Atlanta to have angioplasty, and they and their referring physicians spread the word rapidly. Thousands of the earliest angioplasty operators came to Atlanta to spend a week twice a year learning the technique."[35]

Even before Grüntzig was settled in Atlanta, Hartzler was becoming increasingly restless in Rochester. A cardiologist he helped train recalled, "The contrast between Geoff's pioneer spirit and a conservative setting at Mayo led him to look for an opportunity to join former Mayo colleagues at St. Luke's Hospital in Kansas City, Missouri."[36] Hartzler left Rochester in the spring of 1980 to join the Mid America Heart Institute, which former Mayo cardiologist Benjamin McCallister had helped create a few years earlier.

Vlietstra reflected on Hartzler's decision: "Mayo has strengths and weaknesses as viewed from the perspective of each individual's personality. One of the things we used to say at Mayo was that you had to be a good company man if you're going to enjoy Mayo. For Geoff, who was incredibly inventive, enthusiastic...Mayo, I think, was claustrophobic. It was not really a fault of his or a fault of Mayo's. It was not a good long-term marriage, and I think that's why he left."[37] Hartzler moved from a huge bureaucratic institution where cardiology was considered a subspecialty of internal medicine to a single specialty group that focused on one organ rather than the whole patient. This had implications in terms of his autonomy and income potential.[38]

In the spring of 1981, cardiology chair Robert Frye expressed concern to the Department of Medicine chair about the fact that Hartzler and two other staff members had left Mayo in the past year: "The reasons for their departures are varied and have been discussed in several forums. Financial concerns, professional dissatisfaction in a large diversified group, as well as spouse unhappiness have been identified as contributory to their decisions to leave."[39] But the good news was that seven cardiologists would be joining the staff in the summer, including Mayo fellowship graduates John Bresnahan, Fletcher Miller, and Guy Reeder. Alfred Bove would return to Rochester from Temple University in Philadelphia. Three cardiologists trained elsewhere were also hired: Raymond Gibbons and Stephen Hammill from Duke University, and Michael Mock from the NHLBI. Frye informed the chief of medicine, "We now face the major challenge of providing an environment which will be satisfying for these excellent additions to our staff."[40]

The Rapid Diffusion of Angioplasty into Clinical Practice

University of Pittsburgh epidemiologist Katherine Detre claimed in 1981 that angioplasty was "spreading like wildfire."[41] Several things contributed to the very rapid diffusion of PTCA into practice, but chief among them was the lack of formal training guidelines. It is hard for current-day cardiology trainees to comprehend how easy it once was for doctors who performed diagnostic coronary angiograms to transform themselves into so-called interventional cardiologists, subspecialists who used special catheters as therapeutic tools.[42]

Most American cardiologists who began performing PTCA in the early 1980s learned the technique by attending one or more live demonstration courses at Emory University or from one of their colleagues who was already doing the procedure. The four-day course in Atlanta in February 1981 cost $500 and provided attendees with twenty-six hours of continuing medical education credit. Its main attraction was a series of live demonstrations of patients undergoing PTCA. Real-time fluoroscopic and angiographic images were projected on a large screen in an auditorium filled with several hundred cardiologists.[43] Hospitals, eager to introduce the new therapeutic procedure, had a low threshold for granting privileges to perform angioplasty to cardiologists who were already doing coronary angiograms at their institution.

Grüntzig boasted in 1983 that more than 1,000 cardiologists had attended Emory's live demonstration courses. Acknowledging the value of experience in terms of patient safety and success rates of the procedure, he contrasted "what can be expected from angioplasty in the learning period of a novice" with "what can be achieved by a team with vast experience."[44] When Grüntzig made this point, many novices were performing PTCA, and there were almost no teams with vast experience. It would be several years before academic centers began offering an additional year of formal training in interventional cardiology. David Holmes, the fourth cardiologist to perform PTCA at Mayo, explained how he learned the technique: "I would have scrubbed with Hartzler or Smith or Vlietstra. Sort of as a 'see one, do one, teach one.' All apprenticeship."[45] This was the accepted model (Figure 16.3). Spencer King recalled the early years of angioplasty: "When Andreas began to teach, it was 'see one, do one.' That was it."[46]

Grüntzig gave participants in a 1984 Emory angioplasty course a list of seventy-five questions and answers. "How should a novice get started?" was of interest to many attendees. Grüntzig's answer: "In the dog lab. It is a good idea to insert [a] No. 8 French guiding catheter and the dilatation catheter into the coronary artery of the dog, to become acquainted with the connections, blood pressure measurements, leaks, and techniques to get the system 'bubble-free.' Come to our 'starter courses' or to other courses throughout the world."[47] But most participants had no access to animal laboratories; they were in private practice and worked in community hospitals. The last question and answer in the list related to angioplasty's cost and income implications. At Emory University Hospital the charge was $4,500 to $5,000, of which $1,500 was the interventional cardiologist's fee. Undoubtedly, some

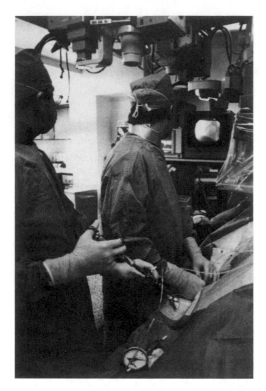

FIGURE 16.3 *Mayo cardiologists David Holmes Jr. and Guy Reeder performing a percutaneous transluminal coronary angioplasty (PTCA), 1981.*

Mayovox, November 1981; used with permission of Mayo Foundation.

heart specialists began performing angioplasty because it could increase their earnings. In 1984 the average annual pretax net income for cardiologists was about $125,000.[48]

The Mayo cardiologists who worked in the catheterization laboratory at Saint Marys Hospital had advantages over most heart specialists with respect to gaining experience with angioplasty and other evolving catheter-based technologies. When Alfred Bove returned to Rochester in 1981, he already had extensive experience with catheterization and animal research. Back at Mayo, he divided his time between the catheterization and research laboratories. He explained that the interventional cardiologists would practice new procedures in animals before attempting them in patients.

Alfred Bove appreciated the camaraderie among the cardiologists who worked in Mayo's catheterization laboratory: "Everybody was close together and helped each other.... You could be in the lab and start to get into something that you weren't quite sure about, and you would just say to the technician: 'Could you ask Dr. Vlietstra to wander in?' The next thing you know there would be three guys in the control room watching what you were doing, and you would hear little voices: 'Try this. Try that.'" Bove explained, "To me the real core value of the clinic is groups of people working together. Not competing with each other...[but] moving forward with innovation and good patient care at the same time."⁴⁹

Surgeons Sit on the Sidelines When Patients Undergo PTCA

The advent of angioplasty forced cardiologists and cardiac surgeons to renegotiate their roles and relationships. Suddenly, the tradition whereby medical heart specialists functioned as diagnosticians who treated patients with pills and referred some of them for surgery was upended. A new type of subspecialist, an interventional cardiologist, used balloon catheters to treat coronary blockages. Post-procedure angiograms revealed a dramatic improvement in blood flow in most patients.

For patients, the contrast between PTCA and CABG was impossible to ignore. Medical science reporter Gina Kolata explained in 1979 that "at least 10 percent of the 100,000 people who have coronary bypass operations each year may be able to have a far simpler treatment instead—one requiring two days rather than two weeks in the hospital and costing $1,000 rather than $12,000 or more."⁵⁰ The percentage of patients with coronary disease who were potential candidates for angioplasty would rise in the early 1980s, when a few individuals who performed the procedure began treating more than one narrowed coronary artery with the balloon catheter technique.

For cardiac surgeons, the advent of angioplasty had implications beyond the loss of operations and income. They were used to being in charge. During the 1970s, cardiac surgeons played a central role in treating hundreds of thousands of patients with angina by performing bypass surgery on them. This changed early in the next decade. If a cardiologist recommended a PTCA, a cardiac surgeon and open-heart surgery team were expected to sit on the sidelines during the catheter procedure—like an ambulance crew at a car race—ready to rush into action if a serious accident occurred. Atlanta cardiologist Spencer King recalled, "After Grüntzig joined our laboratory at Emory, things were not always smooth with the surgeons. Despite a strong camaraderie, all was not smiles when PTCA cases crashed late on Fridays necessitating emergency surgery. As the most desirable surgical candidates began finding their way to the catheterization table for angioplasty, things did get a bit testy."⁵¹

Cardiac surgeon Ellis Jones, who was Andreas Grüntzig and Spencer King's colleague at Emory University, spoke on the surgeon's role in angioplasty at the 1982 annual meeting of the Society of Thoracic Surgeons. The Emory group held the world record for the number of PTCAs performed, and their short-term results and low complication rates were very impressive. Jones attributed this "to careful patient selection, careful planning of the procedure, the superb technical abilities of the three individuals performing the procedure at our institution, and the ready availability of a rather large and experienced anesthesia and surgical staff."[52]

One audience member, North Carolina surgeon Francis Robicsek, said what many of his peers were thinking: "For the past five years, our cardiology colleagues have fought us surgeons, asking us not to operate on single-vessel lesions.... Now they proclaim the same type of lesion an 'ideal' candidate for a procedure that turns the operating room into a terror and has a higher morbidity and mortality rate than elective surgery for single-vessel disease."[53] Jones responded, "We agree with your strong feelings that angioplasty, if not carefully controlled, can disrupt an entire surgical and even hospital service and make life unpleasant for many."[54]

Despite the Mayo Clinic's culture of collaboration and collegiality, it was not immune from angioplasty-induced tensions. Mayo's angiographers were among the pioneers of PTCA, but some of their colleagues—medical and surgical heart specialists alike—thought that things were moving too quickly. Vlietstra recalled a range of responses to the advent and growth of angioplasty from cardiologists, surgeons, and patients. Each individual viewed coronary artery disease and the competing treatment strategies of drugs, bypass surgery, and angioplasty from a unique vantage point. For example, Vlietstra explained that Bruce Kottke, a Mayo vascular specialist who devoted most of his time to atherosclerosis research, opposed angioplasty "because of his certainty that plaque would not yield to such a blunderbuss approach."[55] Moreover, Mayo's cardiac surgery staff was suddenly depleted in 1979, when PTCA was poised to transform their specialty. Dwight McGoon stopped operating that year (at age fifty-four) after he developed a hand tremor caused by early-onset Parkinson's disease. Robert Wallace, who had been on the Mayo staff for fifteen years, left that year to become chief of surgery at Georgetown University in Washington, DC.[56]

Two Mayo Clinic heart surgeons summarized some of the friction points around PTCA in the mid-1980s. James Pluth wrote about self-referral, a thorny issue that some radiologists had raised when they were excluded from performing coronary angiograms. "The physician who evaluates the patient's condition may often be the same person who provides the therapy," Pluth complained, "and the checks and balances of the internist-to-surgeon referral are lacking."[57] Surgeon Jeffrey Piehler, who had trained at Mayo during the early years of angioplasty, claimed that "few subjects will arouse more emotional discussion among cardiac surgeons than the role of PTCA in the treatment of patients with coronary artery disease."[58] Although Mayo's surgeons worked at an institution where the number of procedures they performed did not influence their incomes, they knew that these issues affected most of their peers who practiced elsewhere.

In 1981 Mayo's interventional cardiologists reported their experience with the first thirty-four patients in whom angioplasty had been attempted since the program debuted in the fall of 1979.[59] Strict selection criteria helped explain why it had been done in fewer than 3 percent of the 1,200 patients who had undergone coronary angiograms at Mayo during that interval. Each potential angioplasty patient had to be a candidate for bypass surgery based on a combination of severe angina and a near-total blockage in a single coronary artery. Moreover, many physicians still considered PTCA to be an experimental procedure and did not refer their patients with angina to cardiologists who performed it. When Mayo cardiologist Robert Brandenburg was president of the American College of Cardiology in 1980, he cautioned, "The mature clinician... has learned to be wary of the initial claims for new drugs, new operations and procedures until experience and scientific scrutiny have indicated their probable worth."[60] Although Mayo's interventional cardiologists did not try to predict PTCA's ultimate place in clinical practice, they were impressed by its "potential major therapeutic implications."[61]

Tensions Around the Diffusion of Heart Care Technologies

Massachusetts cardiologist David Spodick characterized the 1981 Mayo article that reviewed angioplasty at the institution as "an excellent description of good work by first-class workers." Then he issued a challenge: "Because the Mayo Clinic has the intellect and skills, the prestige, and the patients to carry out appropriately designed randomized, prospective trials of therapy, it is unfortunate that this was not done.... With facilities unexcelled in the world and prestige unexcelled among the public as well as the profession, the Mayo Clinic should be the leader in this kind of therapeutic investigation."[62] Spodick was a former colleague and disciple of Thomas Chalmers, an academic internist who was one of the earliest and the most persistent promoters of randomized clinical trials.[63] Mayo's angioplasty pioneers agreed with Spodick that randomized trials comparing new treatment strategies for patients with angina were desirable, but they noted the difficulty of designing "a study that is both meaningful scientifically and feasible in practice."[64]

It seemed impossible to tame the multiple technologies that were changing the landscape of heart care as they raced across America during the early 1980s. For example, bypass surgery and angioplasty sprinted from the starting line of conception to the finish line of clinical application in record time. The rapid diffusion of these treatment technologies, combined with the high prevalence of heart disease in adults, had major economic implications for patients, physicians, hospitals, medical industries, government entities, third-party payers, and other segments of society. In this context, a group of Mayo authors added their voices to a small but growing chorus that advocated restraint and a more rational approach to evaluating a hailstorm of new procedures and products.

In a 1980 article in the *New England Journal of Medicine*, Mayo research-ers reported trends in the numbers of catheterizations and coronary angio-grams performed in Olmsted County, Minnesota.[65] The county's stable population of 90,000 and Rochester's relative isolation facilitated the study. So did Mayo's comprehensive medical record system and staff of biostatisti-cians. The authors emphasized that the brief interval between the invention of several diagnostic and therapeutic technologies and their diffusion into practice was problematic because it "resulted in a commitment of financial resources before clinical trials have provided adequate evidence of efficacy."[66]

Wading into the turbulent waters of health policy, they argued that "contin-uous increases in costs have led to the realization that the financial resources available for health care are limited." Then they offered a prescription for the problem: "Ensuring appropriate use of these resources demands careful analysis by the medical profession of the impact on finances and patient care of the introduction of new equipment or procedures. If such an analysis is favorable for a particular service, then guidelines regarding the appropriate number and distribution of medical facilities to provide the new service could be developed."[67] Based on a recent report of the Inter-Society Commission for Heart Diseases Resources, the Rochester researchers recommended that a hospital should perform a minimum of 300 adult catheterizations annually to minimize the procedure's risk and cost and to maintain staff proficiency. But the commission's survey showed that less than half of the 830 hospitals with catheterization laboratories in the United States reached this benchmark.[68]

Arnold Relman, editor of the *New England Journal of Medicine*, praised the Mayo Clinic authors' "experience-based approach" to evaluate catheter-ization, but he warned that "any extrapolation from Olmsted County must be made cautiously, with the realization that the largely white, middle-class, Scandinavian population of the semirural region is not characteristic of the country as a whole." Something else set the clinic's experience apart: "Mayo physicians are salaried and have no personal financial incentives or disincen-tives in the decision to use a procedure." These circumstances led Relman to conclude that the Olmsted County experience was a "conservative but prob-ably good estimate" of the medical need for catheterization.[69]

As more (and more expensive) technologies diffused into practice, it became increasingly apparent that the government would assume a more active role in developing policies that would affect patient care. Mark Brataas chaired Mayo's Division of Public Services and the Medical Group Management Association's Governmental Relations Committee in 1983, when he described the clinic's increasing involvement in legislative activities:

> For many years the healthcare profession ignored public affairs. Preoccupied with its own professional, ethical, and scientific problems, it failed to keep in touch with the public and the politicians and with

what was happening in other segments of the economy. As a result, it was losing the power to shape its own destiny. With a head-in-the-sand attitude, healthcare professionals hoped that politics and politicians would go away and government would leave us alone. We didn't have time to waste on public affairs. We at the Mayo Clinic are as guilty as the rest. We call our political involvement "public affairs," no doubt in the hope that our colleagues won't think we are involved in such a seamy, unprofessional activity as politics. In reality, though, we should be letting everyone know that we are concerned, that we want to participate in shaping the healthcare system. We are knowledgeable in our field and can contribute to the formation of laws and regulations concerning our activities. Little by little we are finding out that political involvement is not as bad as it seemed. Mayo has started a program of "legislative action," and it's working.[70]

When Brataas published this essay, Mayo was doing well financially, but the Board of Governors knew that their institution, and American medicine in general, faced challenges.[71]

Health economist Eli Ginzberg spoke to a large audience in Rochester in 1983. Arguing that American medicine was moving from a "spend-thrift era" into one characterized by a "tighter health care economy," the Columbia University professor outlined contemporary controversies, such as rising health care costs, right-sizing physician and nurse workforces, and pending legislation to establish the diagnosis-related groups (DRG) model for Medicare reimbursement for hospitalizations. The DRG strategy would replace the traditional model that reimbursed hospitals for the inpatient care charges they submitted to a new model that paid them a standardized amount based on a patient's diagnosis.[72]

In a 1984 report on angioplasty prepared for the American College of Cardiology, a market analyst declared, "Given this exceptional opportunity in which the Federal Government is subsidizing the proliferation of PTCA through DRG payments, it is important that the cardiologist and hospital administrator know that this opportunity exists."[73]The following year, Eli Ginzberg claimed that there was "widespread agreement among knowledge-able persons that the rapid and continuing introduction of new technology has been a major contributor to a steady and steep rise in health care costs."[74] But it was very hard to control the scientific and social forces that stimulated the spread of PTCA and other heart care technologies.

Comparing Coronary Bypass Surgery With Angioplasty

The rapid growth of two treatment technologies for patients with angina—CABG and PTCA—attracted attention in the early 1980s as the nation grappled with a serious economic slowdown. In the United States, more than $2 billion was spent on 137,000 CABG operations in 1980, little more than a decade after the procedure's debut.[75] Mayo and ten other centers collaborated in a study comparing the costs of CABG and PTCA in patients with single vessel coronary disease who had undergone either of these procedures in 1980 and 1981. The investigators concluded that the average patient charge for the hospital and professional components of bypass surgery ($15,580 ± $7,281) was three times that for angioplasty ($5,315 ± $2,159). The average hospital stay was also three times longer for surgery (12 ± 2 days) than for angioplasty (4 ± 2 days).[76] The economic implications of PTCA stimulated more insistent calls for controlled trials to compare these catheter-based and surgical approaches for treating patients with angina.

Angioplasty's role in treating patients with angina expanded significantly with the development of multivessel angioplasty. Medical science writer Gina Kolata spoke to Ronald Vlietstra and other participants in an NHLBI-sponsored angioplasty workshop in 1981. Initially, PTCA was limited to a single coronary artery, but some interventional cardiologists were eager to expand its boundaries. Kolata reported that "Vlietstra and others are beginning to use it to push back multiple plaques in two or even all three coronary arteries." She explained that this territorial expansion had implications for patients with angina and for the heart surgeons who treated them: "As PTCA becomes suitable for a wider variety of arterial blockages, it becomes more competitive with bypass surgery."[77]

The Mayo group, among the first to publish results relating to multivessel coronary angioplasty, concluded a 1983 article, "In selected patients with multivessel disease, PTCA can be performed with low morbidity and mortality, and it merits the critical comparison with coronary bypass grafting best achieved in a randomized clinical trial."[78] The clinic's heart specialists argued repeatedly that randomized trials were the only way to sort out the relative merits of various coronary disease treatment strategies.

In 1985 six Mayo cardiologists and a cardiac surgeon coauthored an opinion piece in the *New England Journal of Medicine* advocating randomized trials of angioplasty and bypass surgery. They argued that trials should be designed to consider more than clinical outcomes. The Mayo authors contended that the cost consequences of these competing treatment strategies must be studied because "the continued growth of health care expenditures in the United States has justifiably made the cost of medical care a central issue in cardiovascular practice."[79] Their observations appeared when the so-called outcomes movement was gaining momentum in health care. Arnold Relman, the journal's editor, claimed that the emergence of "a strong new consensus on the need for assessment and accountability" represented a revolution in medical care.[80] Randomized clinical trials would become the main currency of the outcomes movement. And cardiology would provide many opportunities to use the approach to help adjudicate disputes about treatment strategies.

New Heart Attack Treatment Strategies: Racing Against Time

While Andreas Grüntzig was developing angioplasty as a treatment for angina, other cardiologists were evaluating a catheter-based drug treatment for patients with an acute myocardial infarction. Unlike angina, which is a chronic condition, a heart attack is a sudden, life-threatening event.[81] Thrombolytic therapy, a clot-dissolving heart attack treatment strategy introduced into clinical practice in the late 1970s, was the result of decades of research on a substance produced by beta-hemolytic streptococci bacteria.[82] This substance, named streptokinase, could dissolve fresh thrombi (blood clots). German cardiologist Peter Rentrop was the first author of a 1979 article that reported the results of dripping streptokinase through a catheter directly into the coronary arteries of five patients who presented with an acute myocardial infarction.[83]

The intracoronary streptokinase strategy had major implications for men and women who went to a hospital with an acute infarction and for their doctors. It involved rushing an unstable patient into a catheterization laboratory for an emergency coronary angiogram. The catchphrase "Time is Muscle" became a rallying cry for individuals involved in a SWAT team approach to treating patients with a heart attack. This strategy reflected the fact that the longer a fresh clot completely blocked a coronary artery, the more heart muscle died due to a lack of oxygen-rich blood cells. If an emergency angiogram revealed a totally blocked coronary artery, streptokinase was infused through the catheter into the vessel in an attempt to dissolve the blood clot. Successful "reperfusion" could be life-saving and could result in a smaller amount of heart muscle damage, which meant that a patient was less likely to develop heart failure and other complications.[84]

Thrombolytic therapy seemed logical, but it was based on the belief that an acute myocardial infarction was caused by a fresh clot that formed in— and blocked—a major coronary artery. Some influential individuals, notably NHLBI pathology chief William Roberts, argued that this was not always the case. They claimed that a clot in a coronary artery was often the consequence of a heart attack rather than its cause. The controversy about what role blood clots played in acute myocardial infarction and so-called unstable angina had implications for thrombolytic therapy.[85] When this debate raged, cardiologists were splashing around in a sea of uncertainty with respect to coronary disease. They were contending with a host of new diagnostic tests, theories, and treatment strategies. This situation was highlighted in several books that included the word "controversies" in their titles.[86]

Mayo cardiologist Valentin Fuster became interested in the connection between blood platelets, thrombus formation, and coronary artery disease after he arrived at the Mayo Clinic in 1971. Born and trained in medicine in Barcelona, Spain, Fuster had decided to become a cardiologist when his main medical school mentor had a heart attack when he was forty-five years old. His interest in thrombosis matured at Mayo, where was "able to expand investigationally and clinically" as a result of working with cardiologists, hematologists, and vascular specialists.[87] Fuster and Robert Frye were the first authors of a 1975 article describing the angiographic findings in 300 patients with angina or a prior (non-acute) myocardial infarction. Their study showed that total occlusion of at least one coronary artery was more common in patients with a history of a heart attack. Reflecting the ongoing debate about the mechanism of acute myocardial infarction, the Mayo authors acknowledged William Roberts's opinion that coronary thrombosis might be "a secondary event rather than the cause of the infarct."[88]

David Holmes, Geoffrey Hartzler, Hugh Smith, and Valentin Fuster coauthored a 1981 article on sixteen patients with unstable angina who were found to have a coronary artery thrombus at the time of angiography. None of these patients had an acute myocardial infarction, but their angina had become much worse in recent weeks. The authors concluded that the thrombus detected during angiography in these individuals "may have been responsible for the abrupt change in clinical condition or may have been a contributing factor in the patient's course."[89]

An addendum to the Mayo article on coronary thrombosis in unstable angina exemplified the phenomenon of new reports being trumped by even newer reports in the fast-moving field of coronary disease research. "After this article was submitted," the Mayo authors explained, "DeWood et al. published their data on the high incidence (69.8%) of coronary thrombosis in patients undergoing angiography during the early hours of transmural myocardial infarction."[90] They were referring to a 1980 article in the *New England Journal of Medicine* by Spokane, Washington, cardiologist Marcus DeWood and his associates, which appeared to prove that acute coronary thrombosis was responsible for causing a majority of heart attacks.[91]

Science writer Elizabeth González summarized a lecture on thrombolytic therapy with streptokinase that she had heard at the 1980 American Heart Association meeting. Thousands of heart specialists attended these annual gatherings, which buzzed with excitement as new treatment technologies and strategies were reported in packed lecture halls. During one session "the audience emitted a collective gasp," González declared, as she described what hundreds of doctors saw and heard: "On a movie screen in front of them, a nasty clot was high-tailing it through a coronary artery. Within 30 seconds, the clot had dissolved." Los Angeles cardiologist

William Ganz delivered the lecture, which "attracted enormous publicity," according to the science writer. She noted that network television had shown his dramatic film two days later. But the California cardiologist cautioned that thrombolytic therapy was still experimental and "should be done only in centers that are physically and intellectually equipped to perform it."[92] Mayo was such a center.

Mayo Begins to Use Intracoronary Streptokinase

In January 1981, one month after the American Heart Association meeting, the clinic's Cardiovascular Practice Committee approved cardiologist James Chesebro's protocol for a clinical trial of intracoronary streptokinase for acute myocardial infarction. Although Mayo had not been involved in thrombolytic research up to this point, Chesebro and Fuster had published several papers on the role of platelets in atherosclerosis and thrombosis, a subject they would continue to investigate.[93]

The first patient treated with intracoronary streptokinase at Mayo was a thirty-four-year-old man with no prior history of heart disease. His first episode of chest pain occurred on April 12, 1981, under very unusual circumstances. The medical resident who admitted the patient to the coronary care unit explained that the man had been

> in his usual state of excellent health without prior history of heart disease or significant cardiac risk factors until about 12:30 p.m. today when he noted the sudden onset of substernal pressure pain while crawling through a narrow area of a cave (pulling himself forward with his arms). The pain abated some within moments, but then immediately recurred with more severity and was associated with diaphoresis [sweating], some shortness of breath and radiation of the pain into the jaw with a sensation of numbness in both arms down to the fingers. He extracted himself from the narrow area, and his friends carried him from the cave.

The man's friends drove him thirty-five miles to the Saint Marys Hospital emergency room, where an electrocardiogram revealed an acute anterior wall myocardial infarction.[94]

Chesebro, who was contacted immediately, evaluated the patient and explained the rationale and risks of attempting to open an obstructed coronary artery with intracoronary streptokinase to the man and his wife. Noting that the patient wanted to proceed, Chesebro also spoke with Valentin Fuster, David Holmes, and Hugh Smith. The cardiologists agreed that the young man was an ideal candidate for thrombolytic therapy. Smith and Holmes performed an emergency coronary angiogram that revealed complete obstruction of the patient's left anterior descending coronary artery. When repeated injections of streptokinase into the obstructed vessel failed to open it, they tried to perform an emergency angioplasty. But they were unable to thread a balloon catheter through the blocked artery. The man then received standard treatment for a heart attack in the coronary care unit. His recovery was uneventful, and he was discharged seventeen days after he was admitted.[95]

Emergency PTCA as an Alternative to Thrombolytic Therapy

Six months after Geoffrey Hartzler left the Mayo Clinic, he pioneered the use of emergency PTCA as an alternative to thrombolytic therapy to open a blocked coronary artery during an acute myocardial infarction. Hartzler, an angioplasty zealot and a procedural virtuoso, had first performed PTCA on a patient with an acute myocardial infarction at St. Luke's Hospital in Kansas City in November 1980.[96] Three years later, he was the lead author of the first article to report the results of performing emergency angioplasty (with or without intracoronary streptokinase) to treat heart attack patients.[97] The article's list of authors reveals how successful the Mid America Heart Institute in Missouri had been in terms of hiring cardiologists from the Mayo Clinic. Six of the eight authors had trained in Rochester, and five were former Mayo staff members. They had left the nation's largest multispecialty group practice to join one of the first and most successful cardiology-cardiac surgery groups.[98]

Back in Rochester, David Holmes was the first author of a 1985 article that was one of the earliest reports of a series of patients with acute myocardial infarction who had been treated either by emergency angioplasty alone or in combination with intracoronary streptokinase.[99] The Mayo group concluded that PTCA was of considerable value in the treatment of certain heart attack patients, but they cautioned that its effectiveness depended on each person's clinical presentation and coronary angiogram findings. There was another problem. Although an emergency angioplasty often opened an artery that had been totally blocked by a fresh thrombus, most patients who had an acute myocardial infarction did not have ready access to this time-sensitive procedure. Fewer than 20 percent of American hospitals offered angioplasty in 1985.[100]

Most patients who had a heart attack in the United States were admitted to community hospitals. A group of Italian cardiologists who worked in such institutions published the results of a pioneering multi-hospital clinical trial of thrombolytic therapy in 1986. The letters GISSI were an acronym for the long name of the Italian trial that is considered to be the first "megatrial," a term used to describe clinical trials involving more than 10,000 patients. This is another example of the major role that Europeans played in developing new heart care strategies and in organizing multi-institutional clinical trials to evaluate them. GISSI, which involved 11,806 patients at 176 hospitals, showed that thrombolytic therapy with streptokinase was safe and effective when it was dripped into a peripheral vein as an alternative to infusing it directly into a coronary artery through a catheter. Boston cardiologist Eugene Braunwald later characterized GISSI as "more than a landmark trial—it was a bombshell."[101] Because intravenous streptokinase could be administered in any hospital, there was no need to arrange an emergency transfer of a patient to a center staffed to perform angioplasty around the clock. Soon, however, streptokinase faced a formidable competitor in the race to open blocked coronary arteries.

"Biotechnology," a term introduced around World War I, has had various meanings. But it meant very little to cardiologists or heart attack patients until the mid-1980s. That is when Genentech, a pioneering California-based genetic engineering company, produced a novel thrombolytic agent named tissue plasminogen activator (t-PA).[102] Mayo was one of thirteen sites selected in 1984 to participate in the Thrombolysis in Myocardial Infarction (TIMI) trial, a multi-institutional clinical trial designed to compare intravenous t-PA with streptokinase. James Chesebro, principal investigator for the Mayo site, was the lead author of one of the TIMI group's first reports of results. It showed that t-PA opened significantly more infarct-related arteries than streptokinase.[103]

In 1986 the clinic's newsletter reported that more than 100 patients had been treated with t-PA at the institution. The writer explained that the experimental thrombolytic agent "makes it possible to stop heart attacks in their tracks, saving vital heart muscle and, in some cases, saving lives."[104] Bernard Gersh, who had been born in South Africa and had trained in Cape Town and Oxford, England, had been director of Mayo's coronary care unit for one year at this point. He recalled thrombolytic therapy's almost immediate effects: "To be in the coronary care unit in the early hours of the morning and to see what happened to the patient when the artery is opened is unforgettable."[105] What Gersh and other physicians witnessed—and what patients experienced—was very dramatic. A patient's chest pain and other heart attack symptoms often disappeared immediately after streptokinase or t-PA opened his or her blocked coronary artery, allowing blood to nourish the heart muscle once again.

Two Patients Describe Very Different Heart Attack Experiences

The autobiographical accounts of two public figures who had heart attacks in the 1980s underscore the dramatic changes in the management of this life-threatening condition that took place during the first half of the decade.

Norman Cousins, longtime editor of the *Saturday Review*, was in his mid-sixties when he had an acute myocardial infarction in 1980. He had recently joined the faculty of the University of California, Los Angeles, School of Medicine, where his work focused on the emotional aspects of illness. Cousins, who had his heart attack at home, recalled, "Just after lunch, I was hit by a wave of nausea and weakness. I began to pant. I had no chest pain, but pressure in my chest and difficulty in breathing left little doubt that my heart was failing." Paramedics took him to the university hospital's emergency room. "The ride to the hospital was a comparatively leisurely one. At my request, the driver had turned off the siren and drove at ordinary speed."[106] This "minutes-don't-count" scenario reflected the fact that Cousins had his heart attack on the eve of the thrombolytic era, which would be characterized by the "Time is Muscle" SWAT team approach.[107]

Cardiologist Kenneth Shine was waiting in the emergency room to evaluate Cousins, who recalled that "they went into action immediately, blood pressure, oxygen tank, and cardiograph." But then, the pace slowed down. Shine took a history and examined his patient-colleague before Cousins was moved to the coronary care unit. "After about an hour, Dr. Shine came in to discuss my case and to tell me what was expected of me. I was to avoid physical exertion and mental strain." At this point, Cousins still had some lingering chest pressure. His four-day coronary care unit stay was marked by interpersonal conflicts, which he detailed in a book, but there were no medical complications. Before being discharged after three weeks in the hospital, Cousins had a very abnormal treadmill exercise test, which suggested the presence of severe coronary artery disease. The editor and medical school faculty member, who had read extensively about his problem, refused an angiogram because he would not consider bypass surgery. Although Cousins considered it "one of the high points in twentieth-century surgery…it was not a universal remedy and…was contraindicated for some patients."[108]

Cousins's description of his care stands in stark contrast to the aggressive catheter-based treatments that David Rogers received five years later. This physician, former dean of the Johns Hopkins School of Medicine and president of the Robert Wood Johnson Foundation, was at home in Princeton, New Jersey, in 1985, when he had a heart attack. It began with fifteen minutes of chest discomfort that came and went: "I felt I must sit down *very, very* quietly. Although I did so, the pain became a steadily expanding, deep, penetrating ache, spreading from beneath my breastbone, around the sides of my chest, up my neck into my lower jaw, and down the inner aspect of my left arm." The pain fluctuated in severity but was often "absolutely intolerable." Sweating profusely, Rogers sat very still, immobilized by fear. "There was absolutely no doubt in my mind that I was about to die." When he got to the hospital, he was given large doses of morphine with little relief. Unlike Cousins, Rogers was rushed to a catheterization laboratory, where he had a coronary angiogram, which he described as a piece of cake. The physician and former medical school dean watched squirts of contrast enter his coronary arteries, but he was dismayed to "see absolutely no dye going into my left anterior descending coronary artery, which appeared completely blocked."[109]

In the five years that separated the experiences of these two prominent men, the treatment strategy for acute myocardial infarction had shifted radically—from resting quietly in bed to a race to a laboratory for catheter-based therapy. Rogers was awestruck by the aggressive care he received: "My cardiologist catheter artisans had maneuvered their catheter into the stump-like orifice of the left anterior descending coronary and had begun dripping in streptokinase.... Quite suddenly, and after only modest amounts of enzyme, I said...'I think you've dissolved it; I've lost my pain.'" Another injection showed "a threadlike squirt of dye...going through a very tight centimeter-long obstruction close to the origin of the coronary." Despite the ongoing streptokinase infusion, Rogers's pain returned and a repeat injection showed a re-occluded coronary artery. "Then followed the use of the latest in modern medical miracle technologies. My physicians skillfully threaded a tiny wire through the obstruction, guided a collapsed balloon over it...they expanded the balloon, forcing arterial wall, clot, and atheroma outwards. Again, I experienced swift and blissful relief of pain." Rogers marveled at the physiological and anatomical consequences of the catheter treatment. He had no further chest pain after the emergency angioplasty, and the once-blocked coronary artery looked virtually normal when the cardiologist injected more contrast into it.[110]

Rogers's personal experiences influenced his attitude about the complex interrelationships of technology, specialization, and health care costs. He thought he was having another heart attack six years later, but a repeat angiogram showed that his coronary arteries were "fat, full, and perfusing well."[111] The site of his previous PTCA showed no signs of restenosis (recurrent blockage). One day later, a doctor pushed a flexible gastroscope into his stomach and discovered an ulcer. Rogers concluded, "I do not know yet what the bill will be for all the technological reassurance brought to bear on me—but it will be considerable. As one of the major champions of basic generalist care and less technologies, I am troubled by this, but I have to admit, reluctantly, that under the circumstances, two expensive technologies made quite a difference to me and my view of the future." They also shifted the treatment focus from his heart to his stomach.[112]

Mayo's approach to caring for patients with acute myocardial infarction changed dramatically during the early 1980s, mirroring the different experiences described by Norman Cousins and David Rogers. Hugh Smith had been director of the catheterization laboratory for nine years when he wrote a report in 1983 that revealed how quickly catheters had become treatment tools: "Whereas we were essentially a diagnostic laboratory performing no invasive therapeutic procedures at the time of the 1979 triennial review, significant advances have since been made with five separate therapeutic procedures."[113] Two of the five treatment techniques related to coronary artery disease: angioplasty and intracoronary streptokinase infusion. In addition to their implications for patients, these new treatments affected cardiologists who worked in the laboratory. In 1982 they began to share responsibility for covering the laboratory around-the-clock for emergency procedures. Meanwhile, almost $3 million was budgeted to build and equip another catheterization laboratory at Saint Marys Hospital. That was just part of Mayo's ambitious plans.

Endocrinologist Eugene Mayberry was the chair of Mayo's Board of Governors in 1983, when he outlined a long list of projects that were underway or planned. They would cost tens of millions of dollars. It was apparent that additional sources of revenue would help Mayo achieve its goals of enhancing patient care and expanding its programs of research and education. Many academic centers were confronting significant financial problems when Mayberry conveyed a positive message to the Mayo staff.[114] One recent piece of federal legislation, known as the Bayh-Dole Act of 1980, seemed to offer new opportunities to institutions that had productive programs of federally funded research.

Like other academic institutions, Mayo responded positively to the Bayh-Dole Act, which was designed to encourage universities and teaching hospitals to commercialize inventions.[115] In 1986 the clinic formed Mayo Medical Ventures to facilitate and oversee technology transfer. Three years later, clinic administrator Rick Colvin claimed that "the long-term prospects of technology transfer are golden in a place like this."[116] But new technologies were like a double-edged sword. The challenge was to differentiate those that made a difference in patient outcomes from those that simply increased the cost of health care.[117]

Coronary Interventions Expand Beyond Balloon Catheters

During the 1980s, angioplasty was the dominant catheter-based treatment technology, but other innovations were being added to interventional cardiology's armamentarium. Ronald Vlietstra and Robert Frye explained in 1989 that more than 200,000 patients in the United States had undergone PTCA the previous year, and that the procedure was being done in almost 1,000 hospitals.[118] Angioplasty had matured by the end of the decade, when several new tools and techniques were being showcased at national meetings and were discussed and debated in medical periodicals.

In this context, Mayo's heart specialists became increasingly visible behind podiums and in print. For example, twenty-eight authors from the clinic contributed to *Interventional Cardiology*, a 1989 book edited by Holmes and Vlietstra. It contained chapters on several very new technologies and techniques used to treat patients with coronary artery disease, valve disorders, congenital heart defects, and abnormal heart rhythms. The editors were enthusiastic about recent developments, but they were reluctant to predict the future: "Some of these innovative therapeutic procedures may never outgrow infancy and may simply remain historical footnotes, whereas others will mature and become part of the standard therapeutic armamentarium."[119]

Coronary atherectomy was one promising therapeutic approach that Holmes and Vlietstra included in their 1989 book. This catheter-based technology, developed by California cardiologist John Simpson, was designed to open an obstructed coronary artery by shaving off and removing atherosclerotic material from inside the vessel rather than simply compressing it with an inflatable balloon catheter.[120] Vlietstra and Holmes did the first coronary atherectomy in Rochester on October 6, 1988, shortly after the FDA approved the procedure for pre-marketing clinical trials. One of Simpson's colleagues was with them when they performed this first coronary atherectomy, which was successful. At the time, Mayo was the sixth center in the United States and the only one in the Midwest that offered atherectomy as an experimental procedure.

The clinic's newsletter informed staff that atherectomy involved "inserting a catheter carrying a tiny, safety-pin-sized capsule into the artery. Inside the capsule is a small blade that moves at 2,500 rotations per minute while cutting away the blockage." The writer explained, "Dr. Vlietstra foresees that in the future the surgery [atherectomy] could become as common as the 1,000 angioplasties Mayo currently does each year. As many as 100,000 patients in the United States may benefit annually from the procedure, he says."[121] In 1989 the Mayo group reported the results of atherectomy in fifty patients, and it was judged successful in 89 percent of them. The authors concluded that coronary atherectomy seemed to have significant potential, but they emphasized that controlled clinical trials comparing it to angioplasty were being planned to better assess its ultimate role in patient care. Other catheter-based techniques to treat coronary disease would come and go by the end of the twentieth century.[122] One that received a lot of publicity involved the use of a laser.

British science fiction writer Arthur Clarke, best known for *2001: A Space Odyssey*, had proclaimed in 1973 that "any sufficiently advanced technology is indistinguishable from magic."[123] Laser beams, which had already shifted from the realm of science fiction to reality, were first used as an adjunct to balloon angioplasty in 1983. The principle was to use laser energy to vaporize atherosclerotic material in order to reduce the size of a coronary artery plaque or to open a channel through a vessel that had been totally blocked for some time (a so-called chronic total occlusion). Brothers Dennis and John Bresnahan performed the first laser-assisted angioplasty at Mayo on July 24, 1989. Expressing "cautious optimism" about the space-age technology, Dennis explained, "Although the application of lasers to cardiovascular disease has great potential, many problems remain."[124] Laser therapy mesmerized some members of the medical profession and the public.

Social and economic forces push and pull unproven technologies into medical practice. The editors of a 1989 book on lasers in cardiovascular disease acknowledged that media attention and consumer awareness had accelerated the technology's rapid diffusion: "Patient demand and a mystical appeal of the laser methods have created substantial economic pressures for physicians...[and hospitals] to have the technique available."[125] But costly laser technology that many cardiac referral centers bought in the early 1990s would be gathering dust by the end of the decade due to disappointing clinical trial results.

As enthusiasm for lasers faded, a much simpler catheter-based technology took center stage. Intracoronary stents, like many innovations in heart care, were developed in Europe, where they were first used in humans in 1986.[126] Fitted over a special angioplasty catheter, a metal mesh stent could be expanded (by inflating a balloon) in a narrowed coronary artery. The stent remained in place after the balloon catheter was pulled out of the vessel. It was easy to explain a cylindrical stent to patients by comparing it to a ballpoint pen spring, which is about the same size and shape. They also learned that an expanded stent functioned like a tubular scaffold—propping open a diseased artery's wall.

Similar to the situation with PTCA, pre- and post-procedure angiograms provided dramatic visual proof of success. Angiograms of the area of the vessel that had been stented usually revealed wide-open arteries and better blood flow. These images impressed physicians, patients, and the public. Stents seemed to be an ideal approach to prevent (or at least reduce significantly) the likelihood of restenosis—blockage recurring at the site of a previous angioplasty. Restenosis, which had become a significant problem with PTCA, led to more diagnostic coronary angiograms and repeat angioplasties.[127]

David Holmes, assisted by staff cardiologists John Bresnahan and Andre Lapeyre and fellow Kirk Garratt, performed Mayo's first coronary stent procedure on October 26, 1989. The patient, a seventy-two-year-old woman from Wisconsin, had been referred by a LaCrosse cardiologist for possible implantation of a Gianturco-Roubin stent (named for its inventors) that was undergoing pre-market testing. She had had CABG eight years earlier for blockages in her right and left circumflex coronary arteries. Her left anterior descending artery had been treated with PTCA in 1986 and again the following year. After the woman developed recurrent angina in the summer of 1989, an angiogram revealed that her left anterior descending coronary artery was open but both vein grafts had developed severe localized narrowings.[128]

Mayo's Institutional Review Board had approved the stent protocol in September, and the patient signed a consent form that explained, in part, "The purpose of this study is to evaluate the effectiveness of a new stent for holding the artery open and preventing blockage after balloon angioplasty treatment.... The unique feature of this device is that it mechanically holds open the vessel walls and thus may help prevent reblockage."[129] Six months after stents were placed in both vein grafts, the woman returned to Rochester for a follow-up evaluation. Her angina was gone, a treadmill exercise test was reassuring, and an angiogram showed excellent blood flow through the stents.

Kirk Garratt, who assisted with the stent procedure, had completed a general cardiology fellowship in Los Angeles before coming to Mayo for a special two-year interventional cardiology fellowship. In an interview, Garratt later explained that he had been attracted to the clinic "in no small measure because David Holmes was there." Garratt described a mentoring experience he had during an interventional procedure:

> We reached a point in the course of that case when he turned to me, and with complete sincerity, asked me how I thought we should proceed. At first I thought he was just testing me, but I realized that he wasn't. He genuinely wanted to hear what I had to say because he knew that sometimes even a young, relatively inexperienced mind can find solutions to problems that might not be apparent to the veteran practitioner. That rare and unusual philosophy pervades Mayo Clinic, and I think that it really does produce optimum patient care.[130]

Garratt, Holmes, and stent pioneer Gary Roubin from the University of Alabama at Birmingham reported Mayo's early experience with the technology in fifteen patients in 1991. In addition to concluding that stents could treat some immediate complications of PTCA, they proposed that the "elective placement of a stent may be safely undertaken in patients with high-risk coronary lesions or recurrent restenotic lesions." Other clinical investigators reached the same conclusion, which had major implications for the number of patients who might be candidates for a stent. But Garratt, Holmes, and Roubin cautioned that the "long-term outcome in all groups of patients who receive coronary stents is unknown."[131] Despite this uncertainty, demand for stents increased dramatically.

Ronald Vlietstra and Robert Frye claimed in 1989 that cardiology was "on the threshold of a new era" and noted that "never before have there been so many potent tools ready for therapeutic development."[132] But they also raised concerns. Citing the spectacular growth of angioplasty and other treatment technologies developed during the previous decade, the Mayo cardiologists warned, "Unfortunately, there is generally widespread application of these

new techniques before their real contribution has been documented and certainly before reasoned consensus has been established on standards, indications, and training requirements."[133]

Robert Frye issued a challenge to heart specialists in 1992, when he was
president of the American College of Cardiology: "Reducing utilization of
one or another procedure clearly will not solve the overall high cost of medical care, but we have a professional responsibility to provide only those services that are truly in the best interest of the patient."[134] A growing number
of interested observers inside and outside the medical profession shared this
concern.[135]

Interventional cardiologist Eric Topol was chief of cardiology at the
Cleveland Clinic when he wrote an editorial on stents in 1995, one year after
the FDA had approved them for the elective treatment of coronary artery disease in certain situations. Clinical trial results had shown that stents reduced
restenosis rates. This "led to a rapid and major revamping of clinical practice," according to Topol. But the Cleveland Clinic heart specialist claimed
that cardiologists had caught "stent fever." He noted that stent sales exceeded
$1 million a day and that the manufacturer could not keep up with demand.
Echoing concerns raised by Mayo cardiologists and others, Topol argued
that "tens of thousands of patients are receiving a prosthetic metal device
in their coronary arteries without adequate long-term follow-up."[136] But who
decided what long-term follow-up really meant?

Device makers were eager to get data that would allow them to market their products and to claim that their technology offered an advantage
over standard care or competitors' products. In a highly competitive race to
complete clinical trials, analyze the data, and publish the results, so-called
long-term follow-up often meant one or two years. Concerns about corporate profits, consumer demand, and competition for patients among cardiologists and hospitals stimulated demand for stents and other new devices.
The number of clinical trials of devices skyrocketed in the 1990s. Their
results could propel a promising technology into a high orbit or send it
crashing to the ground.[137]

Using Balloon Catheters to Open Obstructed Heart Valves

The very high prevalence of coronary disease encouraged inventors, clinical
investigators, and medical device companies to collaborate in the development of technologies to treat patients afflicted with it. Although congenital heart disease and acquired valve disorders were much less common, a
few individuals tried to develop percutaneous catheter-based interventions
to treat specific non-coronary abnormalities. The goal, analogous to that
of angioplasty, was to offer patients with a certain cardiac problems an

alternative to surgery and all that that implied in terms of risk, cost, and convalescence.

In 1982 a pediatric cardiologist, a cardiac surgeon, and two cardiovascular radiologists at the Johns Hopkins Hospital published an article describing how they had used a percutaneous balloon procedure to treat four children who had been born with a stenotic (obstructed) pulmonary valve. It involved threading a special catheter through the right heart and positioning its poly-ethylene balloon in the narrowed opening of the pulmonary valve. They then inflated the contrast-filled balloon for ten seconds while watching it expand with fluoroscopy. Pressure measurements before and after the procedure proved that it significantly reduced the obstruction across the valve.[138] Shortly after this article was published, Mayo pediatric cardiologist Donald Hagler, cardiologist James Seward, and radiologist Paul Julsrud began performing a similar procedure in Rochester.[139]

In the early 1980s, Japanese cardiologist Kanji Inoue led a group that developed percutaneous balloon valvuloplasty as an alternative to surgery in adults with rheumatic mitral stenosis. In 1984 they reported their results in six patients, five of whom had dramatic improvement after the procedure.[140] One year after Inoue published his article on balloon mitral valvuloplasty, French cardiologist Alain Cribier used a balloon catheter made by a Massachusetts company to dilate the aortic valve in a seventy-eight-year-old woman with severe aortic stenosis. In 1986 his group reported the results of the procedure in three patients, each of whom noted dramatic improvement in their main symptom of shortness of breath with activity. Although Cribier conceded that it was too early to compare the results of balloon valvuloplasty with traditional aortic valve replacement, he predicted that the catheter-based technique would be useful in patients in whom surgery was considered very high risk.[141] Mayo cardiologists David Holmes and Rick Nishimura traveled to France to watch Cribier perform the procedure. On June 11, 1986, five months after the French cardiologist published his results, they performed the first aortic balloon valvuloplasty in Rochester on a very elderly patient with severe aortic stenosis.[142]

In August 1986, Holmes and cardiac surgeon Thomas Orszulak presented a proposal on mitral valve balloon valvuloplasty to Mayo's Cardiovascular Clinical Practice Committee. The two men were aware that some surgeons had raised concerns regarding self-referral and potential conflict of inter-est in the context of PTCA. To address this issue, Holmes and Orszulak emphasized that a patient's clinical cardiologist (at Mayo) rather than an interventional cardiologist in the catheterization laboratory would make the final decision of whether the experimental balloon approach was a reason-able alternative to traditional mitral valve surgery. They explained that the patient's clinical cardiologist, Orszulak (representing cardiac surgery), and one of three interventional cardiologists (David Holmes, Rick Nishimura, or

Guy Reeder) would meet *"prior* to approaching a patient with the possibility of performing the procedure" to discuss whether he or she would be a potential candidate. Holmes indicated that they were prepared to perform the first procedure as soon as they received all the required committee approvals.[143] On September 24, 1987, Holmes and Reeder performed the first mitral balloon valvuloplasty on a seventy-nine-year-old woman from Kentucky who had mitral stenosis.[144]

Holmes and Nishimura acknowledged in a 1992 review article that enthusiasm for aortic balloon valvuloplasty had waned because whatever immediate improvement in the obstruction that resulted from the procedure did not last as long as had been hoped. Although the Mayo cardiologists remained cautiously optimistic, they thought aortic balloon valvuloplasty should be reserved for carefully selected patients.[145] Holmes and Nishimura were more optimistic about mitral balloon valvuloplasty. That procedure seemed to be a good alternative to surgery for patients with mitral stenosis who met specific criteria with respect to the structure and function of the valve leaflets. But they emphasized that mitral valvuloplasty was more complicated than aortic valvuloplasty and warned that "it should be performed only at centers that have extensive experience with the procedure."[146]

Charanjit (Chet) Rihal, who had joined the interventional group after completing his fellowship at Mayo, was the first author of a 1991 article written with Nishimura and Holmes that reported the clinic's experience with fifty patients who had undergone mitral balloon valvuloplasty. Three patients had died during or shortly after the procedure, but the early results were excellent in terms of symptom relief and objective measurement of residual obstruction. They attributed the improvement in procedural success and complication rates over time "to refinement of patient selection criteria, technical advances in the procedure, and operator experience."[147] The Mayo interventional cardiologists had chosen a subtitle that conveyed a concept that any doctor who performed procedures understood: "The Learning Curve." Although this notion appeared in articles related to PTCA and other catheter-based alternatives to cardiac surgery, it was rarely highlighted.

Major clinically oriented cardiac referral centers, such as the Mayo Clinic and the Cleveland Clinic, performed a very large number of interventional cardiology procedures. Along with other academic centers, they had replaced the "see one, do one, teach one" approach with a rigorous training program characterized by close supervision of trainees who were given greater responsibility as they demonstrated competence. One contentious issue, which had arisen with PTCA and persisted, related to the minimum number of interventional procedures that an individual or an institution should perform to gain and maintain competence. Mayo's interventional cardiologists embraced the guidelines for procedures, and they subdivided responsibilities for performing the less common techniques among themselves. This strategy reflected the clinic's tradition of subspecialization.[148]

When Andreas Grüntzig performed the first PTCA in a patient on September 16, 1977, he could not have imagined how profoundly this procedure would change the care of patients with heart disease and the practice of cardiology. The formation of an organization that focuses on a specific organ system or technology is a visible step in the evolution of a new specialty. Six months before Grüntzig performed the world's first coronary angioplasty, eleven cardiologists and radiologists had met in Las Vegas, Nevada, to discuss the need for an organization that would be named the Society for Cardiac Angiography. The first annual meeting of the society was held in Chicago on June 5, 1978.[149] The notion of cardiologists or radiologists actually treating coronary disease with catheters was brand new. In 1993 the governing board of the Society for Cardiac Angiography changed the organization's name to the Society for Cardiac Angiography and Interventions. This acknowledged something that many cardiologists understood: a new cardiology subspecialty—interventional cardiology—had reached adolescence. By the end of the twentieth century, catheter-based techniques would be used regularly to treat a broad range of heart problems.

Analyzing and Managing Abnormal Heart Rhythms

A Boston psychiatrist and a cardiac surgeon who were interested in how patients coped with the knowledge that they had heart disease declared in 1979, "The heart is not only the central organ of the body and historically the seat of emotions, it is the only organ that functions in a dramatic on-off mode. If it beats, one lives; if it stops its beat, one dies."[1] But this on-off switch analogy does not recognize a large middle ground. Every day, millions of individuals feel their hearts skipping beats or racing for no obvious reason. For example, celebrated author Joyce Carol Oates began having occasional spells of tachycardia when she was a teenager: "Basically, it is a quickened heartbeat. It is a 'pounding,' or 'runaway,' heartbeat. It's really quite aston- ishing, and if you experience such an attack, your entire body will rock and vibrate with the maniacal pounding of your heart—as if an angry fist were inside your ribcage, pounding to be released."[2]

Cardiac arrhythmias (heart rhythm disorders) may be mildly annoying, or they may be life-threatening.[3] During the second half of the twentieth century, several drugs and electronic technologies were developed to control the heartbeat in an attempt to alleviate patients' symptoms and save lives. Chicago heart rhythm experts Louis Katz and Alfred Pick wrote in 1956, "Arrhythmias constitute definite symptoms with typical clinical pictures, with definite prognoses and with established therapeutic procedures." But such claims oversimplified a very complex and dynamic area of medical prac- tice and research that Katz and Pick acknowledged had "undergone a renais- sance recently."[4] That renaissance owed much to what cardiologist Howard Burchell termed the "wizardry of new technology."[5] Researchers who used these technologies produced new knowledge about the heart's electrical sys- tem and coined words and phrases to describe their discoveries and innova- tions. This also had implications for electrocardiography.

The electrocardiograph had helped two generations of physicians sort out heart rhythm disorders when cardiology section head Robert Parker told

Mayo's Board of Governors in 1958 that many of the clinic's internists did not "feel capable of properly interpreting [electrocardiograms] and would appreciate a brief indication as to whether the objective record presents changes of clinical significance."[6] Mayo had more than 120 internist-diagnosticians on staff at the time, and 90 percent of them were not cardiologists. Most of these physicians, who were busy trying to keep up with developments in their own medical subspecialties, had little or no interest in electrocardiography. This situation led to a policy change regarding the interpretation and reporting of electrocardiograms in Rochester.

In the late 1950s, Mayo's electrocardiography technicians were recording more than 1,000 tracings in the clinic and its two affiliated hospitals every week. The copy of the tracing that they sent to the internist-diagnostician who had ordered the test included a brief description of abnormal findings. But the report did not include a comment on the potential significance of any abnormal waveforms or rhythms. In 1961 the cardiologists decided that they would add a formal impression to each tracing to help an internist-diagnostician decide if an individual patient's electrocardiogram was normal, borderline, or abnormal.[7] Some cardiologists saw the potential for employing new technologies to help them with this work.

Applying Computers to Electrocardiography

During the second half of the twentieth century, a multitude of technologies (such as transistors and computers) transformed all aspects of American life at an accelerating rate. Their impact on medicine in general and the care of patients with heart disease in particular was huge.[8] Robert Parker informed Mayo's board in 1962 that "tremendous advances in the field of electronics" meant that "in the future electrocardiograms might well be taken on magnetic tape and electronic computer techniques used for objective interpretation as well as duplication and recall." Parker was pleased that Ralph Smith, who had joined Mayo's staff four years earlier, was very interested in the emerging field of computerized electrocardiography.[9]

Ralph Smith, the former chief of cardiology at the Minneapolis Veterans Administration Hospital, had access to the first computer on the Mayo campus. The IBM 1620, a small transistorized computer designed for scientific applications and manufactured at the company's new Rochester plant, was installed in the Medical Sciences building in 1962. An article in the clinic's newsletter explained that Mayo's new computer facility would be "operated as an 'open shop' available for the use by staff members and fellows insofar as time permits." Based on research projects that had been approved or were planned, it was predicted that the 1620 system would be used twenty-four hours a day.[10] Milton Anderson, who succeeded Parker as a cardiology section head, informed the board in 1963 that Smith had made great strides in introducing changes into Mayo's electrocardiographic laboratory, "where a system now is ready to function which will largely solve the problem of storage, will permit interpretation of electrocardiograms for the other clinicians in the Mayo Clinic, and will be a step forward to the possibility of eventually using computer analysis for electrocardiography at the Mayo Clinic."[11]

Smith was eager to develop computerized electrocardiography in order to improve the recording, interpretation, and storage of the 75,000 tracings done each year in Rochester. A 1963 article in *Mayovox* described changes in the equipment and procedures that Smith and laboratory supervisor Mildred Christianson were coordinating. It included photographs of the laboratory's staff using equipment that Mayo had developed with IBM and Medtronic, a Minneapolis-based medical electronics firm. By this time, the standard electrocardiogram consisted of twelve separate tracings recorded from leads placed on both arms, on the left leg, and on six locations across the front of the chest. Medtronic had provided Mayo with new technology that could record six leads simultaneously rather than sequentially. Microfilm and a Xerox copier introduced into the laboratory at the same time also improved efficiency.[12] Medtronic cofounder Earl Bakken, who worked on the Mayo project, recalled: "We did some really very early work with Ralph Smith.... [who] was one of the first ones to get into electrocardiography and computer work."[13]

Cesar Caceres, a cardiologist in Washington, D.C., had become interested in computerized electrocardiography in the late 1950s. A pioneer of the field, Caceres was chief of the US Public Health Service's Instrumentation Field Station in 1964, when he predicted, "In the next few years, computers will handle the processing of all routine electrocardiograms. They will do so at low cost, with precision and rapidity unattainable by physicians." Caceres claimed that "the electrocardiogram bettered the practice of medicine, and computers will better the practice of electrocardiography."[14]

In 1965 *Time* magazine ran a cover story on the computer's impact on society. In a section devoted to the technology's emerging role in health care, the writer explained that hospitals had begun to use computers to monitor the condition of some patients and that "computers now read electrocardiograms faster and more accurately than a jury of physicians." This article stressed how quickly computers were infiltrating American culture: "Popping up across the U.S. like slab-sided mushrooms, they are the fastest growing element in the technical arsenal of the world's most technological nation."[15]

In November 1966 Mayo launched a one-year study designed to explore how computers might be used to support every aspect of medical practice. A team of about twenty physicians and support staff would collaborate with fourteen engineers and other specialists from the Lockheed Missiles and Space Company. The clinic's newsletter explained that the Sunnyvale, California, company had chosen "medical information systems as an area of concentration outside of its traditional defense and space fields." The project had implications for Mayo's main mission of patient care and its academic programs:

> By relieving physicians and associated personnel of many routine tasks, such an information system could be expected to enhance the doctor-patient relationship and generally expedite patient care. Also, a comprehensive store of data would be readily accessible for medical education and research purposes. Mayo officials describe the proposed system as a continuation of efforts that have been made throughout the history of the clinic to provide maximum efficiency consistent with the highest standards of patient care.[16]

Ralph Smith was one of five physicians and two senior administrators on Mayo's Medical Information Systems Committee. He explained at a 1967 symposium on the heart's electrical activity that the clinic's computerized electrocardiography system (developed with IBM, Medtronic, and Milwaukee-based Marquette Electronics) had already been used to record a total of more than 200,000 electrocardiograms at Mayo.[17]

Smith published very little, but he attended meetings with other pioneers of computerized electrocardiography. And they were impressed by innovations in the laboratory that he oversaw in Rochester. In one of the first books on the subject, published in 1970, Canadian cardiologist Josef Wartak claimed that "computers have come to be regarded as one of the basic tools in medical theory and practice." Noting that several institutions were involved in the computer analysis of electrocardiograms, Wartak explained that "the leaders in this field are the Instrumental Field Station, U.S. Public Health Service, Washington, DC, and the Mayo Clinic."[18]

Mayo often imported ideas, techniques, and technologies that were then refined or implemented on a larger scale in Rochester. The trans-telephonic transmission of electrocardiograms is an example of this phenomenon. In 1953 University of Kansas cardiologist Grey Dimond had described custom-built equipment that transmitted a patient's electrocardiogram over a telephone line from a small hospital to a medical center, where it could be analyzed by experienced personnel.[19] Ralph Smith helped launch telephone transmission of multilead electrocardiograms between Saint Marys Hospital and the laboratory in the clinic's Plummer building in 1967.[20]

Smith sent an electrocardiogram over a telephone connection from Sydney, Australia, to Rochester in 1971. The Mayo cardiologist was in Australia to participate in the Computerized Medical Equipment Exhibition, which was sponsored by the US Department of Commerce. A news release from the US Trade Center in Sydney boasted, "The significance of the experiment lies in the fact that if the procedure will work between Sydney, Australia and Minnesota, U.S.A., it will work between any two places on earth."[21]

Mayo launched a telephone computerized electrocardiography service on July 1, 1973. A hospital in Mason City, Iowa, was the first institution to send electrocardiograms over telephone lines to Rochester for interpretation. Mayo's newsletter noted that the service could be provided to any hospital in North America, but the primary targets were small hospitals without a cardiologist on staff. The main benefit of the new outreach electrocardiography service was that it made the "results of tests immediately available to the physician" caring for the patient.[22]

Gerald Gau, who had joined the Mayo staff in 1970 after completing a medical residency in Rochester and a cardiology fellowship at London's Hammersmith Hospital, was in charge of the outreach electrocardiography program. Gau, Smith, and two IBM engineers coauthored a 1973 article on the computer program for analyzing electrocardiograms that Mayo and IBM had developed. They concluded that the commercially available computer programs varied in quality, but all of them had problems evaluating heart rhythm abnormalities.[23] This was a significant issue because of the growing interest in the diagnosis and treatment of cardiac arrhythmias.

Treating Slow Heart Rates With an Electronic Pacemaker

Dutch physiologist Willem Einthoven had published the first electrocardiographic tracings of abnormal heart rhythms in 1906. His review article included tracings that depicted ventricular premature contractions, atrial flutter, and atrial fibrillation. One tracing was recorded from a woman whose heart rate was 29 beats per minute, less than half the rate that is considered to be the lower limit of normal. Her electrocardiogram revealed complete heart block— the heart's electrical impulse was blocked before it reached the ventricles.[24] The cardiac conduction system, which can be thought of as a network of microscopic wires, transmits electrical impulses from the atria to the ventricles, causing them to contract and pump blood through the body and the lungs.

The electrocardiograph made it possible to diagnose complete block, but there was no effective treatment for patients who had symptoms as a result of the slow heart rate that accompanied the conduction abnormality. Fredrick Willius, Mayo's first cardiologist and an electrocardiography pioneer, had published an article on complete heart block in 1925. He told the story of a sixty-two-year-old woman who had come to the clinic because she "suddenly became unconscious and had a convulsion" on three separate occasions. The woman, whose electrocardiogram revealed complete heart block with a ventricular rate of 32 beats per minute, "died suddenly on the seventh day in the hospital, in a Stokes-Adams attack."[25] William Stokes and Robert Adams were nineteenth-century Irish physicians who, along with others, described the association between a very slow heart rate and spells that might range from dizziness to faints to seizures to death. During the second quarter of the twentieth century, various drugs (such as subcutaneous epinephrine or oral ephedrine) were used in an attempt to treat patients with Stokes-Adams attacks. But they were impractical for long-term use.[26]

Boston cardiologist Paul Zoll invented a temporary transthoracic (external) pacemaker to treat patients with symptomatic heart block that was marketed in 1954.[27] This external pacemaker included a thirteen-pound stimulator that generated regular electric impulses. These rhythmic bursts of electricity, which traveled through two wires attached to small electrodes strapped to a patient's chest wall, were strong enough to trigger a heartbeat. The transthoracic pacemaker was used in specific situations for a very short time (rarely more than a few hours) because the chest wall shocks were painful. One patient's story illustrates the challenges of treating symptomatic heart block:

> A 78 year-old man was admitted to the Boston City Hospital because of frequent dizzy spells for two weeks. Electrocardiograms showed varying degrees of partial atrioventricular block, and then complete block with idioventricular rates as slow as 16 beats per minute. Initially he had numerous dizzy spells, then he became unconscious and never fully recovered. External electric stimulation was effective: an adequate circulation was maintained with a blood pressure of 118/60. Continued stimulation was necessary for 36 hours because ventricular standstill was observed whenever stimulation was interrupted. An adequate idioventricular rhythm reappeared following the intravenous administration of epinephrine at a rate of 4 micrograms per minute and simulation was then stopped. Ten hours later, however, the ventricular rate slowed markedly and shock supervened. At this time, stimulation again produced electrocardiographic ventricular complexes, but there were no associated pulse beats. Finally, the electrocardiographic ventricular responses to stimulation also failed and the patient died.[28]

Zoll published his experience with a temporary pacemaker in twenty-five patients (between the ages of sixty-two and eighty-three) in November 1955.[29] When his article appeared, two Minnesota surgeons were the only ones in the world who were performing open-heart surgery on a regularly scheduled basis. Their first patients were children with congenital heart defects. But the surgical pioneers were also concerned about heart block.

A Surgical Complication and the Invention of Pacemakers

C. Walton (Walt) Lillehei at the University of Minnesota and John Kirklin at the Mayo Clinic had performed more open-heart operations than any other surgeons by May 1956. That month they discussed complete heart block as a surgical complication at the annual meeting of the American Society for Thoracic Surgery. Specifically, the problem occurred in some children who had surgery to close a ventricular septal defect, a hole between the heart's two main pumping chambers. Lillehei and Kirklin agreed that sutures used to close the hole between the left and right ventricles could damage the heart's electrical conduction system that runs through the ventricular septum.[30]

Some of the children who developed heart block as a result of the operation died because persistent severe bradycardia (slow heart rate) could trigger a cascade of problems culminating in shock and cardiac arrest. Treatments designed to speed up the heart and raise the blood pressure involved the intravenous infusion of epinephrine, ephedrine, atropine, and lactate. Ideally, this drug cocktail bought time for the heart's conduction system to recover or for the child's circulatory system to adjust to the slow rate. But the treatment strategy did not always work.

Walt Lillehei, adept at solving unexpected intra-operative problems on the spot, imported a solution for heart block from his surgical research laboratory, where surgery residents Vincent Gott and William Weirich were using a commercially available physiologic stimulator to treat heart block that they had created in animals. This technology produced a rhythmic electrical impulse that stimulated the heart muscle to contract. Gott recalled the events of January 30, 1957: "Dr. Weirich and I received a call from Dr. Lillehei in the operating room that complete heart block had developed in a 2-year-old girl with a ventricular septal defect during her open-heart procedure. Dr. Lillehei asked us to bring up the Grass stimulator and the myocardial and skin electrodes. This patient did extremely well in the postoperative period."[31] The stimulator, which was connected to a wire that was attached to the patient's heart, functioned as a temporary pacemaker that sped up its beat. This technology provided vulnerable patients with a postoperative safety net that protected them from the life-threatening consequences of complete heart block.

John Kirklin heard Lillehei's group describe their experience using a temporary pacemaker to treat eighteen children with complete heart block at the annual meeting of the American College of Surgeons in October 1957. The Mayo surgeon had confronted the same complication in some of his patients and was impressed that the technology had produced such dramatic short-term results. Prior to using the temporary pacemaker, the mortality from surgically induced heart block was 50 percent. But only one of eighteen patients that Lillehei had treated with the device died in the hospital. The heart block often resolved in a few days, which meant that the device could be removed and the child could be discharged. Lillehei's group concluded, "This remarkable reduction in mortality associated with complete heart block has been the single most important factor in reducing the overall risk of open-heart surgery to low levels."[32] Swedish surgeon and pacemaker pioneer Åke Senning, who visited Lillehei after the meeting, described this strategy as "the beginning of the era of clinical pacing."[33]

On October 31, 1957, just a few days after the University of Minnesota group reported their experience with temporary pacemakers at the surgery meeting in Atlantic City, New Jersey, the Minneapolis area lost power for several hours. It was Halloween, and the power outage had frightening implications for any child connected to a pacemaker because the device was powered by electricity from a wall outlet. The Variety Club Heart Hospital operating rooms where Lillehei worked had auxiliary power, but the patient rooms did not. Recognizing the risk, he asked Earl Bakken, a self-employed electrical engineer who serviced the university's electronic equipment, to build a battery back-up system to power the external pacemakers.

Bakken's initial idea was to use an automobile battery to power the electrical pulse stimulators. Seeking to simplify and shrink this bulky system, he modified a transistorized metronome circuit that he had recently read about in *Popular Electronics* magazine and connected it to a nine-volt photographic flash battery. This unit generated a rhythmic electrical impulse that triggered a heartbeat. One month after Lillehei asked him for help, Bakken tested the custom-built unit in the university's surgery laboratory. It worked. One day later, Lillehei used it to pace a child's heart. It worked.[34]

Lillehei attached Bakken's prototype pacemaker to a patient just one month after he had presented the heart block problem to the electronics specialist. In the 1950s there were almost no regulatory or bureaucratic speed bumps to slow down the development and diffusion of new treatment technologies. Bakken wrote four decades later: "Nowadays, when it takes an average of seven years for a new medical device to find its way through the regulatory labyrinth in the United States, four weeks seems unbelievable."[35]

When the published version of the lecture that Lillehei's group had presented at the Atlantic City meeting appeared in 1958, it included a sentence that no one in the audience had heard. Without fanfare, the brief article announced the birth of what would become a multibillion dollar industry: "A featherweight transistorized pacemaker activated by a dry cell and taped or attached to the patient's trunk has been developed to facilitate transportation of these patients about the hospital and also to allow them more mobility in their convalescent interval in those cases where early return to sinus rhythm has not occurred."[36] Bakken's "featherweight transistorized pacemaker" also helped transform Medtronic from what had begun as a garage-based Minneapolis electronics repair firm into the world heavyweight champion of the cardiac device industry.

John Kirklin admired Walt Lillehei's surgical team and Earl Bakken's miniaturized life-saving technology. At the fall 1959 meeting of the American Heart Association, the Mayo group reported that the death rate from surgically induced heart block fell dramatically after it adopted the temporary pacing technique.[37] The following summer, the University of Minnesota group published its experience with transistorized Medtronic pacemakers in sixty-six patients, most of whom were children. But they also described using the device in a few adults who had not undergone surgery. The results when the external pacemaker was used to treat men and women who had Stokes-Adams attacks were impressive: "Not only has the threat of sudden death in these patients been removed, but their physical and emotional rehabilitation has been dramatic."[38]

Pacemakers, the Public, and the Medical Profession

The long title of a 1961 *Saturday Evening Post* article on pacemakers sounded like something a carnival barker might shout to attract pass-ersby: "Making a Heartbeat Behave: An Amazing New Pocket-Size Ticker Sparks Hesitant Heartbeats and Provides Added Years of Near-Normal Life for Many Cardiac Patients." Pictures of patients complemented the story about pacemakers that began with a description of the problem they were designed to fix: "In the marvelously integrated pattern of action that maintains life in the human body, one movement is central, paramount and indispensable—the beating of the heart. If it stops for five to fifteen seconds you become lightheaded or fall in a faint. A longer pause, further depriving the brain of oxygen, may produce convulsions. A halt of two minutes or more usually ends in death."[39] A photograph of Lillehei listening to a young boy's heart dominated the first page of the article. David Williams, who was recovering from open-heart surgery, looked directly at the camera as he held a Medtronic external pacemaker that maintained his heartbeat.

Saturday Evening Post writer Steven Spencer declared, "Among the achievements of today's engineering wizards is one of the most dramatic, an electronic 'heart' you can hold in your hand, a transistorized 'spark of life.' " The pacemaker that David Williams held was about the size of a transistor radio, a popular new technology. And Spencer used a musical analogy to explain its rhythmic role: "Day after day, year upon year, the pacemaker, like a tireless orchestra conductor, taps out the vital tempo of life's long and sometimes discordant journey." But there was a problem with the notion of using the external electronic device for years—the lives of patients who were dependent on it "hang by a thin pair of insulated wires attached to a portable pacemaker."[40]

Spencer described a solution to this problem that was very good news for the future of pacemakers and for the future patients who might need one. His *Saturday Evening Post* article included another photograph that showed Buffalo, New York, surgeon William Chardack and engineer Wilson

Greatbatch with a man who was not holding a pacemaker. The device these two men had invented was inside—not outside—the patient's body. Their fully implantable pacing system included an electrode connected to a sealed unit that housed a pulse generator (powered by six thimble-sized batteries) that sent an electrical impulse through a wire connected to a patient's heart. Already, several patients were "wearing their artificial pacemakers under the skin" in a round silicone rubber-covered case about the size of an ice hockey puck. How did they feel? Relieved! "Those who wear the devices today shudder as they recall the blackouts, head-cracking falls and other near-fatal experiences they suffered before they got their hearts on a dependable electric schedule."[41] Spencer knew how to tell a story.

Mayo surgeons John Kirklin and Dwight McGoon and pediatric cardiologist Patrick Ongley were among five dozen doctors and scientists who coauthored papers that were presented at a 1963 pacemaker symposium in New York City. Their talk dealt with how to avoid surgically induced heart block in children undergoing ventricular septal defect closure. The results were excellent, but it was old news.[42] Most of the other presentations described the role of implanting permanent pacemakers in adults with heart block unrelated to any operation. Several speakers discussed recent developments in the technology that Yale University heart surgeon William Glenn attributed "to the application of highly sophisticated electronic circuits, developed primarily for the refinement of communication systems required by the modern space age."[43]

During a discussion period at the conference, an audience member asked William Chardack how much a permanent pacemaker cost. The Buffalo surgeon, who had co-invented the device that Medtronic was now marketing, admitted that the price was high, just over $600. He did not compare it to other expensive consumer products, but this small permanent pacemaker cost about one-fourth as much as a full-size Chevrolet Impala. Instead, Chardack cleverly framed his answer in terms of the cost per heartbeat: "There are eighty thousand beats a day and prorated this way it is quite cheap."[44]

Paul Zoll, who had a financial interest in the Electrodyne Corporation that also manufactured pacemakers, provided another rationale for the cost of the technology: "Patients rarely pay for it. It is usually paid for by some insurance company or Blue Cross. The cost of the instrument really isn't particularly significant in our society." When the Boston cardiologist made these comments in 1963, Medicare did not exist, but about 70 percent of Americans had some form of private health insurance.[45] Despite cost concerns, the new technology gained acceptance. By June 1964, Mayo surgeon Henry Ellis had implanted permanent pacemakers (made by Medtronic or Electrodyne) in thirty-one adults, almost all of whom had a history of Stokes-Adams attacks. Ellis considered pacemaker implantation a "major surgical procedure" and noted that most patients remained in the hospital for seven to ten days after it was performed.[46]

Mayo Imports and Implements Pacemaker Innovations

Mayo cardiologist Howard Burchell had encouraged Benjamin McCallister to focus on cardiac arrhythmias shortly after he began his medical residency in Rochester in 1961. McCallister, who also learned to perform catheterizations during his training, introduced a pacing innovation at Mayo that surgeon Seymour Furman had described in 1959. Working at Montefiore Hospital in the Bronx, Furman had developed a method for installing a pacemaker electrode that did not require opening a patient's chest to attach it to the heart's outer surface. His technique involved inserting an electrode catheter into an arm vein and threading its tip into the right ventricle, where it was positioned against the heart's inner wall.[47] McCallister first used this approach in October 1963, when he placed an electrode catheter in a patient who needed a temporary pacemaker. During the next thirty months, temporary transvenous pacemaker electrodes were inserted in ninety-one patients in the catheterization laboratory at Saint Marys Hospital. Most of these men and women were scheduled for subsequent permanent pacemaker placement by a surgeon.[48]

The volume of permanent pacemaker implantations increased rapidly as the technology improved and spread to community hospitals. Medicare, launched in 1966, stimulated the spread of pacemakers and other hospital-based health care technologies. The following year this new government insurance program reimbursed hospitals $3.4 billion for inpatient care.[49] Medtronic cofounder Earl Bakken wrote three decades later, "Because of Medicare, along with increasing physician acceptance, pacemaker sales (ours and our competitors') really began to take off in the late 1960s. Medicare reimbursement thus ranks with the development of open-heart surgery, the evolution of the transistor and battery technology, and the emergence of new coatings and materials as essential elements that made implantable pacing a viable reality."[50] During the first decade that permanent pacemakers were available at Mayo, there was a tenfold increase in the number of implants per year, from a dozen in 1961 to 138 in 1971.[51]

In 1965 Howard Burchell helped Mayo medical resident John Merideth, who was very interested in electrocardiography, get an NIH-funded postdoctoral fellowship to work with basic electrophysiologist Gordon Moe in Utica, New York. When Merideth returned to Rochester the following year, he considered himself knowledgeable about basic cardiac electrophysiology (the science of the heart's electrical system). But he felt the need "to get clearly established on the clinical side." He joined the staff in 1968 "when the whole business of pacing was just ready to roll."[52] Not only were more pacemakers being implanted, they were becoming increasingly sophisticated as manufacturers competed to invent devices that did more than just send out an electrical impulse at a fixed rate.

The Mayo surgeons and surgical residents who implanted pacemakers worked closely with Merideth as the devices became more complicated. New Jersey heart surgeon and pacemaker pioneer Victor Parsonnet explained in 1966:

> Although the surgeon is temperamentally trained to face complications of his own making, he may find himself annoyed by repeated problems of technologic origin. What is more, often he cannot decipher all the complications by clinical judgment and "routine" laboratory work alone but must resort to an analysis of voltage, resistance, impedance and current, all ghostly terms from his dimly remembered past. All in all, pacemaker complications are nuisances, if not outright dangers.[53]

By the end of the decade, John Merideth routinely advised Mayo's surgeons on what type of pacemaker to implant, helped them test it before they closed the skin incisions, and relieved them of the responsibility of dealing with questions and problems that arose after a patient left the hospital.

The first permanent pacemakers, designed to prevent faints and save lives by sending an electrical impulse to the heart at a fixed rate (like a metronome), could occasionally end lives by triggering ventricular tachycardia or fibrillation. A new type of pacemaker marketed in 1968 was designed to avoid this problem. These so-called demand pacemakers included technology that could "sense" a patient's own spontaneous heartbeat. A pacemaker with this sensing function delivered a stimulus only after a preset period of time (measured in milliseconds) elapsed following a spontaneous or a paced beat. Longer battery life was another advantage of demand pacemakers. Patients welcomed this advance because it increased the interval between operations to replace the pulse generator when its batteries were close to running down.[54]

Merideth established a weekly Pacemaker Clinic at Mayo in 1971 to facilitate the follow-up of patients with the devices. They came to the special clinic (which was located in the Heart Station near the cardiologists' outpatient offices) to have their pacemakers tested for evidence of battery depletion or other problems.[55] Shortly after Robert Frye became head of the Cardiovascular Division in 1974, he appointed Merideth as director of a new pacemaker-electrophysiology group. In addition to Merideth, this subspecialty team that focused on heart rhythm disorders included CCU director Paul O'Donovan and James Maloney, who had just finished his cardiology fellowship. One of these three cardiologists was present for each permanent pacemaker implantation, and they shared responsibility for overseeing the Pacemaker Clinic. Frye informed the chief of medicine in 1975 that this new arrangement was "essential to ensure high quality care for patients requiring permanent pacemakers" and that it had "the strong support of the cardiovascular surgeons, who are responsible for the actual placement of these pacemaker systems."[56]

The importance of routine follow-up of patients with permanent pacemakers had become increasingly clear during the early 1970s, when manufacturers recalled some devices because of problems with the pulse generator or electrodes. This required a patient to undergo an additional, unplanned procedure, which caused concern at several levels.[57] In this context, President Gerald Ford signed the Medical Device Amendments of 1976 into law. When he signed the legislation, the president explained:

> Medical and diagnostic devices have produced a therapeutic revolution, but in doing so they have also become more complex and less easily understood by those who use them. When well designed, well made, and properly used they support and lengthen life. If poorly designed, poorly made, and improperly used they can threaten and impair it. Despite the increasing importance of devices, the Food and Drug Administration has had inadequate authority to deal with them. FDA has had no reliable way of knowing how many devices there are, who is making them, who is selling them, what risks to health and life they may present, and when a manufacturer has found it necessary to remove them from the medical marketplace. In addition, no device was required to be proven safe and effective prior to marketing, no matter how crucial it might be to the person using it, even if that use involved implantation in his body.... The Medical Device Amendments of 1976 eliminate the deficiencies that accorded FDA "horse and buggy" authority to deal with "laser age" problems.[58]

The law had important implications for cardiologists and cardiac surgeons, whose complementary fields were being redefined by new technologies.

Cardiologists Assume More Responsibility for Pacemakers

By the mid-1970s, Mayo's cardiac surgeons were busy performing coronary bypass operations and valve replacements on adult patients in addition to maintaining their high-volume congenital heart disease practice. This contributed to a shift in responsibility for pacemaker implantation from surgeons to cardiologists at the institution. James Maloney and David Holmes, who was in his final year of fellowship, began implanting pacemakers in 1976. They threaded the pacing catheter electrode through a vein and into the right ventricle. Next, they connected the electrode's external end to a pulse generator that was placed in a pocket under the skin. This pocket was fashioned by dissecting the subcutaneous tissue off the dense layer of fascia (fibrous tissue) that covered the anterior chest muscle below the clavicle (collarbone). When the incision was closed, the pacemaker caused a telltale bulge under a patient's skin.

Mayo cardiologist James Broadbent, who began implanting pacemakers in 1977, recalled, "The pacemaker business became onerous for the surgeons. They really didn't want to be involved in it. First of all, they didn't mind the surgery. They didn't mind cutting and sewing. They just didn't want to fiddle with the catheters [electrodes]. They didn't want to program the pacemaker. They didn't want to follow up patients. They wanted to cut and close and turn it over to somebody else."[59]

Dwight McGoon informed Mayo's chief of surgery: "One of the urgent items commanding our attention during 1977 has been an attempt to solve the problem of personnel to accept the responsibility for pacemaker implantation. This has been the function of our surgical residents, which is no longer a satisfactory solution because the demand for services exceeds the requirements for training of residents and because of a lack of continuity in the expertise and practice in this important area."[60] Within a year, cardiologists in Mayo's pacemaker-electrophysiology group had assumed responsibility for implanting the devices.[61]

James Maloney replaced John Merideth as head of the pacemaker-electrophysiology group in 1978. He sent his first annual summary of its activities to cardiology chief Robert Frye the following year. The fifty-eight-page report was filled with data and diagrams detailing the group's recent accomplishments and justifying his requests for more staff, space, and equipment. Maloney boasted that Mayo physicians and surgeons had implanted 336 pacemakers in 1978, which he claimed was the third highest number of any institution in the nation. He also described the challenges of caring for patients with serious heart rhythm disorders and keeping up with new developments in the twin fields of pacing and cardiac electrophysiology.[62] In a 1978 letter to the chair of medicine, Frye praised the pacemaker-electrophysiology group for providing "the most current advances in care for our patients and attracting physician referrals of difficult cardiac rhythm problems."[63]

In a 1980 publication on the analysis of pacemaker functions, Merideth stressed the importance of having a "thorough knowledge of the technical characteristics of the particular pacemaker implanted in a particular patient." But he conceded that this was very difficult because "the field has developed so rapidly that much information is outdated by the time it is published."[64] In fact, cardiologists (to say nothing of internists) found it impossible to keep up with all of the new technologies and concepts that were transforming the care of patients with heart disease. Depending on the doctor and the context, subspecialization seemed to offer a solution. Gerald Lemole, the chief of cardiac surgery at New Jersey's Deborah Heart and Lung Center, claimed in 1983 that the current "age of technology has procreated an era of super specialists."[65]

In 1979 Mayo cardiologists began implanting a new type of pacemaker that incorporated a so-called multiparameter-programmable pulse generator. This tongue-twisting term reflected the increasing flexibility of pacemakers, which made it possible to match some their functions to the specific needs of an individual patient. But no cardiologist could comprehend all of the complex physical, mathematical, and physiological principles that related to the functions or parameters that might be programmed into some new pacemakers, such as rate, voltage/current, pulse width, sensitivity, refractory period, hysteresis, mode, and telemetry.[66]

The problem was compounded by the fact that most doctors who implanted pacemakers had very limited experience with the technology. Victor Parsonnet complained in 1982 that pacemakers were being "implanted by almost any physician who claims to have the technical skills to do so, regardless of specialty or training." A survey suggested that about 5,600 doctors had implanted permanent pacemakers in more than 100,000 patients in the United States the previous year.[67] Pacemakers had become very big business by 1980, when the three largest American manufacturers (Medtronic, Cordis, and Intermedics) had combined sales of almost $500 million.[68]

David Hayes was the first Mayo cardiologist to receive extensive formal pacemaker training from experts in the field. He developed an interest in the technology in 1979 during his cardiology fellowship. Maloney mentored Hayes and encouraged him to evaluate the clinic's early experience with multiparameter-programmable pacemakers. Hayes presented a summary of the initial indications, clinical efficacy, and reliability of the devices in one hundred patients at the 1981 meeting of the North American Society of Pacing and Electrophysiology. The organization had been founded two years earlier by individuals especially interested in heart rhythm disorders. Its creation was a manifestation of progressive subspecialization in cardiology.[69] Hayes's debut before an audience that included many pacing pioneers was auspicious; he won second prize in the 1981 Young Investigator Award Competition.[70]

Maloney helped arrange for Hayes to spend the spring of 1982 with pacemaker pioneer Seymour Furman at Montefiore Hospital in the Bronx. The following year, he spent three months working in Paris with Jacques Mugica, who had the largest experience with pacemakers in Europe.[71] When Hayes returned to Rochester, he assumed a major role in Mayo's pacemaker program. One of his first initiatives involved granting more autonomy to the nurses who worked in the Pacemaker Clinic. Mayo's cardiologists benefited from the institution's tradition of training nurses and other non-physician staff to do specialized tasks under a doctor's supervision. Nurse Sharon

Neubauer had helped Merideth launch a telephone monitoring service for outpatient pacemaker checks in 1977.[72]

The following year, the service was offered around-the-clock to non-Mayo physicians. Patient visits and call volume grew steadily. By 1982, four nurses worked in the Pacemaker Clinic, and they evaluated as many as twenty patients a day. Neubauer explained in an interview for the clinic's newsletter: "This call is from Saint Marys Hospital, but it could have been from Uruguay or Turkey. Our patients are everywhere."[73] By subspecializing, these nurses became educators and troubleshooters in the dynamic field of pacemakers.

Concerns About the Cost of and Indications for Pacemakers

In 1983 Parsonnet summarized concerns that had arisen after two decades of pacemaker development: "Ordinarily such an advance would be a source of pride, much as we have been proud of technologic progress in other fields, from cars to space satellites and from adding machines to supercomputers. However, as with supersonic transport, the space shuttle and home computers, questions now arise concerning usefulness, applicability, and cost."[74] The context was important. That year, two leaders of the Robert Wood Johnson Foundation opened an article on health care costs with a sobering statement: "In American society today, the depressed state of our economy has led government at all levels, industry, labor, and, indeed, all sectors of our society to begin to place or plan for substantial restrictions on spending for medical care."[75] These considerations contributed to a movement to develop clinical practice guidelines as a strategy to rationalize care.[76]

The cost of heart care attracted increasing attention because so many men and women had cardiovascular disease and so many diagnostic tests and treatment technologies had been developed during the 1960s and 1970s. In 1980 the American College of Cardiology partnered with the American Heart Association to form a joint task force to assess cardiovascular procedures. Its charge was *very* ambitious: "The Task Force shall address, where appropriate, the contribution, uniqueness, sensitivity, specificity, indications, and contraindications, and cost-effectiveness of such specific procedures."[77] This general charge was published in a nine-page document, "Guidelines for Permanent Cardiac Pacemaker Implantation, May 1984," which a task force subcommittee chaired by Robert Frye had produced. It was the first of many practice guidelines that the two organizations would develop. The pacemaker guidelines included a date because the subcommittee knew that they would change as the technology evolved.

Two main concerns stimulated the development of the pacemaker guidelines: cost and appropriateness. Indiana University cardiologist Charles

Fisch, who was a member of the joint task force's pacemaker subcommittee, explained in a preamble to the 1984 guidelines: "It is becoming more apparent each day that despite a strong national commitment to excellence in health care, the resources and personnel are finite. It is, therefore, appropriate that the medical profession examine the impact of developing technology on the practice and cost of medical care. Such analysis, carefully conducted, could potentially impact the cost of medical care without diminishing the effectiveness of that care."[78]

During the development of the guidelines, Robert Frye suggested a classification scheme to help a doctor decide whether it was appropriate to implant a permanent pacemaker in a specific patient: "Class I: Conditions in which there is general agreement that permanent pacemakers should be implanted; Class II: Conditions in which permanent pacemakers are implanted but there is divergence of opinion with respect to the necessity of their insertion; and Class III: Conditions in which there is general agreement that pacemakers are not necessary." This basic classification scheme would become a feature of all guidelines developed by the American College of Cardiology and the American Heart Association.[79]

Many references in the pacemaker guidelines related to so-called His bundle studies, a catheter-based technique designed to evaluate how the heart's electrical impulse traveled from the atria to the ventricles. Wilhelm His Jr. was a medical professor at the University of Leipzig in 1893, when he published an article describing his discovery of a muscle bundle that connected the atria and the ventricles. His bundle studies, introduced in the late 1960s, would be a fundamental building block of electrophysiologic testing—a new invasive approach to enhance the diagnosis and management of heart block in selected patients.

Electrophysiologic testing involved placing electrode catheters inside a patient's heart to gather information about arrhythmias that could not be obtained from an electrocardiogram recorded from the body's surface. His bundle studies marked the birth of clinical cardiac electrophysiology. The word "clinical" was important because it highlighted the fact that some tools and techniques that scientists had used for decades to study the heart's electrical system in animals were migrating from research laboratories into the realm of patient care.[80]

Unraveling the Mysteries of Wolff-Parkinson-White Syndrome

Several pioneers of clinical cardiac electrophysiology focused on the problem of heart block, which could cause symptomatic bradycardia. Others were attracted to Wolff-Parkinson-White (WPW) syndrome, a rare condition that was defined by specific electrocardiographic abnormalities and sudden spells of tachycardia. The syndrome is named for Louis Wolff and Paul Dudley White of Boston and John Parkinson of London. These cardiologists coauthored a 1930 article that reported several patients with recurrent episodes of tachycardia (with heart rates above 150 beats per minute) associated with two electrocardiographic abnormalities: a bundle branch block pattern and a short P-R interval.[81]

Mayo cardiologist Fredrick Willius reviewed WPW syndrome in 1946, when he reported on sixty-five electrocardiograms recorded at Mayo that revealed a wide QRS complex and short P-R interval. Noting that many hypotheses had been advanced to explain these electrocardiographic abnormalities, Willius cited compelling evidence that they were a reflection of "accessory pathways of conduction."[82] This is a complicated subject, and the mechanisms were debated for decades. Basically, if the heart's electrical impulse travels through an abnormal accessory pathway rather than through the His bundle, it reaches the ventricles earlier than normal—hence the term "pre-excitation."[83]

Howard Burchell was especially intrigued by the WPW syndrome and concept of pre-excitation. In 1956 he moderated a session on the spread of the electrical impulse through heart muscle at a symposium on cardiac electrophysiology in New York City. His research on the subject had been undertaken in animals, but Burchell was also interested in heart rhythm disorders in patients.[84] The symposium's impact on the embryonic field of clinical cardiac electrophysiology was far greater than he or any other of the participants could have imagined. It played a significant role in stimulating the development of several new technologies and procedures, such as computerized electrocardiography, the "mapping" of abnormal heart rhythms, and arrhythmia surgery.[85]

On May 18, 1967, Howard Burchell and Robert Frye stood in an operating room at Saint Marys Hospital, where Dwight McGoon would perform a novel procedure on a man with WPW syndrome. The forty-three-year-old mail carrier had come to Mayo nine months earlier for evaluation of increasingly frequent episodes of rapid heart action. His spells of tachycardia, which lasted from several minutes to a few hours, always began and ended suddenly. Although the mail carrier had passed out just once, he had almost fainted many times. His doctors in Indiana had diagnosed WPW syndrome. Burchell agreed, but he also concluded that the patient had an atrial septal defect.[86] He recommended an elective operation to close the congenital defect, a procedure that had been performed hundreds of times in Rochester. On August 15, 1966, Burchell wrote in the man's medical record, "I wonder whether [this] situation [is] not ideal to plan exploration of the ventricle and right side of the septum by electrodes at time of surgery. The paroxysmal tachycardia [is] not of sufficient severity to justify an attempt to interrupt the preexcitation pathway in light of present knowledge."[87]

When Burchell wrote this note, no one had published an article describing the procedures he mentioned: recording electrical activity from the outer and inner surfaces of the heart in a patient with WPW syndrome and interrupting the abnormal connection thought to be responsible for the spells of tachycardia. But Burchell had recently become editor of the American Heart Association's journal *Circulation*, and he was aware of an unpublished report of a diagnostic procedure that was relevant to his patient's problem. He had read a manuscript submitted by his friend Dirk Durrer, a Dutch cardiologist who was a world leader of electrophysiology. The article from Amsterdam would be published in the January 1967 issue of the journal, four months before the man from Indiana returned to Rochester for surgery to close his atrial septal defect.[88]

Shortly after McGoon started the operation in the spring of 1967, the anesthetized patient developed short bursts of tachycardia. McGoon moved a recording electrode across the surface of his heart to produce a series of electrograms that Frye recorded on an electrocardiograph machine. Burchell was one of very few cardiologists in the world who knew how to piece the tracings together in his mind in order to create a map of the abnormal path that the heart's electrical impulse traveled. Next, McGoon injected a local anesthetic into the region of the right ventricular wall that Burchell thought contained the abnormal connection (termed a Kent bundle). This resulted in the disappearance of the telltale delta wave on the electrocardiogram. The surgeon then made a one-centimeter incision inside the right atrium in an attempt to cut the Kent bundle. It seemed to be successful—but for just a few minutes.

When McGoon closed the chest incision, the delta wave (reflecting pre-excitation) reappeared on the patient's electrocardiogram. Burchell wrote in the record shortly after surgery, "Tantalizing to have been so close to cure of W.P.W. but it did not seem proper to jeopardize to the least extent the primary surgical objective. Dr. Frye and I will write up an extended report on findings."[89] Their report, published in *Circulation* six months after the operation, concluded, "Our study indicates the feasibility of a surgical approach to the treatment of some varieties of the preexcitation (WPW) syndrome."[90] Although McGoon's small incision did not cure the mail carrier's WPW syndrome, his attempt contributed to a North Carolina surgeon's decision to try the procedure on another patient.

Duke University surgeon Will Sealy performed the first successful operation to treat WPW syndrome in 1968. He described the context and consequences of the procedure three decades later: "The beginnings of clinical electrophysiology and arrhythmia surgery at Duke coincided with the 25 years (1950–1975) that were the golden years of medical research.... Research money was plentiful and seemingly inexhaustible. Space was available and expanding. Clinical demands on doctors were reasonable and controllable."[91]

Sealy's story of the first patient treated surgically for an arrhythmia had a Mayo connection. A thirty-two-year-old commercial fisherman was unable to work because he had frequent spells of tachycardia due to WPW syndrome. During the patient's evaluation at Duke, senior cardiology fellow Frederick Cobb asked Sealy about the possibility of performing a novel operation because all drug treatments had failed to control the man's episodes of rapid heart action. Sealy recalled, "Shortly before this time, at the Mayo Clinic, Doctors Howard Burchell and Dwight McGoon identified an accessory pathway by surface mapping.... Conduction was blocked temporarily with procaine. With this information, Fred presented the case for operating to [cardiologists] Andy Wallace, John Boineau, and me."[92] The operation was a success.

The passion of several individuals at Duke who collaborated in the development of clinical electrophysiology and arrhythmia surgery around 1970 was analogous to the situation that had existed at Mayo in the mid-1950s, when a multidisciplinary team pioneered open-heart surgery. Just as Rochester had become a magnet for patients with congenital heart disease, Durham would become an international center for patients with cardiac arrhythmias. John Boineau recalled that once this reputation spread, "WPW was as common at Duke as the smell of tobacco in the Durham warehouses. Patients came from all over."[93]

What happened to arrhythmia surgery in Rochester? Years later, Burchell wrote to Mayo surgeon Gordon Danielson, "It might be wondered why we did not pursue the problem with surgical treatment at the clinic. The main reason was we did not have the recording and stimulating equipment that they had at Duke, which [as] you know, is important regarding hazards and the need for immediate read-out records. I referred two early Duke cases to them."[94] Burchell focused on the lack of state-of-the-art technology, but he did not mention other local factors, such as individual time pressures and institutional priorities.

At a time when Sealy considered the clinical demands on Duke's doctors "reasonable and controllable," Mayo's cardiologists were still required to perform thousands of general diagnostic examinations each year in addition to their heart-related work. Cardiologists who were hired as full-time faculty members at traditional academic medical centers devoted little (if any) of their time to general medical diagnosis. After completing their training, they had been hired to function as subspecialists. And almost all of these academic cardiologists had protected time for research.[95]

Mayo also lost momentum in the emerging field of clinical electrophysiology when Burchell left Rochester to become chief of cardiology at the University of Minnesota in January 1968, two months after he had coauthored the paper on WPW syndrome with McGoon and Frye.[96] In 1969 cardiologist Thomas James, who worked with former Mayo surgeon John Kirklin at the University of Alabama in Birmingham, declared, "In a very real sense one may look on the Wolff-Parkinson-White (WPW) syndrome as the Rosetta stone of electro-cardiography, since a full understanding of all its features and their possible mechanisms encompasses many fundamentally important principles."[97]

The Development of Clinical Cardiac Electrophysiology

When Will Sealy began operating on patients with WPW syndrome at Duke in 1968, he mapped the heart's electrical activity by moving a recording elec-trode over its outer surface, just as McGoon had done at Mayo. The follow-ing year, physiologist Benjamin Scherlag and his clinical colleagues at the US Public Health Service Hospital in Staten Island, New York, published an article that described a technique for recording the heart's electrical activ-ity from *inside* the beating organ. Their procedure, which did not require opening a patient's chest, heralded the advent of modern clinical cardiac electrophysiology.

The Staten Island group used a specially shaped electrode catheter to record electrical impulses from the His bundle.[98] Scherlag later recalled Burchell's crucial role in getting their article published in the journal *Circulation*:

> The reviewers' comments were highly critical and ranged from too few patients studied [ten] to frank disbelief in the ability to record from such a small structure as the His bundle with an electrode catheter. Dr. Burchell...apologized for the harsh criticism leveled by the reviewers and indicated that the paper on the His bundle technique...would be acceptable for publication with some revisions. In closing, Dr. Burchell prophetically indicated that, contrary to the several reviewers' comments, he believed the His bundle recording technique would become a "standard reference."[99]

Two months before the article appeared in print, Burchell told attendees at the American Heart Association's annual meeting: "As most of you know, I was appointed editor [of *Circulation*] a couple of years ago. Editors may be compared to judges in the courts; they decide on the admission of evidence." Burchell did not mention one major difference: an editor can overrule manu-script reviewers, but under ordinary circumstances a judge cannot overrule a jury verdict. His decision to publish the Staten Island group's manuscript in the world's most prestigious cardiology journal brought the His bundle technique to the attention of a large audience of heart specialists.[100] In 1971 Dutch cardiologist Hein Wellens, a pioneer of clinical cardiac electrophysiol-ogy, claimed that Scherlag's article had very practical implications for patient care because it described "a method to record His bundle activity in man in a systematic reproducible way."[101]

James Maloney launched Mayo's clinical cardiac electrophysiology program in 1972, when he performed the first His bundle study on a patient in Rochester. Pediatric cardiology fellow Ehud Krongrad had planned to perform His bundle studies at Mayo, but he left to begin a research fellowship in New York City before the clinic's Engineering Department had finished building the necessary equipment. When the apparatus was available, Maloney began doing His bundle studies in the operating room on patients who were undergoing surgery for congenital heart disease. The goal of these intra-operative electrophysiology studies, which were done with Dwight McGoon or Gordon Danielson, was to identify areas where a suture might cause heart block. Soon, Maloney began doing His bundle studies in adults in the catheterization laboratory or the coronary care unit's procedure room. The main purpose was to evaluate asymptomatic adults with electrocardiographic evidence of abnormal cardiac conduction to help decide whether an individual patient needed a permanent pacemaker.[102]

As the number of His bundle studies increased at Mayo, Maloney encouraged cardiology fellow Geoffrey Hartzler to join him in the emerging field of clinical electrophysiology. John Merideth, who directed the pacemaker-electrophysiology group, boasted in his 1977 report that "the quality of their work is excellent." He noted that growing experience with new invasive catheter-based electrophysiology techniques was expanding the scope of their studies—beyond the evaluation of patients with heart block and bradycardia to those with ventricular tachycardia, a potentially life-threatening arrhythmia.[103] Hartzler and Maloney had just published their experience with programmed ventricular stimulation, a technique that Hein Wellens and Dirk Durrer had developed in Amsterdam. The Mayo cardiologists' matter-of-fact description of the catheter-based procedure did not reflect its extreme complexity:

> Electrophysiologic studies were performed with standard techniques. The approach was modified for individual cases, although most studies included the following methods. A tripolar electrode catheter was positioned across the tricuspid valve for recording the low septal-right atrial, His bundle, and high right interventricular septal electrograms. A quadripolar electrode catheter was positioned high in the right atrium for stimulating and recording. Bipolar or quadripolar electrode catheters were positioned in the coronary sinus and right ventricular apex for recording and stimulation.[104]

The four special electrode catheters positioned at very specific locations inside a patient's heart told only part of the story. These complex electrophysiology studies usually lasted several hours. If the goal was to try to identify a combination of medications to control spells of ventricular tachycardia, a patient would usually have to spend many hours on a hard X-ray table in the laboratory during repeat visits over two or more days.

Hartzler and Maloney's 1977 jargon-filled article described this complicated drug-testing approach. Seeking an effective combination, they administered lidocaine, procainamide, propranolol, phenytoin, quinidine, and digoxin to a patient sequentially over a 36-hour period.[105] Two years later, Hartzler acknowledged that "drug-resistant, chronic, recurrent ventricular tachycardia is frustrating for both patient and physician. Repeated and prolonged hospital admissions, DC [direct current] cardioversions, and multiple drugs and drug trials with their attendant side effects take a physical, psychologic, and financial toll."[106] These factors contributed to the slow diffusion of clinical cardiac electrophysiology procedures into practice.

Electrophysiology's National and Local Growing Pains

Very few cardiologists wanted to be involved in these extraordinarily time-consuming and complex procedures that involved causing ventricular tachycardia in order to identify a drug regimen that might suppress it. Moreover, the role of these invasive catheter-based tests in patient care was still evolving. The title of a 1982 editorial by Indiana University electrophysiologist Borys Surawicz made the point: "Intracardiac Extrastimulation Studies: How To? Where? By Whom?"[107] He did not ask a question that was on the minds of many physicians: On Whom? These questions were not unique to clinical cardiac electrophysiology. They arose each time innovators pushed a promising new technique or technology out of the close confines of the animal laboratory into the real-world realm of clinical practice.

San Francisco cardiologist Elliot Rapaport, who edited a 1980 book on controversies in cardiology, worked with cardiac electrophysiology pioneer Melvin Scheinman. Speaking of Scheinman, Rapaport confessed that he "admired the sophistication brought to the studies he performs and the information that he has contributed to our understanding of conduction disturbances and arrhythmias." But shifting his gaze away from the local scene, Rapaport complained about the "overutilization of electrophysiologic studies in clinical practice today." He argued that "too many asymptomatic patients have had permanent pacemakers inserted . . . based upon demonstrated electrophysiologic abnormalities, despite the fact that there is lack of proof that such management prolongs life."[108]

In addition to subjective impressions about the role of invasive electrophysiology procedures in patient care, there were objective logistical issues that slowed their diffusion into practice. Compared to coronary angioplasty, for example, clinical electrophysiology testing with multiple electrode catheters required sophisticated electronic recording apparatus and much more training. Like most major innovations in the care of patients with cardiac disease, younger heart specialists developed the field—often as an extension of research or clinical activities they had begun during their cardiology fellowships.

James Maloney and Geoffrey Hartzler were in their early thirties when they launched Mayo's invasive cardiac electrophysiology program. Their peers perceived them as brilliant, ambitious, and very strong willed. Many of the innovators and pioneers of heart care technologies and techniques exhibited these traits. Examples include Earl Wood in catheterization, Walt Lillehei in open-heart surgery, Mason Sones in coronary angiography, and Andreas Grüntzig in coronary angioplasty. This combination of personality traits contributed to Maloney and Hartzler's success in introducing cutting-edge electrophysiology procedures into the Mayo practice, but it also strained their relationship.

Maloney recalled that "some friction and some conflict" had developed between them by 1979, when Robert Frye, hoping "to resolve some of this conflict, came up with the solution that pacing and electrophysiology should be separated." Maloney was frustrated that the scope of his leadership role had been reduced.[109] Before long, both men left the Mayo Clinic. Hartzler, who had become involved in the emerging technique of coronary angioplasty in addition to remaining very active in electrophysiology, joined the Mid-America Heart Institute in Kansas City, Missouri, in 1980. Maloney joined the Cleveland Clinic the following year.

After Hartzler and Maloney left Rochester, Robert Frye appointed David Holmes as the director of Mayo's pacing-electrophysiology group. Shortly thereafter, Duke electrophysiologist Edward Pritchett visited the clinic. When Pritchett (who had gone to college with Holmes) returned to North Carolina, he told Duke junior faculty member Stephen Hammill that Mayo appeared to offer an excellent opportunity for a formally trained electrophysiologist. Hammill visited Rochester and recalls being "thoroughly impressed with Mayo from the start." Coming from a research-oriented academic institution, Hammill was pleasantly surprised by the many systems that the clinic had designed to facilitate efficient patient care.[110]

In 1981 Hammill joined Mayo's busy pacing-electrophysiology group, which included Bernard Gersh, Michael Osborn, and Ronald Vlietstra, all of whom had joined the staff recently. David Holmes directed the arrhythmia program, but he would soon become more involved in coronary angioplasty. Holmes describes this as a magical time when he and his Mayo colleagues were "pushing the envelope in all directions" as they participated in the development of clinical cardiac electrophysiology and coronary angioplasty.[111]

Ronald Vlietstra, who was very interested in cardiac pharmacology, helped Mayo's cardiologists and their patients gain access to experimental drugs that were being developed to treat heart rhythm disorders. The FDA expected pharmaceutical companies to prove that any drug they had developed and hoped to sell was effective *and* safe. Clinical trials were designed to provide the necessary data, and Mayo participated in several of them. Nurse Julianne Osborn was hired in 1981 as a "cardiovascular drug assistant" to help cardiologists involved in investigational drug protocols, to enhance communication with patients enrolled in these studies, and to educate nurses about the medications.[112] These activities were important because some recently released or investigational anti-arrhythmic drugs reduced the frequency of attacks of tachycardia, but they had side effects that ranged from minor issues to potentially life-threatening problems.[113] The lack of drugs that were both effective and safe encouraged a few electrophysiologists to develop new approaches to attempt to cure some arrhythmias.

Treating Spells of Rapid Heart Action With "Catheter Ablation"

In 1982 the Duke electrophysiology group published an article describing a new catheter-based treatment for patients with recurring spells of dizziness due to episodes of supraventricular tachycardia (a phrase that refers to heart rhythm disorders that originate above the level of the ventricles). Some of these patients had WPW, and others had atrial fibrillation or atrial flutter with a very rapid ventricular rate that could cause a drop in blood pressure and a variety of symptoms. The authors explained: "Patients with recurrent supraventricular tachyarrhythmias occasionally become disabled because available pharmacologic agents are ineffective or poorly tolerated, and pacemaker techniques fail to control recurrences."[114]

The new approach, termed catheter ablation, was developed as an alternative to the open-heart operation that Will Sealy had pioneered at Duke a dozen years earlier. It was designed to ablate (permanently interrupt) the His bundle so it could no longer transmit the heart's electrical impulse from the atria to the ventricles. First, an electrophysiologist sent a short burst of strong shocks from a defibrillator through an electrode catheter to a specific region inside the heart to damage the His bundle. If the ablation was successful, the patient developed complete heart block that would be treated with a permanent pacemaker.[115]

A dozen years after electrophysiologists introduced catheter ablation, Will Sealy described its implications: "During the explosive growth of cardiac surgery in the 1960s, I became interested in the surgical treatment of cardiac arrhythmias. Unfortunately, most of the procedures soon became obsolete because of better [catheter-based] operations developed by cardiologists." Some surgeons were frustrated about losing patients to cardiologists who performed catheter-based treatments that were far less invasive than the traditional open-heart surgery alternative. The arrhythmia situation mirrored (on a much smaller scale) the decrease in coronary bypass surgery that resulted from the development of coronary angioplasty. Sealy was philosophical about the rise and decline of arrhythmia surgery: "My experience with an operation that I helped to develop and that became obsolete was the most rewarding event in my life. The information gathered from my studies contributed to the development of a better procedure by my colleagues, the electrophysiologists."[116] But there was an important difference between coronary bypass surgery and arrhythmia surgery. Almost every heart surgeon performed the bypass operation, but very few attempted to treat arrhythmias.

Stephen Hammill performed Mayo's first catheter ablation for an arrhythmia on July 22, 1982, six months after his former Duke colleagues published their results with the procedure. The patient was a twenty-five-year-old woman with a four-year history of fainting spells due to paroxysmal supraventricular tachycardia that had not responded to standard or experimental drugs. The ablation was successful, but as expected she needed a pacemaker. Five cardiologists coauthored an article summarizing Mayo's experience with the new technique in 1983. Its opening paragraph described the problem and a potential solution: "Patients with disabling supraventricular tachycardias refractory to medical treatment or use of antitachycardia pacing devices (or both) may require interruption [ablation] of the atrioventricular conduction system and implantation of a permanent pacemaker for effective control of their arrhythmia. In the past, the only reliable technique for interruption of atrioventricular conduction was a cardiac surgical procedure."[117]

Melvin Scheinman, a catheter ablation pioneer, wrote an editorial to accompany the Mayo article. The San Francisco electrophysiologist noted that the major objection to the procedure was "that the clinician in effect substitutes pacemaker-dependent complete atrioventricular block for drug-refractory tachyarrhythmias." Scheinman thought the trade-off made sense in selected patients: "The report by [Douglas] Wood and associates supports the observations by others of the effectiveness of catheter ablation for control of tachycardia. These reports might well portend the beginning of an exciting new era in interventional electrophysiologic treatment."[118] Scheinman was right—they did.

Mayo's cardiologists responded to the introduction of procedures and technologies for the diagnosis and treatment of heart rhythm disorders in ways that sociologists interested in the diffusion of innovations would predict. For example, James Maloney, Geoffrey Hartzler, David Holmes, and Stephen Hammill were early adopters. Maloney recalled that some of their senior colleagues were "very helpful and very understanding of what we were doing." But others were very skeptical about invasive electrophysiology, believing that it "really didn't have much of a role" in patient care.[119] Hammill considered Ralph Smith one of the hardest individuals to convince: "He was a superb electrocardiographer, great with rhythms, but he just did not see a need for invasive electrophysiology." Hammill also described a phenomenon that stimulated the development of electrophysiology as a subspecialty at Mayo and elsewhere. Some cardiologists "hated arrhythmias, just didn't want to have to deal with them. So they were glad to have you deal with them."[120] This attitude became increasingly prevalent among practitioners as ever more complex diagnostic and treatment technologies for arrhythmias were introduced.

Saving Lives With an Automatic Implantable Defibrillator

Supraventricular arrhythmias could cause unpleasant symptoms, but they rarely resulted in syncope or sudden death. On the other hand, ventricular fibrillation was always fatal unless it was treated immediately. The defibrillator, an electronic device designed to shock a patient's heart out of this life-ending arrhythmia, had been a key catalyst for the development of the coronary care unit concept in the early 1960s.[121] This care model involved placing a vulnerable patient in a unique hospital environment staffed by specially trained personnel and equipped with life-saving electronic technologies. A hospitalized patient who had a cardiac arrest due to ventricular fibrillation would die unless the arrhythmia was identified immediately, cardiopulmonary resuscitation (CPR) was started within about four minutes, and a doctor or nurse shocked his or her heart back into a stable rhythm. If a person who was not hospitalized had a cardiac arrest, he or she had almost no chance of surviving.[122] One man became obsessed with developing a technology to address the deadly problem of spontaneous ventricular fibrillation.

Michel Mirowski, a European-born cardiologist who practiced at Sinai Hospital in Baltimore, a community hospital affiliated with Johns Hopkins, worked tirelessly throughout the 1970s to develop an automatic defibrillator that could be implanted into a patient, much like a permanent pacemaker.[123] The word "automatic" was critical to the concept of an implantable defibrillator, which was designed to deliver a life-saving shock to a patient's heart— anytime, anywhere, and without any human intervention. Two of Mirowski's collaborators described the main challenges he faced: "struggles to obtain development funds, difficulties in finding the scientific talent needed to develop working models, the continuous efforts to gain scientific acceptance of the concept, challenges to the veracity of the research data, and even challenges of the ethics of implanting a defibrillation device in a patient."[124]

The first automatic implantable defibrillator was placed in a fifty-seven-year-old woman at the Johns Hopkins Hospital on February 4, 1980. Levi Watkins Jr., who had completed his surgical training at the institution seven months earlier, performed the procedure with the assistance of Vincent Gott, the chief of cardiac surgery.[125] A 1982 article in *Ebony* magazine focused on Watkins, who was the "first Black to enter and graduate from Vanderbilt University School of Medicine...[and] the first Black to enter and complete a residency at Johns Hopkins."[126] The writer who profiled Watkins in *Ebony* magazine explained the deadly problem that the automatic implantable defibrillator was designed to treat:

> Often it happens without warning. The unknowing victim—standing at a bus stop, sitting at a desk or maybe running around the block—begins to lose consciousness. A curious quiver of the heart has started and it will last only two or three minutes before the person—if left untreated—drops dead. Each year, nearly a half million people are stricken by these strange quivers known as ventricular fibrillation, an arrhythmia which keeps the heart from pumping blood.... Until recently, the only victims who would live to talk about the experience were those who were stricken miraculously near medical professionals with defibrillating pads that can be used to shock a patient back to life. Few have been that lucky.[127]

The original implantable defibrillator operations involved inserting an electrode catheter into a patient's left internal jugular vein and positioning its tip inside the heart and placing a "defibrillating electrode" on the organ's outer surface. The surgeon made a tunnel under the skin so these two electrodes could be connected to a titanium-cased defibrillator generator. This device, the size of a cigarette pack, was inserted in a pocket fashioned under the skin of a patient's abdomen.

The *Ebony* writer explained, "Priced in the neighborhood of a mid-size car, the $7,000 device must be replaced after three years or 100 shocks, whichever comes first."[128] Readers of the magazine were told not to expect it to arrive at their local hospital anytime soon. In 1982, two years after the first defibrillator was implanted at Hopkins, the FDA had approved only one other institution to conduct a clinical trial—Stanford University.

Mayo electrophysiologists Bernard Gersh and Michael Osborn were in a Saint Marys Hospital operating room on October 31, 1984, when cardiac surgeon Hartzell Schaff (who had trained with Vincent Gott at Hopkins) implanted the first automatic defibrillator in Rochester. The patient was a sixty-one-year-old woman from South Dakota who had a history of congestive heart failure and had been resuscitated after several in-hospital cardiac arrests. During her hospitalization at Saint Marys, she was found to have extensive coronary artery disease and severely reduced left ventricular function. Despite receiving anti-arrhythmic drugs, including the experimental agent amiodarone, she continued to have episodes of ventricular tachycardia. The patient underwent coronary bypass surgery, but a postoperative electrophysiology study revealed that she was still very vulnerable to ventricular tachycardia. The defibrillator functioned properly during this study, and she was discharged nine days after surgery. Despite the operation to improve her heart's blood supply and the device to protect her from sudden death, she died in South Dakota six weeks after surgery as a result of congestive heart failure.[129]

A Patient Describes the Challenges of Surviving Sudden Death

Lawyer William Nehmer Jr. wrote a humorous book about the events that culminated in the implantation of his automatic defibrillator in January 1985.[130] The fifty-eight-year-old man's story began the previous April, when he had a cardiac arrest at the Milwaukee airport. He was resuscitated by two cardiologists (who were traveling with him) and three paramedics, who used a portable defibrillator to shock his heart back into rhythm. Nehmer underwent an emergency angioplasty to open a blocked coronary artery and was discharged from the hospital, taking a drug designed to reduce his risk of a recurrent arrhythmia. Just before Christmas, he had a cardiac arrest at a YMCA, where he was resuscitated again. His cardiologists at the Milwaukee County Hospital Complex recommended a trial of investigational anti-arrhythmic drugs. "No point in referring to the specific drugs at this time," Nehmer joked, "because by the time you read this book there will be new drugs with new names."[131]

The research protocols for the experimental drugs that Nehmer's doctors hoped would stabilize his heart rhythm required repeated electrophysiology studies in Milwaukee. During these tests, a cardiologist sent pulses of electricity into his heart through an electrode catheter in an attempt to trigger ventricular fibrillation. If the drug was effective, there would be no fibrillation. Nehmer was not so lucky. "Oops! This time they got the fibrillation started, and my heart was off to the races. I felt a little warm, had a little trouble breathing. Suddenly there was no pulse and I 'died' again! They laid the [defibrillator] 'paddles' on my chest and shocked me back to life." Now, his doctors recommended trying other drugs for longer periods of time, which required ongoing hospitalization for rhythm monitoring and additional invasive tests. The lawyer became frustrated after another electrophysiology study showed that a new drug was not working: "Following this test, I momentarily considered leaving the hospital and taking my chances— and might have done so if they hadn't kept using the term 'sudden death syndrome'...I'm into a new drug again." After more drug failures, his doctors recommended an implantable defibrillator.[132]

Nehmer explained how his defibrillator worked: "When my heart starts to race uncontrollably, the sensors will alert the battery pack, which in turn will send a charge back to the heart and restore the beating or pumping of the heart to its normal rhythm—hopefully!" Two months after his forty-seven day hospitalization, he returned for a follow-up electrophysiology study. His cardiologist was able to trigger ventricular fibrillation, which caused him to pass out. "This time," Nehmer explained, "they relied on my implanted box to fire up, and it did. Now I know what it feels like, and more importantly that it does work (and in all probability will work again) when required." He ended his personal story by admitting, "I still seem to wonder more about tomorrow than I used to."[133] The middle-aged man, who had survived two out-of-hospital cardiac arrests, lived for twenty years after his defibrillator was implanted.

Automatic implantable defibrillators, like pacemakers, shrank in size and grew in sophistication over time. Technological and procedural innovations made it possible for non-surgeons to insert the devices into patients. In Rochester, cardiologist David Hayes implanted the first defibrillator that did not involve surgery to open the chest cavity on February 7, 1991.[134] This marked the beginning of a new era in device therapy for arrhythmias at Mayo. At the same time, new catheter-based techniques for treating other types of tachycardia were being developed. One of these involved sending low power radiofrequency current through a catheter to destroy abnormal electrical connections between the atria and ventricles.

Radiofrequency Ablation: A New Approach to an Old Problem

Douglas Packer had trained in electrophysiology at Duke, where he was on the staff until he joined the Mayo Clinic in 1989. The following year he submitted a protocol for radiofrequency catheter ablation of accessory pathways to the Cardiovascular Division's Clinical Practice and Quality Assurance Committee. Packer referred to the early experience of University of Oklahoma electrophysiologist Warren Jackman and others who had described the procedure's effectiveness. He explained that radiofrequency catheter ablation could benefit patients because it offered "the potential for an arrhythmia 'cure' at less cost, hospitalization time, and probably less risk than currently available surgical techniques. This is particularly critical at a time of increasing cost-consciousness. Furthermore, it allows us to remain competitive in both the regional and national setting."[135] Packer performed the first radiofrequency ablation at Mayo on November 19, 1990. Ten months later, a writer in *Prevention* magazine described the procedure for general readers:

> When you turn to the middle of the AM dial on your radio, all you'll probably hear is static. But for young patients suffering from deadly heart rhythms, it's music to their ears—and hearts. A new therapy

called radiofrequency ablation is...designed for people suffering from a deadly form of tachycardia, in which the organ beats up to 300 times per minute.... During the treatment, a thin wire catheter is inserted into veins in the leg and neck, x-ray images guide the catheter to the precise location in the heart where the problem—an extra tissue strand that causes the fast beats—lurks. There the catheter releases a series of pulses—coming from a generator set on the middle of the AM dial of radio frequency—that burns away the unwanted tissue. Patients feel only a mild sensation.[136]

Packer summarized the status of treating some types of heart rhythm disorders with ablation in 1996: "Judging from the development of techniques over the past five years, substantial further improvement in these treatment modalities can be expected in the near future. This kind of progress should, in turn, result in a decrease in morbidity and mortality from serious ventricular arrhythmias as well as improve the quality of life in patients with supraventricular tachycardias."[137] As the near future unfolded, Packer's optimistic appraisal would prove to be accurate.

Seeing the Heart

ECHOCARDIOGRAPHY AND OTHER
IMAGING TECHNOLOGIES

Cardiac catheterization and coronary angiography were powerful diagnostic tools, as described in earlier chapters. But they were invasive procedures that required putting a catheter into a patient's vein or artery and threading its tip into the heart or the vessels that supply the organ with blood. During the final third of the twentieth century, so-called noninvasive cardiac imaging techniques, such as echocardiography and nuclear cardiology, were developed.[1] Catheterization, although generally safe, could cause complications. In 1968 cardiologists Eugene Braunwald and Jeremy Swan co-edited the report of a multi-institutional study of catheterization. Separate chapters in the document dealt with specific complications, such as abnormal heart rhythms, blood vessel injuries, hemorrhage, stroke, and death. Although these complications were rare, they could not be ignored.[2] Understandably, there was interest in inventing noninvasive tests that provided clinically useful information about the heart's structure and function without the risks associated with catheter-based diagnostic procedures.

Echocardiography: Cardiac Ultrasound as a Diagnostic Tool

In the fall of 1968, four months after Eugene Braunwald and Jeremy Swan's report on cardiac catheterization appeared, Mayo cardiologist Thomas Schattenburg published an article describing how he had used echocardiography (cardiac ultrasound) to confirm the diagnosis of a tumor inside a thirty-three-year-old woman's heart. The non-malignant mass, a myxoma, was subsequently removed surgically, and she made a full recovery.[3] This was the first article published by a Mayo author on the new noninvasive cardiac diagnostic technique. Echocardiography had been inspired by mid-century developments in sonar technology and also by the industrial use of pulsed ultrasound (inaudible high-frequency sound) to detect flaws in manufactured metal products. Before ultrasound was applied to the heart, it had been used in obstetrics and also to create images of the brain, liver, and other organs.[4]

Echocardiography produces pictures of the heart by sending ultrasound waves into the organ from a handheld transducer placed on a patient's chest wall. The same transducer detects reflected ultrasound waves, and an echocardiograph machine transforms them into electrical signals that are displayed as a series of moving dots and lines on an oscilloscope screen. During the final third of the twentieth century, methods to create permanent records of these displays would evolve from Polaroid photographs, to printouts using strip-chart recorders, to videotape.

Cardiologist Inge Edler and physicist Hellmuth Hertz of Lund University in Sweden had published the first article on echocardiography in humans in 1954. Nine years later, cardiologist Claude Joyner and electrical engineer John Reid of the University of Pennsylvania coauthored the first North American article on cardiac ultrasound as a diagnostic tool.[5] Edler and Joyner published several more papers on echocardiography, but neither man had the evangelistic fervor necessary to inspire widespread interest in it. The histories of cardiology and cardiac surgery are replete with individuals who promoted innovations and inventions with missionary zeal. Examples include Mason Sones for coronary arteriography, René Favaloro for coronary bypass surgery, and Andreas Grüntzig for coronary angioplasty.[6]

Echocardiography's earliest and most effective evangelist took the stage in 1965. Harvey Feigenbaum, a thirty-three-year-old cardiologist at Indiana University in Indianapolis, was the first author of an article published that year that promoted cardiac ultrasound as a tool to diagnose pericardial effusion (an accumulation of fluid around the heart). Others had reported similar findings, but Feigenbaum's paper in the widely read *Journal of the American Medical Association* brought echocardiography to the attention of thousands of practitioners.[7] Depending on a pericardial effusion's size and rate of accumulation, it can interfere with cardiac function and, in rare instances, cause death by compressing the heart (pericardial tamponade).

In their article, the Indiana University group emphasized that echocardiography was simpler and safer than "more complicated diagnostic tests, such as cardiac catheterization, intravenous carbon dioxide determinations, angiocardiography, various scanning procedures using radioisotopes, or pericardiocentesis." They described the case of a very sick fourteen-year-old boy who had clinical findings suggestive of cardiac tamponade. The echocardiogram proved that there was a pericardial effusion, and the authors concluded that "the diagnosis was made at the bedside of a desperately ill patient using a procedure that was no more difficult than obtaining an electrocardiogram." The teenager had an operation to remove the fluid (which was due to an infection) and made a good recovery.[8]

Feigenbaum performed echocardiograms with an Ekoline 20 Diagnostic Ultrasonoscope, which the Smith Kline Instrument Company first sold in 1963. The Philadelphia firm's marketing brochure claimed that it was "a practical diagnostic instrument for routine use by the cardiologist and the radiologist." Smith Kline also tried to appeal to academics by describing it as "an important research tool with unique value for studies of the cardiovascular system."[9] Despite such rhetoric, echocardiography spread slowly during the late 1960s. This was due, in large part, to the fact that the reflected ultrasound waves produced unique images of the heart's moving parts that were totally unfamiliar. One of the first tasks for Feigenbaum and other echocardiography pioneers was to produce collections of annotated cardiac ultrasound pictures with captions so doctors could understand what they were seeing.

Thomas Schattenberg Launches Echocardiography at Mayo

Harvey Feigenbaum promoted echocardiography by delivering lectures, publishing papers, and teaching practitioners how to perform the procedure and interpret the images that the technology produced. In 1968 he launched an annual course in Indianapolis that grew in popularity as early echocardiographers demonstrated that cardiac ultrasound could do more than detect a pericardial effusion or diagnose mitral valve stenosis. Thomas Schattenberg, who had joined the Mayo staff in 1964, saw Feigenbaum show slides and speak about echocardiography at a national meeting about three years later. "This is pretty exciting," he recalled thinking, "I'd like to get in on this."[10]

After returning to Rochester, Schattenberg learned that Mayo's neurosurgeons and neurologists were imaging patients' brains with the same Smith Kline instrument that Feigenbaum was using to study hearts.[11] He started to borrow their instrument when he or another Mayo heart specialist thought an echocardiogram might help clarify a patient's cardiac diagnosis. Cardiology section head Milton Anderson informed the Board of Governors in 1969: "Dr. Schattenberg continues to have an interest in echocardiography and is called upon by his colleagues when that device is of diagnostic importance."[12]

The establishment of a formal echocardiography program had to await the purchase of an instrument and the identification of a room in which to use it on a routine basis. The space problem was solved in 1969, when the cardiologists moved to the sixteenth floor of the Mayo Building after an eight-floor addition had been completed. Most of their floor was devoted to dual-purpose physician office-examination rooms, but one wing included a small group of rooms termed the Heart Station. This new facility was separate from the ground floor Electrocardiography Laboratory. Ralph Zitnik, who had joined the staff in 1965 after completing his training at Mayo, was selected to supervise the Heart Station, where treadmill exercise electrocardiogram stress tests, pacemaker checks, phonocardiograms (heart sound recordings), and echocardiograms would be performed.

When Zitnik was finalizing plans for the Heart Station in the summer of 1969, he asked Schattenberg about the equipment, personnel, and time necessary to perform and interpret echocardiograms.[13] Schattenberg responded, "I would foresee our using this machine on an average of four or five patients a day with capabilities of perhaps five times that number, should there develop such a demand. For now, I would see its primary application in patients with mitral stenosis or possible pericardial effusions." In terms of charges, Schattenberg informed Zitnik that Blue Cross paid $15 for the test, but he thought that $25 was more reasonable.[14]

Creating a Formal Echocardiography Program at Mayo

Mayo's first echocardiography instrument, a Smith Kline Ekoline 20, arrived in November 1970. Vernon Weber, an Air Force veteran with electronics training, was the first technician assigned to use it. The clinic's newsletter explained that he was "involved in the development, installation, maintenance and modifications of electronic equipment" and that he assisted "in the several procedures used for cardiac evaluation of patients."[15] Weber would perform the M-mode echocardiograms (where M stood for motion across an oscilloscope screen), and Schattenberg would drop by to interpret them between his routine clinical responsibilities.

When Zitnik left Rochester to practice in suburban Chicago in 1972, Schattenberg and Gerald Gau took charge of the echocardiography portion of the Heart Station. Gau had learned to perform and interpret echocardiograms during the two years he had spent at London's Hammersmith Hospital in the late 1960s.[16] Schattenberg and Gau soon encouraged Emilio Giuliani, who had joined the staff in 1961, to become involved in echocardiography. Schattenberg credits Giuliani with formalizing Mayo's cardiac ultrasound program, especially after cardiology chair Robert Brandenburg appointed him head of the phonocardiography-echocardiography portion of the Heart Station in 1974. An accomplished clinical cardiologist, Giuliani had already published several papers on phonocardiography and had coauthored five articles on echocardiography.[17]

Between 1970 and 1975, the number of outpatient echocardiograms performed annually in the Heart Station increased tenfold, from 188 to 2082. As illustrated in Table 18.1, the number of exercise tests, which were also done in the Heart Station, grew dramatically as well. Because there was no space for expansion on the cardiology floor, the echocardiography laboratory moved to the ground-floor level of the half-century-old Plummer Building in

TABLE 18.1 Echocardiograms and Treadmill Exercise Tests at
Mayo, 1971–1975[a]

Year	1971	1972	1973	1974	1975
Echocardiograms	188	264	848	1,407	2,082
Treadmill exercise electrocardiogram stress tests	720	1,114	1,461	1,899	2,406

[a] Adapted from "Heart Station Workload Report for 1970 through 1977," MCA.

July 1976. Eighteen months later, Giuliani sent a status report on the outpatient program to Robert Frye, who had succeeded Brandenburg as chair of cardiology. Giuliani said that he had wanted "to develop the very best echocardiographic laboratory" and that "the first important step was to design a laboratory that would be both efficient and effective in terms of patient care.... The primary responsibility of this laboratory is clinical, and that is to supply our consulting colleagues with the very best data in the most efficient and effective way possible."[18]

Giuliani stressed the contributions of the laboratory's seven "excellent, competent, and well-qualified" technicians and its two secretaries: "The group is proud of their work, which continues to stimulate improvement in technique and in the quality of the echocardiograms done. It is largely the effort of the paramedical personnel that is responsible for the success of the laboratory."[19] The technicians recorded the M-mode echocardiograms (sometimes working with a cardiology fellow) that were later reviewed by a staff cardiologist. The new ground-floor laboratory contained four separate rooms for performing studies and space for interpreting them. For the first time at Mayo, a cardiologist was given dedicated time to devote to the work that was carried out there. This shortened the delay between the completion of an echocardiogram and the creation of a final report of the findings. Giuliani, who spent much of his time in the laboratory, expected that all reports be sent out within one day.[20]

Giuliani was very interested in echocardiography, but cardiology fellow A. Jamil Tajik became obsessed with it. Tajik had arrived in Rochester in 1968, after graduating from medical school in Pakistan and completing a medical residency in Canada.[21] During a year-long rotation in Mayo's catheterization laboratory (beginning in 1972), he became fascinated by congenital heart disease. Cardiologists who trained with Tajik remember him pushing an echocardiograph machine on a cart through the halls of Saint Marys Hospital in the evening and on weekends. He was tracking down patients who had undergone a catheterization so he could perform an echocardiogram on them for the purpose of correlating the invasive and noninvasive test results.[22] By the end of 1973, Tajik was the first author on nine echocardiography articles. Alexander Nadas, a world expert in congenital heart disease, proclaimed in a review of one of these papers that "the echocardiographic bandwagon is proceeding full speed."[23]

In 1975 Tajik began working with James Seward, a senior cardiology fellow, and Donald Hagler, who had just joined the staff as a pediatric cardiologist. During the next three years, they coauthored more than a dozen articles on the echocardiographic findings in various forms of congenital heart disease. Tajik and Seward, who became very close professional colleagues and personal friends, shared a passion for exploring the heart with emerging ultrasound technologies that soon would provide even more insight into cardiac structure and function than the original M-mode format.[24]

Cross-Sectional or Two-Dimensional Echocardiography

Cross-sectional or two-dimensional (2D) echocardiography was developed during the 1970s, mainly in Europe, Japan, and the United States.[25] The pictures produced by the new technology were cross-sectional or tomographic slices through the heart. Cross-sectional or tomographic images could be explained to patients as being analogous to making thin slices of an apple. The earliest 2D echocardiography images were difficult for physicians to interpret because they were blurry and their relationship to anatomical structures had not been clarified. As more advanced technology was introduced later in the decade, it became obvious that 2D echocardiography offered real advantages for imaging the heart compared to the original M-mode display and older X-ray techniques.

Standard still frame X-rays and fluoroscopy produce silhouette images of the heart, but the resulting shadows conceal the organ's contents—its chambers and valves. Angiocardiography, which involves injecting radiopaque contrast material into the heart, produces a white image of the organ's blood-filled chambers. It takes training and experience to decipher the clues to heart disease that might be hidden in these shadows. During open-heart surgery, cardiac surgeons can look directly inside a patient's non-beating heart for a few minutes. But the operator's field of view is limited, and he or she has very little time to look around. Anatomists and pathologists can spend as long as they like staring at and photographing every part of a human heart, but nothing moves after death. With 2D echocardiography, a pie-piece-shaped slice of the heart is displayed as a moving image on an oscilloscope screen. By tilting and moving the handheld ultrasound transducer over the chest wall, the heart can be sliced in innumerable ways. The result is a moving picture of the organ's walls contracting and valves opening and closing.[26]

Tajik, aware that prototype wide-angle 2D echocardiograph machines were being tested at a few academic centers in 1976, traveled to Palo Alto,

California, to see one (made by the Varian Corporation) that cardiologist Richard Popp's group at Stanford University was using.[27] Very impressed, Tajik returned to Rochester eager to introduce the technology at Mayo. After Giuliani expressed concern that $100,000 was too much to spend on the emerging technology that had no clinical track record, Tajik tried another approach. He got approval for the purchase from pediatric cardiologist Donald Ritter, co-director of the catheterization laboratory, and Robert Frye, who had succeeded Robert Brandenburg as chair of cardiology.[28] In February 1977 Mayo's Board of Governors approved spending $100,000 to buy a Varian V-3000 2D echocardiography instrument for use in the catheterization laboratory at Saint Marys Hospital.[29]

When the Varian 2D instrument arrived early in 1977, Tajik and Seward were ecstatic because they were convinced it would be a valuable tool for patient care, clinical research, and education. Ambitious and curious, the two men captured countless hours of moving cross-sectional slices of the heart on videotape for study, storage, and comparison. Very soon, they were coordinating a team effort that would push Mayo from the sidelines of echocardiography to center stage.

It took almost no time for the Varian instrument to prove itself in the catheterization laboratory. But it was the size of a refrigerator, much too big to transport to Mayo's outpatient building, which was a mile away. Giuliani, who was impressed with the technology once he saw it in action, now recommended that Mayo buy a second Varian instrument for the outpatient laboratory that he directed. The board approved the request, and the machine was delivered early in 1978.[30] Ileen Marxhausen, a technician who had been performing M-mode echocardiograms when the new 2D machine arrived, recalled how it took time for everyone who worked in the laboratory (including the cardiologists) to understand the heart's anatomy as it was displayed on an oscilloscope screen.[31]

Mayo's 2D echocardiography program burst onto the international scene in May 1978, when Tajik and Seward coauthored an article on the technology with pediatric cardiologists Donald Hagler and Douglas Mair and cardiac pathologist Jauw Lie. Published in the *Mayo Clinic Proceedings*, which had a circulation of 75,000, the paper helped propel the institution to the front ranks of echocardiography. The article's impact was due, in part, to the fact that the authors took advantage of Mayo's sophisticated departments of anatomic pathology, photography, and medical illustration. Several of the 2D images were accompanied by a high-resolution photograph of a heart sliced at autopsy in a plane that corresponded to the echocardiographic cross section.[32]

Many cardiologists who read the article noticed that the pie-piece-shaped echocardiogram images were better in quality and bigger than those they were used to seeing in other publications or at meetings.[33] The Varian created an 80-degree arc, whereas the Smith Kline 2D instrument that Feigenbaum used produced a 30-degree arc. Switching from a 30-degree to an 80-degree cross-sectional image of the heart was analogous to taking blinders off a horse. Similar to CinemaScope, a widescreen motion picture technology, the 80-degree sector scanner showed much more of the heart's action than was possible with standard screens. It also made it much easier for all doctors (not just cardiologists interested in echocardiography) to understand what they were seeing.

In an editorial that accompanied the 1978 *Mayo Clinic Proceedings* article, adult cardiologist Robert Frye and pediatric cardiologist Donald Ritter emphasized that 2D echocardiography had already changed heart care at Mayo. It had reduced the number of angiocardiograms done to evaluate patients with congenital heart disease and had occasionally eliminated the need for catheterization altogether. Frye and Ritter also commented on the new technology's cost implications: "It is incumbent on the medical profession to utilize this method as a decisive clinical tool in patient management after careful documentation so that it does not become simply another test added to the patient's bill."[34] When they raised this concern, the total cost of health care in America was attracting ever more attention and cardiology was being inundated by a flood of new technologies.[35]

Frye and Ritter's editorial also revealed a trend toward subspecialization within cardiology at the Mayo Clinic. They explained that the article by Tajik and his coauthors was the "result of an intensive concentration of experience with the instrument on the part of a small group of experienced echocardiographers."[36] In a 1978 letter to the chair of medicine, Frye praised Tajik, Seward, and Hagler for developing 2D echocardiography: "As a result of these efforts, our institution is identified as a leader in this important field that has already made a major impact on the management of our patients."[37] Tajik's identity as one of the pioneers of 2D echocardiography was reinforced when he was selected to serve on an American Society of Echocardiography committee that was charged with developing nomenclature and standards for the technique.[38]

2D Echocardiography: You've Got to See It to Believe It!

"You've Got to See It to Believe It!" was the title of a 1979 talk on 2D echocardiography delivered at Wisconsin's Marshfield Clinic, where an echocardiography laboratory had been established one year earlier. About one hundred doctors in the group practice listened and watched as the speaker (this author) narrated a videotape containing wide-angle 2D echocardiograms of a dozen patients' hearts. The examples had been chosen for their visual impact. Audience members were mesmerized by the moving images of heart walls contracting and valves opening and closing. As hoped, the presentation stimulated a significant increase in the number of requests for echocardio-grams at Marshfield Clinic.[39]

James Warren, a catheterization pioneer and longtime chair of medicine at the Ohio State University, described his first impressions of 2D echocardiog-raphy in 1980: "What a tour de force! It was sensational to see on videotape the opening and then the closing of a normal mitral valve and then the tight little hole of mitral stenosis. Topping this, we saw with remarkable clarity the ball-like vegetation of bacterial endocarditis...the demonstration was over-whelming." Warren also reported on his experience at the annual American Heart Association meeting: "One could see the impact of a tidal wave of high technology on the traditional practice of medicine. The exhibit area was packed with hundreds of expensive, highly sophisticated machines."[40]

Brandenburg asked Giuliani to write a chapter on the role of echocar-diography in evaluating outpatients for a 1980 Mayo-authored book *Office Cardiology*. Giuliani's review focused on M-mode echocardiography, but he concluded that "with improvement in technology and greater clinical expe-rience, two-dimensional ultrasound cardiac imaging will ultimately replace M-mode echocardiography in the noninvasive evaluation of cardiac disor-ders."[41] Neither Giuliani nor Brandenburg worked in the catheterization labo-ratory, where Mayo's 2D echocardiography program was gaining momentum and national visibility. Frye, who had been director of the catheterization laboratory before he succeeded Brandenburg as chief of cardiology, had seen Tajik and Seward working there.

In a 1979 letter to the chief of medicine, Frye praised Giuliani for his "important contributions to making this laboratory responsive to heavy clin-ical demands while maintaining high quality studies." He again applauded Tajik, Seward, and Hagler for their contributions to 2D echocardiography, "establishing the Mayo Clinic as a leading institution in the application of this technique."[42] When the clinic purchased a third Varian machine in that year, no other institution in the world possessed so many state-of-the-art 80-degree 2D instruments.[43]

Giuliani, a respected clinical cardiologist, did not envision continued rapid growth of the echocardiography program when he was asked to pro-vide a three-year projection in 1979. Specifically, he did not think more space or additional professional, technical, or secretarial personnel would be needed.[44] But he enclosed a list of projected equipment needs that Tajik had prepared at his request. "I strongly believe," Tajik declared, "we will need another [fourth] phased-array sector scanner by 1981, if not 1980."[45] Giuliani reassured an administrator that his junior associate's assessment represented "an estimate of maximal needs."[46]

In March 1980 Frye informed the chief of medicine that echocardiogra-phy was "undergoing rapid development and it is important that we maintain our leadership in this area."[47] When he wrote this, Frye was about to make a local leadership change. Giuliani had directed the echocardiography laboratory for four years when Frye appointed Tajik to succeed him in July 1980. This decision surprised some Mayo cardiologists, but it made sense to others. They recognized how an individual's passion for a technology or a procedure could influence its development locally and advance their institution's reputation outside Rochester. Tajik's accomplishments in 2D echocardiography and his ambition (for himself, his associates, and his institution) influenced Frye's decision to place the Pakistani-American in charge of the laboratory that his good friend and longtime colleague Giuliani had directed.[48]

Mayo's decision to invest in expensive 2D technology paid off in terms of enhanced diagnostic power in Rochester and increased respect for its echocardiography program elsewhere as a result of a growing number of publications and presentations. Clinic staff members had spoken at regional, national, and international medical meetings for decades, and they often projected images to complement their words. In 1979 Mayo spent $475,000 on a Genigraphics system that the clinic's Medical Graphics section used to produce very sophisticated slides—unlike anything that most physicians had ever seen. General Electric had just commercialized the expensive technology, which the company had developed for NASA to create high-resolution images for use in flight simulators.[49] The advent of 2D echocardiography also coincided with the commercialization of videotape technology that facilitated the recording, storage, and display of the moving heart images. Videotape also made it easier to create motion pictures that were shown at educational meetings.

Harvey Feigenbaum considered Tajik a "fantastic speaker" and asked him to participate in his echocardiography courses in Indianapolis. The Indiana University cardiologist also acknowledged the educational value of the 80-degree images that Tajik displayed, recalling that "they made a huge impact on acceptability of 2D echocardiography."[50] In 1981 Tajik and Seward gave the first of many Mayo courses on the technology at the American College of Cardiology's new Learning Center in Bethesda, Maryland.[51] The facility's auditorium contained state-of-the-art audiovisual equipment that was ideal for showing videotapes of 2D echocardiograms. Stanford University cardiologist Richard Popp recalled the camaraderie that developed among the academic cardiologists who spoke and socialized at meetings. Frequently lecturing at the same events, they referred to themselves as the "echo gypsies." Vernon Weber, Mayo's first echocardiography technician, helped create videotapes for what he described as "road shows."[52]

Doppler Echocardiography: Blood Flow in Sound and Color

The videotapes of 2D echocardiograms shown at medical meetings in the early 1980s were silent; a speaker narrated the moving images of the heart.

This changed in the middle of the decade with the advent of Doppler echo-cardiography, a technology that produces an audible whooshing sound that varies in pitch depending on the velocity of blood flowing through the heart's valves.[53] Doppler echocardiography had been developed mainly in Europe and Japan during the late 1970s. Norwegian cardiologist Liv Hatle, work-ing with biomedical engineer Bjørn Angelsen and others, published articles describing how it could be used to quantify the severity of mitral stenosis and aortic stenosis.

Harvey Feigenbaum considers Hatle's 1980 article on aortic stenosis "prob-ably the most important development that stimulated interest in Doppler echocardiography."[54] At the time the paper was published, valve replacement for aortic stenosis had become a common cardiac operation. Understandably, a patient's cardiologist and heart surgeon wanted to be sure that the obstruc-tion across the valve was severe enough to justify surgery. Catheterization had been the "gold standard" that doctors depended on to measure the pres-sure gradient across the valve until the approach that Hatle pioneered was validated. She would accomplish this goal in collaboration with cardiologists at Stanford University and the Mayo Clinic.[55]

Mayo cardiologists published several articles in the mid-1980s that dem-onstrated very good correlation between catheterization-derived and Doppler-derived data for pressure gradients across obstructed valves and for right ventricular systolic pressure. In a 1985 editorial on a Mayo article on right ventricular systolic pressure, Richard Popp concluded that "the full potential of Doppler ultrasound will not be known until these ideas are tested using improved equipment and appropriate scientific methods as has been done in the recent study from the Mayo Clinic."[56] Popp's group at Stanford led the effort to assess the severity of aortic stenosis with Doppler, but he later explained that "all of the really good studies were done at Mayo because they had the cath lab set up to do these comparative studies.... They had this great volume and great research impetus to do it, and so their papers are really the classic papers."[57]

In less than a decade, many of Mayo's medical and surgical heart spe-cialists trusted the Doppler-derived data about the severity of aortic steno-sis. They considered the information from this noninvasive test sufficient to decide if heart surgery was indicated, which meant that some patients would not have to undergo cardiac catheterization to measure the valve gradient. In 1992, for example, only one-third of patients who had an aortic valve replace-ment at Mayo underwent preoperative catheterization.[58]

When the next innovation, color flow Doppler imaging, burst onto the scene in the mid-1980s, its visual impact was immediate and impressive. Moving blood, invisible on a 2D echocardiogram, makes a whooshing sound with standard Doppler technology. But color flow Doppler paints the blood's motion on an oscilloscope screen. The main colors are red and blue (depending on the direction of flow). Turbulence caused by blood rushing through an obstructed valve creates a complex multicolored, mosaic-like picture.[59] For first-time observers, the effect of turning on color Doppler is like the scene in the *The Wizard of Oz* where Dorothy steps out of a black and white world into one filled with color. But it is even better. In that movie, you actually see nothing new.

The introduction of color flow Doppler into clinical practice amazed and humbled experienced echocardiographers. A patient's mitral valve might look almost normal with standard 2D echocardiographic imaging, but turning on color Doppler could reveal that it leaked a lot. Severe mitral regurgitation suddenly showed up on the screen as a big burst of blue flooding backward from the left ventricle through the mitral valve and into the left atrium. This new imaging approach had significant implications for the evaluation of aortic and mitral regurgitation. It also led to the recognition of abnormalities that were not always apparent using traditional diagnostic techniques, such as a stethoscope examination or chest X-ray.

Transesophageal Echocardiography: A New View of the Heart

Echocardiography evolved from a noninvasive procedure to a semi-invasive one with the development of transesophageal echocardiography (TEE) in the 1980s.[60] The wedding of two technologies led to an instrument that could be inserted into a patient's mouth and down his or her esophagus relatively simply and safely. TEE provided unique information about the heart and the thoracic aorta. This was made possible by the commercialization of flexible endoscopes and the miniaturization of 2D ultrasound transducers.[61]

Mayo gastroenterologist Eugene DiMagno reported using a custom-made flexible ultrasonic endoscope in twenty-two individuals in 1982. His main interest was imaging the pancreas, but the instrument he used also produced 2D images of the beating heart and the aorta: "In the esophagus, the ultrasonic probe was rotated to face anteriorly to view the heart, coronary sinus, left atrium, mitral valve, and left ventricle.... Next, the aorta could be identified as a double-walled, pulsating large vessel which could be traced into the abdominal cavity."[62]

When DiMagno's article was published, Seward was collaborating with him in an attempt to develop a wide-angle 2D transesophageal system for use in humans. Seward presented their animal research at a 1982 echocardiography symposium in Hamburg, Germany, where cardiologist Peter Hanrath of that city was actively developing TEE technology.[63] This meeting (and similar ones in North America and Europe) provided Seward, Tajik, and other Mayo echocardiographers with opportunities to network with peers and publicize the clinic's high volume, state-of-the-art cardiac ultrasound program.

The first application of TEE in patients at Mayo in the early 1980s was a research project that did not relate directly to patients with heart disease. Seward used a prototype 2D TEE transducer in 1982 as part of a research protocol to identify air embolism in patients undergoing neurosurgical operations performed in the sitting position.[64] Shortly after this experience was published two years later, Mayo anesthesiologists and echocardiographers collaborated in a research study designed to evaluate the use of TEE during coronary artery bypass graft surgery. They found that it was useful for monitoring the overall pumping function of the left ventricle and for identifying left ventricular wall segments that did not contract normally.[65]

When Seward presented a proposal to Mayo's Cardiovascular Clinical Practice Committee to move TEE out of the operating room and into the outpatient practice in 1987, he explained that this semi-invasive procedure was already "fairly routine" in Europe and was being done at Duke University and Stanford University. Seward emphasized that the components for a successful outpatient program, such as sufficient preparation, suitable instrumentation, and adequate staff and paramedical support, were already in place at Mayo.[66] The committee approved the proposal, and outpatient TEE was launched in November 1987.

This new program led to subspecialization among Mayo's echocardiographers. Rather than expecting each one to perform TEE, a few of them would be trained to do it. The initial training, which focused on inserting an endoscope into a patient's esophagus, was supervised by gastroenterologist Rollin Hughes in the clinic's outpatient endoscopy unit.[67] The *Mayo Clinic Heart Book*, written for patients and the public, described the procedure: "You swallow the end of the tube that has the transducer on it (which is easier than it sounds), and the cardiologist manipulates the instrument to obtain the images that are needed. The examination is extremely well tolerated by more than 90 percent of people."[68]

In 1988 Seward and eight Mayo coauthors, including cardiac pathologist William Edwards, published an article titled "Transesophageal Echocardiography: Technique, Anatomic Correlations, Implementation, and Clinical Applications" in the *Mayo Clinic Proceedings*. It included a signature feature of Mayo-authored review articles on 2D echocardiography: high-quality photographs of hearts sectioned at autopsy with the anatomical landmarks labeled to make it easier to understand the cross-sectional ultrasound images. The coauthors' professional identities reflected the collaboration that was involved in launching the TEE program. In addition to cardiologists, two anesthesiologists, a gastroenterologist, a pathologist, and a nurse were listed under the title. Based on their experience with the first one hundred outpatient procedures at Mayo and reports published by other groups, the authors identified several situations in which TEE was especially helpful. These included seeing a blood clot in the left atrium (which may occur in patients with atrial fibrillation), evidence of endocarditis (infection of a heart valve), and a dissection (tear) of the thoracic aorta.[69] Such findings could make a big difference in the care of a patient. For example, an abnormal TEE might be the deciding factor in recommending life-saving surgery for a specific problem, such as an aortic dissection, a deadly condition that took the life of actor John Ritter.

Indiana University cardiologist Thomas Ryan, a Feigenbaum protégé, described the 1988 Mayo article on TEE as an excellent summary by "one of the most active research groups in the country."[70] This was not hyperbole. Feigenbaum explained two decades later: "There is no question that the Mayo echocardiography experience played a huge part in the popularity of the technique…the studies were always very, very well done. There is a standard of excellence that is unmatched anywhere else."[71]

The Mayo Clinic achieved international recognition as a leading center for echocardiography as a result of the staff's steady stream of publications and frequent participation in national and international meetings. Lectures by the clinic's echocardiographers, which targeted practitioners, showcased new technologies and quantitative approaches that were relevant to patient care. Mayo also produced and sold several series of videotaped educational programs on echocardiography.

Echocardiography-Guided Needle Pericardiocentesis

Echocardiography had first gained widespread attention in the United States in 1965, when Harvey Feigenbaum published an article on its value in diagnosing a pericardial effusion. The standard non-surgical treatment for a significant pericardial effusion was to perform a pericardiocentesis. This procedure to drain the fluid involved inserting a needle through the wall of a patient's chest or upper abdomen and into the pericardial space. But this blind approach could be risky—even fatal.

Cincinnati cardiologist Noble Fowler cautioned in 1966: "Needle aspiration of the pericardial space is a major procedure. Laceration of a coronary artery or of the myocardium may cause death from cardiac tamponade. Either ventricular fibrillation or vasovagal arrest is another complication."[72] This warning captured the essence of concerns that others had written about and had passed on by word of mouth. It is understandable that doctors welcomed a test to prove the presence of a pericardial effusion before sticking a needle into a patient's chest in search of fluid around the heart. Despite echocardiography's power to make a definitive diagnosis of a pericardial effusion, blind needle aspiration remained risky. A Los Angeles cardiologist warned in 1980, "Pericardiocentesis is a procedure with great danger to the patient."[73]

Mayo echocardiographers were not the first to use ultrasound to find the safest path for a needle to reach pericardial fluid, but they would become the most persistent promoters of this approach. In 1982 cardiologists at the University of Virginia published an article titled "Traumatic Perica rdiocentesis: Two-Dimensional Echocardiographic Visualization of an Unfortunate Event." The unfortunate event was the inadvertent puncture of a thirty-two-year-old woman's right ventricle during an attempt to withdraw fluid from around her heart. She survived, but the authors pointed out that their use of 2D echocardiography to try to see the needle during the procedure had not prevented this complication. They concluded that "a large series of patients will need to be studied to determine if simultaneous 2D echocardiographic monitoring is useful in actually decreasing the incidence of complications during pericardiocentesis."[74] The Mayo Clinic provided the answer six months later.

In 1983 Mayo cardiologists reported the clinic's experience with 2D echocardiography-guided pericardiocentesis. They explained that, despite ultrasound's critical role in diagnosis, "too little notice has been given to 2D echocardiography as a means of directing the actual pericardiocentesis procedure, and no series of cases has been reported."[75] Their article described performing the combined diagnostic-therapeutic procedure in forty patients without any complications. The technique's benefits included visualizing the fluid-filled pericardial sac, estimating the amount of fluid, identifying structures (such as the liver) that might be between a potential needle insertion site and the pericardial space, and determining the most direct route to the effusion. Many institutions adopted 2D echocardiography-guided pericardiocentesis, and Mayo's cardiologists used it consistently.[76]

Stress Echocardiography and Coronary Artery Disease

During the late 1970s, Feigenbaum's group at Indiana University pioneered the use of 2D echocardiography in conjunction with treadmill exercise testing to evaluate patients with known or suspected coronary disease.[77] But logistical and technological challenges delayed the diffusion of stress echocardiography into practice until the late 1980s. It was very hard to obtain good images of the beating heart by holding a transducer on a patient's chest while he or she walked on a treadmill. Stress echocardiography gained in popularity after the commercialization of better technology (including digital systems for acquiring images) and the publication of studies demonstrating its value as a tool for diagnosis and prognosis. The recognition that valid results could be obtained by imaging the heart immediately after a patient stopped exercising was a major breakthrough because this overcame the challenge of trying to image a moving heart inside a moving patient.

Jamil Tajik asked cardiologist Patricia Pellikka to take the lead in introducing stress echocardiography at Mayo when she joined the staff in 1989. She oversaw the development of a clinical protocol, the acquisition of equipment, and the training of personnel. The test proved to be popular, and the number of treadmill exercise echocardiograms increased from 335 in 1990 to 1,538 in 1993.[78] But some patients cannot walk on a treadmill at all or cannot exercise long enough to increase their heart rate to a point that the test results can be used to predict the likelihood of significant coronary artery disease. This led to the introduction of pharmacological stress testing—using drugs that accelerate the heart or otherwise increase blood flow through the coronary arteries. Stress echocardiography using dobutamine (an adrenalin-like drug that speeds up the heart) rather than exercise, was introduced at Mayo in 1990. Dobutamine echocardiography soon became the preferred alternative to treadmill exercise testing in selected patients.[79]

Mayo cardiologists concluded in a 1995 review that the "versatility of stress echocardiography, rapid availability of results, relatively low cost, and diagnostic yield have brought this procedure to the forefront of noninvasive evaluation of coronary artery disease."[80] On the other hand, they emphasized the importance of special training: "Simply having performed echocardiography previously is inadequate training for stress imaging. For the assessment of ventricular wall motion and the accurate recognition of ischemic changes, a high level of skill and experience is necessary."[81] These comments reflected an ongoing trend in cardiology toward longer and more formal training.[82]

Between 1965, when Feigenbaum published his article on echocardiography in pericardial effusion, and 1995, the length of cardiology fellowship training at the Mayo Clinic had increased from one to four years (after completion of a three-year internal medicine residency).[83] During the 1990s, Mayo heart specialists continued to contribute to the development and implementation of cutting-edge cardiac ultrasound technologies, such as intravascular ultrasound (IVUS) and intracardiac ultrasound.[84]

Nuclear Cardiology: Using Radioisotopes to Image the Heart

Nuclear cardiology, another noninvasive imaging technique popularized during the last third of the twentieth century, involves recording the radiation sent out of the body after a tiny amount of a short-lived radioactive isotope is injected into a vein and circulates through the heart and bloodstream. The sophisticated technology used to record and create images from the emitted radiation is related to a Geiger counter, a simple tool that most individuals have heard and seen in action on television. But nuclear cardiology is a complicated field.[85] Mayo cardiologist Raymond Gibbons, whose career would focus on it, explained in a 1987 textbook that "a complete understanding of the course of events between the injection of an isotope, or radionuclide, into a patient and the display of a nuclear cardiology study for interpretation involves considerable knowledge of nuclear physics, radiation principles, and instrumentation."[86]

The emerging field of nuclear medicine (of which nuclear cardiology would become a subspecialty) had received a big boost from discoveries made and technologies developed during World War II. Radioisotopes that facilitated the development of nuclear medicine were byproducts of the Manhattan Project, a top-secret wartime research program. In 1946, one year after the United States dropped atomic bombs on Japan, the government made synthetic radioisotopes available to investigators at several institutions. Mayo's Board of Governors approved a recommendation from the institution's Research Committee in August 1946:

> Recent developments in nuclear physics have placed a highly important tool for clinical research, diagnosis, and therapy in the hands of investigators; namely, the radioisotope, and its use promises revolutionary advances in fundamental knowledge of the human body in health and disease. So great are the potentialities of its use in research, in accurate diagnostic tests, and in therapy, that the Mayo Clinic and Mayo Foundation should not only support but stimulate research employing radioisotopes. Fortunately, important researches employing radioactive substances carried on both in town and at the Institute of Experimental Medicine have given our institution a background of experience and a reputation in this field.[87]

During the first half of the century, radioactive material had been used in medicine almost exclusively to treat malignant tumors.[88] Radioisotopes would be applied to diagnosis in the 1950s.

Mayo established its first radioisotope laboratory in 1952 in the Section of Clinical Pathology. Laboratory director Charles Owen Jr. published a 425-page book on diagnostic radioisotopes seven years later, but he devoted just three pages to the cardiovascular system.[89] Owen's successor, clinical pathologist Newton Tauxe, considered the use of radioisotopes in medicine "still in the beginning stage" in 1962.[90] The commercialization of an instrument termed a scintillation or gamma camera in the mid-1960s catalyzed the field of nuclear medicine and set the stage for the development of nuclear cardiology. When Mayo acquired a scintillation camera in 1970, the clinic's newsletter summarized how it was used in patient care:

> A small quantity of a radioisotope is injected into a vein. Gamma rays emitted by the isotope from the organ under study enter a detector head

and cause scintillations in a sodium iodide crystal. The scintillations are displayed momentarily as dots of light on an oscilloscope (which resembles a TV screen) within the console and are recorded by still and movie cameras.... Concentration of dots or the pattern of their distribution on the print has diagnostic significance.[91]

At the time this article appeared, clinical investigators at the Johns Hopkins Hospital and a few other medical centers were developing nuclear medicine techniques to evaluate left ventricular function, coronary blood flow, and congenital heart defects.[92] Acknowledging the growing clinical relevance of the field, Mayo created a separate Section of Nuclear Medicine in 1971, the same year that the American Board of Nuclear Medicine was established.[93]

Mayo's Section of Nuclear Medicine introduced techniques to scan bones, brains, and several organs, but it got off to a slow start with respect to using radioisotopes to study the heart. Nuclear medicine section head Heinz Wahner explained in a report to the Board of Governors: "On the national scene, the year 1975 has seen great activities in the area of cardiology and the development of non-traumatic [noninvasive] diagnostic tests, such as myocardial imaging, shunt evaluation, ejection fraction, isotope angiography, and ventricular wall motion analysis." Noting that these heart-related procedures required special scintillation cameras and computer software, he concluded that "the general usefulness of these tests will have to await the test of time."[94] Wahner also provided the board with his opinion as to why the Mayo Clinic was lagging in the development of nuclear cardiology:

> Newer techniques in Nuclear Medicine not only require expertise in technology, but also a familiarity with the medical or surgical specialty involved. For example, the introduction of new cardiology methods requires knowledge of cardiac catheterization, echocardiography, electrocardiography, and clinical cardiology. We should be able to give one [nuclear medicine] staff member the time for obtaining some expertise in a new field while he develops the isotope technique. At the present time the routine schedule is so heavy that this is not possible. The result is that we are relying on clinicians not only for the definition of goals and objectives and for supplying patients, but also on his technical skills. This takes development of new tests completely out of our hands.[95]

Frustrated that a proposed nuclear cardiology program had not gotten underway, Wahner claimed that part of the problem related to whether the focus should be on research or clinical practice. In early 1978 he complained that "on the national scene, newer techniques in cardiology are dominating the frontiers in nuclear medicine.... Several larger medical centers have established cardiac nuclear medicine laboratories as subspecialties of nuclear medicine."[96] Wahner's concern about workload echoed the comments that other Mayo staff members made with respect to the challenge of introducing and developing new technologies and techniques in the context of a very busy clinical practice.

James Chesebro and Valentin Fuster, who joined the Mayo staff in 1975 after completing cardiology fellowships in Rochester, were the first heart specialists to collaborate with the clinic's nuclear medicine group. Their main project was an NIH-funded study of the role that blood platelets played in the development of obstructions in vein grafts that were used in coronary artery bypass surgery. Chesebro explained early in 1977 that he was impressed by recent reports of the use of radioisotopes to evaluate left ventricular function before and after exercise and was convinced that a "gamma camera is an absolute must for our clinical practice and future research."[97] A few weeks later the Board of Governors approved purchasing a portable gamma camera that would be located at Saint Marys Hospital, where it could be used in the coronary care unit and catheterization laboratory.[98]

Like other new technologies introduced at Mayo, nuclear cardiology procedures evolved from being performed on a limited basis to becoming a routine test. In 1978 Mayo's Clinical Practice Committee approved a request from cardiologist Robert Tancredi and nuclear medicine specialist Manuel Brown to begin performing myocardial infarction scans at the institution. It also approved a test to assess left ventricular function that would be known as MUGA, an acronym for multiple-gated acquisition scan. This blood-pool isotope imaging technique was the subject of Mayo's first nuclear cardiology publication, which appeared in 1978.[99]

Wahner, who had expressed frustration about the slow development of nuclear cardiology at Mayo, was delighted that radioisotope techniques for evaluating left ventricular function and heart attacks would now be offered as routine tests. He reported in 1978: "I see these developments with great excitement and with pride in the excellent work of Drs. Brown, Tancredi and colleagues in nuclear medicine and cardiology. This development is in parallel with developments elsewhere in the country and abroad and allows [us] to catch up with major medical centers in the use of radiopharmaceuticals in cardiology."[100]

Two cardiologists played a major role in developing nuclear cardiology at Mayo in the early 1980s. Ian Clements, who was born and trained in Ireland before completing a cardiology fellowship in Rochester, joined the staff in 1979. Two years later, Raymond Gibbons joined the staff after completing a cardiology fellowship at Duke University. He had received extensive training in nuclear cardiology at Duke, where he was mentored by one of the field's pioneers, cardiac surgeon Robert Jones.

Clements and Gibbons oversaw the rapid expansion of exercise testing that incorporated radioisotopes to evaluate patients with known or suspected coronary artery disease. Between July 1980 and November 1982, more than 2,500 patients underwent a test termed an exercise radionuclide ventriculogram that could identify left ventricular wall motion abnormalities. This helped physicians decide whether a patient had significant coronary disease.[101] Gibbons recalls: "Within a few months of establishing a reasonable service, the growth rate compared to what had been done previously was phenomenal.... It was clearly felt by people to be useful in their practice."[102] He would become a prolific contributor to the literature of nuclear cardiology.

In 1980 the *American Journal of Cardiology* published a symposium on "Two Dimensional Echocardiography Versus Cardiac Nuclear Imaging Techniques."[103] This title symbolized tensions between the technologies. The most vocal participants in debates about the relative merits of echocardiography and nuclear cardiology were usually junior faculty members who were trying to establish identities in their respective fields. The same year, three academic cardiologists from California published a book designed to provide a "comparative analysis of the value, indications, and limitations of the two modalities in providing answers to specific clinical questions." Rejecting a common perception, they argued that the two imaging technologies were not in "scrimmage competition." Although they conceded that "for certain conditions, one technique is clearly acknowledged to be the procedure of choice," the authors claimed that "they are usually complementary in providing useful additive information about a given problem."[104] Echocardiography and nuclear cardiology evolved rapidly during the 1980s. In terms of clinical use, however, echocardiography was more popular because the technology was less expensive, more mobile, and did not involve radiation exposure.

New Tomographic Imaging Technologies: CT and MRI

Smaller and more powerful computers that were commercialized in the 1970s were critical for the development of other imaging technologies, such as computed tomography (CT) scans and magnetic resonance imaging (MRI).[105] British computer expert and electrical engineer Godfrey Hounsfield, who would share the Nobel Prize for Physiology or Medicine for his role in the development of the CT scanner, presented the results of using a prototype scanner to image the brain in the spring of 1972.

In August 1972, Mayo's Board of Governors approved spending $302,000 for one of the first production units. The technology was being developed by Electric and Musical Industries Ltd. (EMI), a decades-old London-based electronics company that had gained fame a few years earlier for recording and releasing the Beatles' first hit songs. The first CT scanner in North America (built by EMI) was installed at Mayo in the spring of 1973 and was first used on June 19 to image a patient's brain.[106] Applying CT technology to the heart, however, was very problematic because the organ moved with every cardiac contraction. During the final two decades of the twentieth century, this motion problem and other challenges were overcome, making CT scans practical and clinically useful.[107] In Rochester, this led to the demise of a unique imaging technology that had been developed at Mayo.

In the spring of 1983 Northwest Airlines passengers saw an article in the company's in-flight magazine with the intriguing title "On the Inside Looking Out: The Body in 3-D." It described unique experimental technology that was located in Mayo's Medical Sciences building:

> Imagine watching the human heart beating in quiet rhythmic pattern. Imagine seeing it as if you possessed Clark Kent's x-ray vision and could effortlessly, and with no discomfort to the heart's owner, penetrate the obstructing layers of the chest cavity and view the organ as it functions in its normal environment. Then imagine possessing the additional capability of being able to manipulate the image any way you wished:...isolate one thin slice at any plane for closer scrutiny; measure the rate of blood flow through an artery and the thickness of the walls between the chambers; dissect the organ without disrupting a beat....
>
> At the Mayo Clinic, in Rochester, Minnesota, a team of research scientists has created a machine that possesses these capabilities. It is the Dynamic Spatial Reconstructor (DSR), a fifteen-ton, twenty-foot-long scanning device that takes radiographic motion pictures inside the body and electronically reconstructs pull-apart, three-dimensional video models of targeted organs. The result is the closest thing to x-ray vision for humans that science has yet developed. The DSR is the most advanced scanner in the world.[108]

Freelance writer Patricia Skakla's story sounds like pure science fiction. But the DSR had become operational in 1979 and had already been used to make images of the hearts of eight patients.

Mayo's DSR was a one-of-a-kind machine, and its developers knew it. Skakla quoted Richard Robb, a computer scientist and biomedical engineer who directed the research program, as saying that the DSR was "too expensive, cumbersome, and complex for routine hospital use." He predicted that it would stimulate the development of less expensive technologies that could provide at least some of the information that the massive $3 million machine produced.[109] The unique DSR was dismantled in 1998.

The Mayo Clinic, which had installed the first CT scanner in North America in 1973, was among the earliest institutions to acquire another new noninvasive technology that was initially termed nuclear magnetic resonance imaging. The word "nuclear" was dropped to avoid confusion with procedures that exposed patients to radiation. Magnetic resonance imaging (MRI) creates pictures of structures inside the body by detecting energy signals emitted by atoms that are in its tissues.

In 1980 two Mayo radiologists visited the University of Nottingham in England, where a pioneering clinical MRI program had been launched four years earlier. The December 1982 issue of the clinic's newsletter announced that the new imaging technology had just been installed at Saint Marys Hospital. Thomas Berquist, one of the radiologists who would use it, explained that MRI was at the same point that CT had been eight years earlier: "At the beginning, we didn't know what its potential was either. But we made progress by leaps and bounds."[110] Compared to MRI's use in imaging static organs and structures, MRI of the heart (like cardiac CT) got off to a slow start because the organ moved.

Cardiac applications of CT and MRI at most institutions were also delayed because radiologists controlled the massive immobile units. Meanwhile, cardiologists controlled 2D echocardiography, a powerful and mobile noninvasive technology that was much less expensive and produced clear images of the moving heart. Cardiovascular radiologists Paul Julsrud and Jerome Breen coauthored the chapter on cardiac MRI in the 1996 edition of *Mayo Clinic Practice of Cardiology*. Their opening paragraph put things in perspective: "In the first edition of this textbook [1987], the topic of cardiac magnetic resonance imaging (MRI) was discussed in a few paragraphs, and it was stated that 'the dimensions of its capability as a diagnostic tool have not yet been defined.' MRI of the heart and great vessels has since evolved into a modality of proven clinical utility, yet as this third edition goes to press, the statement remains accurate and appropriate."[111] Collaboration between Mayo's radiologists and cardiologists would increase in subsequent years, as advances in CT and MRI technology led to their expanded use in cardiovascular diagnosis.

British cardiologist John Goodwin claimed in 1991 that "all cardiologists have welcomed with open arms the benefits of high technological diagnostic methods." But he expressed concern that this trend had led to an erosion of traditional clinical skills, such as taking a detailed history and listening to a patient's heart with a stethoscope. Goodwin understood the phenomenon: "Of course, the appeal of high technological investigation is irresistible. The keen young cardiologist, vibrating with passionate desire to analyze the instrumental results cannot always see the point of laborious clinical examination. He or she can hardly be blamed. After all, the pressures are intense. Is not the echocardiogram so much more accurate in assessing mitral stenosis than the human ear?"[112] Others expressed nostalgia over the decline of interest in (and skill in using) the stethoscope.[113]

The cost of heart-related diagnostic technologies, such as echocardiography, that had become available during the final third of the twentieth century generated concern, but they seemed to be unstoppable. Patients and their physicians shared an interest in accurate diagnosis as a critical step toward appropriate treatment. Moreover, insurance shielded most patients from much of the cost associated with having these tests, and it provided payments to doctors and hospitals that provided them.

Eric Cassell, a New York City internist and public health professor, spoke on the implications of technology at Mayo in 1990. He claimed that "the seemingly irresistible spread of technology into every level of medicine—irresistible to doctors, patients, and nations alike" was the main "engine of the medical economic inflation now occurring everywhere in the world." He drew an analogy to the broom in the *Sorcerer's Apprentice*, Goethe's poem popularized in Walt Disney's motion picture *Fantasia*: like the brooms, "technologies come to have a life of their own."[114] The challenge was choosing between them and applying them in a way that provided information that was useful. Mayo cardiologists contributed to an ongoing effort to help clinicians make informed decisions about which imaging tests were most useful in certain specific situations.[115]

Treating Heart Failure and Preventing Cardiovascular Disease

Heart failure, rather than being a specific disease, is a term that describes a cluster of subjective symptoms and objective signs that reflect impairment of the heart's vital pumping function. The most common symptoms of heart failure are breathlessness with exertion, reduced exercise tolerance, and fatigue. Patients with it often retain fluid, which may accumulate in the legs (edema) or the lungs (pulmonary congestion). In the medical literature, heart failure is often described as left-sided or right-sided and as systolic or diastolic. But these concepts are of little interest to patients, who seek relief from their symptoms and reassurance that progressive disability and death are not inevitable.[1]

At the midpoint of the twentieth century, Boston cardiologist Paul Dudley White listed the most common causes of heart failure as aortic and mitral valve disease, chronic hypertension, and left ventricular muscle damage due to one or more acute myocardial infarctions (heart attacks).[2] At the same time, Mayo cardiologist Thomas Dry outlined the standard heart failure treatments: rest, a low salt diet, digitalis (an eighteenth-century remedy), sedatives, and diuretics to remove excess fluid. But the only effective diuretics in 1950 were mercury-containing compounds that could cause kidney damage. Another problem was that these drugs had to be administered by vein or by deep muscular injection, which meant that a patient had to make regular visits to his or her physician's office, or the doctor had to make frequent house calls.[3]

The first effective oral diuretics that did not have distressing or dangerous side effects were developed in the mid-1950s. Chlorothiazide, marketed as Diuril in 1958, was the breakthrough drug. Originally designed to treat hypertension, it also relieved some heart failure symptoms, such as leg swelling and shortness of breath. Kidney specialist Garabed Eknoyan explains that Diuril marked a new era in the history of diuretics because it was "designer developed, industry financed, chemically modeled, thoroughly

investigated and aggressively marketed."[4] This drug and other diuretics introduced around 1960 had very visible effects in terms of treating edema. Most
patients who were breathless as a result of heart failure found that these new
diuretics also led to improvement in this very bothersome (and sometimes
disabling) symptom.

Cardiac Transplantation: A Radical Heart Failure Treatment

Despite the introduction of effective diuretics, some patients progressed to
severe "end-stage" heart failure. South African cardiologist Velva Schrire, who
had helped transform Cape Town's Groote Schuur Hospital into his nation's
leading heart center, cared for such a patient in 1967. Fifty-four-year-old
Louis Washkansky had suffered three heart attacks in the past eight years.
Schrire explained that his patient "remained in intractable congestive heart
failure, with fatigue and dyspnea on the slightest effort" despite very aggressive treatment in the hospital.[5] He discussed Washkansky's rapidly deterio-
rating condition with heart surgeon Christiaan Barnard, who had done part
of his training with C. Walton (Walt) Lillehei at the University of Minnesota.
Schrire and Barnard decided to offer the dying patient, who was "bedridden and totally incapacitated, with inadequate perfusion of all body tissues,"
an experimental procedure—replacing his diseased and failing heart with
another person's healthy one.[6]

Christiaan Barnard performed the world's first human heart transplant
on December 3, 1967, at Groote Schuur Hospital. A dozen days later, *Life*
magazine published a cover photograph of Washkansky lying in bed and
smiling. Barnard and a nurse were leaning over him wearing surgical masks
and gowns. The text on the cover emphasized that this was no ordinary surgical scene: "Gift of a Human Heart: A Dying Man Lives with a Dead Girl's
Heart." Inside, pictures of twenty-five-year-old Denise Darvall, the organ
donor, and Washkansky were accompanied by a caption: "She died violently,
hit by a car.... But her heart beats on in his body."[7]

The operation itself was a success, but the *Life* article ended on a cautionary note: "Though his new heart went on beating steadily, it was his own
body—and the possibility that his system would reject as foreign tissue the
very heart that was keeping it alive—that was causing the greatest worry for
his doctors. But as long as it continued, Washkansky's heartbeat would represent a gift of life from one human being to another, and a triumph of modern
surgery."[8] The entire December 30, 1967, issue of the *South African Medical
Journal*, published less than a month after Barnard replaced Washkansky's
weak heart with Darvall's strong one, was devoted to various aspects of the
case. But the story did not have a happy ending. The last article summarized

Washkansky's autopsy. He had died of pneumonia eighteen days after receiving a new heart.[9]

Barnard was not deterred. On January 2, 1968, he transplanted the heart of twenty-four-year-old Clive Haupt, who was in a coma after a massive brain bleed, into fifty-eight-year-old Philip Blaiberg. The retired dentist lived for one and a half years, long enough for him to publish an autobiography. In *Looking at My Heart*, Blaiberg explained that he had had his first heart attack when he was forty-six. A dozen years later, he had another one that resulted in congestive heart failure. In the months before his transplant, Blaiberg had received progressively larger doses of diuretics to combat the fluid buildup in his lungs. "I gasped for breath," he recalled, "and the coughing spells racked me more than before." Blaiberg welcomed the operation and celebrated its success: "Only a few months ago I lay in the hospital, a dying man with a stricken heart. It had deteriorated until it scarcely beat. I gasped for breath. I could barely lift a hand or foot. The nurses wondered how soon my bed would be ready for the next patient. Then came the miracle: I was given a new heart." Blaiberg spent ten weeks in the hospital. He gradually regained strength and resumed activities that were impossible before his transplant.[10]

Walt Lillehei was in South Africa in July 1968 to participate in the Cape Town Heart Transplantation Symposium. Looking to the future, the bold American surgeon warned the international audience that it was foolish to predict that something could *not* be done in the field of cardiovascular surgery "because it is quite likely that you may be interrupted by your radio in the operating room telling you that somebody has just finished doing it."[11]

Heart Transplantation Faces Scientific and Social Challenges

One thing a surgeon could not do was control the human immune system. When a patient receives a heart transplant, his or her body identifies the organ as foreign tissue and mounts an intense immune response in an attempt to reject it. Early attempts to blunt this immunologic reaction with drugs that were available greatly increased the likelihood that a patient would die as a result of infection.[12] British cardiologists John Goodwin and Celia Oakley wrote in the spring of 1969 that "the recipient of a new heart steers a perilous course between the Scylla of rejection and the Charybdis of infection." They also noted that philosophical, religious, and medicolegal issues surrounding heart transplantation had "aroused controversial and acrimonious discussions which have not been aided by massive publicity."[13]

In his book on the history of organ transplantation, Scottish surgeon David Hamilton terms 1968 as the "Year of the Heart." He argues that the publicity surrounding Barnard's experience in Cape Town stimulated surgeons "in places not known for transplant innovation or notable cardiac surgery" to begin transplanting hearts. Hamilton explains that "immediate death was the result of most of the first, and often only, heart transplants carried out in Bombay, São Paulo, Buenos Aires, Prague, Sapporo, Caracas, Madrid, Leningrad, Ankara, Istanbul, and Warsaw."[14] Enthusiasm for the procedure had already waned when the *New York Times* announced on August 18, 1969, that Philip Blaiberg had died as a result of organ rejection nineteen months after Barnard performed his "historic heart transplant."[15]

On September 17, 1971, not quite three years after *Life* magazine celebrated Barnard's first heart transplant operation, the popular weekly told a very different story. The cover depicted five men and a woman standing together. But the headline did not match their smiling expressions: "The Tragic Record of Heart Transplants: A New Report on an Era of Medical Failure." A caption above the group photograph put things in perspective: "Six Recipients of Transplants, Shown Here against a Picture of the Heart, Were All Dead within Eight Months of Being Photographed Together."[16] Houston pediatric cardiologist James Nora, who worked with heart surgeon Denton Cooley, told *Life* reporter Thomas Thompson: "I went into the transplant program with great hope.... What more noble purpose could there be in medicine than to return dying people to useful life?"[17] Within a few weeks, however, Nora had become disillusioned.

James Nora, like others who had helped pioneer heart transplantation, was troubled by the very high percentage of patients who died as a result of rejection of the donor organ. He urged Cooley to stop transplanting hearts that did not pass new tests designed to predict rejection. The *Life* magazine reporter explained that "Nora tried to point out that two of America's most distinguished heart surgeons, John Kirklin of Alabama and Dwight McGoon of the Mayo Clinic, did not attempt a single transplant."[18] One reason that McGoon and his colleagues did not launch a transplant program in Rochester was that they were overwhelmed by the volume of standard cardiac surgery procedures they were performing. McGoon informed Mayo's Board of Governors early in 1968: "It is increasingly apparent that this field of surgery is an extremely demanding one and is made still more difficult by the fact that the present staff cannot comfortably handle the volume of patients coming to the Mayo Clinic requiring this type of care."[19]

Readers of the 1971 *Life* magazine article learned that the American Heart Association had tallied the results on the third anniversary of the first cardiac transplant. Only 23 of the 166 patients who had undergone the procedure (anywhere in the world) were still alive. Norman Shumway at Stanford University, who had helped to lay the scientific and technical foundations of the operation, persisted after almost every other surgeon who had transplanted a heart had stopped. The *Life* article explained, "Shumway had been the man who American medicine thought would usher in the era of transplanted hearts. Instead he became the principal surgeon to survive it. Mercifully, the race was no longer a race. The spectators had gone home; all the runners save one had dropped out. He could afford to take all the time he needed to reach the finish line."[20] This was only a slight exaggeration. Between 1967 and 1974, 263 heart transplants had been performed by sixty-four surgical teams in twenty-two countries. But in 1974, only twenty-seven patients in the world had heart transplants, and Shumway did half of them. His Stanford team attributed this decline to general recognition of the challenges associated with organ rejection.[21]

In a 1981 review of the experimental basis for cardiac transplantation, Shumway described the development of methods to identify and manage rejection. He highlighted animal experiments that had been done in Rochester two generations earlier.[22] Between 1931 and 1933, Mayo physiologist Frank Mann had led a team of researchers who transplanted the heart of one dog onto the neck of another one in order to study how the organ functioned after its connections to the nervous system were cut. The transplanted hearts contracted for an average of four days before failing. Postmortem microscopic examination revealed that the heart muscle was "completely infiltrated with lymphocytes, large mononuclears and polymorphonuclears." These are white blood cells associated with an intense immunological reaction. The Rochester researchers concluded that "the failure of the homotransplanted heart to survive is not due to the technic of transplantation but to some biologic factor which is probably identical to that which prevents survival of other homotransplanted tissues and organs."[23]

Mann and his team emphasized the potential role of human organ transplantation in their Depression-era article: "The subject of transplantation of various tissues or organs is important since great practical value might come from the development of a successful method. This applies particularly to the transplantation of an organ such as the kidney, whereby a normal organ might be exchanged for a diseased one."[24] Norman Shumway, reflecting on this research at the Mayo Clinic, explained that "immune suppression did not exist at that time, and the field of experimental heart transplantation came to a halt for another twenty years."[25] Surgeon and historian Stephen Westaby considers the Mayo article to be a "landmark in transplantation research" because it was the first description of acute organ rejection.[26]

Cardiomyopathy: Defining Diseases of the Left Ventricle

The development of effective drugs to combat rejection in the late 1970s did not address another major problem with heart transplantation—the huge gap between the number of donor organs available and the number of patients who were considered suitable recipients (based on their symptoms, associated medical conditions, and age). Severe heart failure due to a poorly functioning left ventricle was the main problem that heart transplantation was designed to treat. Two years before Christiaan Barnard performed the first human heart transplant, epidemiologists estimated that about 3 percent of Americans over the age of forty-five had heart failure.[27] A 1974 article in the *New York Times Magazine* declared that "as many as 50,000 people with heart disease might be saved yearly by transplantation." But the article's subtitle put the nation's organ supply-demand mismatch in perspective: "The 'bottleneck in bodies' has created the agonizing ethical dilemma: Who shall live and who shall die?"[28] It was obvious that transplantation was not a realistic treatment solution for the vast majority of patients with severe heart failure.

During the 1970s, there was increasing interest in trying to understand the basic mechanisms that caused heart failure and to develop new drugs to treat it. Boston cardiologist Eugene Braunwald wrote in 1974, "If we liken the conquest of heart failure and myocardial infarction to the climbing of a mountain, then we might say that we have now assessed its height, assembled the team at the base, and have even climbed a small portion of the way up. Now we are on the first plateau and the terrain ahead looms steeper and rougher."[29] When Braunwald wrote this, a few teams of scientists and clinical investigators were seeking new ways to save, or at least improve, the lives of patients who were sick or dying as a result of heart failure.

As more patients underwent coronary angiography in the 1970s, it became clear that heart failure was often the result of left ventricular muscle damage caused by coronary artery disease and myocardial infarction. But experience had also shown that a significant percentage of patients with severe heart failure had normal or minimally diseased coronary arteries. The term "cardiomyopathy," which had been proposed in the mid-1950s to describe heart muscle disorders that were not associated with coronary disease, was becoming increasingly popular. In 1980 the World Health Organization and the International Society and Federation of Cardiology's Joint Task Force on the Definition and Classification of Cardiomyopathies formalized a scheme that British cardiologist John Goodwin had developed. It included three main categories: dilated cardiomyopathy, hypertrophic cardiomyopathy, and restrictive cardiomyopathy.[30] These technical terms meant nothing to patients with heart failure. And regardless of which category a patient might fit, his or her symptoms were basically the same.

In 1981 Mayo cardiologist Valentin Fuster and five of his colleagues published a review of the clinical course of 104 patients with "idiopathic dilated cardiomyopathy" who had been evaluated in Rochester between 1960 and 1972. The three-word phrase was shorthand for a group of conditions (of unknown cause) that was characterized by an enlarged, poorly contracting left ventricle. These patients had been followed an average of eleven years, and two-thirds of those who had died succumbed within two years of their initial evaluation in Rochester. Predictors of death included older age, an enlarged heart on X-ray, and objective evidence that the heart's pumping function was reduced (low cardiac output proved by cardiac catheterization).[31] When the Mayo article appeared, it was considered a valuable contribution to knowledge about cardiomyopathy. Three decades later, Cleveland Clinic heart failure specialist Gary Francis characterized it as a "time-honored classic."[32]

Bernard Gersh, one of the authors of the dilated cardiomyopathy article, had begun to help plan a heart transplant program at Mayo in 1979. He was very familiar with the surgical treatment strategy, having been an intern at Groote Schuur Hospital until a few months before Barnard performed the world's first human heart transplant there in 1967. After spending three years at Oxford University as a Rhodes Scholar, Gersh had returned to the Cape Town hospital, where he completed his cardiology training and remained on the staff until he joined the Mayo Clinic in 1978.[33] The following year, Gersh, cardiovascular surgical research director Michael Kaye, and cardiac surgeon James Pluth began planning a heart transplant program in Rochester. Kaye had relevant laboratory experience. Prior to joining the clinic, he had directed the Artificial Heart Testing Facility at the Illinois Institute of Technology Research Institute. Pluth had just succeeded Dwight McGoon as head of cardiac surgery.

Gersh, Kaye, and Pluth presented their proposal for establishing a heart transplant program to Mayo's Clinical Practice Committee in January 1980. During this meeting, Gersh reviewed the recent experience at Stanford University where the three-year survival rate exceeded 65 percent. This statistic reflected, in large part, advances in the early identification and treatment of rejection that the Stanford group had pioneered. In Rochester, Pluth estimated that Mayo's cardiologists were evaluating about forty potential recipients each year. The three men also discussed the logistics of obtaining donor hearts and providing postoperative patient follow-up.[34] The committee supported the proposal, and the Board of Governors approved the heart transplant program in October 1980. *Mayovox*, the clinic's newsletter, announced the decision the following month.[35]

Mayo's Cautious Entry into the Field of Cardiac Transplantion

Valentin Fuster admitted a fifty-two-year-old man to Saint Marys Hospital in January 1981. The patient, who had been diagnosed with a dilated cardiomyopathy a dozen years earlier, was transferred from a Nebraska hospital for consideration of a heart transplant. He had been seen previously at Mayo, where an echocardiogram had shown that he had a severely dilated left ventricle that barely contracted. This finding explained his heart failure symptoms. The man understood the implications of the diagnosis—his father and brother had died as a result of dilated cardiomyopathy. Progressively disabled by the condition, he had been bedridden for a month; any activity caused severe breathlessness. When the middle-aged man was admitted to Saint Marys Hospital, he was taking eight cardiac drugs, two of which were investigational. By any measure, he was receiving maximal medical therapy. Fuster, who wrote in the record that the patient "wants us to consider transplantation," asked Pluth and Gersh to evaluate him. The surgeon and cardiologist agreed that the man was an appropriate candidate for transplantation. Now, the wait for a donor heart began. As soon as a donor heart became available on February 7, 1981, Pluth operated. The patient did not survive surgery. His death was attributed to acute failure of the right side of the transplanted heart.[36]

Before Pluth operated on the man from Nebraska, he had submitted an editorial to the *Mayo Clinic Proceedings*. The surgeon opened his essay "Cardiac Transplantation: Foolhardy or Farsighted?" by noting that Mayo had announced its decision to launch a heart transplant program just after the trustees of the Massachusetts General Hospital had decided not to authorize one. "It appears paradoxical," Pluth proclaimed, "that two prestigious institutions in the field of medical care delivery could have arrived at opposite conclusions."[37]

Alexander Leaf, chief of medicine at the Boston hospital, provided a perspective on the trustees' decision: "The unproved ability of the procedure to benefit a large number of the many patients at risk, the unsolved problem of tissue rejection, and the diversion of limited resources to a procedure that at present has little impact on the all-too-common health problem that it addresses presumably weighed heavily in the final decision of the trustees." Leaf, an internist and kidney physiologist, argued that "the rapid proliferation of expensive medical technology" had led the Massachusetts General Hospital's trustees to reflect on a larger societal issue—the need "to evaluate new procedures in terms of the greatest good for the greatest number."[38]

Pluth pointed out in his editorial in the *Proceedings* that Mayo had decided to enter the field because the introduction of new drugs to combat organ rejection had resulted in improved survival of transplant recipients. Shifting his gaze from individual patients to American culture, the Rochester surgeon wrote: "In this day of rising health care costs and concern for cost/benefit ratios, surgical survivorship alone does not appear to justify a procedure. The cost of transplantation, not only to the patient but also in terms of its impact on the total national expenditure for health-related activities, must be considered as well." Pluth argued that the nation had "already embarked on many expensive programs," citing coronary artery bypass graft surgery as an example. Claiming that bypass surgery "absorbs a major portion of the national health dollar," the Mayo surgeon compared cardiac transplantation with the coronary bypass procedure, which was little more than a dozen years old. Pluth pointed to relative costs, survival statistics, and the potential

for patients returning to work to support his conclusion that "in competing for 'effective' national health dollars, cardiac transplantation becomes a
bargain."[39]

It was debatable whether heart transplantation was a bargain, but heart
failure certainly was not—for society or for an individual patient. In 1982
Eugene Braunwald emphasized that more than 4 million Americans had
heart failure. Turning from statistics to social consequences, the Boston cardiologist declared that heart failure "causes much personal suffering and
places enormous economic burdens on the patient, on his family, and on
society at large."[40]

Pluth, blending the needs of individual patients with institutional pride,
emphasized that Mayo was "a tertiary care center, not only for southeastern Minnesota but for the entire nation." He estimated that as many as fifty
patients with heart failure and cardiomyopathy who met the criteria for
transplantation were seen at the clinic each year. Pluth argued that Mayo
must be able to provide these individuals with "the most advanced medically
accepted modes of therapy." Citing the clinic's culture of collaboration, the
surgeon predicted: "We are confident that with the close cooperation that has
developed among our medical colleagues, further enhancement of the results
of this procedure can be accomplished." In his editorial, Pluth explained that
recent experience elsewhere showed that about two-thirds of patients who
underwent the operation were alive at one year.[41]

In March 1982, thirteen months after Pluth performed Mayo's first heart
transplant, he met with the Clinical Practice Committee to discuss the program's status after four patients had undergone the procedure. Robert Frye,
chief of the Cardiovascular Division, Sister Jean Keniry, director of nursing
at Saint Marys Hospital, and Michael Myers, the hospital's new administrator, accompanied the surgeon. They reported that "three of the four transplants were unsuccessful and the length of time required to accomplish the
four procedures was disappointing."[42]

Pluth and Frye agreed that a minimum of one transplant per month was
necessary to establish a viable cardiac transplantation program. Because
donor organs were so scarce and so perishable, the surgeon stressed the
importance of developing an efficient system to transport them from distant
hospitals. The committee discussed the benefits of having a surgeon with special expertise run Mayo's program, but this was problematic. The projected
volume of twelve transplants a year was minuscule, considering the fact that
Mayo's surgeons performed 1,355 open-heart operations in 1981.[43]

Better heart transplant outcomes required more than surgical expertise. When Frye met with the Clinical Practice Committee, he argued
that a specific cardiologist must be identified and given time to devote
to transplantation in order to help meet the needs of individual patients
and the overall program. Mayo would have to make "a long term major

commitment" to ensure success. "After considerable discussion," the committee unanimously supported a continued commitment to the concept of a heart transplant program.[44] The word "concept" in their minutes was significant. Mayo's Board of Governors came to a similar conclusion in November 1982, when it "approved in principle" a plan to "seek out a surgeon to engage primarily" in cardiac transplantation. But the main goal of the mission would be to gather information rather than to recruit a surgeon: "Discussions with that individual should develop the total needs for the initiation of an appropriate cardiac transplant effort. The board will reassess the proposed program before a final decision is made to activate the cardiac transplant program."[45]

Despite growing knowledge about heart failure, many challenges remained. Michael Mock, who had joined Mayo's Cardiovascular Division in 1981, edited a book on congestive heart failure with Eugene Braunwald the following year. It was based on a conference that the NIH had sponsored when Mock was chief of the Cardiac Diseases Branch of the National Heart, Lung, and Blood Institute. He closed his chapter on the future of clinical investigation with a plea for cooperation and coordination:

> The challenge for the future is in the development of effective methods to detect the occurrence of congestive heart failure at an early stage. Then innovative therapies must be hypothesized that are designed to reverse the process and to prevent the relentless progression to severe symptoms. To perfect such diagnostic techniques, develop newer effective therapies, and establish the relationship of advanced technology and therapies to the current state of the art will require the joint effort of physiologists, pharmacologists, biomedical engineers, cardiologists, and surgeons. This type of multi-disciplined research activity can be stimulated by the development of clinical research units with a special targeted emphasis on the study and treatment of patients with congestive heart failure.[46]

When Mock joined the Mayo staff in 1981, none of the cardiologists focused on heart failure. Nor was it his interest.

The situation was different in Minneapolis, where Jay Cohn had succeeded Howard Burchell as head of cardiology at the University of Minnesota seven years earlier. Cohn, who had an international reputation as a leader in heart failure research, had played a major role in the university's decision to launch a cardiac transplantation program in 1978. The authors who reviewed the university program's results six years later acknowledged that "skepticism about cardiac transplantation persists, both within and outside the medical profession because it is perceived to be too expensive in this era of rapid increase in health care costs." But they argued that most patients who received transplants could "be expected to return to productive roles in society."[47]

Treating End-Stage Cardiac Failure With an Artificial Heart

Heart transplantation, and human organ transplantation in general, raised complex ethical questions. Major concerns related to a shortage of potential donor organs and to decisions about who should be eligible to receive them. Two weeks after Christiaan Barnard transplanted Denise Darvall's heart into Louis Washkansky in 1967, *Newsweek* magazine noted that "even if the success of organ transplants were guaranteed, surgeons would still face a serious shortage of organs." The writer, who had interviewed several surgeons for the story, explained that "an artificial heart that could be mass-produced would alleviate the shortage of hearts."[48]

A few individuals, notably biomedical engineer Willem Kolff and surgeon Michael DeBakey, aggressively promoted the concept of an artificial heart as a treatment strategy for patients with end-stage cardiac failure. Kolff had invented an artificial kidney before he emigrated from Holland to America in 1950, when he joined the Cleveland Clinic's Division of Research. Eight years later, he and his colleague Tetsuzo Akutsu reported the first implantation of an artificial heart in an animal. In 1964, before any such device had been placed in a patient, Kolff predicted that "the irreparably sick human heart will be replaced in the near future by a mechanical pump. Although I have been told that nobody will want such a machine inside his chest, I think that the person who said this did not realize that for the person who really needs it, the alternative is not popular either."[49]

Kolff moved from the Cleveland Clinic to the University of Utah in 1967 as a result of increasing interpersonal tensions and decreasing institutional support for his work.[50] Two years later, he and William DeVries, a medical student who worked in his laboratory, attended the National Heart Institute's first Artificial Heart Conference. Two men from the Mayo Clinic, Robert Tancredi and Giancarlo Rastelli, were among the 750 doctors, scientists, engineers, and industry representatives who participated.[51]

Tancredi was a thirty-one-year-old cardiology fellow. Rastelli, thirty-five years old, directed the Cardiovascular Surgical Research Laboratory, where he focused on inventing or improving operations for specific types of congenital heart disease. But when Rastelli attended the 1969 conference, he had had Hodgkin's disease for five years. He would die a few months later. Mayo had pioneered the clinical use of the heart-lung machine in the mid-1950s, but it would not play any role in the development of an artificial heart.[52] In fact, very few institutions would actively participate in this very complex initiative.

Houston surgeon Denton Cooley did not attend the Artificial Heart Conference in June 1969, but most participants knew that he had made history two months earlier when he implanted a prototype device in a patient as a stopgap measure. Sixty-four hours after the initial operation, Cooley replaced the artificial heart with a human donor organ, but his patient died of pneumonia less than two days later. The procedure ruptured the relation-ship between Cooley and his mentor Michael DeBakey. Cooley had not asked the senior surgeon's permission to use the experimental device that was being tested in his animal laboratory. *Life* magazine showcased the rift in 1970 when it published a story with a provocative headline on the cover: "A Bitter Feud: Two Great Surgeons at War over the Human Heart."[53] It would be more than a decade before another attempt was made to implant an artificial heart.

In September 1981 another *Life* magazine cover proclaimed, "The Artificial Heart Is Here." The article described an operation that Cooley had performed on a thirty-six-year-old Dutch bus driver who was awaiting a heart transplant. The man had the mechanical device in his chest for two days before Cooley replaced it with a human heart.[54] A second story in the same issue of *Life* added to the drama: "Two Great Surgical Teams Race for the Man-Made Heart." One large color photograph depicted Cooley in an operating room with his hand on the patient's head and surrounded by more than a dozen surgical team members. The opposite page contained a similar staff-filled picture, but there was no patient on the operating table. The cap-tion explained, "Dr. William DeVries (arms folded) and his team stand ready to implant the Jarvik-7 heart."[55]

Willem Kolff, who was head of artificial heart program at the University of Utah, where DeVries and biomedical engineer Robert Jarvik worked, sent a telegram to Cooley that was quoted in the *Life* article: "Congratulations. Well done. Save the patient's life while you are blazing the trail. Best wishes for your patient, my fellow Dutchman, and for you from all of us in Utah."[56] The Texas surgeon's patient died of infection and other problems one week after he received the human heart.

The following year the focus shifted to DeVries, Jarvik, Kolff, and a retired dentist. "In December 1982, after decades of research and amid the dramatization of world press coverage, physicians at the University of Utah placed a permanent artificial heart in Dr. Barney Clark, heralding a new era in the practice of cardiovascular medicine." This was the opening sen-tence of an essay on the history of the artificial heart published in the *New England Journal of Medicine* in 1984.[57] Clark survived 112 days, and his air compressor-powered artificial heart beat 12,912,499 times before he died as a result of multiple organ failure.[58]

DeVries, who had moved to Louisville, Kentucky, to work at the new Humana Hospital-Audubon, would remain at the center of the tiny but awe-inspiring artificial heart universe. The cover of the May 1985 issue of *Life* magazine showed him with an arm around his patient William Schroeder. DeVries had implanted an artificial heart in the fifty-nine-year-old man on November 25, 1984. But the article's title, "Bill's Heart: The Troubling Story Behind a Historic Experiment," hinted at tensions surrounding the operation.[59]

DeVries recognized that ever since Barnard had performed the first human heart transplant seventeen years earlier that "physicians with a 'spectacular' case have found themselves in the unwavering spotlight of the press." He was not surprised that "the idea of a man-made replacement for the human heart caught the imagination of the storytellers of today— the press." The surgeon knew that the artificial heart story included many themes, such as the influence of government in biomedical research, the role of private enterprise in clinical investigation, the right to life, and the right to die.[60]

When the National Heart, Lung, and Blood Institute's Working Group on Mechanical Circulatory Support submitted its report in June 1985, William Schroeder's artificial heart had kept him alive for six months. The report's title, "Artificial Heart and Assist Devices: Directions, Needs, Costs, Societal and Ethical Issues," revealed its broad scope. Mayo cardiologist Robert Frye and cardiac surgeon Dwight McGoon were members of the fourteen-person working group. In addition to physicians, it included individuals involved in biomedical engineering, clinical decision-making, health policy, medical ethics, and patient relations.[61] One portion of the report addressed how many Americans might be candidates for an artificial heart. Extrapolating from a population-based study of Olmsted County, Minnesota, which Mayo researchers had undertaken, the working group concluded that each year between 17,000 and 35,000 individuals under the age of seventy would be candidates for such a device.[62]

The Working Group on Mechanical Circulatory Support estimated that the annual total cost to society of the devices would range from $2.5 to $5 billion. It stressed that "issues of cost, distributive justice, and patient selection are not unique to artificial heart and ventricular assist device development, but highlight the need to direct attention to the issues often associated with increasingly complicated medical care."[63] The group urged the National Heart, Lung, and Blood Institute to resume funding for the development of a permanent implantable artificial heart. The institute followed this recommendation.[64] Meanwhile, the release of better anti-rejection drugs in the early 1980s led several major institutions to establish (or re-establish) human cardiac transplantation programs.

Mayo Cardiologists Want a New Heart Transplant Program

Robert Frye stepped down as chair of Mayo's Cardiovascular Division in the fall of 1984. His successor, catheterization laboratory director Hugh Smith, sent a letter to the chair of Mayo's Department of Surgery in June 1985 expressing his colleagues' frustration that their institution did not have a heart transplant program. Smith included an attachment that contained a clear message: "The Cardiovascular Division strongly supports the active recruitment of a clinical cardiac surgeon with appropriate training, interest and commitment to cardiac transplantation and artificial heart development. The desire for seeing this program established is stronger and the feelings much more uniform now than during the period that our transplantation program was active." Smith cited several reasons for the cardiologists' sense of urgency, including the fact that the number of surgical procedures performed at Mayo on patients with congenital heart defects and valve disease had leveled off in the face of competition from other referral centers. Coronary artery bypass surgery showed "definite signs of slacking off," especially in "areas where aggressive coronary angioplasty programs exist." Smith listed four such locations, including Kansas City, Missouri, where former Mayo cardiologist Geoffrey Hartzler had established an international reputation as an innovator in angioplasty.[65]

Smith explained that the recent release of cyclosporine, a very effective drug to combat rejection, and the development of a computerized nationwide donor search system had led to the "continued development in cardiac transplantation at multiple centers (other than Mayo Clinic) in the United States." Frustrated that cardiologists at one of the nation's top medical centers had to send their patients elsewhere for a heart transplant, Smith reported that his colleagues had referred men and women with severe heart failure to Stanford University, Washington University in St. Louis, the University of Pittsburgh, and the University of Minnesota. His message was simple—Mayo must act. In addition to emphasizing the importance of recruiting an experienced cardiac surgeon who could re-establish a transplantation program in Rochester, Smith acknowledged the need to enhance the preoperative evaluation, postoperative care, and long-term follow-up of patients who would undergo the procedure. To achieve these goals, the Cardiovascular Division wanted to recruit one or more cardiologists with formal training in transplantation or to "send several current consultants with a strong interest in participating in this field to Stanford or other centers for further specialized training." In the meantime, the division was developing a heart failure working group to "provide a more sophisticated uniform approach to those patients currently presenting to us with refractory heart failure."[66]

Hugh Smith knew that Mayo had not been involved in heart failure research to any significant degree. A 1985 institutional review noted that the Cardiovascular Division "maintains an active and productive research program in diverse areas, ranging from lipid biochemistry to cardiac electrophysiology." Although fifteen of the division's fifty-four staff members had 10 percent or more protected time for research, the total commitment represented the equivalent of just 4.25 full-time individuals. In contrast, most leading academic cardiology programs placed much greater emphasis on research because a significant portion of their budgets came from NIH funding that supported this activity.[67]

Mayo had always focused on patient care, and many of the staff members' publications were clinically oriented. This was evident in 1987, when the group produced an eleven-pound textbook: *Cardiology: Fundamentals and Practice*. It was very comprehensive, and each chapter included a long list of references. Some sections, especially those on congenital heart disease, reflected Mayo's major contributions to knowledge and practice. But close inspection of the book reveals some gaps. For example, James Chesebro's chapter on the management of heart failure listed 286 references, but only five were by Mayo authors (and one of those references was an unpublished manuscript and two were brief abstracts rather than full articles).[68]

Robert Anderson of the Cardiothoracic Institute at London's Brompton Hospital wrote in his review of the volume, "Any new textbook encompassing just over 2000 pages and containing 64 chapters is an important event in cardiologic publishing. Perhaps it is the more important when the book represents the combined experience of the world-renowned Mayo Clinic." The four editors (Robert Brandenburg, Valentin Fuster, Emilio Giuliani, and Dwight McGoon) had considered writing all of the chapters themselves, but they concluded that this was unrealistic in the context of an ever-accelerating avalanche of new cardiological knowledge, techniques, and technologies. Anderson explained that the editors had asked their colleagues to contribute to the effort, "hoping to benefit from the production of a textbook by 'a single clinical unit which functioned in a highly integrated and cooperative manner.'" Although Anderson acknowledged the advantages of this approach, he described one disadvantage: "No matter how renowned and good the unit involved, it cannot be best at everything. It is certainly the case that some areas could have received better coverage by venturing outside the Mayo Clinic in the search for authors but, taken overall, the editors have achieved an impressive result."[69]

Mayo Begins to Build a Heart Failure Team

The chapter on diuretic therapy for congestive heart failure in the 1987 cardiology textbook was coauthored by kidney physiologist Franklyn Knox, who was dean of the Mayo Medical School, and two staff members who had worked in his laboratory.[70] One of them, John Burnett Jr. had trained in internal medicine, renal physiology, and cardiology at Mayo before joining the staff in 1982. His research focused on atrial natriuretic peptide, a newly recognized substance produced in the atrial wall and secreted into the bloodstream. Burnett led a team effort to develop a method for measuring the serum level of the peptide and to try to evaluate how it related to heart failure.[71]

Thomas Schwab was a nephrology fellow working in Burnett's laboratory in 1986, when he suggested that it would be interesting to measure atrial natriuretic peptide levels in a unique group of humans—those with artificial hearts. Schwab and cardiology fellow Brooks Edwards visited William DeVries in Louisville and studied the second and third patients in the world who had artificial hearts. Their article "Atrial Endocrine Function in Humans with Artificial Hearts" reported that elevations of right atrial pressure stimulated the release of atrial natriuretic peptide into the circulation. These findings lent support to the notion that the peptide levels were elevated in patients with heart failure.[72]

Although this technical article was of limited interest to most readers of the *New England Journal of Medicine*, it signaled Mayo's entry into the growing field of heart failure research. Burnett's laboratory became an incubator for cardiologists whose careers at Mayo would focus on heart failure. In addition to Edwards, his earliest trainees included Margaret Redfield and Wayne Miller. They formed the core of a heart failure group at the clinic with Richard Rodeheffer, who had been the medical director for cardiac transplantation at Vanderbilt University prior to joining the Mayo staff in 1987.

An article in *Mayovox* informed staff in the fall of 1987 that the institution was preparing to resume cardiac transplantations after surgeon Christopher McGregor arrived in Rochester. McGregor had trained in his native Scotland and in England before completing fellowships in cardiac surgery and heart and lung transplantation under Norman Shumway at Stanford. Mayo's newsletter explained that he had launched the United Kingdom's third approved cardiac transplant program (at Newcastle upon Tyne) and that fifteen of the first sixteen patients who had undergone the procedure there were still alive.[73] McGregor arrived in December 1987 and performed his first heart transplant at Mayo on June 1, 1988. The patient was a thirty-year-old man from Rochester who had progressive symptoms of heart failure due to severely reduced left ventricular function (less than 20 percent of normal). The operation was successful, and the man was discharged one month after he received a new heart.[74]

During the 1990s, advances in the drug treatment of heart failure would improve and prolong the lives of patients with this distressing and disabling condition. Mayo cardiologists Lyle Olson and Wayne Miller summarized the use of newer heart failure drugs in the 1996 edition of *Mayo Clinic Practice of Cardiology*. Large multicenter randomized clinical trials had shown that two classes of drugs (angiotensin-converting enzyme inhibitors and beta-adrenergic receptor blockers) improved heart failure symptoms and reduced hospitalization rates. But Olson and Miller emphasized that heart failure was the only major cardiovascular disease that was increasing in prevalence. More than 400,000 Americans were found to have heart failure each year, and ten times that many carried the diagnosis. It was the most frequent hospital discharge diagnosis in patients over the age of sixty-five.[75] The real challenge was preventing heart failure's most common cause—coronary disease.

Preventing Coronary Disease and Treating Hypertension

During the middle third of the twentieth century, the focus of heart disease prevention shifted gradually from rheumatic fever–related valve disorders to atherosclerosis and coronary artery disease. Fredrick Willius, Mayo's first cardiologist, had opened a 1929 article on the prevention of heart disease with wording that highlighted the problem: "The greatest individual cause of death in the United States today is heart disease. Other diseases have shown decreased morbidity over a period of years; heart disease has shown a steady increase. The fact is a direct challenge to the medical profession and can no longer be ignored." Willius discussed diseases of the heart muscle, noting that long-standing hypertension caused the left ventricle to hypertrophy (grow thicker) and to stop functioning efficiently. Coronary artery disease also caused heart failure, and modernity was contributing to its increasing incidence: "Never before in the history of mankind has the pace of industrial, business, professional and even social life been so rapid." Other lifestyle issues, such as diet, also mattered in terms of coronary disease. Noting that "the average American is largely carnivorous," the Mayo cardiologist recommended "reasonable restriction of animal proteins as persons approach middle life, especially when their occupations are sedentary."[76]

The American life insurance industry had collected data that demonstrated an association between high blood pressure and excess mortality from heart disease and stroke.[77] Blood pressure cuffs, which had been introduced at the turn of the century, made diagnosis possible; but therapy was very problematic. President Franklin Roosevelt's doctors had no effective drugs to treat the severe hypertension that contributed to his death in 1945 at the age of sixty-three. Five years later, Boston internist and blood pressure expert Robert Wilkins began his lecture at a hypertension symposium at the University of Minnesota with a simple statement: "There is no satisfactory pharmacologic treatment for hypertension."[78] But this was about to change.

Seven Mayo vascular specialists opened a 1954 article on hypertension therapy by contrasting the current situation with "that which existed three years ago." To highlight the hailstorm of antihypertensive drugs that had been marketed recently, they cited advertisements for thirteen drugs that had appeared in a recent issue of the journal *Circulation* (veralba, serpasil, rautensin, rauvera, methium, raudixin, semphyten, thesodate, vertavis, vertavis-phen, serpiloid, apresoline, and hexameton). The Mayo physicians complained, "Advertisements commonly indicate that the treatment of essential hypertension is easy, actually it is often complicated and difficult."[79] Ray Gifford, one of the article's coauthors, had just finished his medical residency at Mayo when, in his words, "the explosion of antihypertensive pharmacotherapy began." In 1957 Gifford arranged for the clinic to get early samples of the investigational antihypertensive drug chlorothiazide (Diuril) from the Merck pharmaceutical company.[80]

Mayo's two vascular sections established an outpatient hypertension therapy service in July 1958 in response to the introduction of several new antihypertensive drugs. Most of these medicines had significant side effects, especially when two or more of them were combined. Before the advent of this outpatient program, patients who were started on multiple antihypertensive drugs were usually hospitalized in Rochester for about two weeks. This gave the hypertension specialists time to adjust each person's regimen and to assess both its beneficial and undesirable effects.

Early in 1959, vascular section head Edgar Hines summarized the status of the new hypertension therapy service for Mayo's Board of Governors: "It has enriched our experience in the treatment of hypertension as well as providing patients with a superior form of antihypertensive therapy. In addition, the cost of such care appears to be less for patients managed in this manner because the expense of hospitalization is avoided. Many hypertensive patients now remain for outpatient treatment whereas they refused to do so in the past when we required hospitalization."[81] Shortly after the hypertension therapy service was established, it was renamed the Hypertension Clinic.

A 1963 article in Mayo's staff newsletter described the Hypertension Clinic, where about 500 patients were receiving care annually. Over a week and a half, each patient came to the subspecialty clinic four times a day to have his or her blood pressure measured by a specially trained technician. Many patients were taught to take their own blood pressure and to record the results on graph paper. Using this information, a hypertension specialist assigned to the clinic adjusted their drug doses. The new care model also included a research component. Mayo's Section of Biometry and Medical Statistics collected information on patients seen in the new clinic, including clinical and laboratory data and blood pressure responses to various drugs. The newsletter article explained that "these data, recorded on IBM cards, will eventually be analyzed through use of the computer and will serve as a baseline for detailed follow-up studies related to survival, incidence of complications [related] to high blood pressure, and effectiveness of therapy."[82] Mayo had pioneered population-based research, and this statistical study was one of many epidemiological projects undertaken at the institution.[83]

In January 1975 *Time* magazine ran a cover story titled "Hypertension: Conquering the Quiet Killer." The article revealed that there were many problems. Hypertension was prevalent, and "most hypertensives are not even aware that they are being stalked by a quiet killer that often produces no symptoms until it is too late." Citing statistics from the American Heart Association, the article explained that fewer that half of patients with hypertension were aware that their blood pressure was high. "Even worse...only half of hypertensives who are aware of their illness are under treatment to control their blood pressure, and of these, only half are getting the proper therapy. For the remainder, the consequences can be fatal." The *Time* article outlined an alternative scenario, noting that many deaths that were a complication of hypertension were avoidable: "Doctors may not be able to cure cancer or the common cold, but modern medicine can now treat virtually every case of hypertension, from the mildest to the most severe, effectively and relatively inexpensively."[84] Most physicians would have regarded this assessment as overly optimistic.

The chapter on hypertension in a 1980 Mayo-authored book on outpatient cardiology began with statements designed to attract attention: "Hypertension is the chief epidemic of the twentieth century.... At least 35 million Americans of all ages are afflicted." After noting that high blood pressure contributed to 1 million fatal heart attacks and strokes each year, the authors claimed that "treatment is effective in preventing these complications, and it is much less expensive to treat hypertension than to treat its complications."[85] This message for physicians echoed what *Time* magazine had told the public five years earlier. But hypertension was just one of several factors that contributed to heart attacks and strokes.

High Cholesterol, Smoking, and the Risk Factor Concept

The most influential ongoing study of the epidemiology of coronary heart disease was launched in Framingham, Massachusetts, in 1948. Located twenty miles west of Boston, the small town became the centerpiece of a long-term project designed to evaluate the role that hypertension, high serum cholesterol, and other variables played in the development of coronary disease. When the leaders of the Framingham Heart Study introduced the phrase "risk factors" in 1961, the concept was controversial. In part, this was because they used so-called inferential statistics rather than more standard approaches, such as laboratory research, to test their hypotheses and draw their conclusions.[86]

The Framingham group's observations complemented research that University of Minnesota physiologist and epidemiologist Ancel Keys had begun at mid-century. *Time* magazine ran a cover story on diet and health in 1961 that featured him as the head of a $200,000-a-year experiment on diet involving subjects in seven countries. The article also noted that Keys had recently coauthored the best-selling book *Eat Well and Stay Well*. His message in *Time* magazine was simple: "Americans eat too much fat…and most of that is saturated fat—the insidious kind, says Dr. Keys, that increases blood cholesterol, damages arteries, and leads to coronary disease." The article described cholesterol as "a mysterious yellowish, waxy substance, chemically a crystalline alcohol" that was vital for some bodily functions but posed a significant risk for others. Keys explained how cholesterol that became embedded in the walls of the coronary arteries contributed to heart attacks: "As cholesterol piles up, it narrows, irritates and damages the artery, encouraging formation of calcium deposits and slowing circulation."[87]

Keys outlined two life-threatening scenarios that could occur in a coronary artery. The cholesterol-induced damage might cause a clot to form inside the vessel, triggering a heart attack, or "the deposits themselves get so big that they choke off the artery's flow to the point that an infarct occurs: the heart muscle is suffocated, cells supplied by the artery die, and the heart is permanently, perhaps fatally injured." Keys preached prevention, but he was pessimistic about the public's response. The *Time* writer explained, "It is difficult for a physician to convince a patient who feels fine that he must give up something he likes to preserve his health. Yet, says Dr. Keys, that is exactly what many Americans should do." Regarding the effect of diet on cholesterol, the Minnesota scientist declared: "People should know the facts…. Then if they want to eat themselves to death, let them."[88]

Meanwhile, the search was on for drugs to treat high cholesterol in an attempt to delay the development of atherosclerosis. *Newsweek* magazine's medical editor Marguerite Clark had claimed in 1958 that when the average American gets sick he "demands a wonder drug that will cure him."[89] A host of medicines had been introduced since World War II that could cure or at least control certain diseases and the symptoms associated with them. These included antibiotics, tranquilizers, and oral anti-diabetic agents, among others. In this context, some scientists and pharmaceutical companies were trying to develop cholesterol-lowering drugs. The 1961 *Time* article on diet and health noted that nicotinic acid (a B vitamin) lowered serum cholesterol. But there was a catch: "Nicotinic acid, to be effective, must be administered in massive doses. The result: flushing, itching, nausea, headaches, changes in the blood."[90] This summary in *Time* was based mainly on nicotinic acid research that had been done recently at the Mayo Clinic.

Two Mayo internists were responsible for their institution's early involvement in the evaluation of nicotinic acid as a cholesterol-lowering drug. Richard Achor and Kenneth Berge would have been considered cardiologists in many contexts by virtue of their training and interests, but they were members of the clinic's only general medicine section. Their practices were confined to patients from Rochester, which made it possible for them to arrange regular follow-up visits to assess the effects of cholesterol-lowering drugs.

Shortly after Berge joined the staff in 1955, Achor encouraged him to participate in a local clinical trial that involved administering high-dose nicotinic acid to thirteen patients with elevated cholesterol.[91] Nine patients' cholesterol levels fell significantly, and the side effects of flushing and itching tended to decrease after a few days of taking the drug. The Mayo internist-investigators placed their study in perspective in 1956: "The search continues for a simple, safe and effective method for correcting abnormalities of lipid metabolism, although admittedly there is no positive evidence that such therapy would prevent the development or arrest the progress of clinical atherosclerosis."[92]

Achor opened a 1960 article on "the cholesterol problem" by refashioning Hamlet's familiar soliloquy: "To restrict fats or not to restrict fats: that is the question: whether 'tis nobler on the arteries to use corn oil instead of butter or to suffer the flush caused by nicotinic acid? Ay, there's the rub."[93] Achor considered high cholesterol a contributing factor to the development of atherosclerosis, and he claimed that an increasing number of patients wanted their cholesterol level checked when they came to the Mayo Clinic.

Although Achor advocated a low saturated fat diet and exercise in patients with elevated cholesterol, he acknowledged that these lifestyle changes rarely had a significant effect on its serum level. Turning to possible drug therapy, he mentioned several agents but admitted that evidence about their effectiveness was lacking and that side effects were common. Achor's cholesterol research and promising career ended prematurely in 1962, when he died of acute leukemia at the age of forty.[94]

Achor's protégé Kenneth Berge was among six clinical investigators invited to help design a protocol for a National Heart Institute–sponsored study of cholesterol-lowering drugs in 1962. Jeremiah Stamler, a Chicago cardiologist and atherosclerosis researcher, chaired the Coronary Drug Project's Steering Committee. It was an ambitious study, and Berge's role would be significant. Mayo's Board of Governors approved his request to devote 45 percent of his time to the project for up to seven years. But there was a catch. As always, the clinic's leaders wanted to be sure that sufficient staff were available to fulfill the institution's main mission of patient care. The board's approval was contingent on the assumption that "this research can be conducted without interfering with the clinical load of the section and without replacement."[95]

Berge, who had the support of his colleagues, was appointed vice chair of the Coronary Drug Project's Steering Committee, and Mayo was one of four sites chosen to participate when the project was launched in December 1965. Eventually, fifty-three institutions and more than eight thousand individuals would be involved in the randomized, double-blind, placebo-controlled clinical trial. The results of the Coronary Drug Project were published over several years. Of the five drugs tested, nicotinic acid was the only one recommended as a cholesterol-lowering agent on the basis of this national trial.[96]

When Mayo began enrolling patients in the Coronary Drug Project, the public heard mixed messages about cholesterol. Popular British-American journalist and television personality Alistair Cooke spoke at the clinic in 1965. In his lecture "The Patient Has the Floor," he addressed the issue of diet as a cardiac risk factor. "Four or five years ago," Cooke told his Rochester audience, "it was established, at least to the satisfaction of a panicky populace...that cholesterol was as fatal as silt along a riverbed." The suave middle-aged man then recounted some remarks that he had made recently at an annual dinner of the Massachusetts Heart Fund:

> If animal fats and carbohydrates were certain prescriptions for heart attacks, then they would have to explain the miracle whereby fifty-five million Britons were still alive...with their morning toast and eggs bubbling in bacon fat, their biscuits at eleven o'clock, their lunch of more meat and potatoes and (worse) suet, then tea and more biscuits and cake, and dinner and meat and bread again, and potatoes and pudding.... How to explain the endurance, the ignorant but cheerful survival, of the British?[97]

When Alistair Cooke spoke at Mayo, British physicians and scientists were less interested in the cholesterol debate than were their American counterparts.[98] Cooke would outlive most of the men and women who heard him speak in Rochester in 1961. He died a half-century later at the age of ninety-five.

In 1964, during Lyndon Johnson's first full-year as president, an advisory committee (that US Surgeon General Luther Terry had appointed) published a 387-page report, *Smoking and Health*. The authors emphasized that about one-third of the 1.7 million Americans who died each year lost their lives as a result of "atherosclerotic heart disease including coronary disease." This number far exceeded the annual deaths from lung cancer, estimated to be about 39,000.[99] In the section on smoking and coronary heart disease, the committee cited a quarter-century-old Mayo article for perspective. Fredrick Willius and his coauthors had used statistics and a sample of 2,000 men who had been seen at the clinic to conclude in 1940 that there was a significant relationship between smoking and coronary disease in patients under the age of fifty.[100] Decades later, Boston cardiologist Oglesby Paul and catheterization pioneer Richard Bing cited this paper as the first to link cigarette smoking to coronary heart disease. There would be many others.[101]

The 1964 Surgeon General's report on smoking declared: "Over the last two decades a considerable number of epidemiologic studies on different populations, employing different techniques, have shown with remarkable consistency a significant relationship between cigarette smoking and

an increased death rate from coronary heart disease in males, particularly
in middle life." Despite growing evidence, controversy continued to swirl
around the role of smoking and sickness in the early 1960s—just as smoke
continued to fill the air at most social settings, including medical meetings.
The authors of the report concluded cautiously: "Male cigarette smokers
have a higher death rate from coronary artery disease than non-smoking
males, but it is not clear that the association has causal significance."[102]
They also acknowledged that high serum cholesterol and hypertension
were associated with an increased death rate from coronary heart disease.
Meanwhile, the tight-knit community of preventive cardiologists was growing impatient with those who refused to acknowledge that some risk factors
contributed to coronary disease with its consequences of heart failure and
sudden death.

The Minnesota Symposium on Prevention in Cardiology

The Mayo Clinic, the Minnesota Heart Association, and the American
Heart Association cosponsored "The Minnesota Symposium on Prevention
in Cardiology: Reducing the Risk of Coronary and Hypertensive Disease"
in May 1968. Mayo vascular specialist John Juergens, who was president of
the state association, welcomed a large audience to the two-day program
held at Rochester's Kahler Hotel. He proclaimed with missionary zeal, "At
a time when coronary heart disease has reached epidemic proportions in the
western world, it is particularly appropriate to spread the gospel of preventive medicine and to disseminate all available information about reducing
the risks of atherosclerosis." Juergens demanded a change in philosophy and
practice: "We are beyond the stage when this type of information can be
regarded as of interest only to the epidemiologist or the clinical investigator.
It must be made available to, and used by, the medical practitioner who now
spends his time almost exclusively with diagnosis and treatment rather than
prevention. And that is what this symposium is all about."[103]

Cardiologist Henry Blackburn, who had begun working with Ancel Keys
at the University of Minnesota in the mid-1950s, chaired the committee
that had organized the Rochester symposium. Speaking after Juergens,
he declared, "It is appropriate to sound this call in Minnesota, where so
many have been concerned with preventive cardiology, and in Rochester,
where the Mayo Clinic holds the respect of all for its practice of diagnostic and therapeutic medicine."[104] In a memoir written three decades later,
Blackburn explained that his committee "saw the Mayo conference as crys-
tallizing the status of prevention at the peak of the North American coronary epidemic, and as a platform to launch research and policy initiatives
for prevention."[105]

Several pioneers and promoters of preventive cardiology spoke at the Rochester symposium, including William Castelli, Thomas Dawber, William Kannel, Ancel Keys, Jeremiah Stamler, and Paul Dudley White. Keys applauded recent advances in the treatment of patients with heart disease with drugs and devices, such as pacemakers and external defibrillators. Speaking a few months after Christiaan Barnard had performed the world's first human heart transplant, Keys made a cynical comment about that aggressive approach to the treatment of end-stage cardiac disease: "Finally, when all else fails, we look at Dr. Blaiberg walking around with his new heart and we read a forecast that before long a thousand teams of surgeons may be busy installing nuclear-powered contraptions to replace hearts diseased beyond redemption." Then the Minnesota epidemiologist put things in perspective: "In spite of all advances in diagnosis and treatment, prevention is essential for any real control over most of the heart disease problem...[because] in the majority of cases of heart disease specific treatment has great limitations."[106] No one could dispute this.

One presentation at the preventive cardiology symposium in Rochester described a new subspecialty clinic that Mayo had launched recently. John Fairbairn, head of one of the clinic's two vascular sections, had informed the Board of Governors early in 1967 that he was enthusiastic about establishing a Lipid Clinic. He thought it was important "because we handle these problems on a clinic-wide basis rather haphazardly and without uniformity."[107] The Lipid Clinic was inaugurated in July 1967, and John Juergens directed it. Participants in the Rochester symposium learned that the Mayo group had seen several hundred patients with elevated cholesterol levels in the Lipid Clinic in less than a year. Each one underwent an evaluation that included dietary and family histories, in addition to determinations of their cholesterol, triglyceride, and lipoprotein levels. Treatment recommendations were individualized on the basis of this information.[108]

Jeremiah Stamler, who had invited Kenneth Berge to help organize and direct the Coronary Drug Project, spoke last at the 1968 symposium. He reminded the Rochester audience that very few doctors shared the speakers' passion for prevention: "The overwhelming bulk of our medical practitioners today, generalists and internists, the army who must contend with this problem [of cardiovascular disease], are preoccupied with the care of people who are ill."[109]

Stamler's assessment applied to most of Mayo's cardiologists, who were busy incorporating new diagnostic tests and treatments into patient care. Like their peers across the country, the clinic's heart specialists devoted little time or energy to prevention. On the other hand, a few of them thought that Mayo should develop an atherosclerosis research program. Cardiovascular Division chief Robert Brandenburg informed the chief of medicine in the spring of 1971 that recent attempts to recruit lipid expert Robert Levy from the National Heart Institute to become head of atherosclerosis research had been unsuccessful.[110] Instead, Mayo vascular specialist Bruce Kottke, who had joined the staff a decade earlier, would run the program. His PhD thesis had focused on cholesterol metabolism in animals, and he was actively involved in the Lipid Clinic and lipid research.

In the summer of 1971 a *Rochester Post-Bulletin* headline announced, "Clinic Gets $2.1-Million Grant for Arteries Project." Kottke would direct an NIH-funded Specialized Center of Research (SCOR) project designed to "develop new knowledge relevant to the prevention, diagnosis and treatment of atherosclerosis and to hasten the clinical application of this knowledge."[111] A *Mayovox* article explained that the clinic was one of twenty-nine institutions chosen to receive grants under the new program. About forty Mayo staff members would participate in the project in Rochester, including internists, cardiologists, pediatricians, radiologists, nutritionists, biochemists, physiologists, pathologists, microbiologists, and epidemiologists.[112] Although Mayo's SCOR grant was not renewed in 1977, Robert Frye had some good news to share with the chair of medicine. Valentin Fuster's research on atherosclerosis was "attracting national and international attention."[113]

Promoting Physical Activity and Cardiac Rehabilitation

Herman Hellerstein, a cardiologist at Western Reserve University in Cleveland, Ohio, spoke on the benefits of physical activity at the 1968 preventive cardiology symposium in Rochester. He described a six-year study designed to evaluate the effects of a program of increased physical activity for middle-aged men who either had evidence of coronary artery disease or were considered "coronary-prone" on the basis of their risk factors. Hellerstein painted an unflattering picture of a typical study subject when he explained that the goal was to "determine the feasibility and efficacy of activating habitually sedentary, lazy, hypokinetic, hypercholesterolemic, cigarette-smoking, hypertensive, overweight males, with or without manifest coronary artery disease, to participate in and adhere to a program of enhanced physical activity."[114] Based on his group's research, the Cleveland cardiologist concluded that a supervised program of physical conditioning was safe and resulted in improved exercise tolerance. Published reports by Hellerstein and others inspired a few institutions to launch similar programs in the late 1960s.

In 1968 Ralph Spiekerman and Charles Kennedy, members of Mayo's general medical section that cared for Rochester residents, launched a small study of the effects of exercise on men in their forties who had angina pectoris. Four years later, a *Mayovox* article "You've Had a Coronary? Maybe You Can Join the Club" publicized an exercise program that had evolved from Spiekerman and Kennedy's initiative. It explained that several men met at 6:30 a.m. at the Rochester YMCA three days a week: "These stalwarts are gym-suited and jogging around the basketball court, which is preliminary to jumping jacks, leg lifts, and other muscle stretching exercises." Each forty-five minute session ended with a volleyball game. "Sure, it's an early hour for exercise, but what makes it so special you say? What makes it so special is that nearly all of these men have 'unequivocal angina pectoris' (a serious heart ailment), that many, maybe most, have suffered a 'myocardial infarction' (heart attack), and several have undergone open-heart surgery. It's an exercise program tailored for heart patients."[115]

Before entering the exercise program, each patient underwent a physical examination and a treadmill exercise test. A photograph in the *Mayovox* article depicted six men exercising. An impressive array of life-saving technology was between them and the camera. An oxygen tank, an open medicine case, a blood pressure cuff, and a portable defibrillator sat on the floor of the basketball court. This juxtaposition of animated men and inanimate objects conveyed a powerful message. If one of the men collapsed, a trained team was ready to rush into action with resuscitation paraphernalia. One of the participants commented on this display of technology: "I look at it when I run by, but I'm glad it's there and I'm glad there's someone here who knows how to handle it." Another man explained that he considered it "kind of a visual insurance policy." The article quoted a fifty-two-year-old participant: "Probably the thing that I appreciate most about the program...is the group therapy it provides. It would take a great deal of self discipline or dedication to do this on my own."[116]

When the article describing Mayo's small outpatient exercise program appeared in 1972, both Saint Marys Hospital and Rochester Methodist Hospital were establishing inpatient cardiac rehabilitation programs for men and women recovering from heart attacks. They used a team-based approach that involved cardiologists, nurses, dieticians, physical therapists, occupational therapists, and a psychiatrist.[117] The practice of keeping patients in bed for more than a month after a heart attack was gradually changing as experience showed that earlier ambulation was safe. Spiekerman recalled that when prolonged bed rest was the norm "it was harder to get their leg muscles going than it was to get their heart muscle going."[118] Outpatient cardiac rehabilitation programs became increasingly popular as post–heart attack hospital stays shortened from a month to two weeks or less. Mayo's program grew in size and sophistication in the 1970s and 1980s.[119] Around the same time, there was growing interest in developing primary prevention programs for individuals without evidence of heart disease.

In 1979 Mayo cardiologist George Gura met with the Cardiovascular Practice Committee to present a proposal to establish a "Cardiovascular Fitness Clinic" that would focus on individuals who were apparently healthy, as well as those who were considered "coronary-prone." The program, which would be open to patients and clinic employees, included a cardiac risk factor analysis, a fitness assessment, and a prescription for exercise. In addition to a cardiac examination, participants would have a resting electrocardiogram, pulmonary function tests, and a treadmill exercise test.[120]

The committee endorsed Gura's proposal, and he launched the program in the summer of 1979. Six months later he proposed changing its name to the Cardiovascular Health Clinic and extending it to include monitored exercise sessions for patients with known heart disease.[121] Gerald Gau, who had been involved in Mayo's inpatient cardiac rehabilitation program since its inception in 1973, took over the Cardiovascular Health Clinic in 1980, when Gura left Rochester to join the Mid America Heart Institute in Kansas City, Missouri.[122]

Treadmill exercise testing (with electrocardiography) gained a prominent place in the evaluation of patients with known or suspected coronary disease in the 1970s. The number of treadmill tests performed on Mayo outpatients skyrocketed from 720 in 1971 to 3,338 in 1978.[123] Harold Mankin, who directed the exercise test laboratory, summarized the procedure's indications and usefulness in a 1980 Mayo-authored book on outpatient cardiology. He described how an exercise test could help a doctor decide how to manage individual patients and how it might be useful in counseling asymptomatic men and women who were planning to "embark on a 'flight into health' with a program of physical training." An experienced clinical cardiologist, Mankin emphasized that a "test is but a test" and argued that it "does not relieve the clinician of his responsibility to exercise clinical judgment." Still, a very abnormal treadmill test might lead directly to coronary angiography. Alternatively, a totally normal test was reassuring and might eliminate the need for a trial of medical therapy or a more extensive cardiac evaluation.[124]

The Preventive Cardiology Movement Gains Momentum

Mayo cardiologist Robert Brandenburg was president of the American College of Cardiology in 1980, when he welcomed more than eighty physicians, scientists, nurses, and others to a coronary disease prevention conference in Bethesda, Maryland.[125] Jeremiah Stamler, a pioneer of preventive cardiology, followed Brandenburg on the program. The Chicago cardiologist was pleased that substantial progress had been made during the 1970s in "controlling the epidemic of premature coronary heart disease in the United States." He claimed that millions of Americans were being treated effectively for hypertension, and millions more had changed their eating habits in an attempt to address their personal coronary risk factors. Stamler applauded the 25 percent reduction in mortality rates from coronary disease in the past decade, but he reminded participants that the nation's "rates of sickness, disability, and death from this modern plague still remain high."[126]

Despite the huge toll that coronary artery disease took in terms of death and disability, some physicians envisioned a time when prevention would prevail. In 1980 academic internist Paul Beeson spoke at the first meeting of the Council of Medical Societies of the American College of Physicians. He had been a physician for almost fifty years when he discussed the history of medical subspecialties with a group of individuals that represented them. Most of Beeson's talk described the rise of subspecialties, but one section dealt with how some fields had declined or even disappeared. For example, the advent of antibiotics for the treatment of tuberculosis had revolutionized the management of patients with this common communicable disease and had disrupted the careers of physicians who had helped care for them: "Before the advent of chemotherapy in 1947, we had hundreds of doctors treating patients in sanatoriums, by prolonged bed rest and [lung] collapse therapy. What happened to those hundreds of specialists and those scores of sanatoriums? Something of the same has happened to rheumatic fever, rheumatic heart disease, and the treatment of syphilis."[127]

At one point, Beeson challenged his audience to consider the future of specialists whose careers focused on the care of patients with heart disease: "Just contemplate what would happen to both medical cardiology and cardiac surgery if better methods to prevent or reverse the course of coronary artery sclerosis become available. Most of the business of managing angina pectoris, either medically or surgically, would go, and with it would disappear those income-producing angiograms, exercise tolerance tests, and bypass procedures. The coronary care units in our hospitals would have to be put to other uses."[128]

Mayo surgeon Dwight McGoon made the same point in 1987. Like Beeson, he used tuberculosis as an example of how new knowledge and effective treatments had totally transformed the care of patients with this communicable disease. Turning to heart disease and the future, McGoon predicted that true prevention would become a reality once the underlying causes and basic mechanisms of its various forms were understood. This would have major implications for patients, but it would also affect institutions and individuals involved in heart care: "Thereafter, many hospitals, catheterization laboratories, and cardiac operating rooms will become used for other purposes, and cardiologists, surgeons, nurses, and technicians will become dedicated to other pursuits.... The surgery of heart disease will return whence it was born—to the repair of the traumatized heart—and cardiology will be absorbed into the sphere of preventive medicine."[129]

In 1987, the same year that Dwight McGoon championed prevention, the US Food and Drug Administration approved the release of a new type of drug that had been shown to significantly lower cholesterol. Lovastatin

(Mevacor) was the first "statin" approved for clinical use; others marketed during the next decade included pravastatin (Pravachol), simvastatin (Zocor), and atorvastatin (Lipitor).[130] Prescriptions for statins surged after the results of the Scandinavian Simvastatin Survival Study (4S trial) that involved 4,444 patients were published beginning with a 1994 paper in the *Lancet*. The article's first sentence acknowledged the ambivalence that surrounded older cholesterol-lowering medicines: "Drug therapy for hypercholesterolemia has remained controversial mainly because of insufficient clinical trial evidence for improved survival." But the 4S trial results provided proof that patients who had been given simvastatin had fewer heart attacks and better survival rates than those who had been given a placebo.[131]

William Roberts, America's leading cardiac pathologist and a strong proponent of preventive cardiology, proclaimed in 1996 that "statin drugs are to atherosclerosis what penicillin was to infectious diseases" and argued that these "miracle drugs" were underused.[132] Physicians' attitudes about cholesterol were changing, and the public's awareness of new drugs was increasing. The 2000 edition of the *Mayo Clinic Heart Book* informed general readers that "several large studies done in several parts of the world" had shown that statins reduced the risk of a heart attack.[133] Pharmaceutical companies that sold statins used clinical trial results to promote their products on television and radio after the FDA approved direct-to-consumer advertising of drugs in the broadcast media in 1997. During the next decade, statins became the best-selling class of prescription drugs in the United States. In 2010 Lipitor topped the list with sales of $7.2 billion.[134]

Mayo cardiologists Véronique Roger and Robert Frye and members of the clinic's Department of Health Sciences Research reported trends in deaths from cardiovascular disease in Olmsted County, Minnesota, between 1979 and 2003. During the quarter-century period they studied, there was a 50 percent decline in cardiovascular disease mortality in the county that contained Rochester. The Mayo authors described a "marked annual decrease" of 3.3 percent for deaths attributed to coronary heart disease. They authors acknowledged that there was controversy about the relative contributions of primary prevention (risk factor modification before a cardiac event), acute cardiac care, and secondary prevention (risk factor modification after a cardiac event).[135]

In 2013 the *New England Journal of Medicine* published the results of a study of the decrease in deaths due to coronary disease in the United States between 1980 and 2000. The authors explained that "these two decades saw rapid growth in costly medical technology and pharmaceutical treatments for coronary heart disease, as well as substantial public health efforts to reduce the prevalence of major cardiovascular risk factors." They concluded that reductions in major cardiac risk factors and therapies (such as coronary bypass surgery, angioplasty, and statins) contributed almost equally to the decline of more than 40 percent in the mortality rate from coronary heart disease.[136]

Despite the marked reduction in the mortality rate from cardiovascular diseases during the past half-century, about one-third of Americans still die as a result of them.[137] Heart failure, especially, continues to be a major problem. Véronique Roger emphasized in a 2013 editorial that heart failure represents a "staggering clinical and public health problem, associated with significant mortality, morbidity, and healthcare expenditures." She noted that almost 6 million persons in the United States have heart failure and that the five-year mortality rate is about 50 percent, despite advances in treatment.[138]

Mayo heart failure specialist Richard Rodeheffer had asked rhetorically in 2011, "Are we facing a tsunami of heart failure?" Reminding readers that the prevalence of heart failure increases with age and that the Baby Boom generation would soon swell the ranks of the elderly, he declared, "You do the math." Rodeheffer explained that this "tidal wave" had implications for individuals and the nation because "heart failure brings with it personal suffering and disability, lost productivity, and a growing burden on an already excessively US per capita medical care expenditure." He was cautiously optimistic, however, because a half-century of epidemiological research had revealed the importance of risk factor modification, and recent clinical trial results had provided insight into what strategies were more likely to reduce the impact of those risk factors.[139] In their editorials, Mayo cardiologists Roger and Rodeheffer pointed out that many challenges remained, despite impressive progress in preventing and treating heart disease during the past half-century. It is impossible to say whether it will take decades or generations before Dwight McGoon's 1987 prediction that prevention will ultimately prevail comes true.

Challenges and Opportunities Around the New Millennium

During the past two generations, the care of patients with heart disease has been totally transformed by new diagnostic and treatment technologies and procedures. Meanwhile, powerful social, economic, and political forces have buffeted health care delivery in the United States.[1] In this context, Mayo Clinic's leaders (at an institutional level and in cardiology) worked to maintain the clinic's longtime reputation as a regional, national, and international center of excellence.

Eugene Mayberry, chair of the Board of Governors, informed the staff in November 1983 that Mayo was on track to have its most successful year ever. Demand for services was strong, hospital admissions were up, and the full-time professional staff had grown to 819. Mayo's postgraduate training program was also thriving, with more than 800 residents and fellows. But Mayberry explained that the board had recently debated five scenarios for the future: maintaining the status quo, continuing current growth rates, becoming more like traditional academic medical centers, launching another group practice elsewhere, and diversifying. The board favored diversification, but it had no interest in reinventing the institution or reordering its priorities.[2]

The following year, Mayberry described Mayo's mission in terms of a tricycle, "where the large front wheel is the practice of medicine with compassionate care for the individual patient and the two smaller rear wheels are research and education. Research and education are very important—the tricycle will not go without them—but the steering force in the institution remains that of the large front wheel of patient care."[3] Mayberry could have used a tricycle analogy to describe the clinic's vital relationships with the two hospitals where its staff cared for patients.

The officers of the Mayo Foundation, Saint Marys Hospital, and Methodist Hospital signed an agreement on May 28, 1986, that would unite their organizations under a common governance and management structure. A press release explained that the merger (which involved 1,700 doctors, 14,000 employees, 1,800 hospital beds, and assets of $1 billion) would result in a new organizational structure that would be "better able to manage every aspect of our operation more efficiently and to plan effectively for the future." The Mayo Foundation Board of Trustees would be the overarching governing body, and Saint Marys Hospital would continue to be a Catholic institution.[4]

St. Paul health reporter Walter Parker exclaimed in 1986 that "over the past year, the traditionally reclusive clinic has been in the news again and again announcing major business developments aimed at keeping itself steaming along through a second century." Among other things, he noted the recent formation of Mayo Medical Ventures, which was designed "to make money from ideas and technology developed at the clinic," and plans to launch practices in Florida and Arizona.[5] Mayo opened a branch in Jacksonville, Florida, with thirty-five physicians on October 13, 1986, and one in Scottsdale, Arizona, with forty-two physicians on June 29, 1987. *New York Times* health reporter Milt Freudenheim explained in 1988, "As one of the largest and richest medical centers in the world, the Mayo Clinic has been in a class by itself for much of its... history. But in recent years, even the prestigious clinic has been affected by the cost pressures and competition buffeting the health-care industry." Its leaders had decided to expand into Florida and Arizona "rather than retrench as many in the health-care industry have been forced to do."[6]

The new Sun Belt practices did not address competition that was intensifying much closer to Rochester. Minneapolis and St. Paul, less than ninety miles away, were serving as an early proving ground for what would be called the managed care movement. According to the authors of the 1987 book *The Best Hospitals in America*, the Twin Cities area was "one of the most competitive hospital markets in the country." Turning to Rochester, they claimed that "the Mayo Clinic is one of the few medical institutions in the United States whose status can legitimately be called legendary."[7] Despite such accolades, Mayo's leaders and its heart specialists recognized the risks of ignoring trends that were transforming the market for health care.

Mayo's Cardiologists Confront Increasing Competition

In 1989 Hugh Smith, who had chaired the Cardiovascular Division for five years, summarized the status of its programs of clinical practice, research, and education. Looking to the future, Smith predicted that demand for Mayo's outpatient cardiology services was "likely to remain high if we can effectively compete against private cardiovascular practices in the Twin Cities' area, western Wisconsin, and northern Iowa. Part of our strategy has involved our Cardiovascular Outreach practice."[8]

The division had launched an outreach consultation program in 1978, when Gerald Gau began seeing patients in Charles City, Iowa, eighty miles south of Rochester. An outreach echocardiography program (which involved a technician transporting an echocardiograph machine in a van) was inaugurated in 1989. Two years later, cardiologist Andre Lapeyre began performing coronary angiograms in a mobile catheterization laboratory that was housed in a customized semi-tractor trailer. By the fall of 1993, the outreach consultation program had expanded to fifteen sites. Cardiologist Donald Johnston inaugurated a mobile nuclear cardiology program two years later.[9] The main incentive for developing this comprehensive program of outreach heart care services was to identify patients who might be referred to Rochester for more specialized diagnostic tests and treatments. Robert Frye and Douglas Wood, cardiologists who led the Department of Medicine, claimed in 1997 that the outreach program "has been a critical component of the continued success" of the Cardiovascular Division.[10]

The division's outreach program was part of a strategy to make it possible for Mayo's cardiologists to devote more time to the care of patients with heart disease. Smith had informed the Board of Governors in the spring of 1988 that the Cardiovascular Division's eleven-member Executive Committee supported the creation of a general internal medicine division in the Department of Medicine. This reflected the cardiologists' desire to decrease the number of general medical evaluations they were expected to do.[11] Robert Frye, who had become chair of the Department of Medicine in 1987, supported the concept. Mayo's Division of General Medicine, which was established early in his tenure, made it possible for physicians in technology-intensive medical subspecialties, such as cardiology and gastroenterology, to devote more time to the types of patients and procedures that were related to their chosen fields. But the shift would be gradual.[12]

Hugh Smith emphasized in 1989 that cardiology had evolved from a largely outpatient practice into a "laboratory and hospital-based subspecialty." The fact that he had been co-director of the catheterization laboratory at Saint Marys Hospital informed his perspective. "It is vital," he insisted, "that we keep our hospital and laboratory practices on the forefront in terms of quality of care rendered, rapidity of access, and full utilization of available technology." Referring to Mayo's catheterization, electrophysiology, echocardiography, and nuclear cardiology laboratories, Smith claimed that each one "holds a position of national and international prominence. Maintaining this prominence, along with the prominence of cardiovascular research at the Mayo Clinic, is the best mechanism available for guaranteeing continued growth of our practice." One sentence in his report to the board was highlighted: *"It is in the institution's best interest to make efficient use of cardiovascular specialists; that is, cardiovascular specialists should be utilized to handle cardiovascular diseases."*[13] The clinic responded. Between 1988 and 1995, twenty-one internists would be added to the Division of Internal Medicine.[14]

Mayo's leaders implemented another strategy in the early 1990s to help maintain the flow of patients who needed specialized services to Rochester. As managed care continued to gain momentum, they decided to create a primary care network by acquiring selected small physician practices and hospitals. Other referral centers in the region and around the nation were employing similar strategies for the same reason.

The Mayo Health System had its origins in a 1992 agreement between the clinic and a six-physician practice in Decorah, Iowa, 75 miles southeast of Rochester. In a 1995 article in *Modern Healthcare*, writer Lisa Scott proclaimed that "the Mayo Clinic, long a fountainhead of medical miracles, is becoming a powerhouse of primary care." She explained that in the past three years Mayo had acquired nine hospitals and forty-one clinics (with 345 physicians) within a 120-mile radius of Rochester. Scott's article included portions of her interview of the physician who was coordinating the development of the Mayo Health System: "As managed care wrapped its arms around more patients, Twin Cities health systems reached toward Mayo territory, and Iowa providers established outposts near its border. Fearing a bleak future, Mayo decided to build 'the very best delivery system that would be very, very attractive to payers,' said Michael O'Sullivan, chairman of its Regional Strategy Working Group."[15]

When Mayo was taking steps to maintain its position as a major referral center in 1995, University of California health policy analyst Stephen Shortell coauthored an article describing the national context: "American health care is in a state of hyper-turbulence characterized by accumulated waves of change in payment systems, delivery systems, technology, professional relations, and societal expectations."[16] That year, Mayo's Department of Medicine (chaired by Frye and comprising fifteen subspecialty divisions) developed a business plan. One section, termed "Critical Success Factors," included a list of things that were considered vitally important if the department was to maintain its position as "the premier provider of health care in the region and the country" and was to extend its lead over competitors:

- Recruiting and retaining high quality staff
- Maintaining staff satisfaction and morale during restructuring where change is the norm
- Increasing demands for service by becoming a high quality, low cost provider
- Ability to sustain innovation in research and practice that provides services unavailable in many other referral centers
- Ability to sustain and enhance the intellectual performance of our physician and scientific staff
- Ability to enhance physician productivity through practice innovation

- Ability to improve service to referring physicians and to take advantage of new system-wide opportunities for delivery of secondary and tertiary level internal medicine services
- Ability to improve our financial performance
- Ability to understand and address the needs of payers and purchasers.[17]

Several of these themes had appeared in older documents prepared by the department or the clinic, but some bullet points reflected recent changes in health care that affected how physicians practiced in other contexts.[18] In terms of heart care, one national trend involved the formation or expansion of single-specialty cardiology groups. Between 1972 and 1992, the percentage of cardiologists in the United States that practiced in single specialty-groups tripled, from 15.3 to 46 percent.[19]

The Mayo Model of Care: Meeting the Needs of the Patient

Throughout the twentieth century, the Mayo Clinic remained the world's largest private physician-led health care institution. A 2000 statistical summary illustrated just how big the multispecialty group practice had become: Rochester, Jacksonville, Scottsdale, and the Mayo Health System included 2,708 full-time staff physicians and scientists; 1,893 residents, fellows, and predoctoral students; and 44,186 allied health staff. That year, just over 500,000 unique patients were seen at Rochester, Jacksonville, and Scottsdale.[20] Although Mayo's 2000 annual report indicated that the institution generated just over $3 billion from patient care, it warned that "income from current activities fell short of projection for the year and did not meet the level of income needed to fund growth and support all operational activities, including education, research and non-practice operations."[21]

Another booklet published in 2000, *Mayo Clinic Model of Care*, declared that throughout its history Mayo had "embraced change, new ideas and new ways of working, whenever and wherever necessary, to provide the highest quality care possible." It emphasized that the clinic's primary focus was "meeting the needs of the patient." This message, which paraphrased a statement clinic founder Will Mayo had made in 1910, was very familiar to the staff.[22] In 2000 Mayo president and CEO Michael Wood published an abridged version of the institution's strategy for meeting the needs of the patient. This included "collegial, cooperative staff teamwork...unhurried examination...compassion and trust...respect for the patient, family, and the patient's local physician...most advanced, innovative diagnostic and therapeutic technology...valued professional allied health staff...scholarly environment of research and education...physician leadership."[23] The one thing on the list that was proving difficult to preserve was an unhurried examination.

Physicians at Mayo and elsewhere were expected to become more efficient as reimbursement for services declined. During the 1990s, the Cardiovascular Division increased the use of non-physicians in the inpatient and outpatient practices as national regulations reduced the hours that residents could work in a week and concerns about an oversupply of cardiologists led to a reduction in the number of cardiology fellows trained at Mayo and other centers. In this context, certified nurse practitioners and physician assistants were hired and were identified as physician extenders or mid-level providers.[24]

Robert Frye and Douglas Wood, who had served on local and national committees dealing with health policy and quality improvement, wrote an editorial on the business of medicine in 1997. It opened with a blunt assessment of the contemporary scene: "Like it or not, the business of medicine is forcing a focus on economic realities that were never an issue for academic medicine, or medicine in general, from the end of World War II until the 1980s. Monies from clinical practice flowed in abundance, the academic enterprise flourished, and an extraordinary [number] of well-trained specialists spread across the country." Frye and Wood identified the implementation of Medicare in 1966 as the beginning of a boom that was ending. They expressed concern that the end of this three-decade boom posed a serious threat to academic medicine because "the flow of funds from clinical practice to support research and education is severely constrained." The new and unstable environment required academic cardiology divisions to be proactive and innovative if they hoped to succeed when there was a growing expectation that they deliver the right care to the right patient at the right time.[25]

Eugene Braunwald Chairs a Committee to Review Research at Mayo

In 1999 Harvard Medical School professor Eugene Braunwald, America's most influential academic cardiologist, chaired a five-man committee that reviewed the Cardiovascular Division's research program. Braunwald and Frye had been medical residents together at Johns Hopkins four decades earlier, and Frye was the first person that Braunwald had hired after he returned to the NIH as director of the catheterization laboratory.[26]

The so-called Braunwald Report, prepared after the site visit, acknowledged the division's "long tradition of excellent patient care and the high quality and importance of its clinical research." Noting that the division (in Rochester) had 107 full-time clinicians and the equivalent of 11.5 full-time researchers, the report speculated that its clinical revenues, which exceeded $90 million, were the highest of any cardiovascular division in the nation.

But Braunwald's committee raised concerns about the balance between clinical responsibilities and research productivity at Mayo. The Cardiovascular Division's "immense clinical load" meant that "many of the faculty are left with little time for scholarly activity or for mentoring young cardiologists (fellows or junior staff) in research."[27] This conclusion did not surprise Mayo's heart specialists because they knew that their institution's primary mission was patient care. But the five site visitors had spent their careers in traditional academic medical centers, where the main mission was research.[28]

The Braunwald Report included several recommendations designed to enhance Mayo's cardiovascular research program. One of the most striking suggestions was that the Department of Medicine or the institution should provide sufficient resources to the chair of the Cardiovascular Division to hire twenty new faculty members "and guarantee these individuals up to 30 percent protected time for research (depending upon their abilities and desire)."[29] This was impossible at Mayo because new staff positions were approved centrally and had to be justified by proof of patient demand.

Several other steps were taken to increase the size, scope, and significance of Mayo's cardiovascular research programs. A 2003 strategic planning retreat focused on three themes: promoting excellence in clinical and basic research; fostering training, mentoring, and career development of researchers; and identifying funding sources for disease-oriented research and translational (so-called bench-to-bedside) research. Between 1999, the year of the site visit, and 2007, the total amount of cardiovascular research funding at Mayo almost doubled, from about $14 million to about $26 million.[30]

In a 2005 interview, Braunwald described a fundamental distinction between traditional research-oriented academic medical centers and the academically oriented but patient-centered Mayo Clinic:

> The mission and the value systems are significantly different. I think that in an academic medical center the highest value is placed on the creation of new knowledge, so on the research arm. There are a lot of tugs and pressures within an academic medical center, but I think many people believe that the clinical mission is there to support the educational arm and to support the research. And here it is exactly the opposite. I think the perspective here at the Mayo Clinic is that the way to serve the patient best is to have very strong education and very strong research, but these are support functions.[31]

Braunwald compared the situation at his own institutions, Harvard Medical School and the Brigham and Women's Hospital, with Mayo: "We've got a lot of prima donnas and people who are superb. And institutional practices go around these people. They are built to retain and to attract superstars. I think at the Mayo Clinic there is much more of an institutional feeling."[32] Cardiologist Bernard Gersh had made the same point in a 1993 interview, shortly after he had left Mayo to become chief of cardiology at Georgetown University in Washington, D.C. He characterized Mayo as "an extraordinarily self-sustaining institution. No matter what the prestige of an individual, if he or she leaves, the institution will carry on without missing a beat."[33] Gersh, who returned to Rochester in 1998, explained later, "Georgetown was experiencing financial constraints, and the shape it would take in the future was uncertain.... I was attracted back to Mayo by the strength and stability of the institution and the translational research opportunities."[34]

Promoting More Subspecialization within Cardiology

During the last quarter of the twentieth century, the number of cardiologists and cardiac surgeons in the United States increased significantly. As they completed training, these medical and surgical heart specialists facilitated the transfer of new technologies and techniques from large academic centers and teaching hospitals to medium-sized institutions, including community hospitals. Between 1993 and 2004, for example, 301 new open-heart surgery programs opened in the United States. This increase of about 30 percent occurred in the context of an overall decline in the number of coronary artery bypass operations performed nationally. The authors of the article explained that this growth spurt may have stimulated "competition based on quality, price, or both, but it may also have increased surgical rates, with unknown results."[35]

Cardiologists also began providing new services in many smaller community hospitals. Between 2001 and 2006, for example, the number of US hospitals capable of providing coronary angioplasty and stenting increased from 1,176 to 1,695.[36] More patients with common heart problems were able to get care close to home. Faced with this reality, Mayo's medical and surgical heart specialists emphasized their ability to diagnose and treat less common problems.

Jamil Tajik, who had succeeded Hugh Smith as chair of Mayo's Cardiovascular Division in 1993, actively promoted subspecialization among the cardiologists. The minutes of a 1999 meeting of the division's Executive Committee reflect this strategy:

> Of particular interest was the discussion on the further subspecialization of the division's activities. There is a proposed plan to establish a Valvular Heart Disease Clinic, an Atherosclerosis Clinic, and a Marfan's Clinic.... It was noted that Cleveland Clinic and others with whom Mayo competes are marketing their subspecialty care quite heavily. These marketing techniques provide high visibility to

these programs which in turn attract patients, physician referrals, and financial resources to support clinical and translational research.[37]

Tajik's successors as division chair, David Hayes (2002–2011) and Charanjit (Chet) Rihal (2011–), also encouraged these ventures. Between 1996 and 2013, sixteen subspecialty clinics were established, as summarized in Table 20.1. Meanwhile, cardiology subspecialties were also achieving formal recognition nationally, as evidenced by the creation of new organizations, journals, and certifying examinations.[38]

Tajik and his successors also encouraged the expansion of the Cardiovascular Division's continuing medical education courses. These courses had become relevant to a much larger number of board-certified cardiologists after 1990, when the American Board of Internal Medicine instituted a policy that their certificates in general medicine and medical subspecialties (including cardiology and its subspecialties) would be valid for ten years. Physicians who wanted to maintain their certified status would have to take examinations on a recurring basis.[39]

TABLE 20.1 Cardiology Subspecialty Clinics Founded at Mayo, 1971–2013

Subspecialty Clinic and Year of Fouding	First Director
Pacemaker [later Implantable Device] Clinic (1971)	John Merideth
Cardiovascular Health Clinic (1979)	George Gura
Adult Congenital Heart Disease Clinic (1988)	Carole Warnes
Heart Failure Clinic (1991)	Richard Rodeheffer
Pulmonary Hypertension Clinic (1996)	Michael McGoon
Arrhythmia [later Heart Rhythm] Clinic (1997)	Stephen Hammill
Thrombophilia [Hypercoagulability] Clinic (1997)	John Heit
Cardiomyopathy Clinic (1998)	Rick Nishimura
Women's Heart Clinic (1998)	Sharonne Hayes
Valvular Heart Disease Clinic (2000)	Maurice Sarano
Long QT-Syndrome/Genetic Heart Rhythm Clinic (2000)	Michael Ackerman
Marfan Syndrome [and Thoracic Aortic Aneurysm] Clinic (2002)	Heidi Connolly
Chest Pain and Coronary Physiology Clinic (2002)	Amir Lerman
Interventional Cardiology [later Coronary Artery Disease] Clinic (2003)	Henry Ting
Early Atherosclerosis Clinic (2004)	Iftikhar Kullo
Sports Cardiology Clinic (2009)	Thomas Allison
	Todd Miller
Statin Intolerance Clinic (2010)	Stephen Kopecky
Cardiac Amyloid Clinic (2012)	Martha Grogan
Pericardial Disease Clinic (2012)	Jae Oh
Cardiology-Oncology Clinic (2013)	Joerg Herrmann

In 1997 Mayo's cardiologists published a 724-page board review textbook that was an outgrowth of the lectures they had developed for educational courses. San Francisco cardiologist William Parmley, who edited the *Journal of the American College of Cardiology*, considered the book "a 'must' for those planning to take the cardiovascular board certification examination."[40] In 2000 the Cardiovascular Division sponsored or co-sponsored thirty-two courses in Rochester and other several other locations.[41] Reflecting the introduction of certification in more cardiology subspecialties, Mayo sponsored board review courses in general cardiology, echocardiography, electrophysiology, heart failure, and interventional cardiology in 2013.[42]

Five Decades of the "War on Heart Disease"

Physician-historians David Jones and Jeremy Greene argued in 2012 that "at some unnoticed moment in the mid-1960s, mortality from coronary heart disease in the United States peaked and then began to decline." The decline was significant. Since it peaked, mortality from coronary heart disease has fallen 60 percent. Claiming that "this achievement may represent the greatest public health accomplishment of the twentieth century," Jones and Greene acknowledged that "it is not clear who or what deserves credit." The challenge has been to sort out the relative contributions to the decline of the "therapeutic power of modern medicine," lifestyle changes, and the management of coronary risk factors.[43]

After President Lyndon Johnson established the Commission on Heart Disease, Cancer and Stroke in 1964, the *Boston Globe* ran a story "LBJ Declares War on 3 Killer Diseases."[44] Johnson, a heart attack survivor, described the commission's task to its members at a White House meeting: "You are here to begin mapping an attack by this Nation upon the three great killers.... We must conquer heart disease, we must conquer cancer, we must conquer strokes. This Nation and the whole world cries out for this victory.... When this occurs—not 'if,' but 'when,' and I emphasize 'when'—we will face a new challenge and that will be what to do within our economy to adjust ourselves to a life span and a work span for the average man or woman of 100 years." The president told the commission's members: "I want to thank you very much for beginning the work that I think will ultimately win the hardest fight that we have ever fought." Johnson put their mission in perspective by mentioning several of his other priorities: "While we are interested in the food stamp plan... Medicare for the aged... the civil rights bill... the immigration bill that will allow families to join each other... [and] the poverty bill... there is nothing that really offers more and greater hope to all humanity...than the challenge...you have undertaken."[45]

Political fights would undermine the ambitious program that the commission proposed. But research did result in a notable increase in new knowledge about cardiovascular disease during the final quarter of the twentieth century. Meanwhile, many new technologies were developed and marketed as tools to care for patients with heart disease. University of Arizona cardiologist and journal editor Joseph Alpert marked the new millennium by creating a list of the top ten developments in heart care during the second half of the twentieth century. He ranked cardiac catheterization first; followed by open-heart surgery, basic research that increased understanding about cardiovascular disease, noninvasive tests (such as echocardiography and nuclear scans), intensive care units, innovative heart attack treatments (such as thrombolytic therapy), preventive cardiology, heart rhythm technologies (such as pacemakers and implantable defibrillators), interventional (catheter-based) treatment procedures, and improved heart failure therapies.[46]

Cardiologists were not the only ones impressed by developments in heart care. In 2001 health economist Victor Fuchs and academic internist Harold Sox reported the results of a survey of 225 general internists. They asked these doctors to assess the relative importance of thirty medical innovations introduced into practice during the final three decades of the twentieth century. Four of the six top-ranked innovations related to cardiovascular disease: angiotensin-converting enzyme (ACE) inhibitors for treating heart failure, percutaneous transluminal coronary angioplasty, statins, and coronary artery bypass graft surgery. Fuchs and Sox speculated that the high rankings of heart care innovations reflected "both the high incidence of cardiovascular disease...and the greater efficacy of new cardiovascular procedures and medications relative to innovations that address other major diseases such as malignant neoplasms."[47]

It is true that much more progress has been made in treating heart disease than most types of cancer during the past half century. Harvard economist David Cutler was the first author of a 2006 article in the *New England Journal of Medicine* that reviewed the gains in life expectancy and the increasing cost of care in the United States during the final four decades of the twentieth century. The life expectancy for a baby born in 2000 was seven years longer than one born in 1960. Cutler and his coauthors concluded that 70 percent of this increased life expectancy (almost five years) had resulted from a reduced rate of death from cardiovascular disease. Only 3 percent of this increased life expectancy (about ten weeks) had resulted from a reduced rate of death from cancer. They acknowledged that their approach had limitations, but their study and several others have demonstrated the uneven progress in the wars that Lyndon Johnson declared against heart disease, cancer, and stroke in 1964.[48]

Public Figures Living With or Dying From Heart Disease

Heart disease, because of its high prevalence, has affected many public fig-ures. One prominent person's series of health problems illustrates the cen-tral role that technology has come to play in heart care in recent decades. In 2012 *New York Times* medical writer Lawrence Altman declared: "Mr. Cheney's medical history could almost be the history of medical progress against heart disease, the leading cause of death in this country and many others. Most of the advances have come during his lifetime, through taxpayer investment in research financed by the National Institutes of Health and through private investment by industry and entrepreneurs."[49] Altman, who was trained as a physician but had spent four decades as a health reporter, was not exaggerating. He understands that the course of history changes to varying degrees depending on whether a national leader dies or whether he or she survives a life-threatening disease as a result of developments in diagnosis and treatment.[50]

Dick Cheney was thirty-seven years old when he had his first heart attack in 1984. Four years later, he had another heart attack followed by qua-druple coronary artery bypass surgery at George Washington University Hospital in Washington, DC. Cheney's next major cardiac event occurred in November 2000, just after the presidential election. Controversy surround-ing the vote count in Florida put the outcome in limbo—it was unclear whether Al Gore and Joe Lieberman or George Bush and Dick Cheney would win. Cheney recalled, "I awoke in the middle of the night with an uncomfortable sensation in my chest." Secret Service agents rushed him to George Washington University Hospital where a cardiologist performed a coronary angiogram and "inserted a stent made of stainless steel mesh in an artery that was 90 to 95 percent blocked." He spent Thanksgiving Day in the hospital.[51]

David Sanger, the chief Washington correspondent for the *New York Times*, reported in July 2001 that doctors had implanted "a sophisticated pacemaker and defibrillator" in Cheney's chest. The article also noted that the vice presi-dent had focused on improving his coronary risk factors by changing his diet, by losing weight, and by exercising on a stationary bicycle about 30 minutes a day.[52] Jonathan Reiner, his cardiologist, later described the implantable car-dioverter defibrillator (ICD) as a device "less than half the size of a deck of cards and the price of a small Lexus."[53] Cheney's defibrillator first went off in 2009, shortly after his second vice presidential term ended: "While I was backing my car out of the garage of our house in Wyoming, everything went blank. I had gone into ventricular fibrillation. Somebody else would likely be telling the story right now if the ICD hadn't kicked in."[54]

Cheney survived sudden death, but his heart's pumping function continued to deteriorate: "By the beginning of June 2010, I was approaching end-stage heart failure. As I went through the month, I found it increasingly difficult to carry out any tasks around the house.... I could no longer climb the stairs to get to the second floor."[55] Reiner explains that an echocardiogram in early July showed "a huge heart, easily twice the normal size, which barely moved."[56] Cheney was hospitalized in preparation for the implantation of a left ventricular assist device (LVAD) to keep him from dying from progressive heart failure.

An LVAD is a mechanical pump that helps the weakened left ventricle propel blood through the body. "By this time," Cheney recalls, "we had used nearly all the technology and medical procedures available for dealing with my disease.... Under ordinary circumstances, the idea of putting a device operating at nine thousand RPM into my chest, attached to my heart and to a driveline running through a hole in my chest wall would have seemed a little off-putting. But it was an option, and I was out of other options."[57] The LVAD kept him alive until March 2012, when he had a heart transplant. The *Washington Post* reported that this operation was "the latest chapter in the semi-public chronicling of Cheney's life with coronary heart disease, the leading cause of death in the United States for more than half a century."[58]

Cheney credits technology and the care he has received from medical and surgical heart specialists with saving his life several times. He was also lucky several times—because a significant percentage of individuals who have a heart attack die before they get to a hospital. The former vice president, who was seventy-one when he received a heart transplant, also had excellent health insurance and ready access to the latest technologies.

In 2008 *New York Times* medical science reporter Denise Grady told another person's story that had a very different ending. "A doctor's care is not a protective bubble," she declared, "and cardiology is not the exact science that many people wish it to be." Grady made these observations in an article about a middle-aged man who "took blood pressure and cholesterol pills and aspirin, rode an exercise bike, had yearly stress tests and other exams and was dutifully trying to lose weight. But he died of a heart attack anyway."[59] This man had known Dick Cheney for several years.

In 2001, two months after Cheney's doctors had implanted a defibrillator in his chest, Tim Russert interviewed him on *Meet the Press*. The program attracted a lot of viewers, but it had nothing to do with Cheney's heart disease. Russert interviewed the vice president at Camp David, Maryland, five days after the terrorist attacks of September 11. On June 14, 2008, Russert, himself, was the subject of an *NBC* news bulletin. Former *NBC Nightly News* anchor Tom Brokaw interrupted afternoon programming to announce that his fifty-eight-year-old friend and colleague had just died. The network reported the circumstances:

> Russert was recording voiceovers for Sunday's *Meet the Press* broadcast when he collapsed. He was rushed to Sibley Memorial Hospital in Washington, where resuscitation attempts were unsuccessful. Russert's

physician, Michael Newman, said cholesterol plaque ruptured in an artery, causing sudden coronary thrombosis. Russert had earlier been diagnosed with asymptomatic coronary artery disease, but it was well-controlled with medication and exercise, and he had performed well on a stress test in late April, Newman said.[60]

A *New York Times* article published four days after Russert's death described interviews with Newman and George Bren, his cardiologist. The physicians explained that an autopsy had revealed significant coronary artery disease. " 'What is surprising,' Dr. Newman said, 'is that the severity of the anatomical findings would not be predicted from his clinical situation, the absence of symptoms and his performing at a very high level of exercise.' "[61]

Six weeks after Russert died, *New York Times* health writer Jane Brody interviewed Mayo cardiologist Todd Miller about treadmill exercise testing. Based on her conversation with him, she explained, "This test is unable to detect the kind of problem that caused Mr. Russert's death—a plaque within the wall of a coronary artery that ruptured, resulting in a clot that set off a rapidly fatal heart rhythm abnormality."[62] Most adults are familiar with sudden death, based on the unexpected loss of a family member or friend. The media regularly report the toll it takes on public figures like Tim Russert. Fifty-one-year-old actor James Gandolfini won major awards for his portrayal of a Mafia boss in the popular television series *The Sopranos*. No one was with him in June 2013, when he had a cardiac arrest in Rome. But tens of millions of viewers have seen Don Vito Corleone, a Mafia boss played by Marlon Brando, drop dead in a garden while playing with his grandson in the 1972 movie *The Godfather*.

Despite the word and picture images of sudden cardiac death and the sobering statistics about lives shortened by heart disease, there are many success stories. Minnesota-born Garrison Keillor, host of the popular radio program *A Prairie Home Companion*, recounted his experience with open-heart surgery at the Mayo Clinic in a *Time* magazine article "I Just Needed a Valve Job." The humorist provided a historical perspective on a heart procedure he had undergone in Rochester: "Fifty years ago, in my boyhood, a guy who blew out his mitral valve was sent home to sit in a sunny corner and play cribbage until congestive heart failure swept him away." But Keillor's experience was different: "I've always had a slight heart murmur...and when the valve came loose at the moorings, there wasn't much doubt about it. So my wife drove me to the Mayo Clinic." He reflected on what happened later: "Heart surgery is an artistic performance to benefit an audience that is sound asleep at the time. A man you've met only once slices open your chest so your heart can be stopped and chilled so a loose flap in your mitral valve can be sewn up. No big deal when it goes right, which, with an ace surgeon, it should."[63] Rather than replacing Keillor's leaking mitral valve, his Mayo surgeon repaired it at Saint Marys Hospital.

Valve repair rather than replacement is now the preferred procedure in most cases of mitral regurgitation. Mayo surgeon Dwight McGoon had published a pioneering article on mitral valve repair back in 1960, the same year that Nina Braunwald and Andrew Morrow of the National Heart Institute performed the first successful mitral valve replacement. But there was little interest in mitral repair until the 1980s, when French surgeon Alain Carpentier took the lead in developing procedures that corrected leaks but preserved a patient's own valve. Shortly thereafter, a few surgeons in the United States began performing and promoting mitral valve repair.[64]

During the 1990s, Mayo researchers reported that patients who had severe mitral regurgitation detected by echocardiography derived long-term benefit if their leaking valve was repaired before rather than after they developed symptoms. Cleveland Clinic surgeon Toby Cosgrove, a pioneer of mitral valve repair, claimed that a 1996 article in the *New England Journal of Medicine* by Mayo authors had "a major impact in increasing mitral valve surgery throughout the United States."[65] Physicians and surgeons who subspecialize in heart valve disease remain concerned that many patients who are candidates for mitral valve repair are not offered that option. This is especially true in hospitals where the number of valve operations is relatively low.

The *U.S. News & World Report* special issue on America's Best Hospitals for 2000 included an article "Higher Volume, Fewer Deaths: For a Risky Operation Head for a Hospital That Does It Regularly." Health science writer Avery Comarow recommended that patients "request [procedural] volume information from the surgeon and from the hospital where an operation will be done." Although he predicted that "most surgeons won't be caught short by the question," Comarow expressed concern that "most people facing surgery don't ask."[66]

Another article in the same issue of *U.S. News & World Report* addressed the plight of patients enrolled in managed care plans that limited their choices in terms of hospitals and doctors. In her article "To Get Top Care, Get Pushy," staff writer Susan Brink suggested steps that patients could take: "If it comes down to fisticuffs with the insurer, line up your allies, starting with your local doctor. Most top hospitals have physician-to-physician referral lines, and your local doctor might help find a specialist at Mayo Clinic, for example."[67] By the time Brink wrote this, managed care policies were becoming less restrictive in the face of legal challenges, legislation, and a backlash from the public and physicians.[68]

Rising Health Care Costs and Health Care Reform

Concerns about health care costs in the United States have been raised for decades, but calls for action have become more insistent as evidence mounts that the cost trajectory is unsustainable. Health economist Victor Fuchs reports that the share of America's GDP related to health care increased from 4.4 percent in 1950 to 17.9 percent in 2011.[69] The Robert Wood Johnson Foundation published a report in 2008 showing that health care spending had increased by an average of 7.7 percent per year between 1985 and 2006, while the nation's GDP had increased 5.6 percent per year. The authors also pointed out that spending on health care as a percentage of GDP was six percentage points higher in the United States than the average for other developed countries. They identified technology as the key driver of health care spending, accounting for one-half to two-thirds of spending growth.[70] This was certainly not a new notion. For decades, health policy analysts have emphasized the cost consequences of the development and diffusion of technologies. What continues to change is that there are many more (and more expensive) medical technologies being applied to a growing number of patients and potential patients.[71]

In June 2009 Boston surgeon and best-selling author Atul Gawande published "The Cost Conundrum" in the *New Yorker* magazine. His article, which attracted a lot of attention, focused on McAllen, Texas, a city of 120,000 near the Mexican border. Gawande explained that McAllen is in a county with "the lowest household income in the country" but "is one of the most expensive health-care markets in the country." Turning from one city to the whole nation, he declared: "Our country's health care is by far the most expensive in the world.... The financial burden has damaged the global competitiveness of American businesses and bankrupted millions of families, even those with insurance."[72]

Gawande backed up the impressions he had gained from interviews of doctors, patients, and others in Texas with data from the Dartmouth Institute for Health Policy and Clinical Practice and two private firms. He concluded that overuse of medical care explained the situation: "Compared with patients in El Paso and nationwide, patients in McAllen got more of pretty much everything—more diagnostic testing, more hospital treatment, more surgery, more home care." In terms of heart care, patients in McAllen "received two to three times as many pacemakers, implantable defibrillators, cardiac-bypass operations...and coronary-artery stents" than those in El Paso.[73]

A Harvard Medical School faculty member who practices surgery at Brigham and Women's Hospital, Gawande declared, "Americans like to believe that, with most things, more is better. But research suggests that where medicine is concerned it may actually be worse. For example, Rochester, Minnesota, where the Mayo Clinic dominates the scene, has fantastically high levels of technological capability and quality, but its Medicare spending is in the lowest fifteen percent of the country."[74]

Gawande had drawn some of his conclusions from a trip to Rochester as a visiting surgeon. While there, he had spoken to Denis Cortese, a lung specialist who was Mayo's president and CEO. The Boston surgeon, who characterized Mayo as one of the highest-quality, lowest-cost health care systems in America, described some of the human interactions he observed. He was impressed with "how much time the doctors spend with the patients. There was no churn—no shuttling patients in and out of rooms while the doctor bounces from one to the other." Gawande explained that all Mayo physicians are salaried "so that the doctors' goal in patient care couldn't be increasing their income. Mayo promoted leaders who focused first on what was best for patients, and then on how to make this financially possible."[75]

Denis Cortese had helped push Mayo into the spotlight as an actor in the national debate about health care reform, which was intensifying. This effort had been formalized with the creation of the Mayo Clinic Health Policy Center in 2006. That spring, former Minnesota congressman Timothy Penny participated in the Mayo Clinic Symposium on Health Care Reform. He told an interviewer, "When Mayo talks, people listen. . . . It will be noticed and respected by lawmakers."[76] On June 6, 2009, five days after Gawande's essay appeared in the *New Yorker*, President Barack Obama delivered his weekly address. In the course of outlining his goals for health care reform, he said, "There are places like the Mayo Clinic in Minnesota, the Cleveland Clinic in Ohio, and other institutions that offer some of the highest quality of care in the nation at some of the lowest costs in the nation. We should learn from their successes and promote the best practices, not the most expensive ones."[77]

Three months later, two *Washington Post* writers raised some questions: "Few dispute the prowess of Mayo, which brings in $9 billion in revenue a year and hosts 250 surgeries a day. But a battle is underway among health-care experts and lawmakers over whether its success can be so easily replicated. Before embracing a fundamentally new approach to health care, dissenting experts and lawmakers say, Congress should scrutinize the assumption that a Mayo-type model is the answer."[78] The *Washington Post* writers' claim that the Mayo Clinic model represented "a fundamentally new approach to health care" overlooked the institution's role in inventing multi-specialty group practice a century earlier. For perspective, a Canadian surgeon's observations, published after he visited Rochester in 1906, are worth repeating:

> When one has seen the various activities centered here, the degree of excellence to which diagnostic methods are carried, the extreme pains to which the large staff of specialists take in their various departments, and the master minds controlling this huge machine, he can understand why the hotels. . . of Rochester find it difficult to accommodate those who wish to be relieved from their burden of pain and those who seek relief from their burden of ignorance [about their illness]. Specialization

and cooperation, with the best that can be had in each department, is here the motto. Cannot these principles be tried elsewhere?[79]

Several multispecialty group practices formed during the early twentieth century were modeled after the Mayo Clinic, including the Geisinger Clinic in Pennsylvania (1915), the Marshfield Clinic in Wisconsin (1916), and the Cleveland Clinic in Ohio (1921).[80]

The Committee on the Costs of Medical Care, formed in 1927 and funded by eight philanthropic foundations, concluded six years later that "group practice in one form or another seems essential if the mode in which medical service is rendered is to be consonant with the demands of modern medical science and technology."[81] In 1963 Isadore Falk, an influential member of the Depression-era committee, claimed that "group practice is [the] pattern of the future."[82] Group practice would become more popular during the last quarter of the century. For years, Mayo's leaders had claimed that the multispecialty group practice model offered certain advantages in terms of efficiency, cost, and outcomes. Some studies done in the early twenty-first century support this assertion.[83]

Mayo Clinic Announces the Destination Medical Center Concept

Neurologist John Noseworthy, who replaced Denis Cortese as Mayo's president and CEO in 2009, cautioned three years later, "Our competitors are making strategic moves to replicate our model and, in many cases, they are partnering with state and local governments to enhance their medical centers, bolster the medical economy, and create...enhanced patient experiences."[84] Early in 2013, Mayo announced a bold plan to address this concern. The Destination Medical Center concept generated a lot of discussion because it involved major financial commitments from Rochester, Olmsted County, and Minnesota. Mayo proposed spending $3.5 billion over twenty years to expand its Rochester campus if various government entities were willing to invest in improvements in the city's infrastructure. In May 2013 the Minnesota Legislature approved a $585 million public funding plan that was described as the largest economic development project in the state's history.[85]

Passengers on Delta Airlines could read an article "The Domestic Medical Tourist" in the July 2013 issue of *Delta Sky Magazine*. The long subtitle included a question and an answer: "Why would you travel out of state for a medical procedure that could be done closer to home? Lots of reasons." The writer noted that medical tourism was not new and mentioned that Johns Hopkins and the Mayo Clinic "have long drawn patients in dire straits." Today, patients do not have to be that sick. He described a "new class of health traveler seeking more economical or speedier care" and included a table listing six destination medical centers that "seek to serve patients from almost anywhere, domestic or foreign."[86] In addition to Mayo, they included Cleveland Clinic, Johns Hopkins Hospital, Massachusetts General Hospital, New York-Presbyterian Hospital, and Texas Medical Center.

Although the writer did not discuss heart care, the 2014 Best Hospitals issue of *U.S. News & World Report* ranked Cleveland Clinic first (with a score of 100/100), Mayo Clinic second (with a score of 95.8/100), and New York-Presbyterian Hospital third (with a score of 78.2/100).[87] In an article on how the magazine ranks hospitals, Avery Comarow, editor of the annual Best Hospital issue, explained its purpose:

> We provide patients who need unusually skilled inpatient care and have time to seek out the best with a tool to help them find it.... Why focus on such individuals, who number as many as 2 million a year but only account for 2 or 3 percent of all hospital patients? Because the majority of hospitals may not be good choices for them. Just one example: a man in his 90s who needs a faulty heart valve replaced. Most hospitals would either decline to perform such major surgery on elderly patients (as they should if they aren't up to speed on the special techniques and precautions required and don't see many such cases) or, worse, they would operate and subject them to great risk. A hospital ranked in cardiology and heart surgery is likely to have the necessary experience and expertise.[88]

The example Comarow chose to help explain the magazine's approach to rankings, "a man in his 90s who needs a faulty heart valve replaced," surely shocked some readers.

The "Technological Imperative" and Changing Demographics

Jack Copeland, a prominent heart transplant surgeon, coauthored a 1999 article from the University of Arizona Medical Center with a title designed to attract attention: "The Oldest Patient to Undergo Aortic Valve Replacement." It summarized the case of a ninety-eight-year-old man with a history of aortic stenosis who was asymptomatic when he had come to their outpatient clinic recently to establish routine care. He was seen again two months later, after having almost fainted. The patient's physical examination was consistent with aortic stenosis, and an echocardiogram documented severe valve obstruction (with a mean aortic valve gradient of 81 mmHg and an aortic valve area of 0.5–0.6 cm^2). About two weeks later, the patient returned after having almost fainted three more times and having developed breathlessness that was slowly progressive. Catheterization confirmed the diagnosis of severe aortic stenosis. An angiogram revealed normal coronary arteries.[89]

About fourteen weeks after this ninety-eight-year-old patient was described as having no cardiac symptoms, he underwent aortic valve replacement. The authors explained that the man had been discharged from the hospital six days after surgery and that "he has done very well since discharge and has returned to his usual independent lifestyle." Based on this one man's hospital experience and short-term follow-up, they emphasized two points: "The oldest documented patient to undergo aortic valve replacement demonstrates the benefits of cardiac surgery in the elderly...[and] aortic valve replacement should be strongly considered in the majority of octogenarians and even in nonagenarians with symptomatic aortic valve disease, as long as their underlying medical condition presents no contraindication." These sweeping conclusions seem hard to justify, considering the fact that the authors acknowledged that they were based on the short-term outcome of a single patient.[90]

This ninety-eight-year-old man had been born at the very beginning of the twentieth century, and he had his aortic valve replaced at the very end of the century. When he was born, the average life expectancy for US males was forty-eight years. But he had lived twice that long and still had "an independent lifestyle." In fact, he was older than 99.9 percent of the US population. In their case report, the Arizona authors noted that "life expectancy at age 80 is greater than eight years." They did not mention that in 1998 the average life expectancy of a ninety-eight-year-old US male was about two and a half years.[91] The decision to replace his aortic valve (which had opened about 3.5 billion times during his long life) is an example of what health economist Victor Fuchs termed the "technological imperative." When he coined the phrase in 1968, Fuchs used history to explain the concept: "Medical tradition emphasizes giving the best care that is technically possible; the only legitimate and explicitly recognized constraint is the state of the art." One thing missing in medicine, he argued, was willingness to weigh costs against benefits.[92]

Fuchs had first written about the technological imperative two years after Medicare was launched in 1966. That program, and the growth of private insurance, would insulate the majority of patients from the costs of a significant amount of the care they received. Fuchs wrote in 2011, "New drugs, new devices, new imaging equipment, new surgical procedures have proliferated, as would be expected in a system in which approximately 90 percent of the cost of the new technology at the time of use is paid by third parties other than the patient and the revenues from their use enhance the incomes of the providers of care," which include hospitals as well as physicians.[93]

The print and broadcast media disseminate news of medical breakthroughs on a regular basis. They report what scientists, clinical investigators, or institutions have told them. These stories raise the expectations of some patients or members of their families. As a result, a patient may request a procedure or technology that has not been proven to provide any benefit in his or her specific situation.[94] For example, the cover of a 2001 issue of *Newsweek* magazine featured a color photograph of an implantable artificial heart and a headline "How Technology Will Heal Your Heart." In the article on the artificial heart, the chief scientific officer of the company that manufactured the device declared, "This opens a whole new chapter in cardiac medicine." But the authors of the story asked, "Will it be a happy one?"[95]

The late twentieth and early twenty-first centuries have witnessed the introduction of heart treatment technologies that have attracted the attention of the public, physicians, health policy analysts, and ethicists, among others. Transcatheter aortic valve implantation or replacement (TAVI or TAVR) is a compelling example. French cardiologist Alain Cribier, who pioneered this catheter-based alternative to open-heart surgery for treating severe aortic stenosis, first performed it in a human in 2002. Transcatheter aortic valve implantation involves placing an artificial valve inside a patient's own severely obstructed aortic valve.[96] In 2011 the FDA approved one manufacturer's model for use in patients who were not considered candidates for standard surgical aortic valve replacement because of advanced age or other serious medical problems.

The day after the FDA announced its decision, the *New York Times* published an Associated Press article with the headline "Less Invasive Heart Valve Replacement is Approved." It contained language that glorified the new technology and painted a disturbing picture of the standardized half-century-old valve operation: "Every year about 50,000 people in the country undergo open-heart surgery to replace the valve, which involves sawing the breastbone in half, stopping the heart, cutting out the old valve and sewing a new one into place. Thousands of other patients are turned away, deemed too old or ill to survive the operation." The article quoted Mayo's senior interventional cardiologist David Holmes as characterizing the new catheter-based technique as a "game changer" for patients who are not considered candidates for open-heart surgery.[97] Transcatheter aortic valve implantation was new, but some not-so-new heart care technologies continued to make news.

In 2008 *New York Times* reporter Anemona Hartocollis told the story of a woman who had had a "specialized pacemaker and defibrillator that synchronizes her heartbeat and can administer a slight shock to revive her if her heart falters" implanted four years earlier. This device combines so-called cardiac resynchronization therapy, which may improve heart failure symptoms, with an automatic defibrillator, which is designed to prevent sudden death from ventricular fibrillation. The *Times* reporter explained that the procedure, which had been performed one month before the woman's 100th birthday, "reflects what some doctors are hailing as a new frontier in medicine: successful surgery for centenarians. But others say that such aggressive treatment for what are euphemistically known as the late elderly can be wasteful and barbaric, warning that the rush to test the limits of technology can give patients false hope and compound their health challenges with surgical complications."[98]

In a subsequent article, Hartocollis reported that the woman's cardiologist replaced her device in 2010, when she was 105. The *Times* reporter explained that this same cardiologist had implanted the original one when she was 99 after "several other doctors" had advised against the procedure, claiming that "she was too old and the risks were too great." One month after the replacement (which was presumably done because of battery depletion), the woman was hospitalized for dehydration. "After dialysis, she seemed to be improving until March 22, when her blood pressure dropped and there seemed to be internal bleeding. The doctor said he could put her in intensive care, but he was not sure she would be herself again." With this news, the patient's eighty-three-year-old daughter said, "O.K., let her go." Her mother died within minutes. "I was there, holding her hand. There was no struggling. Nobody dismissed her in any way, and she got the best of treatment."[99]

"Do Not Try to Live Forever: You Will Not Succeed"

Irish playwright and author George Bernard Shaw wrote in 1911, "Do not try to live forever. You will not succeed."[100] Dallas heart surgeon Michael Mack was president of the Society of Thoracic Surgeons in 2011, when he wrote an editorial to accompany an article about patients aged eighty-five and older who had undergone catheter-based coronary interventions (mainly stent implantations): "This study again raises the age old question of 'just because we can do it does that mean we should do it?'"[101] Several trends have resulted in this question being asked more often. These include the ongoing introduction of new technologies, an aging population, changing attitudes about old age, growing concerns about health care costs, and the development of new methods to evaluate the risk-benefit ratio of medical or surgical interventions.[102]

Howard Spiro, an academic internist at Yale University, was eighty-five in 2009, when he published "An Old Doctor Grows Older." He reflected on how attitudes toward aging had changed during his half-century career: "Once physicians comfortably limited their therapeutic suggestions to those over 65, but ethical niceties have displaced our comfortable paternalism. Doctors now offer therapy to the aged that we may not need and should not want. When does treatment equal to that for the young lead to over-treatment for the old? We want to be treated as individuals. Yet, there is something vaguely indecent for a man of 80 to get a new kidney, or for a defibrillator to be inserted into a 90-year-old-woman's chest."[103] Victor Fuchs, who had coined the phrase "technological imperative" in 1968, argued in 2011,

"When escalating health care expenditures threaten the solvency of the federal government and the viability of the U.S. economy, physicians are forced to reexamine the choices they make in caring for their patients."[104]

Mayo internist and bioethicist Jon Tilburt has coauthored articles on providing patient-centered care in an era of increasing technological capability and of growing concern about undertaking treatments that may be more harmful than helpful to an individual.[105] He and Christine Cassel, a geriatrician and past president and CEO of the American Board of Internal Medicine, wrote an editorial in 2013 in which they distinguished the ethics of parsimonious medicine from the ethics of rationing. They defined parsimonious medicine as "delivering appropriate health care that fits the needs and circumstances of patients and that actively avoids wasteful care—care that does not benefit patients."[106] This advice echoed a challenge that Robert Frye had issued to heart specialists two decades earlier, when he was president of the American College of Cardiology: "Reducing utilization of one or another procedure clearly will not solve the overall high cost of medical care, but we have a professional responsibility to provide only those services that are truly in the best interest of the patient."[107]

Tilburt and Cassel pointed to the Choosing Wisely campaign that the American Board of Internal Medicine Foundation had launched in 2012. They explained that "the ethical rationale for rationing appropriately rests on a concern for distributive justice.... To the extent that health care helps citizens obtain health, health care should be distributed fairly throughout society, especially where supported by public funding. Expenditures of health care resources that are only modestly more effective but far more expensive represent a barrier to achieving this basic right for all."[108]

The American College of Cardiology and the American Society of Nuclear Cardiology were among the first nine specialty organizations to join the Choosing Wisely campaign, which *Consumer Reports* also joined and promotes.[109] The leadership of the Society of Thoracic Surgeons, which joined the Choosing Wisely campaign in 2013, ended a special report on partnering with patients: "Responsible use of health care resources is one of the key principles of professionalism that cardiothoracic surgeons and other physicians advocate and adhere to. Patients need to know when to say 'whoa' to doctors, and physicians need to be empowered to avoid tests or procedures that are not supported by evidence."[110] By 2014 several dozen specialty organizations had joined the campaign.

The Growth of Social Media and the Empowerment of Patients

The Choosing Wisely campaign acknowledges that patients are now playing a much more active role in decisions regarding their health care. The rapid development and diffusion of social media (such as Facebook, Twitter, and YouTube) and powerful search engines (such as Google) have revolutionized the way individuals get information about health and disease. In 1912 Ellen Firebaugh, whose husband had been a general practitioner in Robinson, Illinois, for more than two decades, declared that "the telephone has revolutionized the doctor's life."[111] Twenty-first century communication and information technologies have revolutionized patients' lives. For example, in a growing number of contexts, personal health records that were traditionally controlled by hospitals and physicians and were off limits to patients are now accessible to them over secure Internet connections.[112]

Mayo's president and CEO John Noseworthy wrote the foreword to *Bringing Social Media #Revolution to Health Care*, a book published in 2012 by the Mayo Clinic Center for Social Media. He explained that it was designed to "explore how social tools can improve patient care, catalyze medical research, strengthen medical education and promote continuous professional development." Reflecting on the role that Will and Charlie Mayo had played in developing the group practice model a century earlier, Noseworthy declared, "As stewards of their legacy and early adopters of modern social networking tools, we see an opportunity and feel a responsibility to help the broader health care system harness social tools safely and effectively."[113]

Groups tracking the adoption of social media by health care organizations have cited the Mayo Clinic as a leader in promoting the use of this transformational technology by patients and staff. MHADegree.org, an online forum for aspiring health care administrators, gathered social media use statistics for all of the hospitals that *U.S. News & World Report* ranked nationally in at least one adult specialty. MHADegree.org ranked Mayo Clinic first and Cleveland Clinic second in a list of the top fifty most social media friendly hospitals for 2013.[114] Cardiologist Farris Timimi, medical director of the Mayo Clinic Center for Social Media, explains that a major incentive for the clinic to develop a robust electronic presence was that "patients are spending more and more of their time online seeking health care information."[115] This statement comes as no surprise to readers of this book, nor does the fact that health care organizations are adopting social media applications at very different speeds.

Mayo was also an early adopter of the electronic medical record as an alternative to traditional paper records. The earliest stages involved electronic access to some laboratory reports in 1993 and to outpatient clinical notes the following year. In 2013 *U.S. News & World Report* ranked the clinic first (among all the institutions in its Best Hospitals list) in terms of the implementation of electronic health records.[116] Mayo has a secure website that allows patients to review their clinical notes, test results, hospital summaries, and more. The site explains, "As part of our continuing initiative toward greater medical transparency, we've recently built online access to several parts of your medical record."[117] Mayo is also using the Internet to provide general health information and descriptions of specific diseases to the public and to health care professionals.

A Cardiovascular Division project exemplifies how social media can be used to promote heart health. In 2012 Mayo produced a *YouTube* video that encouraged women and men to know their cardiac risk factor numbers. The music video (complete with central characters, a live band, and an energized audience) paired new risk reduction lyrics to Tommy Tutone's 1981 hit song "867-5309/Jenny." The upbeat Mayo version replaced the song's original refrain, "Jenny don't change your number: 867-5309," with a heart-healthy message: "Jenny please watch your numbers, blood pressure, lipids, and BMI."[118] The high-energy video surprised some Mayo insiders because it seemed to represent a bold break from the institution's conservative image. But the goal of the "Watch Your Numbers" video was laudable: to present a heart disease prevention message in a way designed to resonate with the social media-savvy public.

The Cardiovascular Division used a more traditional approach to promote prevention when it published the book *Mayo Clinic Healthy Heart for Life* in 2012. In their introduction, written for the general public, cardiologists Martha Grogan and Chet Rihal explained, "Heart disease affects all of us, either directly or indirectly. It is the leading cause of death in the United States. You may feel bombarded with conflicting information about heart health: What's good, what's bad, and what do you really need to know? That's the reason we've written this book—to provide a clear program to help you have a healthy heart for life."[119] One section includes ten steps to heart health: eat healthy, be active, sleep well, deal with tobacco and weight, know your numbers, know your history, set your targets, take your medications, plan for emergencies, and enjoy life.

In 2011 the American Heart Association predicted that the prevalence of cardiovascular disease and the costs associated with it would increase substantially in the United States over the next two decades.[120] Historians recognize the perils of trying to predict the future. But it is inevitable that the debate over the rational use of technology will intensify as more new tools and techniques are developed, the population ages, and health care costs continue to rise. This book has demonstrated how heart care has been characterized by an ever-growing array of impressive diagnostic and treatment technologies since World War II. Ultimately, however, the phrase "caring for the heart," the book's main title, must have a broader meaning. Caring for the heart must focus on prevention—taking actions before this vital organ becomes damaged to the point that it is in need of repair or replacement.

{ Appendix: Interviews }

I interviewed sixty-three individuals (including physicians, surgeons, scientists, nurses, and technicians) for this project. These oral histories (subjects listed alphabetically below, were done to complement the insights gained from published and manuscript sources as well as from my own personal experiences. They provided unique perspectives that helped me understand and explain developments in heart care at the Mayo Clinic and in general. Audiotapes of the interviews, which lasted thirty to ninety minutes, are stored in the Mayo Archives.

Earl Bakken. Co-founder of Minneapolis-based Medtronic, a leading developer and manufacturer of pacemakers and other devices. Minneapolis, MN, August 28, 2007.

Kenneth H. Berge. General internist with a special interest in lipids who joined the Mayo staff in 1955. Rochester, MN, January 26, 2011.

Lawrence I. Bonchek. Cardiac surgeon who trained with heart valve pioneer Albert Starr around 1970. New Orleans, LA, November 11, 2004.

Alfred A. Bove. Cardiologist who trained at Mayo with Earl Wood, was on the Mayo staff (1981–1986) and was president of the American College of Cardiology (2009–2010). New Orleans, LA, November 9, 2004.

Robert O. Brandenburg. Cardiologist who joined the Mayo staff in 1951, was the first chair of Mayo's combined cardiology sections (1965–1974), and was president of the American College of Cardiology (1980–1981). Orlando, FL, March 18, 2001.

Eugene Braunwald. America's leading academic cardiologist, who has spent the majority of his half-century career in Boston. Rochester, MN, May 3, 2005.

James Broadbent. Cardiologist who joined the Mayo staff in 1953 and was involved in the management of patients with kidney failure until a nephrology section was established in 1963. Rochester, MN, January 29, 2008.

Howard B. Burchell. Cardiologist who joined the Mayo staff in 1940 and helped organize the cardiac catheterization and open-heart surgery programs. He left to become chief of cardiology at the University of Minnesota in 1968. St. Paul, MN, June 17–18, 2000; Minneapolis MN, October 19, 2004, and June 30, 2007.

John A. Callahan. Cardiologist who joined the Mayo staff in 1955 and helped organize the coronary care unit. Rochester, MN, October 22, 2001.

James H. Chesebro. Cardiologist who joined the Mayo staff in 1975. Jacksonville, FL, March 15, 2006.

Delos M. Cosgrove. Cardiac surgeon at the Cleveland Clinic, who became that institution's CEO in 2004. Cleveland, OH, September 20, 2007.

James W. DuShane. Pediatric cardiologist who joined the Mayo staff in 1946. Rochester, MN, September 26, 2001.

Jesse E. Edwards. Cardiac pathologist who joined the Mayo staff in 1946. He left in 1960 to become director of laboratories, Charles T. Miller Hospital, St. Paul, MN. Rochester, MN, December 20, 2005.

Titus C. Evans Jr. Cardiologist who joined the Mayo staff in 1972. Rochester, MN, October 26, 2004.

Harvey Feigenbaum. Cardiologist at Indiana University who was a pioneer of echocardiography. Chicago, IL, March 29, 2008.

James Fellows. Technician who began working at Mayo in 1952. He was a member of the original open-heart surgery team and then was coordinator of the catheterization laboratory. Rochester, MN, December 7, 2011.

Robert L. Frye. Cardiologist who joined the Mayo staff in 1964. He was chair of the Cardiovascular Division (1974–1984), chair of the Department of Medicine (1987–1999), and president of the American College of Cardiology (1991–1992). Rochester, MN, June 8, June 11, July 2, July 6, July 20, 2001.

Valentin Fuster. Cardiologist who joined the Mayo staff in 1975. He left Mayo in 1981 to become chair of cardiology at Mt. Sinai Hospital in New York City and was president of the American Heart Association (1998–1999). Atlanta, GA, March 12, 2006.

Gerald T. Gau. Cardiologist who joined the Mayo staff in 1970. Rochester, MN, July 27, 2006.

Bernard J. Gersh. Cardiologist who joined the Mayo staff in 1979. He left in 1993 to become chief of cardiology at Georgetown University, Washington, DC, and returned to Mayo five years later. Rochester, MN, October 24, 2005.

Raymond J. Gibbons. Cardiologist who joined the Mayo staff in 1981. Rochester, MN, April 3, 2002.

Vincent L. Gott. Cardiac surgeon who trained at the University of Minnesota in the mid-1950s, during the advent of open-heart surgery. He later became chief of cardiac surgery at Johns Hopkins. Minneapolis, MN, December 13, 2007.

George M. Gura. Cardiologist who joined the Mayo staff in 1974. He left in 1980 to join a single-specialty practice in Kansas City, MO, but returned to Mayo thirteen years later. Rochester, MN, December 26, 2005.

Stephen C. Hammill. Cardiologist who joined the Mayo staff in 1981 and was president of the Heart Rhythm Society (2004–2005). Rochester, MN, July 12, 2005.

Maurine K. Hardke. A registered nurse who began working at Rochester Methodist Hospital in 1964. She was the head nurse of the hospital's coronary care unit. Rochester, MN, July 8, 2005.

Liv Hatle. Norwegian cardiologist and pioneer of Doppler echocardiography who was a visiting scientist at Mayo in 1986. Rochester, MN, January 18, 2005.

David L. Hayes. Cardiologist who joined the Mayo staff in 1982, was chair of the Cardiovascular Division (2002–2011), and was president of the North American Society of Pacing and Electrophysiology (1998–1999). Rochester, MN, October 14, 2005.

H. Frederic Helmholz Jr. Internist and pulmonary physiologist who joined the Mayo staff in 1943 and worked with catheterization pioneer Earl Wood. Rochester, MN, July 19, 2006.

Morrison Hodges. Cardiologist trained at Johns Hopkins who moved to Minneapolis in 1974. Minneapolis, MN, November 28, 2007.

David R. Holmes Jr. Cardiologist who joined the Mayo staff in 1976. He was president of the Society for Cardiovascular Angiography and Interventions (1995–1996) and the American College of Cardiology (2011–2012). Snowmass, CO, August 7, 2004.

J. Willis Hurst. Cardiologist who served as chair of medicine at Emory University (1957–1986) and was president of the American Heart Association (1971–1972). Atlanta, GA, March 11, 2006.

Marcia Jackson. Long-time leader of continuing medical education at the American College of Cardiology. New Orleans, LA, November 7, 2004.

Allan S. Jaffe. Cardiologist who joined the Mayo staff in 1999, after spending two decades at other academic medical centers. Rochester, MN, November 6, 2004.

Bijoy Khandheria. Cardiologist who joined the Mayo staff in 1987 and was president of the American Society of Echocardiography (2005–2006). Scottsdale, AZ, January 4, 2007.

Spencer B. King III. Atlanta cardiologist who was an American pioneer of coronary angioplasty at Emory University and was president of the American College of Cardiology (1998–1999). Chicago, IL, March 29, 2008.

Francis J. Klocke. Chicago cardiologist who was president of the American College of Cardiology (1987–1988). Chicago, IL, March 28, 2008.

Robert A. Kyle. Hematologist who joined the Mayo staff in 1959. Rochester, MN, May 7, 2008.

Richard P. Lewis. Cardiologist at Ohio State University who was president of the American College of Cardiology (1996–1997). New Orleans, LA, November 7, 2004.

Jane A. Linderbaum. Nurse practitioner and supervisor of the mid-level practitioners on the inpatient cardiology service at Saint Marys Hospital. Rochester, MN, August 22, 2005.

Malcolm I. Lindsay Jr. General internist who joined the Mayo staff in 1967. Rochester, MN, February 2, 2011.

Benjamin D. McCallister. Cardiologist who launched coronary angiography at Mayo in 1965, the year he joined the staff. He left Mayo four years later to join a single-specialty practice in Kansas City, MO. Atlanta, GA, March 12, 2006.

Michael D. McGoon. Cardiologist who joined the Mayo staff in 1983 and was chair of the Pulmonary Hypertension Association's Board of Trustees (2006–2008). His father, Dwight McGoon, was a cardiac surgeon at Mayo. Rochester, MN, October 24, 2005.

James D. Maloney. Cardiologist who joined the Mayo staff in 1973 and pioneered the clinic's cardiac electrophysiology program. He joined the Cleveland Clinic in 1981. Washington, DC, September 12, 2004.

Ileen Marxhausen. Joined Mayo as an electrocardiography technician in 1967 and became one of the clinic's first echocardiography technicians (sonographers) in 1976. Rochester, MN, September 13, 2005.

Charlene May. American College of Cardiology staff member who has been involved in the production of practice guidelines for two decades. New Orleans, LA, November 7, 2004.

John M. Merideth. Cardiologist who joined the Mayo staff in 1968. Rochester, MN, August 25, 2000.

Robert L. Parker. Cardiologist who joined the Mayo staff in 1938. Rochester, MN, September 18, 2000.

Richard L. Popp. Cardiologist at Stanford University who was a pioneer of echocardiography and was president of the American College of Cardiology (1997–1998). Chicago, IL, March 29, 2008.

William L. Proudfit. Cardiologist who joined the Cleveland Clinic staff in 1946. Cleveland, OH, July 21, 2005.

William C. Roberts. Cardiac pathologist and longtime editor of the *American Journal of Cardiology.* Dallas, TX, November 14, 2005.

Robert E. Safford. Cardiologist who joined the Mayo staff in 1982 and transferred to Mayo in Jacksonville, FL, four years later. Jacksonville, FL, March 16, 2006.

Thomas T. Schattenberg. Cardiologist who joined the Mayo staff in 1963 and introduced echocardiography at the institution. Rochester, MN, May 28, 2003.

Earl K. Shirey. Cardiologist who joined the Cleveland Clinic staff in 1957 and collaborated with Mason Sones Jr. in pioneering coronary angiography. Cleveland, OH, July 21, 2005.

Ralph Spiekerman. General internist who joined the Mayo staff in 1961 and helped organize the coronary care unit. Rochester, MN, February 2, 2011.

H. J. C. (Jeremy) Swan. Physiologist and cardiologist who joined the Mayo staff in 1951 and helped pioneer cardiac catheterization at the institution. He left in 1965 to become the first full-time director of cardiology at Cedars-Sinai Medical Center in Los Angeles. San Diego, CA, October 7, 2000.

A. Jamil Tajik. Cardiologist with a focus on echocardiography who joined the Mayo staff in 1973 and was chair of Cardiovascular Division (1993–2002). Scottsdale, AZ, January 6, 2007; Rochester, MN, July 24, 2007.

Henry H. Ting. Cardiologist who joined the Mayo staff in 1997 after having been on the staff of the Harvard-affiliated Brigham and Women's Hospital in Boston. Rochester, MN, September 10, 2005.

Ronald E. Vlietstra. Cardiologist who joined the Mayo staff in 1976 and left thirteen years later to join the Watson Clinic in Lakeland, FL. Orlando, FL, March 8, 2005.

Carole A. Warnes. Cardiologist who joined the Mayo staff in 1987. Rochester, MN, December 29, 2005.

Vernon Weber. Trained in electronics, he became Mayo's first echocardiography technician (sonographer) in 1970. Rochester, MN, February 17, 2008.

Arnold M. Weissler. Cardiologist who joined the Mayo staff in 1989 after having been chief of cardiology at several academic medical centers. Rochester, MN, October 31, 2004.

Earl H. Wood. Physiologist who launched Mayo's catheterization program and was a member of the original open-heart surgery team. Rochester, MN, February 5, 2001.

Yang Wang. University of Minnesota cardiologist who had done part of his training at Mayo in the early years of open-heart surgery. Minneapolis, MN, November 29, 2007.

{ NOTES }

Preface and Introduction

1. See W. B. Fye, *The Development of American Physiology: Scientific Medicine in the Nineteenth Century* (Baltimore: Johns Hopkins University Press, 1987); and W. B. Fye, *American Cardiology: The History of a Specialty and Its College* (Baltimore: Johns Hopkins University Press, 1996).

2. Most patient stories in the book came from published autobiographical accounts. Those derived from unpublished sources are used in accordance with the Health Insurance Portability and Accountability Act of 1996. See S. C. Lawrence, "Access Anxiety: HIPAA and Historical Research," *J. Hist. Med. Allied Sci.*, 2007, *62*: 422–460.

3. W. C. Roberts, "Wallace Bruce Fye III, MD, MA, MACC: A Conversation with the Editor," *Am. J. Cardiol.* 2005; *95*: 55–83.

4. W. B. Fye and J. A. Callahan, "The Division of Cardiovascular Diseases," in *A History of the Department of Internal Medicine at the Mayo Clinic*, ed. J. Graner (Rochester, MN: Mayo Foundation, 2002), 257–271.

5. T. R. Frieden and D. M. Berwick, "The 'Million Hearts' Initiative: Preventing Heart Attacks and Strokes," *N. Engl. J. Med.*, 2011, *365*, e27: 1–4.

6. "America's Best Hospitals," *U.S. News & World Report*, April 30, 1990, 52–86. My conclusions are drawn from a review of each annual Best Hospitals issue published between 1990 and 2013. See also W. C. Roberts, "The Best Hospitals in the USA for Patients with Heart Disease," *Am. J. Cardiol.*, 1993, *72*: 626–627.

7. R. Stevens, *American Medicine and the Public Interest*, rev. ed. (Berkeley: University of California Press, 1998), ix. See also G. Weisz, *Divide and Conquer: A Comparative History of Medical Specialization* (New York: Oxford University Press, 2006).

8. In this book I use the term "cardiac surgeon" to refer to doctors who operate on patients with heart disease, although many of these individuals perform other types of surgical procedures and may describe themselves as cardiothoracic or cardiovascular surgeons.

9. See Stevens, *American Medicine*, 115–131; and *Physicians of the Mayo Clinic and the Mayo Foundation* (Minneapolis: University of Minnesota Press, 1937).

10. General readers can obtain information about the technical terms and procedures mentioned in this book by using Google or a similar search engine. Health care sites developed for the public include http://www.nlm.nih.gov/medlineplus/ and http://www.mayoclinic.com/health-information/. Video descriptions and depictions of technologies and procedures may be found on *YouTube*. A state-of-the-art review for medical professionals is J. G. Murphy and M. A. Lloyd, eds., *Mayo Clinic Cardiology: Concise Textbook*, 4th ed. (New York: Oxford University Press, 2013).

11. A. Gawande, "The Cost Conundrum," *The New Yorker*, June 1, 2009, 36–44, quotation from 39.

Chapter 1

1. For the origins and early growth of the Mayo Clinic, see H. Clapesattle, *The Doctors Mayo* (Minneapolis: University of Minnesota Press, 1941); *Sketch of the History of the Mayo*

Clinic and the Mayo Foundation (Philadelphia: W. B. Saunders, 1926); W. F. Braasch, *Early Days at the Mayo Clinic* (Springfield, IL: Charles C Thomas, 1969); and W. B. Fye, "The Origins and Evolution of the Mayo Clinic from 1864 to 1939: A Minnesota Family Practice Becomes an International 'Medical Mecca,'" *Bull. Hist. Med.*, 2010, *84*: 323–357. A memoir by Charles W. Mayo, the son of Charles H. Mayo and the nephew of William J. Mayo, who joined the practice as a surgeon in 1931, provides an insider's perspective. C. W. Mayo, *Mayo: The Story of My Family and My Career* (Garden City, NY: Doubleday, 1968). Short biographies (and complete bibliographies) of more than 1,500 trainees and staff members up to 1936 are in *Physicians of the Mayo Clinic and the Mayo Foundation* (Minneapolis: University of Minnesota Press, 1937).

2. J. Hartzell, *I Started All This: The Life of Dr. William Worrall Mayo* (Greenville, SC: Arvi Books, 2004).

3. R. J. Carlisle, *An Account of Bellevue Hospital with a Catalogue of the Medical and Surgical Staff from 1736 to 1894* (New York: Society of the Alumni of Bellevue Hospital, 1893), quotation from 42.

4. See W. F. Norwood, *Medical Education in the United States before the Civil War* (Philadelphia: University of Pennsylvania Press, 1944). Sources on frontier medicine include M. E. Pickard and R. C. Buley, *The Midwest Pioneer: His Ills, Cures & Doctors* (Crawfordsville, IN: R. E. Banta, 1945); V. Steele, *Bleed, Blister, and Purge: A History of Medicine on the American Frontier* (Missoula, MT: Mountain Press, 2005); C. B. Valencius, *The Health of the Country: How American Settlers Understood Themselves and Their Land* (New York: Basic Books, 2002); J. K. Crellin, *Medical Care in Pioneer Illinois* (Springfield, IL: Pearson Museum, 1982); S. C. Lawrence, "Iowa Physicians: Legitimacy, Institutions, and the Practice of Medicine. Part I: Establishing a Professional Identity, 1833–1886," *Ann. Iowa*, 2003, *62*: 1–47; and R. L. Numbers and J. W. Leavitt, eds., *Wisconsin Medicine: Historical Perspectives* (Madison: University of Wisconsin Press, 1981). A comprehensive overview of the region is R. Sisson, C. Zacher, and A. Cayton, eds., *The American Midwest: An Interpretive Encyclopedia* (Bloomington: Indiana University Press, 2007). Surveys of nineteenth-century medicine include J. S. Haller Jr., *American Medicine in Transition, 1840–1910* (Chicago: University of Illinois Press, 1981); and L. S. King, *Transformations in American Medicine: From Benjamin Rush to William Osler* (Baltimore: Johns Hopkins University Press, 1991).

5. For Louise Wright Mayo's role in her family's success, see Hartzell, *I Started All This*.

6. W. W. Mayo, "Report on the Pathological Indications of the Urine," *Proc. Annual Meeting Indiana State Med. Soc.*, 1854, *5*: 68–77. See also D. J. Warner, "The Campaign for Medical Microscopy in Antebellum America," *Bull. Hist. Med.*, 1995, *69*: 367–386.

7. See M. L. Wingerd, *North Country: The Making of Minnesota* (Minneapolis: University of Minnesota Press, 2010); and T. C. Blegen, *Minnesota: A History of the State* (Minneapolis: University of Minnesota Press, 1963).

8. W. W. Finch, "Physicians, the Climate, and Diseases, in Minnesota Territory," *Boston Med. Surg. J.*, 1853, *49*: 213–214. See also P. D. Jordan, "Salubrious Minnesota," in *The People's Health: A History of Public Health in Minnesota to 1948* (St. Paul: Minnesota Historical Society, 1953), 1–16.

9. Mrs. W. B. Meloney, "Mrs. Mayo, Wilderness Mother," *Delineator*, 1914, *84*: 9, 46; Mayo Clinic Archives, Mayo Historical Unit, Rochester, MN (hereafter MCA).

10. K. Carley, *Minnesota in the Civil War: An Illustrated History* (St. Paul: Minnesota Historical Society Press, 2000).

11. See H. Severson, *Rochester: Mecca for Millions* (Rochester, MN: Marquette Bank & Trust, 1979); and M. W. Raygor, *The Rochester Story* (Rochester, MN: Schmidt, 1976).

12. See J. O. Anfinson, *The River We Have Wrought: A History of the Upper Mississippi* (Minneapolis: University of Minnesota Press, 2003); D. L. Hofsommer, *Minneapolis and the Age of Railways* (Minneapolis: University of Minnesota Press, 2005); and D. Blanke, *Sowing*

the American Dream: How Consumer Culture Took Root in the Rural Midwest (Athens: Ohio University Press, 2000).

13. G. E. Shrady, "The Country Practitioner," *Med. Rec.*, 1868, *3*: 229–230. See also C. E. Rosenberg, "The Practice of Medicine in New York a Century Ago," *Bull. Hist. Med.*, 1967, *41*: 223–253.

14. *Rochester Post*, November 6, 1869, quoted in: Harzell, *I Started All This*, 80.

15. "Half a Century of Anæsthetics," *Northwestern Lancet*, 1896, *16*: 416–417. See also B. M. Duncum, *The Development of Inhalation Anesthesia: With Special Reference to the Years 1846–1900* (London: Oxford University Press, 1947); T. E. Keys, *The History of Surgical Anesthesia* (New York: Schuman's, 1945); and M. S. Pernick, *A Calculus of Suffering: Pain, Professionalism, and Anesthesia in Nineteenth-Century America* (New York: Columbia University Press, 1985).

16. W. W. Mayo, "The Relations of Physicians to the Public and Each Other," *Trans. Minn. Med. Soc.*, 1873, *5*: 24–37.

17. H. W. Davenport, *Not Just Any Medical School: The Science, Practice and Teaching of Medicine at the University of Michigan, 1850–1941* (Ann Arbor: University of Michigan Press, 1999).

18. Mayo, W. J. "Recollections of the Medical School of the University of Michigan in 1880–1883," June 1937, MCA. See also H. W. Davenport, *University of Michigan Surgeons, 1850–1970: Who They Were and What They Did* (Ann Arbor: University of Michigan, 1993); O. H. Wangensteen and S. D. Wangensteen, *The Rise of Surgery from Empiric Craft to Scientific Discipline* (Minneapolis: University of Minnesota Press, 1978); and I. M. Rutkow, *American Surgery: An Illustrated History* (Philadelphia: Lippincott-Raven, 1998).

19. W. J. Mayo to Sister Trude [Gertrude Mayo Berkman], May 5, 1883, MCA.

20. See S. L. Jones, "History of Northwestern University Medical School (Chicago Medical College)," in *Medical and Dental Colleges of the West*, ed. H. G. Cutler (Chicago: Oxford Publishing, 1896), 155–198; and L. B. Arey, *Northwestern University Medical School 1859–1959: A Pioneer in Educational Reform* (Evanston, IL: Northwestern University, 1959).

21. W. W. Mayo and W. J. Mayo, "Report of Drs. W. W. & W. J. Mayo," *Trans. Minn. Med. Soc.*, 1885, *17*: 43–51.

22. See J. J. Walsh, "Post-Graduate Medical School and Hospital," in *History of Medicine in New York* (New York: National Americana Society, 1919), 2: 573–593; and W. M. Hartshorn, *New York Polyclinic Medical School and Hospital* (New York: privately printed, 1942). Clinician-historian Steven Peitzman writes, "The most famous polyclinic students were undoubtedly the Mayo brothers." S. J. Peitzman, "'Thoroughly Practical': America's Polyclinic Medical Schools," *Bull. Hist. Med.*, 1980, *54*: 166–187, quotation from 182. See also C. C. Lee, "The Necessity for Post-Graduate Instruction in the Present State of American Medical Education," *Maryland Med. J.*, 1888, *20*: 121–124; and T. N. Bonner, *American Doctors and German Universities: A Chapter in International Intellectual Relations, 1870–1914* (Lincoln: University of Nebraska Press, 1963).

23. A valuable bibliography of the history of specialization is R. Stevens, "Update to the Bibliography, 1998," in *American Medicine and the Public Interest*, rev. ed. (Berkeley: University of California Press, 1998), 557–561. A collection of contemporary articles is C. E. Rosenberg, ed., *The Origins of Specialization in American Medicine: An Anthology of Sources* (New York: Garland, 1989). See also G. Weisz, *Divide and Conquer: A Comparative History of Medical Specialization* (New York: Oxford University Press, 2006).

24. M. P. Jacobi, "Specialism in Medicine," *Arch. Med.*, 1882, *7*: 87–97, quotation from 88.

25. See G. H. Brieger, "American Surgery and the Germ Theory of Disease," *Bull. Hist. Med.*, 1966, *40*: 135–145; A. S. Earle, "The Germ Theory in America: Antisepsis and Asepsis (1867–1900)," *Surgery*, 1969, *65*: 508–522; M. Worboys, "Was There a Bacteriological Revolution in Late Nineteenth-Century Medicine?" *Stud. Hist. Phil. Biol. & Biomed. Sci.*, 2007, *38*: 20–42;

and N. Tomes, *The Gospel of Germs: Men, Women, and the Microbe in American Life* (Cambridge, MA: Harvard University Press, 1998).

26. S. Smith, "Preface to the Second Edition," in *The Principles and Practice of Operative Surgery*, 2nd ed. (Philadelphia: Lea Brothers, 1887), iii–iv.

27. Ibid. See also G. H. Brieger, "A Portrait of American Surgery: Surgery in America, 1875—1889," *Surg. Clin. North Am.*, 1987, *67*: 1181–1216.

28. J. H. Dunn, "A Decade of Observation and Experience in Antiseptic Surgery," *Trans. Minn. Med. Soc.*, 1887, *19*: 56–81, quotation from 61–62. See also T. P. Gariepy, "The Introduction and Acceptance of Listerian Antisepsis in the United States," *J. Hist. Med. Allied Sci.*, 1994, *49*: 167–206; M. A. Crowther and M. W. Dupree, *Medical Lives in the Age of Surgical Revolution* (Cambridge: Cambridge University Press, 2007); and C. Lawrence and R. Dixey, "Practising on Principle: Joseph Lister and the Germ Theories of Disease," in *Medical Theory, Surgical Practice: Studies in the History of Surgery*, ed. C. Lawrence (New York: Routledge, 1992), 153–215.

29. C. H. Mastin, "The Past, the Present, and the Future of Our Association," *Trans. Am. Surg. Assoc.*, 1891, *9*: 1–13, quotation from 6. See also C. R. Hall, "The Rise of Professional Surgery in the United States: 1800–1865," *Bull. Hist. Med.*, 1952, *26*: 231–262.

30. C. E. Rosenberg, *The Care of Strangers: The Rise of America's Hospital System* (New York: Basic Books, 1987).

31. A. Worcester, *Small Hospitals: Establishment and Maintenance* (New York: John Wiley & Sons, 1894), quotations from 2, 4–5. See also J. S. Billings and H. M. Hurd, eds., *Hospitals, Dispensaries and Nursing* (Baltimore: Johns Hopkins Press, 1894).

32. Minneapolis physician Richard Hill applauded the impact of technology and science on medicine. R. J. Hill, "Medical Advancement in the Past Twenty Years," *Northwestern Lancet*, 1898, *18*: 6–8. See also R. S. Cowan, *A Social History of American Technology* (New York: Oxford University Press, 1997); T. P. Hughes, *American Genesis: A Century of Invention and Technological Enthusiasm, 1870–1970* (Chicago: University of Chicago Press, 2004); J. H. Lienhard, *Inventing Modern: Growing Up With X-rays, Skyscrapers, and Tailfins* (New York: Oxford University Press, 2003); and T. J. Misa, P. Brey, and A. Feenberg, eds., *Modernity and Technology* (Cambridge, MA: MIT Press, 2003).

33. E. Whelan, *The Sisters' Story: Saint Marys Hospital—Mayo Clinic, 1889 to 1939* (Rochester, MN: Mayo Foundation, 2002).

34. "The Cyclone," *Rochester Record & Union*, August 24, 1883, MCA. Eventually, it was judged to have been an F5 tornado. See M. W. Seeley, *Minnesota Weather Almanac* (St. Paul: Minnesota Historical Society Press, 2006), 180–198.

35. Whelan, *The Sisters' Story*, 35–56.

36. C. Kraman, *Odyssey in Faith: The Story of Mother Alfred Moes* (Rochester, MN: Sisters of St. Francis, 1990).

37. See B. M. Wall, *Unlikely Entrepreneurs: Catholic Sisters and the Hospital Marketplace, 1865–1925* (Columbus: Ohio State University Press, 2005); S. Nelson, *Say Little, Do Much: Nurses, Nuns, and Hospitals in the Nineteenth Century* (Philadelphia: University of Pennsylvania Press, 2001); and C. J. Kauffman, *Ministry and Meaning: A Religious History of Catholic Health Care in the United States* (New York: Crossroad Publishing, 1995).

38. W. W. Mayo, "Address," in *Memorial of St. Mary's Hospital* (Rochester, MN: St. Mary's Hospital, 1894), 7–8.

39. See Rosenberg, *Care of Strangers*; M. J. Vogel, *The Invention of the Modern Hospital: Boston 1870–1930* (Chicago: University of Chicago Press, 1980); J. D. Thompson and G. Goldin, *The Hospital: A Social and Architectural History* (New Haven, CT: Yale University Press, 1975); and T. Schlich, "Surgery, Science and Modernity: Operating Rooms and Laboratories as Places of Control," *Hist. Sci.*, 2007, *45*: 231–256.

40. "St. Mary's Hospital," *Rochester Record & Union*, July 19, 1889, MCA. The number of beds is from *Eleventh Annual Report of St. Mary's Hospital* [for 1900] (Rochester, MN: St. Mary's Hospital, 1901).

41. Worcester, *Small Hospitals*, 6–7.

42. Ibid., 41.

43. J. Hartzell, *Mrs. Charlie: The Other Mayo* (Gobles, MN: Arvi, 2000). Useful overviews of nursing history are P. D'Antonio, "Revisiting and Rethinking the Rewriting of Nursing History," *Bull. Hist. Med.*, 1999, *73*: 268–290; and J. W. James, "Writing and Rewriting Nursing History: A Review Essay," *Bull. Hist. Med.*, 1984, *58*: 568–584.

44. For the closed-staff model at St. Mary's Hospital, see Whelan, *Sisters' Story*, 57–75. See also E. Cowles, "The Relations of the Medical Staff to the Governing Bodies in Hospitals," in Billings and Hurd, *Hospitals*, 69–76. See also A. J. Ochsner and M. J. Sturm, *The Organization, Construction and Management of Hospitals* (Chicago: Cleveland Press, 1907).

45. "The Doctors Mayo to the St. Mary's Hospital Board of Trustees, July 1892," published in Whelan, *Sisters' Story*, 71.

46. *Annual Report of St. Mary's Hospital* [for 1894] (Rochester, MN: St. Mary's Hospital, 1895).

47. L. D. Boynton "Address," in *Memorial of St. Mary's Hospital* (1894), 15–17.

48. Ibid.

49. W. J. Mayo "Address," in *Memorial of St. Mary's Hospital* (1894), 20.

50. A. M. Chesney, *The Johns Hopkins Hospital and the Johns Hopkins School of Medicine: A Chronicle. Volume 1. Early Years, 1867–1893* (Baltimore: Johns Hopkins Press, 1943).

51. W. J. Mayo, "John[s] Hopkins, May 1895," handwritten notebook, MCA. See also W. J. Mayo, "What We Owe to Johns Hopkins University," *Proc. Staff Meetings of Mayo Clinic*, 1932, *7*: 32–34, hereafter *PSMMC*. For descriptions of the operating rooms and aseptic techniques at Johns Hopkins when Mayo visited, see H. A. Kelly, "The Gynecological Operating Room in the Johns Hopkins Hospital, and the Antiseptic and Aseptic Rules in Force," *Johns Hopkins Hosp. Reports*, 1890, *2*: 131–139, and H. Robb, *Aseptic Surgical Technique* (Philadelphia: J. B. Lippincott, 1894).

52. *Annual Report of St. Mary's Hospital* [for 1893] (Rochester, MN: St. Mary's Hospital, 1894), 4.

53. W. T. Adams, "The Southern Minnesota Medical Association: A Historical Sketch," *St. Paul Med. J.*, 1911, *13*: 54–59, quotation from 54–55. See also W. Osler, "On the Educational Value of the Medical Society," *Boston Med. Surg. J.*, 1903, *148*: 275–279; and W. J. Mayo, "The Value of the Medical Society to the Practitioner of Medicine," *PSMMC*, 1934, *9*: 38–40.

54. W. J. Mayo, "An Address Delivered to the Graduating Class of the Medical Department of the Minnesota State University, May 5, 1895," *Northwestern Lancet*, 1895, *15*: 221–225, quotations from 224.

55. W. J. Mayo, "The Preliminary Examination of Surgical Patients," *Northwestern Lancet*, 1897, *17*: 87–90. See also J. H. Warner, *The Therapeutic Perspective: Medical Practice, Knowledge, and Identity in America, 1820–1885* (Cambridge, MA: Harvard University Press, 1986); and K. D. Keele, *The Evolution of Clinical Methods in Medicine* (London: Pitman, 1963).

56. Newspaper quotation in N. H. Guthrey, *Medicine and Its Practitioners in Olmsted County Prior to 1900* (St. Paul: Minnesota Medicine, 1951), 196. See also J. R. Watson, "The Mayo's First Partner: Augustus White Stinchfield," *Mayo Alumnus*, 1970, *6*: 16–18.

57. Charlie Mayo discussed hiring Stinchfield in an interview. C. H. Mayo, interviews by Richard Beard, June 29–30, 1932, MCA

58. A. W. Stinchfield, "Casebook," 1892, MCA. See J. Gillis, "The History of the Patient Since 1850," *Bull. Hist. Med.*, 2006, *80*: 490–512. William Osler's textbook is the best source for

contemporary concepts about the causes, diagnosis, natural history, prognosis, and treatment of non-surgical diseases. W. Osler, *The Principles and Practice of Medicine* (New York: D. Appleton, 1892).

59. Stinchfield, "Casebook," 1892, 8. See also C. H. Goodwin, *The Hospital Treatment of Diseases of the Heart and Lungs with Over 350 Formulae and Prescriptions as Exemplified in the Hospitals of New York City* (New York: Goodwin, 1883); and W. B. Fye, "Cardiology in 1885," *Circulation*, 1985, *72*: 21–26.

60. Stinchfield, "Casebook," 1892, 91. Stinchfield did not mention the man's heart rate.

61. These data are from the *[Fourth] Annual Report of St. Mary's Hospital* [for 1893] (Rochester, MN, 1894); and the *Sixth Annual Report of St. Mary's Hospital* [for 1895] (Rochester, MN, 1896).

62. Hartzell, *Mrs. Charlie*, 21–28.

63. Mayo, "Examination of Surgical Patients," 87–88.

64. *The Standard Medical Directory of North America, 1903–4* (Chicago: G. P. Engelhard, 1903). For how the editors chose the doctors included in their list of specialists, see 697.

65. For population growth and railroad expansion, see J. R. Borchert and D. P. Yaeger, *Atlas of Minnesota Resources and Settlement* (St. Paul: Minnesota State Planning Agency, 1969).

66. W. Osler, "Internal Medicine as a Vocation," *Med. News*, 1897, *71*: 660–663, quotation from 660. See also W. Osler, "The Study of Internal Medicine," *Med. News*, 1901, *78*: 645–647; R. C. Maulitz and D. E. Long, eds., *Grand Rounds: One Hundred Years of Internal Medicine* (Philadelphia: University of Pennsylvania Press, 1988); and K. Faber, *Nosography: The Evolution of Clinical Medicine in Modern Times*, 2nd ed. (New York: Paul B. Hoeber, 1930).

67. F. A. Willius, *Henry Stanley Plummer: A Diversified Genius* (Springfield, IL: Charles C Thomas, 1960).

68. F. Billings, "The Relation of General Medicine to the Specialties," *Chicago Med. Recorder*, 1898, *14*: 93–100, quotation from 97.

69. Ibid., 99–100. See also E. F. Hirsch, *Frank Billings: A Leader in Chicago Medicine* (Chicago: University of Chicago Press, 1966). For a prominent Boston internist's perspective, see F. C. Shattuck, "Specialism in Medicine," *JAMA*, 1900, *35*: 723–726.

70. For the organization of specialties, see Stevens, *American Medicine and the Public Interest,* 218–266; and Weisz, *Divide and Conquer*, 63–83.

71. W. J. Mayo, "The Work of Dr. Henry S. Plummer," *PSMMC*, 1938, *13*: 417–422. For a perspective on blood diseases, see R. C. Cabot, *A Guide to the Clinical Examination of the Blood for Diagnostic Purposes*, 4th ed. (New York: William Wood, 1901).

72. Mayo, "Examination of Surgical Patients," 90.

73. Mayo, "Henry S. Plummer." See also J. A. Wyeth, "The Value of Clinical Microscopy, Bacteriology, and Chemistry in Surgical Practice," *JAMA*, 1901, *36*: 1611–1617; and W. D. Foster, *A Short History of Clinical Pathology* (Edinburgh: E. & S. Livingstone, 1961).

74. For Cross, see Clapesattle, *Doctors Mayo*, 366–368. See also F. H. Williams, *The Roentgen Rays in Medicine and Surgery* (New York: Macmillan, 1901); L. R. Brown, "History of Diagnostic Radiology at the Mayo Clinic," *Am. J. Radiol*, 1993, *161*: 1321–1325; E. R. N. Grigg, *The Trail of the Invisible Light* (Springfield, IL: Charles C Thomas, 1965); R. Brecher and E. Brecher, *The Rays: A History of Radiology in the United States and Canada* (Baltimore: Williams and Wilkins, 1959); J. D. Howell, *Technology in the Hospital: Transforming Patient Care in the Early Twentieth Century* (Baltimore: Johns Hopkins University Press, 1995), 103–132; and M. Lavine, "The Early Clinical X-Ray in the United States: Patient Experiences and Public Perceptions," *J. Hist. Med. Allied Sci.*, 2012, *67*: 587–625.

75. W. W. Keen, "The Clinical Application of the Röntgen Rays. II. In Surgical Diagnosis," *Am. J. Med. Sci.*, 1896, *111*: 256–261.

76. C. H. Mayo, "Removal of Open Buckle Impacted in the Esophagus, With X-Ray Skiagraph," *Northwestern Lancet*, 1897, *17*: 92–93.

77. Clapesattle, *Doctors Mayo*, 717–719. This book includes descriptions of the Mayo brothers' personalities, surgical practices, and relationships based on interviews of their family members, colleagues, and former trainees.

78. See H. J. Harwick, *Forty-four Years with the Mayo Clinic* (Rochester, MN: Whiting, 1957). See also G. W. Broome, *Rochester and the Mayo Clinic: A Fair and Unbiased Story Calculated to Aid Physicians to Greater Cures and Larger Incomes* (New York: Shakespeare Press, 1914).

79. C. W. Mayo, *Story of My Family*, 24–25.

80. Harry J. Harwick, interview by Helen Clapesattle, January 26, 1940, Clapesattle papers, MCA.

81. Braasch, *Early Days at the Mayo Clinic*, 102.

Chapter 2

1. E. A. Hall, "Echoes from St. Mary's Clinic, Rochester, Minn.," *Canada Lancet*, 1906, *40*: 289–303, quotations from 291–292.

2. A. J. Ochsner, "One Year's Clinical Observations on the Surgery of the Gall-Bladder," *Northwestern Lancet*, 1902, *22*: 109–113, quotation from 113.

3. N. Senn, "Travel as a Means of Post-Graduate Medical Education," *JAMA*, 1904, *43*: 261–263, quotation from 263.

4. The number of operations performed at St. Mary's Hospital in 1903 (2,640) was similar to the number done at much larger and older hospitals, such as Boston's Massachusetts General Hospital (3,109), New York City's Roosevelt Hospital (2,719), and New York City's New York Hospital (1,680). See *Fourteenth Annual Report of St. Mary's Hospital* [for 1903] (Rochester, MN: St. Mary's Hospital, 1904); and table 3, "Growth of Operative Work [and Patients Registered in the Clinic, 1889–1925]," in *Sketch of the History of the Mayo Clinic and the Mayo Foundation* (Philadelphia: W. B. Saunders, 1926), 31. For the Boston and New York hospitals, see W. S. Halsted, "The Training of the Surgeon," *Bull. Johns Hopkins Hosp.*, 1904, *15*: 267–275.

5. H. Cushing, "The Society of Clinical Surgery in Retrospect," *Ann. Surg.*, 1969, *169*: 1–9, quotation from 2, paper presented in Baltimore, MD, November 16, 1922. See also H. B. Shumacker Jr., *History of the Society of Clinical Surgery* (Indianapolis: Benham Press, 1977).

6. Harvey Cushing to Henry K. Cushing, October 15, 1905, Harvey Cushing Papers, Yale University, Harvey Cushing/John Hay Whitney Medical Library.

7. R. O. Beard, "Scientific Methods in Medical Education," *Northwestern Lancet*, 1904, *24*: 318–321, quotation from 320–321. See also W. W. Keen, "Surgery," in *The Progress of the Century* (New York: Harper & Brothers, 1901), 217–260.

8. S. H. Adams, "Modern Surgery," *McClure's Magazine*, 1905, *24*: 482–492, quotation from 482.

9. Ibid., 483.

10. J. H. Cassedy, "Muckraking and Medicine: Samuel Hopkins Adams," *Am. Quart.*, 1964, *16*: 85–99. See also P. J. Kernahan, "'A Condition of Development': Muckrakers, Surgeons, and Hospitals, 1890–1920," *J. Am. Coll. Surg.*, 2008, *206*: 376–384.

11. Adams, "Modern Surgery," 485.

12. See *Fifteenth Annual Report of St. Mary's Hospital* [for 1904] (Rochester, MN: St. Mary's Hospital, 1905), 18; and *Sixteenth Report of the Superintendent of the Johns Hopkins Hospital for the Year Ending January 31, 1905* (Baltimore: Johns Hopkins Press, 1905), 56, 82.

13. W. J. Mayo, "The Medical Profession and the Issues Which Confront It," *JAMA*, 1906, *46*: 1737–1740, quotations from 1740.

14. W. L. Conklin, "A Visit to the Doctors Mayo, St. Mary's Hospital, Rochester, Minnesota," *Am. J. Nursing*, 1909, *9*: 395–399, quotations from 395–396.

15. S. C. Baker, "The Mayo Clinic at Rochester Minnesota," *J. SC Med. Assoc.*, 1909, *5*: 124–130, quotation from 125. Emil Beckman, a resident at St. Mary's Hospital who joined the Mayo practice in 1911, described the operating rooms. See E. H. Beckman, "Operating-Room Technic," *Old Dominion J. Med. Surg.*, 1909, *9*: 171–179.

16. A. C. Bernays, "A Visit to the Mayos at Rochester, Minnesota. A Feuilleton," *N. Y. Med. J.*, 1906, *83*: 808–810.

17. R. B. H. Gradwohl, "The Mayo Surgical Clinic at Rochester," *Med. Brief*, 1908, *36*: 475–504, quotations from 478–479.

18. A. L. Smith, "Notes on the Mayos' Surgical Clinic," *Montreal Med. J.*, 1908, *37*: 323–333, quotation from 324–325.

19. J. E. Owens, "Discussion of the Papers of Drs. Monks, Ochsner and Harrington," *Trans. Am. Surg. Assoc.*, 1904, *22*: 52–57, quotation from 55. See also Halsted, "Training of the Surgeon."

20. For a list of operations and staff, see *Fifteenth Annual Report of St. Mary's Hospital*.

21. Bernays, "Visit to the Mayos," 808–809.

22. Gradwohl, "Mayo Surgical Clinic," 476.

23. Baker, "Mayo Clinic," 127.

24. Hall, "Echoes from St. Mary's Clinic," 292.

25. Callie to Mrs. Benson, March 15, 1909, postcard in the author's possession.

26. *Twentieth Annual Report of St. Mary's Hospital* [for 1909] (Rochester, MN: St. Mary's Hospital, 1910), 18, 30.

27. Ollie to C. K., Washta, IA, January 1, 1909, postcard in the author's possession.

28. *Twentieth Annual Report of St. Mary's Hospital*. For the consumer movement and health care, see N. Tomes, "Merchants of Health: Medicine and Consumer Culture in the United States, 1900–1940," *J. Am. Hist.*, 2001, *88*: 519–547.

29. W. C. Abbott, Editorial accompanying article by W. F. Church, "A Visit to the Mayos's Clinic," *Am. J. Clin. Med.*, 1908, *15*: 649–652, quotations from 651–652, emphasis in the original. See also D. C. Smith, "Modern Surgery and the Development of Group Practice in the Midwest," *Caduceus*, 1986, *2, no. 3*: 1–39.

30. Hall, "Echoes from St. Mary's Clinic," 302.

31. W. J. Mayo, "Commencement Address," in *Collected Papers of the Staff of St. Mary's Hospital, Mayo Clinic, 1910* (Philadelphia: W. B. Saunders, 1911), 557–566, quotation from 561, paper presented at Rush Medical College in Chicago in 1910. The paper was reprinted as W. J. Mayo, "The Necessity of Cooperation in Medicine," *Mayo Clin. Proc.*, 2000, *75*: 553–556.

32. Ibid., 562.

33. Bernays, "Visit to the Mayos," 809.

34. D. W. Cathell and W. T. Cathell, *Book on the Physician Himself and Things That Concern His Reputation and Success* (Philadelphia: F.A. Davis, 1903), 41.

35. C. A. Wood, "Advantages and Disadvantages of Co-operation and Business Partnership among Medical Men," *Chicago Med. Recorder*, 1909, *31*: 255–262. For medical practice in the Progressive Era, see D. L. Madison, "Preserving Individualism in the Organizational Society: 'Cooperation' and American Medical Practice, 1900–1920," *Bull. Hist Med.*, 1996, *70*: 442–483; G. Rosen, *The Structure of American Medical Practice, 1875–1941* (Philadelphia: University of Pennsylvania Press, 1983); and G. H. Brieger, "Medicine and Surgery in 1909," *Trans. Stud. Coll. Physicians Phila*, 1985, *ser. 5, vol. 7*: 17–25. For the Progressive Era, see R. H. Wiebe, *The Search for Order, 1877–1920* (New York: Hill and Wang, 1967); and J. D. Buenker, J. C. Burnham, and R. M. Crunden, *Progressivism* (Cambridge, MA: Schenkman, 1977).

36. L. S. King, "Medical Practice: Making a Living," *JAMA*, 1984, *251*: 1887–1892.

37. T. Hatch, "The Doctor's Fees," *Northwestern Lancet*, 1900, *20*: 328–329, quotation from 328.

38. S. M. Hohf, "Medical Fees," *J. Minn. State Med. Assoc. NW Lancet*, 1908, *28*: 73–77, quotation from 75. See also G. Rosen, *Fees and Fee Bills: Some Economic Aspects of Medical Practice in Nineteenth Century America* (Baltimore: Johns Hopkins Press, 1946).

39. P. D. Olch, "William S. Halsted and Private Practice: A Re-Examination," *Surgery*, 1972, *72*: 804–811, quotation from 806. See also G. Imber, *Genius on the Edge: The Bizarre Double Life of Dr. William Stewart Halsted* (New York: Kaplan, 2010).

40. C. H. Mayo and W. J. Mayo, "A Review of 1000 Operations for Gallstone Disease, with Special Reference to the Mortality," *Am. J. Med. Sci.*, 1905, *129*: 375–380. See also B. G. A. Moynihan, *Gall-Stones and Their Surgical Treatment* (Philadelphia: W. B. Saunders, 1905).

41. Bernays, "Visit to the Mayos," 809.

42. James J. Walsh to W. J. Mayo, April 1, 1910, Mayo Clinic Archives, Mayo Historical Unit, Rochester, MN (hereafter MCA). See also J. J. Walsh, *Makers of Modern Medicine* (New York: Fordham University Press, 1907); and C. H. Mayo to James J. Walsh, April 4, 1910, MCA.

43. J. J. Walsh, "A Medical Pilgrimage Westward," *Independent*, 1911, *71*: 189–197, quotation from 191.

44. Ibid., 192. See also T. M. Stewart, "Medical and Surgical Fees," *Lancet-Clinic*, 1915, *113*: 624–628.

45. R. M. Harbin, "Notes on the Mayo Clinic," *Atlanta J. Rec. Med.*, 1910, *51*: 459–465, comments about Keen on 460.

46. Keen's description of his illness is from a memoir he prepared in 1915 that was published by his great-grandson. See W. W. K. James, ed., *Keen of Philadelphia: The Collected Memoirs of William Williams Keen Jr.* (Dubkin, NH: William L. Bauhan, 2002), quotation from 188.

47. Ibid., 189–191.

48. A. W. Davis, *Dr. Kelly of Hopkins: Surgeon, Scientist, Christian* (Baltimore: Johns Hopkins Press, 1959), 207–208.

49. W. Osler to H. A. Kelly, September 1911, published in W. E. Goodwin, "William Osler and Howard A. Kelly: 'Physicians, Medical Historians, Friends.'" *Bull. Hist. Med.* 1946, *20*:611–652, quotation from 639.

50. W. Osler, "Remarks on the Medical Library in Postgraduate Work," *Br. Med. J.*, 1909, *2*: 925–928.

51. Davis, *Dr. Kelly of Hopkins*, 208.

52. For Johnson's illnesses and death, see F. A. Day and T. M. Knappen, *Life of John Albert Johnson: Three Times Governor of Minnesota*, (St. Paul, MN: Day & Knappen, 1910), 248–258; H. Clapesattle, *The Doctors Mayo* (Minneapolis: University of Minnesota Press, 1941), 487–491; and W. G. Helmes, *John A. Johnson: The People's Governor* (Minneapolis: University of Minnesota Press, 1949), 88–91, 115, 303–305.

53. *Twentieth Annual Report of St. Mary's Hospital*, 31.

54. For the staff, see H. J. Harwick, *Forty-four Years with the Mayo Clinic* (Rochester, MN: Whiting Press, 1957), 37–40.

55. W. J. Mayo to Max Brödel, February 1, 1913, MCA. See also W. C. MacCarty, *The Early History of Surgical Pathology and the Laboratories in the Mayo Clinic* (Rochester, MN: privately printed, 1953).

56. See *Collected Papers of the Staff of St. Mary's Hospital, Mayo Clinic, 1910* (Philadelphia: W. B. Saunders, 1911). Will Mayo tried repeatedly to recruit Brödel, who was the best medical illustrator in North America. See R. W. Crosby and J. Cody, *Max Brödel: The Man Who Put Art into Medicine* (New York: Springer-Verlag, 1991), 120–128; and *Scalpel to Sketch: The Science and Beauty of Medical Illustration at Mayo Clinic* (Rochester, MN: Mayo Clinic, 2007).

57. W. J. Mayo to Maud Mellish, January 1, 1907, MCA. See also "In Memoriam: Maud H. Mellish Wilson," *PSMMC*, 1933, *8*: 1–12.

58. H. L. Foss to W. J. Mayo, March 9, 1916, MCA. See also M. H. Mellish, *The Writing of Medical Papers* (Philadelphia: W. B. Saunders, 1922).

59. Unsigned review of W. J. Mayo and C. H. Mayo, *A Collection of Papers, Published Previous to 1909* (Philadelphia: W. B. Saunders, 1912), *Bull. Johns Hopkins Hosp.*, 1912, *23*: 349. See also J. L. Dusseau, "Rochester, Minneapolis and Boston: Serendipity," in *An Informal History of W. B. Saunders Company*, (Philadelphia: W. B. Saunders, 1988), 89–100.

60. R. O. Beard, "The Mayo Clinic Building at Rochester," *Journal-Lancet*, 1914, *34*: 425–434, quotation from 432.

61. "The Mayo Clinic Building is Formally Opened," *Rochester Daily Bulletin*, March 7, 1914, MCA. See also "Formal Opening of Clinic Building Attracts Hundreds of People Friday," *Rochester Daily Post & Record*, March 7, 1914, MCA.

62. H. S. Plummer to F. A. Washburn, October 18, 1913, MCA. See also F. A. Washburn, *The Massachusetts General Hospital: Its Development, 1900–1935* (Boston: Houghton Mifflin, 1939).

63. W. J. Mayo to F. A. Washburn, October 30, 1913 (with Plummer's marginal note), MCA.

64. W. F. Braasch, *Early Days at the Mayo Clinic* (Springfield, IL: Charles C Thomas, 1969), 58. For Plummer's profound impact on the Mayo Clinic, see W. J. Mayo, "The Work of Dr. Henry S. Plummer," *PSMMC*, 1938, *13*: 417–422.

65. F. A. Willius, *Henry Stanley Plummer: A Diversified Genius* (Springfield, IL: Charles C Thomas, 1960), 68.

66. B. Foster, "The Importance of Keeping Records of Cases," *St. Paul Med. J.*, 1902, *4*: 339–340, quotation from 339.

67. Examples of these forms are in the MCA. For the evolution of the Mayo's record-keeping system, see "Division of Records," in *History of the Mayo Clinic*, 100–103; C. L. Camp, R. L. Smoot, T. N. Kolettis, C. B. Groenewald, S. M. Greenlee, and D. R. Farley, "Patient Records at Mayo Clinic: Lessons Learned from the First 100 Patients in Dr Henry S. Plummer's Dossier Model," *Mayo Clin. Proc.*, 2008, *83*: 1396–1399; and L. T. Kurland and C. A. Molgaard, "The Patient Record in Epidemiology," *Sci. Am.*, 1981, *245*: 54–63. A general overview is D. L. Kurtz, *Unit Medical Records in Hospital and Clinic* (New York: Columbia University Press, 1943).

68. R. Fitz, "The Case History," in *Practice of Surgery*, ed. D. Lewis (Hagerstown, MD: W. F. Prior, 1929), 1:1–12, quotation from 1–2. Fitz's chapter included a 20¼ by 9½ inch folded fac-simile of the Mayo Clinic general history form.

69. See S. J. Reiser, "The Quest to Unify Health Care Through the Patient Record," in *Technological Medicine: The Changing World of Doctors and Patients* (New York: Cambridge University Press, 2009), 74–104.

70. W. C. Rucker, "Public Health Administration: The Factors upon Which Efficiency Depends," *Public Health Rep.*, March 6, 1914, *29*: 555–559.

71. See F. W. Taylor, *The Principles of Scientific Management* (New York: Harper & Brothers, 1911); H. B. Drury, "Scientific Management: A History and Criticism" (PhD diss., Columbia University, 1915); S. Haber, *Efficiency and Uplift: Scientific Management in the Progressive Era, 1890–1920* (Chicago: University of Chicago Press, 1964); and S. J. Kunitz, "Efficiency and Reform in the Financing and Organization of American Medicine in the Progressive Era," *Bull. Hist. Med.*, 1981, *55*: 497–515.

72. G. Rosen, "The Efficiency Criterion in Medical Care, 1900–1920," *Bull. Hist. Med.*, 1976, *50*: 28–44, quotation from 39–40. See also B. B. Perkins, "Shaping Institution-Based Specialism: Twentieth-Century Economic Organization of Medicine," *Soc. Hist. Med.*, 1997, *10*: 419–435; T. Goebel, "American Medicine and the 'Organizational Synthesis': Chicago Physicians and the Business of Medicine, 1900–1920," *Bull. Hist. Med.*, 1994, *68*: 639–663; S. Reverby, "Stealing the Golden Eggs: Ernest Amory Codman and the Science and Management of Medicine," *Bull. Hist Med.*, 1981, *55*: 156–171; and Madison, "Preserving Individualism in the

Organizational Society." A collection of contemporary articles with an introduction and bibliography is E. T. Morman, ed., *Efficiency, Scientific Management, and Hospital Standardization: An Anthology of Sources* (New York: Garland, 1989).

73. *Program Presented by the Mayo Foundation Chapter of Sigma Xi in Honor of Dr. Louis Blanchard Wilson* (Rochester, MN: Mayo Clinic, 1941).

74. L. B. Wilson, "Laboratory Efficiency," *Indianapolis Med. J.*, 1913, *16*: 512–517, quotations from 514.

75. L. B. Wilson to Francis Peabody, August 26, 1916, MCA.

76. R. C. Cabot, "Better Doctoring for Less Money," *American Magazine*, April 1916: 7–9, 77–78, May 1916: 43–44, 76–79, quotation from 43, emphasis in the original. Cabot is discussed in a newspaper article that detailed the Mayo system of diagnosis; see "Boston's Growing Approval for a New Advance by the Mayo Brothers," *Boston Evening Transcript*, December 10, 1913, MCA. See also C. Crenner, *Private Practice: In the Early Twentieth-Century Medical Office of Dr. Richard Cabot* (Baltimore: Johns Hopkins University Press, 2005). Lewellys Barker, former physician-in-chief of the Johns Hopkins Hospital, described the Mayo Clinic as "a notable example of an institution in which an elaborate diagnostic study can be obtained at moderate cost." L. F. Barker, "The Development of the Science of Diagnosis," *J. SC Med. Assoc.*, 1917, *13*: 278–284, quotation from 284.

77. V. C. Vaughan, "A Preliminary Report on the Reorganization of Clinical Teaching," *Am. Med. Assoc. Bull.*, 1915, *10*: 244–268. Bevan's remarks are on 266–267.

78. J. T. Mason, "Impressions Received from a Visit to Some Eastern Surgical Clinics," *Northwest Med.*, 1914, *6*: 246–248, quotation from 248.

79. For an overview of the evolution of a "clinic" as a teaching event, see I. M. Rutkow, "A History of *The Surgical Clinics of North America*," *Surg. Clin. North Am.*, 1987, *67*: 1217–1239. Will Mayo described John Murphy as the greatest surgeon of his day. See W. J. Mayo, "The Laying of the Corner Stone of the John B. Murphy Memorial Building," *Surg. Gynecol. Obstet.*, 1924, *18*: 282–284. For the history (and changing meaning) of the Osler Clinic at Johns Hopkins, see L. F. Barker, "Osler as Chief of a Medical Clinic," *Johns Hopkins Hosp. Bull.*, 1919, *30*: 189–193.

80. American artist Thomas Eakins memorialized the surgical amphitheater clinic model in his paintings *The Gross Clinic* (1875) and *The Agnew Clinic* (1889). See G. H. Brieger, "A Portrait of American Surgery: Surgery in America, 1875–1889," *Surg. Clin. North Am.*, 1987, *67*: 1181–1216.

81. L. C. Von Der Heidt to Western Engraving & Embossing Co., November 2, 1913, and L. C. Von Der Heidt to E. H. Schlitgu, [1964], MCA. E. Starr Judd served as an intern at St. Mary's Hospital and as Charlie Mayo's first assistant in the operating room before joining the practice in 1904. He married a niece of the Mayo brothers four years later.

82. W. J. Mayo to J. F. Highsmith, January 24, 1931, MCA.

Chapter 3

1. See K. M. Ludmerer, *Learning to Heal: The Development of American Medical Education* (New York: Basic Books, 1985); W. G. Rothstein, *American Medical Schools and the Practice of Medicine: A History* (New York: Oxford University Press, 1987); L. E. Miller and R. W. Weiss, "Medical Education Reform Efforts and Failures of U.S. Medical Schools, 1870–1930," *J. Hist. Med. Allied Sci.*, 2008, *63*: 348–387; and T. N. Bonner, *Becoming a Physician: Medical Education in Britain, France, Germany, and the United States, 1750–1945* (New York: Oxford University Press, 1995).

2. Rosemary Stevens describes the Mayo Clinic's seminal influence on physician training in the United States. See R. Stevens, *American Medicine and the Public Interest* [rev. ed.] (Berkeley: University of California Press, 1998), 129–131.

3. *Report of Addresses at the Dinner Given in Honor of Dr. D. B. St. John Roosa* (New York: privately printed, 1904). Osler's quotation from 15. See also S. J. Peitzman, "'Thoroughly Practical': America's Polyclinic Medical Schools," *Bull. Hist. Med.*, 1980, *54*: 166–187.

4. *Report of Addresses at the Dinner*. Mayo's quotation from 18.

5. Ibid.

6. W. S. Halsted, "The Training of the Surgeon," *Bull. Johns Hopkins Hosp.*, 1904, *15*: 267–275, quotation from 271.

7. See G. Imber, *Genius on the Edge: The Bizarre Double Life of Dr. William Stewart Halsted* (New York: Kaplan, 2010), and H. Markel, *An Anatomy of Addiction: Sigmund Freud, William Halsted, and the Miracle Drug Cocaine* (New York: Pantheon, 2011).

8. H. Cushing, "William Stewart Halsted, 1852–1922," *Science*, 1922, *56*: 461–464. See also I. M. Rutkow, "William Stewart Halsted and the Germanic Influence on Education and Training Programs in Surgery," *Surg. Gynecol. Obstet.*, 1978, *147*: 1–5.

9. W. J. Mayo, "American Surgery," in *The "Guinea Pig": A Year Book, Being the First of Its Kind Published... [at] the University of Minnesota*, ed. M. C. Piper (Minneapolis: University of Minnesota, 1906), Mayo Clinic Archives, Mayo Historical Unit, Rochester, MN (hereafter MCA). See also W. J. Mayo, "Medical Notes of a Recent Trip Through Germany and France," *St. Paul Med. J.*, 1900, *2*: 725–733.

10. For the history of post-medical school training in America, see R. Stevens, "Graduate Medical Education: A Continuing History," *J. Med. Educ.*, 1978, *53*: 1–18; D. K. Wentz and C. V. Ford, "A Brief History of the Internship," *JAMA*, 1984, *252*: 3390–3394; J. A. Curran, "Internships and Residencies: Historical Backgrounds and Current Trends," *J. Med. Educ.*, 1959, *34*: 873–884; and W. D. Holden, "Graduate Medical Education," in *Advances in American Medicine: Essays at the Bicentennial*, ed. J. Z. Bowers and E. F. Purcell, 2 vols. (New York: Josiah H. Macy Jr. Foundation, 1976), 1:313–344.

11. *Sixteenth Report of the Superintendent of the Johns Hopkins Hospital for the Year Ending January 31, 1905* (Baltimore: Johns Hopkins Press, 1905), [4–6]. See also A. M. Harvey, "The Influence of William Stewart Halsted's Concepts of Surgical Training," *Johns Hopkins Med. J.*, 1981, *148*: 215–236. William Osler organized a similar program for training internists; see W. Osler, "The Medical Clinic: A Retrospect and a Forecast," *Br. Med. J.*, 1914, *1*: 10–16.

12. Halsted, "Training of the Surgeon," 273.

13. E. Whelan, *The Sisters' Story: Saint Marys Hospital—Mayo Clinic, 1889 to 1939* (Rochester, MN: Mayo Foundation, 2002).

14. For Wilson's career, see L. B. Wilson, "Notes on Talk at Staff Meeting, Mayo Clinic, November 15, 1937," MCA; and *Program Presented by the Mayo Foundation Chapter of Sigma Xi in Honor of Dr. Louis Blanchard Wilson* (Rochester, MN: Mayo Clinic, 1941). Contemporary perspectives on the role of the laboratory in diagnosis include F. F. Wesbrook, "Relation Between Pathology and General Medicine," *J. Minn. State Med. Assoc. NW Lancet*, 1906, *26*: 459–463; and J. B. Herrick, "The Relation of the Clinical Laboratory to the Practitioner of Medicine," *JAMA*, 1907, *48*: 1915–1919. For the perspective of the longtime director of clinical laboratories at the Mayo Clinic, see A. H. Sanford, "Clinical Laboratories: Their Place in Hospital Functions," *Hosp. Prog.*, 1920, *1*: 302–304; and A. H. Sanford, "The Clinical Laboratories of the Mayo Clinic," [1955], MCA.

15. L. B. Wilson, "A Method for the Rapid Preparation of Fresh Tissues for the Microscope," *JAMA*, 1905, *45*: 1737. See also J. R. Wright Jr., "The Development of the Frozen Section Technique, the Evolution of Surgical Biopsy, and the Origins of Surgical Pathology," *Bull. Hist. Med.*, 1985, *59*: 295–326; A. A. Gal and P. T. Cagle, "The 100-Year Anniversary of the Description of the Frozen Section Procedure," *JAMA*, 2005, *294*: 3135–3137; and L. B. Woolner, "Surgical Pathology at the Mayo Clinic," in *Guiding the Surgeon's Hand: The History of American Surgical Pathology*, ed. J. Rosai (Washington, DC: Armed Forces Institute of Pathology, 1997), 145–179.

16. A. C. Bernays, "A Visit to the Mayos at Rochester, Minnesota. A Feuilleton," *N. Y. Med. J.*, 1906, *83*: 808–810, quotation from 809.

17. L. B. Wilson, "The Hospital Laboratory, With Special Reference to Diagnosis in Surgical Cases," *St. Paul Med. J.*, 1910, *12*: 233–238, quotation from 235.

18. Compare *Fifteenth Annual Report of St. Mary's Hospital* [for 1904] (Rochester, MN: St. Mary's Hospital, 1905) with *Twenty-first Annual Report of St. Mary's Hospital* [for 1910] (Rochester, MN: St. Mary's Hospital, 1911). The terminology of postgraduate training in the decades around 1900 is problematic because labels such as house officer, intern, resident, and clinical assistant were used inconsistently and interchangeably in various contexts. In Rochester, for example, doctors listed as clinical assistants in the annual reports of St. Mary's Hospital were termed residents when the Association of Resident and Ex-Resident Physicians of the Mayo Clinic was founded in 1915. See H. L. Foss, "The Mayo Clinic and Its Alumni," *Trans. Assoc. Resident Ex-Resident Physicians Mayo Clinic*, 1920, *1*: 20–25. These individuals were described as fellows in the institution's definitive bio-bibliographical book, *Physicians of the Mayo Clinic and the Mayo Foundation* (Minneapolis: University of Minnesota Press, 1937).

19. W. J. Mayo, "The Medical Profession and the Issues Which Confront It," *JAMA*, 1906, *46*: 1737–1740, quotation from 1739. The American Medical Association council began on-site evaluations of the nation's medical schools in 1906. See J. G. Burrow, *Organized Medicine in the Progressive Era: The Move Toward Monopoly* (Baltimore: Johns Hopkins University Press, 1977), 33–42.

20. Johnson's operations by Will Mayo (in 1897, 1898, and 1903) are described in W. G. Helmes, *John A. Johnson: The People's Governor* (Minneapolis: University of Minnesota Press, 1949), 88–90, 115.

21. "Dr. Wm. J. Mayo, Regent," *J. Minn. State Med. Assoc. NW Lancet*, 1907, *27*: 35. See also W. J. Mayo, "The Clinical Needs of the Medical College," *J. Minn. State Med. Assoc. NW Lancet*, 1909, *29*: 50–51. Mayo's address was part of a symposium; see "Medical Education and Medical Educators in Minnesota," *J. Minn. State Med. Assoc. NW Lancet*, 1909, *29*: 23–54.

22. See W. B. Fye, *The Development of American Physiology: Scientific Medicine in the Nineteenth Century* (Baltimore: Johns Hopkins University Press, 1987), 205–230; S. Hewa, "Rockefeller Philanthropy and the 'Flexner Report' on Medical Education in the United States," *Int. J. Sociol. Soc. Policy*, 2002, *22*: 1–47; and S. C. Wheatley, *The Politics of Philanthropy: Abraham Flexner and Medical Education* (Madison: University of Wisconsin Press, 1988).

23. A. Flexner, *Medical Education in the United States and Canada* (New York: Carnegie Foundation for the Advancement of Science, 1910), 216. See also T. N. Bonner, *Iconoclast: Abraham Flexner and a Life of Learning* (Baltimore: Johns Hopkins University Press, 2002).

24. Flexner, *Medical Education*, 248. See also L. G. Wilson, *Medical Revolution in Minnesota: A History of the University of Minnesota Medical School* (St. Paul: Midewiwin Press, 1989); and J. A. Myers, *Masters of Medicine: An Historical Sketch of the College of Medical Sciences, University of Minnesota, 1888–1966* (St. Louis: Warren H. Green, 1968).

25. "The Carnegie Foundation," *J. Minnesota State Med. Assoc. NW Lancet*, 1910, *30*: 276–283, quotation from 283.

26. A. Flexner, "The Postgraduate School," in *Medical Education*, 174–177, quotation from 176.

27. Ibid., 177.

28. L. B. Wilson, "Graduate Instruction in Medicine," *St. Paul Med. J.*, 1912, *14*: 287–295, quotation from 288. For a list of postgraduate schools, see *Polk's Medical Register and Directory of North America*, 12th ed. (Detroit: R. L. Polk, 1912), 183–185.

29. Wilson, "Graduate Instruction in Medicine," 294.

30. B. Foster, "Post Graduate Medical Schools," *St. Paul Med. J.*, 1912, *14*: 310–312, quotation from 311.

31. Ibid. Concerns about poorly trained surgeons contributed to the creation of the American College of Surgeons in 1913. Charlie Mayo played a role in founding the organization. See L. Davis, *Fellowship of Surgeons: A History of the American College of Surgeons* (Springfield, IL: Charles C Thomas, 1960); R. Stevens, "Surgeons, Physicians, and General Practitioners: The Rebirth of the College System, 1900–1916," in *American Medicine and the Public Interest*, 77–97; and P. J. Kernahan, "'A Condition of Development': Muckrakers, Surgeons, and Hospitals, 1890–1920," *J. Am. Coll. Surg.*, 2008, *206*: 376–384.

32. See *George Edgar Vincent, 1864–1941* (Stamford, CT: Overbrook Press, 1941). See also S. M. White, "Some Problems of Medical Education in Minnesota," *J. Minn. State Med. Assoc. NW Lancet*, 1911, *31*: 53–60.

33. Wilson, *Medical Revolution in Minnesota*, 124–140.

34. "Increased Requirements," *J. Minn. State Med. Assoc. NW Lancet*, 1910, *30*: 388.

35. F. F. Wesbrook to H. E. Young, 1913, excerpts in W. C. Gibson, *Wesbrook and His University* (Vancouver: Library of the University of British Columbia, 1973), 56.

36. George Vincent. University of Minnesota College of Medicine and Surgery, General Faculty Minutes, March 1, 1913, quoted in Wilson, *Medical Revolution in Minnesota*, 148–149. See also B. Foster, "A Reorganization of the Medical Department of the University of Minnesota," *St. Paul Med. J.*, 1913, *15*: 137–139; J. L. Gunn, "'The First Adequate Graduate School of Medicine in America': A Brief History of the University of Minnesota-Mayo Graduate School of Medicine," *Minn. Med.*, 2003, *86*: 63–68; and Wilson, "Affiliation of the University with the Mayo Foundation, 1915–1917," in *Medical Revolution in Minnesota*, 159–212.

37. O. H. Wangensteen, ed., *Elias Potter Lyon: Minnesota's Leader in Medical Education* (St. Louis: Warren H. Green, 1981).

38. There were approximately 170 part-time faculty members before the cuts. See Wilson, *Medical Revolution in Minnesota*, 141–158; and D. C. Smith and L. G. Wilson, "The Education of Physicians to Practice Scientific Medicine," in Wangensteen, ed., *Elias Potter Lyon*, 172–195.

39. James E. Moore to W. J. Mayo. February 21, 1914, MCA. For a discussion of criteria that might be used to define a specialty, see H. Cabot, "Is Urology Entitled to Be Regarded as a Specialty?" *Trans. Am. Urol. Assn.*, 1911, *5*: 1–20. For a comprehensive list of specialty societies, see J. B. Kirsner, *The Development of American Gastroenterology* (New York: Raven, 1990), 146–150.

40. G. S. Ford, *On and Off the Campus. With a Biographical Introduction by George E. Vincent* (Minneapolis: University of Minnesota Press, 1938). See also G. E. Vincent, "The University and Higher Degrees in Medicine," *JAMA*, 1915, *64*: 790–794.

41. W. J. Mayo to George E. Vincent, November 30, 1914, published in *Sketch of the History of the Mayo Clinic and the Mayo Foundation* (Philadelphia: W. B. Saunders, 1926), 146–147.

42. George E. Vincent to W. J. Mayo, December 2, 1914, published in *History of the Mayo Clinic*, 147. The Mayo brothers created the foundation in an era when several philanthropists focused on medical education and health care. See R. E. Kohler, "Science, Foundations, and American Universities in the 1920s," *Osiris*, 1987, *2d ser. 3*: 135–164; Hewa, "Rockefeller Philanthrophy;" and Wheatley, *Politics of Philanthropy*.

43. See P. C. English, *Shock, Physiological Surgery, and George Washington Crile: Medical Innovation in the Progressive Era* (Westport, CT: Greenwood, 1980); and M. Bliss, *Harvey Cushing: A Life in Surgery* (New York: Oxford University Press, 2005).

44. W. J. Mayo, "Contributions of the Nineteenth Century to a Living Pathology," *Boston Med. Surg. J.*, 1912, *167*: 751–754, quotation from 753. For a prominent surgeon's response to the antivivisection movement, see W. W. Keen, *Animal Experimentation and Medical Progress* (Boston: Houghton Mifflin, 1914).

45. Mayo, "Contributions of the Nineteenth Century to a Living Pathology," 754.

46. F. C. Mann, "To the Physiologically Inclined," *Ann. Rev. Physiol.*, 1955, *17*: 1–16.

47. C. H. Mayo, "Hyperthyroidism: Primary and Late Results of Operation," *Surg. Gynecol. Obstet.*, 1914, *19*: 351–359. See also R. B. Welbourn, *The History of Endocrine Surgery* (New York: Praeger, 1990), 19–64.

48. D. J. Ingle, "Edward C. Kendall," in *Biographical Memoirs. National Academy of Sciences* (Washington, DC: National Academy of Sciences, 1975), 47: 248–290. See also R. E. Kohler, *From Medical Chemistry to Biochemistry: The Making of a Biomedical Discipline* (New York: Cambridge University Press, 1982).

49. E. C. Kendall, *Cortisone* (New York: Charles Scribner's Sons, 1971), 29. This autobiography emphasizes Kendall's research on adrenal cortical hormones, which ultimately led to his sharing the Nobel Prize in Physiology or Medicine.

50. E. C. Kendall, "The Isolation in Crystalline Form of the Compound Containing Iodin, Which Occurs in the Thyroid," *JAMA*, 1915, *64*: 2042–2043. See also L. G. Wilson, "Internal Secretions in Disease: The Historical Relations of Clinical Medicine and Scientific Physiology," *J. Hist. Med. Allied Sci.*, 1984, *39*: 263–302.

51. G. S. Ford, "The Mayo Foundation from the Standpoint of the Graduate School," *Journal-Lancet*, 1915, *35*: 148–149, quotations from 148. The building contained more than 40,000 pathological specimens and about 150,000 patient records. See L. B. Wilson to Richard Cabot, May 24, 1916, MCA.

52. *History of the Mayo Clinic*, 158–159. For background on the foundation movement, see B. D. Karl and S. N. Katz, "The American Private Philanthropic Foundation and the Public Sphere, 1890–1930," *Minerva*, 1981, *19*: 236–270.

53. L. B. Wilson, "The Affiliation of the Mayo Foundation with the Graduate Medical School of the University of Minnesota: A Review of Graduate Medical Education and Research," paper presented to the General Alumni Association of the University of Minnesota, Minneapolis, February 18, 1915, MCA.

54. Ibid. See also R. L. Thompson, *Glimpses of Medical Europe* (Philadelphia: J. B. Lippincott, 1908); and T. N. Bonner, *American Doctors and German Universities: A Chapter in International Intellectual Relations, 1870–1914* (Lincoln: University of Nebraska Press, 1963).

55. For the fellowship system at the Johns Hopkins University in 1876, see H. Hawkins, *Pioneer: A History of the Johns Hopkins University, 1874–1889* (Ithaca, NY: Cornell University Press, 1960), 79–93.

56. For a detailed description of the facilities at the Mayo Clinic and its affiliated hospitals, see L. B. Wilson, "A Concise Statement of Facts Relating to the Proposed Affiliation Between the Mayo Foundation and the University of Minnesota," March 23, 1915, MCA. See also *Report of the Special Committee of the Board of Regents of the University of Minnesota upon the Establishment of Graduate Medical Work at Rochester, Minnesota*, June 5, 1915, MCA.

57. G. E. Vincent, E. P. Lyon, J. E. Moore, J. C. Litzenberg, and R. O. Beard, "The Medical School of the University of Minnesota and the Mayo Foundation for the Promotion of Medical Education and Research," *Journal-Lancet*, 1915, *35*: 135–141, quotation from 136.

58. C. L. Greene, "University-Mayo Affiliation," *Journal-Lancet*, 1915, *35*: 142–147, quotations from 142.

59. Ibid. An accompanying editorial questioned the motives and the process. See "The Affiliation Tangle," *Journal-Lancet*, 1915, *35*: 155–156. For a prominent Chicago internist's perspective on tensions between solo general practitioners, specialists, and group practices, see J. B. Herrick, "Relation Between the Specialist and the Practitioner," *JAMA*, 1921, *76*: 975–978.

60. Benjamin M. Randall to George W. Broome, September 5, 1912, published in G. W. Broome, *Rochester and the Mayo Clinic: A Fair and Unbiased Story Calculated to Aid Physicians to Greater Cures and Larger Incomes* (New York: Shakespeare Press, 1914), 146–147.

61. For the incorporation of the foundation, see *History of the Mayo Clinic*, 158–177. Historian Merle Curti concludes, "The Rockefeller Institute for Medical Research and the

Rockefeller Foundation, the Carnegie Institution of Washington, the Carnegie Corporation of New York, and the Mayo Foundation at Rochester, Minnesota, were by 1915 generously endowing investigation and research." M. Curti, *The Growth of American Thought* (New York: Harper & Row, 1964), 570. See also R. L. Geiger, *To Advance Knowledge: The Growth of American Research Universities, 1900–1940* (New York: Oxford University Press, 1986); and A. Flexner and E. S. Bailey, *Funds and Foundations: Their Policies Past and Present* (New York: Harper & Brothers, 1952).

62. W. B. Fye, "The Origin of the Full-Time Faculty System: Implications for Clinical Research," *JAMA*, 1991, *265*: 1555–1562.

63. W. Osler to Ira Remsen, "Whole-Time Clinical Professors," September 1, 1911, published in A. M. Chesney, *The Johns Hopkins Hospital and the Johns Hopkins University School of Medicine: A Chronicle*, vol. 3 (Baltimore: Johns Hopkins Press 1963), 176–183.

64. J. Keegan, *The First World War* (New York: Vintage Books, 2000).

65. H. Cushing, *From a Surgeon's Journal, 1915–1918* (Boston: Little, Brown, 1936), 78.

66. W. L. Beebe, "Report of the Representative to National Legislative Council," *Journal-Lancet*, 1915, *35*: 598–601, quotation from 598. See also R. O. Beard, "An Inventory of the Progress of Medical Education in America and in Minnesota," *Journal-Lancet*, 1915, *35*: 607–609; and "Graduate Work in Medicine in the Medical School and the Mayo Foundation," *Bull. Univ. Minn.*, April 5, 1917, 19–27.

67. "The Mayo Brothers, Who Have Given $2,000,000 For Science," *The Sun* (New York), May 30, 1915, MCA.

68. L. B. Wilson to Francis Peabody, August 26, 1916, MCA. See also O. Paul, *The Caring Physician: The Life of Francis W. Peabody* (Boston: Francis A. Countway Library of Medicine, 1991).

69. "Mayo Foundation Hit by State Physicians as Disturbing Force," *Minneapolis Tribune*, March 24, 1917, MCA.

70. Ibid.

71. M. D. Dacy, *A Passion for the River: Mayo and the Mississippi* (Rochester, MN: Mayo Foundation, 2004). For the Mayo brother's homes, see C. W. Nelson, *Mayo Roots: Profiling the Origins of Mayo Clinic* (Rochester, MN: Mayo Foundation, 1990), 56–59.

72. L. B. Wilson to Richard Cabot, May 24, 1916, MCA.

73. The subheadings are from "Educators Deplore Possible Break in Mayo Affiliation," *St. Paul Pioneer Press*, April 4, 1917, MCA; and "Mayo Foundation Friends Victors in House Contest," *St. Paul Pioneer Press*, April 5, 1917, MCA.

74. The Welch letter is quoted in "Educators Deplore Possible Break in Mayo Affiliation." Other individuals quoted in the article include Nicholas Murray Butler, Walter B. Cannon, Abraham Flexner, William W. Keen, and Samuel W. Lambert.

75. The Janeway letter is quoted in "Mayo Foundation Friends."

76. "A New Mayo Plan," *Journal-Lancet*, 1917, *37*: 449.

77. *History of the Mayo Clinic*, 171–177.

78. W. J. Mayo quoted in the *Minneapolis Tribune*, September 14, 1917, published in H. Clapesattle, *The Doctors Mayo* (Minneapolis: University of Minnesota Press, 1941), 557–558. See also Clapesattle, "The Clinic and the First World War," in *Doctors Mayo*, 560–580; W. Walters, "The Doctors Mayo and Their Military Medical Activities," *Military Med.*, 1965, *130*: 331–341; and M. C. Gillett, *The Army Military Department 1917–1941* (Washington, DC: Government Printing Office, 2009).

79. C. H. Mayo, "War's Influence on Medicine," *JAMA*, 1917, *68*: 1673–1677.

80. W. J. Mayo quoted in Clapesattle, *Doctors Mayo*, 591. See also C. H. Mayo, "Jaundice and Its Surgical Significance," *Surg. Gynecol. Obstet.*, 1920, *30*: 545–549.

81. W. J. Mayo to Major J. F. Binnie, December 24, 1918, MCA.

82. E. C. Rosenow, "Studies in Influenza and Pneumonia IX.," *J. Infect. Dis.*, 1920, *26*: 567–596. See also B. M. Baruch, *The Great Influenza: The Epic Story of the Deadliest Plague in History* (New York: Viking Penguin, 2004); and N. K. Bristow, *American Pandemic: The Lost Worlds of the 1918 Influenza Epidemic* (New York: Oxford University Press, 2012).

83. H. J. Harwick, *Forty-four Years With the Mayo Clinic* (Rochester, MN: Whiting Press, 1957), 14.

84. "Certificate of Incorporation of Mayo Properties Association," October 8, 1919, published in *History of the Mayo Clinic*, 127–132. See also G. S. Schuster, "The Organization of the Mayo Clinic, the Mayo Foundation, and the Mayo Properties Association." November 1945, MCA.

85. W. J. Mayo, "Address of Welcome," *Trans. Assoc. Resident Ex-Resident Physicians Mayo Clinic*, 1920, *1*: 16–17. See also "Permanency of Clinic Insured," *Clinic Bulletin*, October 11, 1919, MCA.

86. "Income Tax Applied to Physicians," *JAMA*, 1913, *61*: 1833–1834. The Mayo brothers' tax bills were still very high. A New York newspaper published a list of individual federal income taxes paid by "prominent people from all over the country" in 1925 that included Thomas Edison ($3,340), Babe Ruth ($3,432), William Randolph Hearst ($42,239), Charlie Mayo ($69,255), Will Mayo ($75,669), Douglas Fairbanks ($182,190), and Henry Ford ($2.6 million). "List of Taxes Paid by Prominent People from All Over the Country," *The Sun* (New York), September 1, 1925, MCA.

87. W. J. Mayo to Victor Vaughan, February 4, 1921, MCA.

88. Ibid.

89. Ibid. See also "Present Organization of the Mayo Clinic," in *History of the Mayo Clinic*, 117–132.

90. See Wilson, *Medical Revolution in Minnesota*, 235–250.

91. F. Billings, J. M. T. Finney, and V. C. Vaughan, "Survey Committee Report on the Medical School of the University of Minnesota," *Journal-Lancet*, 1921, *41*: 501–506, quotation from 503.

92. Ibid.

93. L. B. Wilson, "Report to the Board of Regents of the University of Minnesota by the Director of the Mayo Foundation. July 16, 1924," *Coll. Papers Mayo Clinic*, 1925, *16*: 1270–1274.

94. Ibid., 1274.

Chapter 4

1. W. J. Mayo to Henry Ogden, May 22, 1918, Mayo Clinic Archives, Mayo Historical Unit, Rochester, MN (hereafter MCA). See also L. Weistrop, *The Life & Letters of Dr. Henry Vining Ogden, 1857–1931* (Milwaukee: Milwaukee Academy of Medicine Press, 1986); M. W. Ireland, "The Achievement of the Army Medical Department in the World War in the Light of General Medical Progress," *JAMA*, 1921, *76*: 763–769; and R. Cooter, M. Harrison, and S. Sturdy, eds., *War, Medicine and Modernity* (Phoenix Mill, England: Sutton, 1998).

2. Anon, "Why Is It So?" *J. Tenn. State Med. Assoc.*, 1919, *12*: 147–148. See also M. Bliss, *William Osler: A Life in Medicine* (New York: Oxford University Press, 1999).

3. W. Osler, "'Why Is It So?' Is It So?" *J. Tenn. State Med. Assoc.*, 1919, *12*: 222. See also W. Osler, "The Medical Clinic: A Retrospect and a Forecast," *Br. Med. J.*, 1914, *1*: 10–16.

4. Osler, "'Why Is It So?' Is It So?"

5. W. J. Mayo to Leon L. Sheddan, March 5, 1921, MCA. Will was responding to Sheddan's letter to Dear Doctor, February 19, 1921, MCA. An internal medicine textbook would soon appear with contributions by 130 authors. R. L. Cecil, ed., *A Text-Book of Medicine by American Authors* (Philadelphia: W. B. Saunders, 1927).

6. Mayo to Sheddan, March 5, 1921.

7. F. A. Willius, *Henry Stanley Plummer: A Diversified Genius* (Springfield, IL: Charles C Thomas, 1960).

8. L. G. Rowntree, *Amid Masters of Twentieth Century Medicine* (Springfield, IL: Charles C Thomas, 1958), 297. See also J. L. Graner, "Leonard Rowntree and the Birth of the Mayo Clinic Research Tradition," *Mayo Clin. Proc.*, 2005, *80*: 920–922; and S. W. Moss, "Dr. Leonard Rowntree of Camden," *New Jersey Med.*, 1995, *92*: 596–600.

9. See L. G. Rowntree, "John Jacob Abel, Decade 1903–1913," *Bull. Johns Hopkins Hosp.*, 1957, *101*: 306–310; J. Parascandola, *The Development of American Pharmacology: John J. Abel and the Shaping of a Discipline* (Baltimore: Johns Hopkins University Press, 1992); J. S. Cameron, *A History of the Treatment of Renal Failure by Dialysis* (New York: Oxford University Press, 2002), 33–41.

10. Rowntree, *Amid Masters*, 126–132. See also W. B. Fye, "The Origin of the Full-Time Faculty System: Implications for Clinical Research," *JAMA*, 1991, *265*: 1555–1562.

11. L. G. Wilson, "Affiliation of the University with the Mayo Foundation, 1915–1917," in *Medical Revolution in Minnesota: A History of the University of Minnesota Medical School* (St. Paul: Midewiwin Press, 1989), 159–212.

12. T. C. Janeway on Rowntree in "Biographies of Men Considered, Medical School, 1915. Selection of Head, Dept. of Medicine [Univ. Minnesota]," MCA. See also Rowntree, *Amid Masters*, 185–204.

13. "Dr. Rowntree in the Mayo Foundation," *Clinic Bulletin*, April 6, 1920, MCA.

14. For perspectives on the role of laboratories by two Mayo clinical pathologists, see W. C. MacCarty, "The Relation of Pathologists to the Institutional Practice of Medicine," *J. Clin. Lab. Med.*, 1921, *6*: 331–334; A. H. Sanford, "Clinical Laboratories: Their Place in Hospital Functions," *Hosp. Prog.*, 1920, *1*: 302–304. See also A. M. Harvey, "Clinical Science at the Mayo Clinic: The Concept of Team Research," in *Science at the Bedside: Clinical Research in American Medicine, 1905–1945* (Baltimore: Johns Hopkins University Press, 1981), 368–392.

15. W. J. Mayo to Frank Billings, July 9, 1920, MCA.

16. W. B. Cannon to L. G. Rowntree, [October 4] 1920, quoted in J. C. Aub and R. K. Hapgood, *Pioneer in Modern Medicine, David Linn Edsall of Harvard* (Boston: Harvard Medical Alumni Association, 1970), 215–216.

17. W. B. Cannon to C. H. Mayo, October 11, 1920, quoted in E. L. Wolfe, A. C. Barger, and S. Benison, *Walter B. Cannon, Science and Society* (Cambridge, MA: Boston Medical Library, 2000), 79. See also W. B. Fye, "Henry P. Bowditch: The Prototypical Full-Time Physiologist and Educational Reformer," in *The Development of American Physiology: Scientific Medicine in the Nineteenth Century* (Baltimore: Johns Hopkins University Press, 1987), 92–128.

18. W. J. Mayo to W. B. Cannon, October 20, 1920, MCA.

19. See E. R. Brainard, "History of the American Society for Clinical Investigation, 1909–1959," *J. Clin. Invest.*, 1959, *38*: 1784–1864; and J. D. Howell, "A History of the American Society for Clinical Investigation," *J. Clin. Invest.*, 2009, *119*: 682–-697.

20. L. G. Rowntree, "The Spirit of Investigation in Medicine," *Science*, 1921, *n.s. 54*: 179–183, quotation from 180.

21. Ibid., 181.

22. See J. J. Drummond, "'The Kahler' Offers Triple Service: Newest Addition to Buildings at Rochester, Minn., for Service to Mayo Clinic Patients is Hospital, Convalescent Home and Hotel, All under One Roof," *Hosp. Management*, 1921, *12*: 36–38; and C. J. Pahlas, *The Unique Voice of Service: The Story of the Kahler Corporation, Rochester, Minnesota* (Rochester, MN: Kahler Corperation, 1964).

23. W. J. Mayo, "Mortality and End-Results in Surgery," *Surg. Gynecol. Obstet.*, 1920, *32*: 97–102, quotation from 102. See also A. D. Bevan, "Borderland Cases and Team Work in Surgery," *J. Iowa State Med. Soc.*, 1914, *4*: 187–194.

24. Mayo, "Mortality and End-Results," 102.

25. W. J. Mayo, "Diseases of the Spleen," *Ann. Clin. Med.*, 1922, *1*: 141–145, quotation from 141. For the American Congress of Internal Medicine, see G. M. Piersol, *Gateway of Honor: The American College of Physicians, 1915–1959* (Philadelphia: American College of Physicians, 1962), 1–37.

26. In 1922 surgeons at the Mayo Clinic performed 1,983 thyroid operations with a mortality rate of one percent. See C. H. Mayo and H. S. Plummer, *The Thyroid Gland* (St. Louis: C. V. Mosby, 1926), 15.

27. See C. T. Sawin, "Henry S. Plummer (1874–1936), Iodine for Hyperthyroidism, and Plummer's Disease," *Endocrinologist*, 2003, *13*: 149–152; and R. B. Welbourn, *The History of Endocrine Surgery* (New York: Praeger, 1990), 19–64.

28. F. C. Mann, "Relation of Experimental Research to Medicine and Surgery," *Ann. Clin. Med.*, 1922, *1*: 331–332, quotation from 331. See also W. W. Keen, *Animal Experimentation and Medical Progress* (Boston: Houghton Mifflin, 1914); and S. E. Lederer, "The Controversy over Animal Experimentation in America, 1880–1914," in *Vivisection in Historical Perspective*, ed. N. A. Rupke (London: Croom Helm, 1987), 236–258.

29. S. R. Miller to W. J. Mayo, April 13, 1922, MCA.

30. J. M. Anders, "The President's Address at the Seventh Annual Convocation of the American College of Physicians," *Ann. Clin. Med.*, 1922, *1*: 1–9, quotation from 6. See also J. L. Gunn, "Science and Skill: Educating the Medical Practitioner at the Graduate School of Medicine of the University of Pennsylvania." (PhD diss., University of Pennsylvania, 1997).

31. *Collected Papers of the Mayo Clinic*, vol. 14 [for] 1922, (Philadelphia: W. B. Saunders, 1923).

32. Minutes, MC Committee on Medical Education, Research, and Scientific Progress, March 28, 1923, MCA.

33. Minutes, MC BOG, April 13, 1923, MCA.

34. *A Souvenir of Saint Mary's Hospital* (Rochester, MN: St. Mary's Hospital, 1922), 82. This booklet describes and illustrates the hospital's facilities and physician staff.

35. *Thirty-fourth Annual Report of St. Mary's Hospital* [for 1923] (Rochester, MN: St. Mary's Hospital, 1924), 58–62.

36. See H. M. Marks, *The Progress of Experiment: Science and Therapeutic Reform in the United States, 1900–1990* (New York: Cambridge University Press, 1997); J. P. Swann, *Academic Scientists and the Pharmaceutical Industry: Cooperative Research in Twentieth-Century America* (Baltimore: Johns Hopkins University Press, 1988); J. Liebenau, *Medical Science and Medical Industry: The Formation of the American Pharmaceutical Industry* (Baltimore: Johns Hopkins University Press, 1987); and M. Weatherall, *In Search of a Cure: A History of Pharmaceutical Discovery* (New York: Oxford University Press, 1990).

37. L. G. Rowntree, "The Role and Development of Drug Therapy," *JAMA*, 1921, *77*: 1061–1065, quotations from 1064.

38. *History of the American Physiological Society Semicentennial, 1887–1937* (Baltimore: 1938), 119–124.

39. See M. Bliss, *The Discovery of Insulin* (Toronto: University of Toronto Press, 1982); and C. Feudtner, *Bittersweet: Diabetes, Insulin, and the Transformation of Illness* (Chapel Hill: University of North Carolina Press, 2003).

40. "Preface" [to the Insulin Issue], *J. Metabolic Res.*, 1923, *2*: [i–ii].

41. R. M. Wilder, W. M. Boothby, C. J. Barborka, H. D. Kitchen, and S. F. Adams, "Clinical Observations on Insulin," *J. Metabolic Res.*, 1923, *2*: 701–728, quotation from 727. See also R. M. Wilder, "Recollections and Reflections on Education, Diabetes, Other Metabolic Diseases, and Nutrition in the Mayo Clinic and Associated Hospitals, 1919–1950," *Perspect. Biol. Med.*, 1958, *1*: 237–277; and F. G. Banting, "The History of Insulin," *Edinb. Med. J.*, 1929, *36*: 1–18.

42. "Professor Macleod's Lecture," *Clinic Bulletin*, February 12, 1923, MCA. For Banting's lecture, see "Staff Report," *Clinic Bulletin*, February 10, 1923, MCA.

43. Bliss, *Discovery of Insulin*, 160–161.

44. Frederick T. Gates to John D. Rockefeller Jr., April 28, 1923, published in K. M. Ludmerer, *Learning to Heal: The Development of American Medical Education* (New York: Basic Books, 1985), 202. See also F. T. Gates, *Chapters in My Life* (New York: Free Press, 1977). Randall Sprague, a protégé of Russell Wilder's who became an endocrinologist at the Mayo Clinic, described his experience as one of the first patients to receive insulin in 1922. R. G. Sprague, "Convocation in Toronto: An Address," *Diabetes*, 1965, *14*: 37–43. See also Sprague, "Development of Endocrinology at the Mayo Clinic, 1913–1951," January 11, 1967, MCA.

45. R. M. Wilder, "How Is the Overworked General Practitioner to Use Insulin?" *Minn. Med.*, 1923, *6*: 524–529, quotation from 529.

46. Bliss, *Discovery of Insulin*, 188.

47. W. J. Mayo, "Problems Underlying Public Hospital Administration," *Boston Med. Surg. J.*, 1923, *189*: 736–740, quotations from 736, 740. See also F. W. Peabody, "Thorndike Memorial Laboratory," in *Methods and Problems of Medical Education*, 1st ser. (New York: Rockefeller Foundation, 1924), 113–121.

48. W. J. Mayo to Harvey Cushing, December 4, 1923, MCA.

49. Minutes, MC BOG, July 30, 1924, MCA.

50. Ibid.

51. J. L. Miller to W. J. Mayo, December 19, 1925, MCA.

52. W. J. Mayo to J. L. Miller, December 23, 1925, MCA.

53. J. M. Anders, "Idealism in American Medicine," *Ann. Clin. Med.*, 1926, *5*: 129–135, quotation from 131.

54. R. J. Godlee to W. J. Mayo, January 21, 1923, MCA.

55. "Know the Clinic. Let the Clinic Know You," *Clinic Bulletin*, August 6, 1923, MCA.

56. For hospitals built in Rochester during the first quarter of the twentieth century, see *Sketch of the History of the Mayo Clinic and the Mayo Foundation* (Philadelphia: W. B. Saunders, 1926), 22–39. For the nursing schools, see V. S. Wentzel, *Sincere et Constanter, 1906–1970: The Story of Saint Marys School of Nursing* (Rochester, MN: Mayo Foundation, 2006); and A. W. Keeling, *The Nurses of Mayo Clinic: Caring Healers* (Rochester, MN: Mayo Foundation, 2014).

57. W. F. Braasch, *Early Days at the Mayo Clinic* (Springfield, IL: Charles C Thomas, 1969), 102.

58. Minutes, MC BOG, October 3, 1923, MCA.

59. *Mayo Clinic Desk Book: Written by the Various Sections and Edited by the Coordinating Committee* (Rochester, MN: Mayo Clinic, 1927), 3, MCA.

60. Minutes, MC BOG, October 22, 1924, MCA.

61. "Pertinent Knowledge: Remember," *Clinic Bulletin*, October 10, 1923, MCA. See also Minutes, MC BOG, July 25, 1923, MCA.

62. E. Whelan, *The Sisters' Story: Saint Marys Hospital—Mayo Clinic, 1889 to 1939* (Rochester, MN: Mayo Foundation, 2002).

63. R. Stevens, "Technology and Institutions in the Twentieth Century," *Caduceus*, 1996, *12*: 9–18, quotation from 14.

64. R. Stevens, *In Sickness and in Wealth: American Hospitals in the Twentieth Century* (New York: Basic Books, 1989), 138. See also T. L. Savitt, *Race and Medicine in Nineteenth- and Early-Twentieth Century Medicine* (Kent, Ohio: Kent State University Press, 2007).

65. L. B. Wilson to Richard Pearce, March 24, 1927, MCA. This letter was in response to Pearce to Wilson, March 18, 1927, MCA.

66. Wilson to Pearce, March 24, 1927.

67. Richard Pearce to L. B. Wilson, March 29, 1927, MCA. Harvey Cushing was surgeon-in-chief of Boston's Peter Bent Brigham Hospital in 1929, when he informed a Cleveland public health official: "We have a good many Southern women who are patients here, and that they should be given a physical examination by a Negro, however well educated, is simply unthinkable. This, I am sure, you can understand." H. Cushing to Dudley S. Blossom, December 19, 1929, published in Michael Bliss, *Harvey Cushing: A Life in Surgery* (New York: Oxford University Press, 2005), 502–503.

68. For perspectives on presentism in historical writing, see A. Wilson and T. G. Ashplant, "Whig History and Present-Centered History," *Historical J.* 1988, *31*: 1–16; J. Burnham, *What Is Medical History?* (Malden, MA: Polity, 2005), 99–103; and N. Tosh, "Anachronism and Retrospective Explanation: In Defence of a Present-Centered History of Science," *Stud. Hist. Phil. Sci.*, 2003, *34*: 647–659.

69. See J. D. Holmquist, *They Chose Minnesota: A Survey of the State's Ethnic Groups* (St. Paul: Minnesota Historical Society, 1981); *The WPA Guide to Minnesota* [1938] (Minneapolis: Minnesota Historical Society, 1985), 74–80, 270–277; and L. Nelson, C. E. Ramsey, and J. A. Toews, *A Century of Population Growth in Minnesota* (Minneapolis: University of Minnesota Agricultural Experiment Station. Bulletin 423, 1954). For segregation in Baltimore, see A. Pietila, *Not in My Neighborhood: How Bigotry Shaped a Great American City* (Chicago: Ivan R. Dee, 2010).

70. In 1924 the newsstand sold newspapers published in Boston, Chicago, Cincinnati, Cleveland, Dallas, Denver, Des Moines, Detroit, Duluth, Fargo, Indianapolis, Kansas City, Los Angeles, Louisville, Memphis, Minneapolis, New York City, Oklahoma City, Omaha, Philadelphia, St. Louis, St. Paul, Sioux City, Sioux Falls, Tulsa, and Washington, DC. See "Papers at the Clinic News Stand," *Clinic Bulletin*, February 26, 1922, MCA. In 1924 Rochester was served by the Chicago Great Western Railroad and the Chicago and Northwestern Railroad. For Rochester railroad and bus schedules, see *Clinic Bulletin*, March 19, 1924, MCA. See also H. Severson, *Rochester: Mecca for Millions* (Rochester, MN: Marquette Bank & Trust, 1979).

71. "Ford Plane for Rochester-Twin City Service," *Rochester Bulletin*, March 30, 1928, MCA.

72. Minutes, MC BOG, July 11, 1928, MCA. See also "Mayo Association to Establish New Rochester Airport," *Minneapolis Evening Tribune*, July 13, 1928, MCA.

73. *Mayo Clinic Desk Book,* 1927, 36.

74. Minutes, MC BOG, July 18, 1928, MCA.

75. R. I. Haddy and T. B. Haddy, "113 Letters From the Mayo Clinic: A Pattern of Medical Referrals in the Early 20th Century," *Mayo Clin. Proc.*, 2002, *77*: 213–215. See also L. Nelson, "Distribution, Age, and Mobility of Minnesota Physicians, 1912–1936," *Am. Sociological Rev.*, 1942, *7*: 792–801. Mayo's context was unique, but the widespread growth of specialization around World War I led to new relationships between doctors in many settings. See L. F. Barker, "The Specialist and the General Practitioner in Relation to Team-Work in Medical Practice," *JAMA*, 1922, *78*: 773–779.

76. "Miscellaneous Information," *Clinic Bulletin*, August 23, 1923, MCA.

77. Anon. to Ruth, February 12, 1934, postcard in the author's possession.

78. Martha to Mrs. Frank A., September 6, 1922, postcard in the author's possession.

79. Millie to Abner L., June 8, 1926, postcard in the author's possession.

80. "Compend of Clinical Examinations at the Mayo Clinic," Rochester, MN, 1924, quotation from [3], MCA.

81. Ibid, [4]

82. Ibid., 5–45.

83. Marie to Julia G., March 3, 1924, postcard in the author's possession. Contemporary perspectives by visiting health care professionals include G. B. Lake, "The Mayo Clinic," *Clin. Med.*, 1925, *32*: 675–680; and "Visit to Mayo Clinic High Spot for Many A.H.A. [American Hospital Association] Members," *Hosp. Management*, 1927, *24*: 45.

84. The facilities are described in detail in M. O. Foley, "The Mayo Clinic and Its Work," *Hosp. Management*, 1923, *16*: 28–40.

85. Minutes, MC BOG, February 10, 1926, MCA. See also Minutes, MC BOG, March 25, 1925, MCA; and L. B. Wilson, "Coordinating the Relations of the Laboratory and Clinical Staffs," *Mod. Hosp.*, 1928, *31*: 49–56.

86. Minutes, MC BOG, April 28, 1926, MCA.

87. Minutes, MC BOG, May 12, 1926, MCA.

88. Ibid.

89. _History of the Mayo Clinic_, 117–123.

90. Willius, _Henry Stanley Plummer_, 47. See also T. F. Ellerbe, _The Ellerbe Tradition: Seventy Years of Architecture and Engineering_ (Minneapolis: Ellerbe, 1980).

91. "3,000 Tons of Steel Used in New Clinic Building at Rochester, Minn.," _St. Paul Pioneer-Press_, April 7, 1929, MCA.

92. "Notice," _Clinic Bulletin_, July 6, 1928, MCA. See also C. S. Fischer, _America Calling: A Social History of the Telephone to 1940_ (Berkeley: University of California Press, 1992).

93. "Dedication of the Carillon," _PSMMC_, 1928, _3_: 284–285, quotation from 285. See also "10,000 Attend Dedication of New Clinic Building and Carillon," _Rochester Post-Bulletin_, September 17, 1928, MCA.

94. Data from _American Medical Directory: A Register of Legally Qualified Physicians of the United States_ (Chicago: American Medical Association, 1929).

Chapter 5

1. R. O. Beard, "The Mayo Clinic Building at Rochester," _Journal-Lancet_, 1914, _34_: 425–434.

2. For my interpretation of the factors that contributed to the development of cardiology in the United States, see W. B. Fye, _American Cardiology: The History of a Specialty and Its College_ (Baltimore: Johns Hopkins University Press, 1996), 13–50.

3. W. J. Mayo, "Pre-Existing Heart Disease in Reference to Surgical Operations," _Am. J. Med. Sci._, 1901, _122_: 141–146, quotation from 143.

4. See W. B. Fye, "A History of the Origin, Evolution, and Impact of Electrocardiography," _Am. J. Cardiol._, 1994, _73_: 937–949; and G. E. Burch and N. P. DePasquale, _A History of Electrocardiography_, with a New Introduction by J. D. Howell (San Francisco: Jeremy Norman, 1990).

5. A. D. Hirschfelder, L. F. Barker, and G. M. Bond, "The Electrocardiogram in Clinical Diagnosis," _JAMA_, 1910, _55_: 1350–1353. The older procedures the authors referred to involved using a sphygmograph or polygraph, tools that produced tracings of the arterial and venous pulse waves. See S. W. Moss, "The Sphygmograph in America: Writing the Pulse," _Am. J. Cardiol._, 2006, _97_: 580–587; and P. Reichert and L. F. Bishop Jr., "Sir James Mackenzie and His Polygraph: The Contribution of Louis Faugeres Bishop Sr.," _Am. J. Cardiol._, 1969, _24_: 401–403.

6. A. D. Hirschfelder, _Diseases of the Heart and Aorta_ (Philadelphia: J. B. Lippincott, 1910).

7. A. D. Hirschfelder, "Recent Studies upon the Electrocardiogram and upon the Changes in the Volume of the Heart," _Interstate Med. J._, 1911, _18_: 557–600, quotation from 557.

8. Anon., "Foreword," in _Recent Studies of Cardio-Vascular Disease: A Reprint of Articles Published in the Interstate Medical Journal_ (St. Louis: Interstate Medical Journal, 1911), [5].

9. A. D. Hirschfelder, _Diseases of the Heart and Aorta_, 2nd ed. (Philadelphia: J. B. Lippincott, 1913), ix.

10. T. Lewis, _Clinical Electrocardiography_ (London: Shaw & Sons, 1913), ii. See also T. Lewis, _Collected Works on Heart Disease,_ ed. W. B. Fye (New York: Gryphon Editions, 1991); and A. Hollman, _Sir Thomas Lewis: Pioneer Cardiologist and Clinical Scientist_ (London: Springer-Verlag, 1997).

11. C. L. Greene, _Medical Diagnosis for the Student and Practitioner_, 4th ed. (Philadelphia: P. Blakiston's Son, 1917), 488–507. Charles Greene, the chief of medicine at the University of Minnesota, was especially interested in heart disease. Ralph Morris operated the institution's electrocardiograph, which was located in the medical clinic. Hirschfelder's training and experience could have placed him in the front ranks of first-generation cardiologists, but he chose not to practice in Minnesota. His appointment in pharmacology at the university was a full-time position, and he did not obtain a medical license. See A. M. Harvey, "Arthur D. Hirschfelder: Johns Hopkins's First Full-Time Cardiologist," _Johns Hopkins Med. J._, 1978, _143_: 129–139.

12. About 20 percent of America's hospitals were staffed with interns, and fewer than 10 percent of them possessed an electrocardiograph. See J. M. Dodson, "Report of the Council on Medical Education," *JAMA*, 1919, *72*: 1751–1757, table 3, "Equipment and Records of Hospitals Using Interns." See also J. D. Howell, *Technology in the Hospital: Transforming Patient Care in the Early Twentieth Century* (Baltimore: Johns Hopkins University Press, 1995), 122–125.

13. E. M. Rogers, "Innovativeness and Adopter Categories," in *Diffusion of Innovations*, 5th ed. (New York: Free Press, 2003), 267–299.

14. J. Burnett, "The Origins of the Electrocardiograph as a Clinical Instrument," *Med. Hist.*, 1985, *suppl. 5*: 53–76.

15. Robert Whipple to Drs. Mayo, Graham, Plummer & Judd, October 3, 1912, Mayo Clinic Archives, Mayo Historical Unit, Rochester, MN (hereafter MCA). The company also forwarded a catalogue: *Electro-Cardiographic Apparatus, Including Full Descriptions and Cost of Outfits Suitable for Taking Electro-Cardiograms and Phono-Cardiograms. Cambridge, England, Cambridge Scientific Instrument Co.* (Rochester, NY: Taylor Instrument Companies, 1913), MCA.

16. The date of the first electrocardiogram is from F. A. Willius, "The Heart in Old Age: A Study of 750 patients 75 Years of Age and Older," *Am. J. Med. Sci.*, 1931, *182*: 1–12. For a description of the apparatus and how it was used, see F. A. Willius, *Clinical Electrocardiography* (Philadelphia: W. B. Saunders, 1922).

17. The modest changes in the treatment of patients with heart disease over a two-decade period are evident from a comparison of the sections devoted to cardiovascular disorders in two editions of the most popular textbook of medicine. See W. Osler, *The Principles and Practice of Medicine* (New York: D. Appleton, 1892), 581–683; and Osler, *The Principles and Practice of Medicine*, 8th ed. (New York: D. Appleton, 1912), 760–862.

18. The data are from table 3, "Growth of Operative Work [and Patients Registered in the Clinic, 1889–1925]," in *Sketch of the History of the Mayo Clinic and the Mayo Foundation* (Philadelphia: W. B. Saunders, 1926), 31; and F. A. Willius, "Statistical Records of the Electrocardiographic Laboratory from August, 1914, to January 1, 1951," in F. A. Willius, "As I Lived It," MCA.

19. W. B. Fye, "Fredrick A. Willius," *Clin. Cardiol.*, 2001, *24*: 751–752.

20. A. M. Harvey, *The Interurban Clinical Club (1905–1976): A Record of Achievement in Clinical Science* (n.p.: Interurban Clinical Club, 1978).

21. J. M. Blackford and F. A. Willius, "Chronic Heart-Block," *Am. J. Med. Sci.*, 1917, *154*: 585–592.

22. W. J. Mayo, "The Laying of the Corner Stone of the John B. Murphy Memorial Building," *Surg. Gynecol. Obstet.*, 1924, *18*: 282–284, quotation from 283.

23. Willius, *Clinical Electrocardiography*, 13.

24. W. J. Mayo to F. A. Willius, January 19, 1922, in Fredrick Willius Scrapbook, in the posession of David L. Holmes Jr., Rochester, MN, copy in the author's posession (hereafter Willius Scrapbook). See also W. B. Fye, "Medical Authorship: Traditions, Trends, and Tribulations," *Ann. Intern. Med.*, 1990, *113*: 317–325.

25. W. B. Saunders Co., "Just Ready: Willius' Electrocardiography," *Boston Med. Surg. J.*, 1922, *186*, advertisement on the cover of the January 12, 1922 issue.

26. F. A. Willius, "Abnormalities of the T Wave," in *Clinical Electrocardiography*, 120–134. See also J. D. Howell, "Early Perceptions of the Electrocardiogram: From Arrhythmia to Infarction," *Bull. Hist. Med.*, 1984, *58*: 83–98.

27. "Lane Told of Ordeal as Death was Near," *New York Times*, May 18, 1921, MCA. See also K. W. Olson, *Biography of a Progressive: Franklin K. Lane, 1864–1921* (Westport, CT: Greenwood, 1979).

28. A. W. Lane and L. H. Wall, eds., *The Letters of Franklin K. Lane: Personal and Political* (Boston: Houghton Mifflin, 1922) (hereafter *Letters of Lane*).

29. F. K. Lane to Hall McAllister, September 25[?], 1920, in *Letters of Lane*, 356–357.

30. W. D. Andrews, "Dr. John George Gehring and His Bethel Clinic: Pragmatic Therapy and Therapeutic Tourism," *Maine History*, 2008, *43*: 188–216.

31. Lane to Elizabeth Ellis, December 27, 1920, in *Letters of Lane*, 397–398.

32. Lane to J. G. Gehring, December 31, 1920, in *Letters of Lane*, 377–380.

33. Lane to Lathrop Brown, January 3, 1921, in *Letters of Lane*, 402–403.

34. Lane to Gehring, January 13, 1921, in *Letters of Lane*, 410–411.

35. Lane to Gehring, February 18, 1921, in *Letters of Lane*, 415–421.

36. W. Heberden, "Some Account of a Disorder of the Breast," *Medical Transactions Published by the College of Physicians of London*, 1772, *2*: 59–67, quotation from 59–60. See also J. O. Leibowitz, *The History of Coronary Heart Disease* (London: Wellcome Institute of the History of Medicine, 1970).

37. W. B. Fye, "Vasodilator Therapy for Angina Pectoris: The Intersection of Homeopathy and Scientific Medicine," *J. Hist. Med. Allied Sci.*, 1990, *45*: 317–340.

38. Lane to "Several Friends," January 10, 1921, in *Letters of Lane*, 408–410.

39. Ibid.

40. F. Billings, *Focal Infection* (New York: D. Appleton, 1916). See also R. V. Gibbons, "Germs, Dr. Billings, and the Theory of Focal Infection," *Clin. Infect. Dis.*, 1998, *27*: 627–633; T. J. Pallasch and M. J. Wahl, "Focal Infection: New Age or Ancient History?" *Endodontic Topics*, 2003, *4*: 32–45; and P. Libby, "Inflammation in Atherosclerosis," *Arterioscler. Thromb. Vasc. Biol.* 2012, *32*: 2045–2051.

41. Billings, *Focal Infection*, vi. Historian Gerald Grob considers Rosenow "one of the most important advocates of the belief that many diseases were the result of dissemination of pathogens through the bloodstream from a local focus." G. N. Grob, "The Rise and Decline of Tonsillectomy in Twentieth-Century America," *J. Hist. Med. Allied Sci.*, 2007, *62*: 383–421, quotation from 388. See also E. C. Rosenow, "Focal Infection and Elective Localization of Bacteria in Appendicitis, Ulcer of the Stomach, Cholecystitis, and Pancreatitis," *Surg. Gynecol. Obstet.*, 1921, *33*: 19–26.

42. See, for example, C. H. Mayo, "Local Foci of Infection Causing General Systemic Disturbances," *Med. Herald*, 1913, *n.s. 32*: 370–373; and C. H. Mayo, "Focal Infection in Chronic and Recurring Disease," *Virginia Med. Monthly*, 1923, *49*: 557–560.

43. W. S. Thayer, "Reflections on Angina Pectoris with Special Regard to Prognosis and Treatment," *Internat. Clin.*, 1923, ser. 33, 1: 1–26, quotation from 21–22.

44. Lane to William Wheeler, January 13, 1921, in *Letters of Lane*, 407.

45. Lane to Mrs. Frederic Peterson, April 26, 1921, in *Letters of Lane*, 440–441.

46. Lane to Alexander Vogelsang, May 4, 1921, in *Letters of Lane*, 451.

47. Lane to Eleanor Roosevelt, May 5, 1921, in *Letters of Lane*, 455–456.

48. Lane to "Friends," May 11, 1921, in *Letters of Lane*, 456–462.

49. "Former Secretary of Interior in Wilson Cabinet Victim of Heart Disease following an Operation," May 18, 1921. Clipping from an unidentified Rochester newspaper, MCA.

50. "Franklin K. Lane Dies: End Comes at an Early Hour Here," *Rochester Daily Post & Record*, May 18, 1921, MCA.

51. *Thirty-second Annual Report of St. Mary's Hospital* [for 1921] (Rochester, MN: St. Mary's Hospital, 1922), 41.

52. F. A. Willius and J. M. Fitzpatrick, "The Relationship of Chronic Infection of the Gall-Bladder to Disease of the Cardiovascular System," *J. Iowa State Med. Soc.*, 1925, *15*: 589–592, quotation from 591.

53. C. H. Mayo, "Focal Infection," *Proc. Inter-State Postgrad. Assembly North Am.*, 1927, *1927*: 435–441, quotation from 435. See also W. L. Bierring, "Focal Infection: Quarter Century Survey," *JAMA*, 1938, *111*: 1623–1627; and R. L. Cecil, "The Rise and Fall of Focal Infection," *Proc. Inter-State Postgrad. Assembly North Am.*, 1941: 301–304. The decline of the focal infection theory was gradual. Kenneth Roberts, best known for his novel *Northwest Passage*, wrote

a humorous account of his encounter with it. See K. Roberts, *It Must Be Your Tonsils* (Garden City, NY: Doubleday, Doran, 1936).

54. W. J. Mayo, "Seventieth Birthday Anniversary of William J. Mayo," *Ann. Surg.*, 1931, *94*: 799–800. Pathologist and historian Lester King made the same point a half century later: "The leading physicians, of whatever era, offered treatment that accorded with their theories, and these reflected the prevalent notions of cause. But theories conflict; explanations change; concepts of cause vary from one era to another." L. S. King, *Medical Thinking: A Historical Preface* (Princeton NJ: Princeton University Press, 1982), 192. See also P. B. Beeson, "Fashions in Pathogenetic Concepts during the Present Century: Autointoxication, Focal Infection, Psychosomatic Disease, and Autoimmunity," *Perspect. Biol. Med.*, 1992, *36*: 13–23.

55. L. A. Conner, "Cardiovascular Section," in *The Medical Department of the United States Army in the World War. Volume I. The Surgeon General's Office*, ed. C. Lynch, F. W. Weed, and L. McAfee (Washington, DC: Government Printing Office, 1923), 377–381, quotation from 379. See also C. F. Wooley, D. Schneider, and A. A. Lerner, "Lewis Atterbury Conner: Appreciation and Bibliography," *Circulation*, 1998, *98*: 1449–1455.

56. See C. F. Wooley, *The Irritable Heart of Soldiers and the Origins of Anglo-American Cardiology* (Burlington, VT: Ashgate, 2002); and J. D. Howell, "'Soldier's Heart': The Redefinition of Heart Disease and Speciality Formation in Early Twentieth-Century Great Britain," *Med. Hist.*, 1985, *suppl. 5*: 34–52. Cardiology was considered a specialty in the United States in the 1920s, but (as discussed in Chapter 6) it was formally designated as a subspecialty of internal medicine in the late 1930s. The terms "specialty" and "subspecialty" were (and remain) problematic because they had (and have) different meanings depending on the time, place, and context. See G. Weisz, *Divide and Conquer: A Comparative History of Medical Specialization* (New York: Oxford University Press, 2006).

57. Minutes, MC BOG, October 25,1923, MCA.

58. For a list of personnel, see "Schedule of Operative, Diagnostic and Laboratory Work for the Quarter Beginning April 7, 1924," *Clinic Bulletin*, April 3, 1924, MCA.

59. F. A. Willius, Cardiology Section Report to MC BOG for 1924. MCA.

60. R. D. Pruitt, "Arlie Ray Barnes, 1892–1970," *Trans. Assoc. Am. Phys.*, 1970, *83*: 12–13.

61. See F. A. Willius, "Angina Pectoris: An Electrocardiographic Study," *Arch. Int. Med.*, 1921; *27*: 192–223; F. A. Willius, "Angina Pectoris and Surgical Conditions of the Abdomen," *Ann. Surg.*, 1924, *79*: 524–532; and F. A. Willius and G. E. Brown, "Coronary Sclerosis: An Analysis of Eighty-Six Necropsies," *Am. J. Med. Sci.*, 1924, *168*: 165–180. See also W. B. Fye, "A Historical Perspective on Atherosclerosis and Coronary Artery Disease," in *Atherothrombosis and Coronary Artery Disease*, ed. V. Fuster, E. J. Topol, and E. G. Nabel (Philadelphia: Lippincott Williams & Wilkins, 2005), 3–14.

62. The details of the patient's case are from F. A. Willius, "Acute Coronary Obstruction," *Med. Clin. North Am.*, 1925, *8*: 1181–1187.

63. Ibid., 1181.

64. Ibid., 1183. See also J. B. Herrick, "Acute Obstruction of the Coronary Artery," *Northwest Med.*, 1925, *24*: 593–601; and W. B. Fye, "The Delayed Diagnosis of Acute Myocardial Infarction: It Took Half a Century," *Circulation*, 1985, *72*: 262–271; C. Lawrence, "'Definite and Material': Coronary Thrombosis and Cardiologists in the 1920s," in *Framing Disease*, ed. C. E. Rosenberg and J. Golden (New Brunswick, NJ: Rutgers University Press, 1992), 50–82; and A. B. Weisse, "The Elusive Clot: The Controversy over Coronary Thrombosis in Myocardial Infarction," *J. Hist. Med. Allied Sci.*, 2005, *61*: 66–78.

65. See A. R. Cushny, *The Action and Uses in Medicine of Digitalis and Its Allies* (London: Longmans, Green, 1925); and W. B. Fye, "Cardiovascular Pharmacology: A Historical Perspective," in *Cardiovascular Therapeutics*, ed. W. H. Frishman, E. H. Sonnenblick, and D. A. Sica (New York: McGraw-Hill, 2003), 57–63.

66. See S. A. Levine, *Coronary Thrombosis: Its Various Clinical Features* (Baltimore: Williams & Wilkins, 1929), 97–98.

67. H. A. Christian, "Cardiac Infarction (Coronary Thrombosis): An Easily Diagnosable Condition," *Am. Heart J.*, 1925, *1*: 129–137, quotation from 135. See also J. Parkinson and D. E. Bedford, "Successive Changes in the Electrocardiogram after Cardiac Infarction (Coronary Thrombosis)," *Heart*, 1928, *14*: 195–239.

68. W. T. Longcope, "The Effect of Occlusion of the Coronary Arteries on the Heart's Action and Its Relationship to Angina Pectoris," *Wis. Med. J.*, 1922, *20*: 449–455, quotation from 449.

69. W. B. Fye, "Organizing the American Heart Association," in *American Cardiology*, 51–84.

70. "Minnesota Cardiologic Club," *Clinic Bulletin*, December 3, 1924, MCA. Henry Ulrich of Minneapolis, one of the group's founders, described Willius as "the leading spirit in the organization" for three decades. H. L. Ulrich, "Minnesota Society for the Study of Diseases of the Heart and Circulation: An Indoctrination." December 1953, typescript in Willius Scrapbook.

71. "Society for the Study of Heart Diseases," *Clinic Bulletin*, December 5, 1924, MCA. For comparison, see F. W. Madison, "The Wisconsin Heart Club," *Wis. Med. J.*, 1976, *75*: 18–20.

72. F. A. Willius, "A Plan for the Organization of Preventive Cardiology in Minnesota," *Coll. Papers Mayo Clinic*, 1925, *17*: 1020–1024, quotations from 1021. See also H. Emerson, "The Prevention of Heart Disease: A New Practical Problem," *Boston Med. Surg. J.*, 1921, *184*: 587–607.

73. F. A. Willius, "The Progress of Cardiology during 1924: A Review of the Works of Clinicians and Investigators in the United States," *Minn. Med.*, 1925, *8*: 165–170, 230–236, 293–297. Willius adopted a format that Boston cardiologist and AHA founder Paul Dudley White had developed. The topics, which reflected subjects of interest to America's first heart specialists, included prevention of heart disease; endocardium; myocardium; the coronary arteries and angina pectoris; pericardium; blood pressure; arteries; congenital heart disease; size of the heart; cardiac response to exercise; treatment; surgical procedures; physiology; electrocardiography; metabolism and vital capacity; X-ray examination of the heart; and miscellaneous. See P. D. White, "Progress in the Study and Treatment of Cardiovascular Disease in 1922," *Boston Med. Surg. J.*, 1923, *188*: 331–338, 439–446, 644–652.

74. Willius, "Progress of Cardiology," 165.

75. J. A. Tobey, "Heart Disease," *American Mercury*, 1925, *4*: 462–465, quotation from 462. See also F. L. Hoffman, "Recent Statistics of Heart Disease," *JAMA*, 1920, *74*: 1364–1371; and M. E. Teller, *The Tuberculosis Movement: A Public Health Campaign in the Progressive Era* (New York: Greenwood, 1988).

76. F. A. Willius and S. F. Haines, "The Status of the Heart in Myxedema," *Am. Heart J.*, 1925, *1*: 67–72.

77. L. G. Rowntree to E. Libman, April 22, 1926, Emanuel Libman Papers, MS C406, Modern Manuscripts Collection, National Library of Medicine, Bethesda, MD, hereafter Libman Papers.

78. F. A. Willius to E. Libman, May 21, 1926, Libman Papers. See also E. R. Brainard, "History of the American Society for Clinical Investigation, 1909–1959," *J. Clin. Invest.*, 1959, *38*: 1784–1864; and J. D. Howell, "A History of the American Society for Clinical Investigation," *J. Clin. Invest.*, 2009, *119*: 682–697.

79. See L. D. Thompson, "Early History of the Central Society for Clinical Research," *J. Lab. Clin. Med.*, 1953, *41*: 3–5; and W. B. Bean, "Origins and Early Days of the Central Society for Clinical Research," *J. Lab. Clin. Med.*, 1978, *91*: 750–759.

80. Minutes, MC EC, March 28,1923, MCA.

81. Willius Scrapbook.

82. F. A. Willius, "Cardiology in the Mayo Clinic and the Mayo Foundation for Medical Education and Research," in *Methods and Problems of Medical Education*, 8th ser. (New York: Rockefeller Foundation, 1927), 193–197.

83. R. M. Pearce, "Prefatory Note," in *Methods and Problems of Medical Education*, 1st ser. (New York: Rockefeller Foundation, 1924), [3].

84. See P. D. White and C. Thacher, "Cardiac Department, Massachusetts General Hospital," in *Methods and Problems of Medical Education*, 8th ser. (New York: Rockefeller Foundation, 1927), 217–223; S. A. Levine, "Heart Work in the Peter Bent Brigham Hospital," in *Methods and Problems of Medical Education*, 8th ser. (New York: Rockefeller Foundation, 1927), 177–180; and F. N. Wilson and P. S. Barker, "The Heart Station of the University of Michigan Hospital," in *Methods and Problems of Medical Education*, 18th ser. (New York: Rockefeller Foundation, 1930), 89–93.

85. See R. D. Pruitt, "Norman M. Keith, 1885–1976," *Trans. Assoc. Am. Phys.*, 1976, *89*: 23–25; and *George Elgie Brown, M.D., F.A.C.P.* (Rochester, MN: Whiting Press, 1937).

86. "Staff Report, Wednesday, July 5," *Clinic Bulletin*, July 8, 1922, MCA. The Mayo Clinic paid for the purchase of the electrocardiograph at St. Mary's Hospital, which was the third machine that Willius oversaw. By comparison, there were just five electrocardiographs in Minneapolis and St. Paul at this time. See H. E. Richardson, "The Instrumental Recognition of Cardiac Irregularities," *Minn. Med.*, 1924, *7*: 638–642.

87. "Mississippi Valley Medical Association: Mayo Clinic Program, October 10–11, 1922," *Clinic Bulletin*, October 3, 1922, MCA.

88. Minutes, MC Committee on Medical Education, Research, and Scientific Progress, January 9, 1923, MCA.

89. The lectures are listed in the *Clinic Bulletin* issues of June 7, 1923, and June 11, 1923 (Wenckebach); January 24, 1924 (Libman); February 27, 1924 (Swift); June 17, 1924 (Thayer); and June 23, 1924 (Aschoff), MCA.

90. Einthoven's lectures are listed in the *Clinic Bulletin* issues of November 10, 1924, and November 21, 1924, MCA. Einthoven's host was Minneapolis cardiologist George Fahr, his first American pupil. See G. E. Fahr, "Einthoven—'Ik Wilde Weten,'" in *Festschrift: George E. Fahr, M.D.*, ed. A. C. Kerkhof (Minneapolis: Lancet Publications, 1962), 15–25.

91. Minutes, MC EC, March 1, 1922, MCA.

92. F. A. Willius, Cardiology Section Report to MC BOG for 1925, MCA.

93. J. L. Graner, ed., *A History of the Department of Internal Medicine at the Mayo Clinic* (Rochester, MN: Mayo Foundation, 2002), esp. chapters 13 (nephrology), 14 (endocrinology), 17 (gastroenterology), and 22 (rheumatology).

94. Physicians recognized that there was no uniform terminology to describe cardiac diseases in this era. See P. D. White and M. M. Myers, "The Classification of Cardiac Diagnosis, with Especial Reference to Etiology," *Am. Heart J.*, 1925, *1*: 87–95.

95. Two influential textbooks provide perspective on the etiology, diagnosis, and treatment, and terminology of various types of heart disease from an American and a British point of view: P. D. White, *Heart Disease* (New York: Macmillan, 1931); and J. Mackenzie, *Diseases of the Heart*, 4th ed. (London: Oxford University Press, 1925).

96. L. A. Conner to E. Libman, May 15, 1925, Libman Papers.

97. L. A. Conner, "The American Heart Journal," *Am. Heart J.*, 1925, *1*: 115–116, quotation from 116.

98. *A Directory of Heart Associations, Committees, Convalescent Homes and Cardiac Clinics in the United States and Canada* (New York: American Heart Association, 1928).

99. Ibid. The limited-hour cardiac clinics placed emphasis on the social and economic consequences of heart disease. See Fye, *American Cardiology*, 36–44.

Chapter 6

1. Minutes, MC BOG, August 21, 1929, Mayo Clinic Archives, Mayo Historical Unit, Rochester, MN (hereafter MCA).

2. C. H. Mayo to W. J. Mayo, November 21, 1929, MCA.

3. M. Klein, *Rainbow's End: The Crash of 1929* (New York: Oxford University Press, 2001), xiii. See also A. J. Badger, *The New Deal: The Depression Years, 1933–1940* (New York: Noonday Press, 1989).

4. Minutes, MC BOG, January 29, 1930, and July 30, 1930, MCA.

5. W. J. Mayo, "Remarks Regarding Financial Adjustments," Faculty Meeting, August 11, 1930, typescript, MCA.

6. Ibid.

7. H. L. Mencken, "What Is Going on in the World," *American Mercury*, 1933, *28*: 257–265, quotation from 257. See also H. Cabot, *The Doctor's Bill* (New York: Columbia University Press, 1935). Very few Americans had health insurance when Mayo and Mencken made their observations. See "Health Insurance," in *American Medicine: Expert Testimony Out of Court*, ed. E. E. Lape, 2 vols. (New York: American Foundation, 1937), *2*: 976–1100.

8. Mayo, "Financial Adjustments."

9. H. J. Harwick, *Forty-four Years with the Mayo Clinic* (Rochester, MN: Whiting Press, 1957), 28. For the new patients in 1927–1928, see W. C. Alvarez, "Peculiarities in the Sex and Age Distribution of the Clientele of the Clinic," *Proceedings of the Staff Meetings of the Mayo Clinic* (hereafter *PSMMC*), 1930, *5*: 225–228.

10. "Mayo Clinic Bookings Data, 1929–1977," Patrick McCarty to Nicole Babcock, May 2007, MCA.

11. A. S. Bower, Annual Report of Collection Department, December 31, 1931, MCA.

12. E. Whelan, *The Sisters' Story: Saint Marys Hospital—Mayo Clinic, 1889 to 1939* (Rochester, MN: Mayo Foundation, 2002), 141. See also C. J. Pahlas, *The Unique Voice of Service: The Story of the Kahler Corporation, Rochester, Minnesota* (Rochester, MN: Kahler Corporation, 1964).

13. Minutes, MC BOG, December 4, 1929, MCA.

14. Minutes, MC Personnel Committee, December 23, 1931, MCA. More salary cuts were imposed in August 1930 and January and May 1932. See Minutes, MC BOG, January 5, 1932, and May 19, 1932, MCA.

15. Minutes, MC BOG, July 20, 1932, MCA.

16. *Clinic Bulletin*, August 30, 1932, MCA.

17. "Incomes of Physicians," *JAMA*, 1938, *111*: 2311.

18. R. L. Sanders to W. J. Mayo, October 5, 1932, MCA. The letterhead of their group practice, the Polyclinic, listed a dozen doctors in seven specialties. See also R. L. Sanders to W. J. Mayo, April 12, 1932; and W. J. Mayo to R. L. Sanders, October 10, 1932, MCA. For a contemporary review of group practice, see C. R. Rorem, *Private Group Clinics* (Chicago: University of Chicago Press, 1931).

19. H. J. Harwick to W. J. Mayo, March 2, 1933, MCA.

20. H. J. Harwick to W. J. Mayo, March 9, 1933, MCA.

21. W. J. Mayo to G. G. Turner, May 31, 1933, MCA.

22. "Roosevelt Lauds Mayos, Stresses Public Service," *Washington Post*, August 9, 1934, MCA. The Mayo brothers were Democrats. See H. Clapesattle, *The Doctors Mayo* (Minneapolis: University of Minnesota Press, 1941), 686–687.

23. "Mayo Clinic Bookings Data, 1929–1977."

24. E. Tuohy to W. J. Mayo, January 27, 1928, MCA.

25. For the internal medicine groups at St. Mary's Hospital, see *Mayo Clinic Desk Book: Written by the Various Sections and Edited by the Coordinating Committee* (Rochester, MN: Mayo Clinic, 1927), 87, MCA; and L. G. Rowntree, "Progress in Medicine in Rochester," *PSMMC*, 1926, *1*: 143–144.

26. L. G. Rowntree to W. J. Mayo, August 18, 1929, MCA. Evanston Hospital was being reorganized as a teaching institution affiliated with Northwestern University. See L. B. Arey, *Northwestern University Medical School 1859–1959: A Pioneer in Educational Reform* (Evanston, IL: Northwestern University, 1959), 288.

27. Minutes, MC BOG, August 21, 1929, MCA.

28. W. J. Mayo to H. J. Harwick, November 4, 1929, MCA.

29. Ibid. Arthur Sanford directed the clinical laboratories, and Edward Kendall was in charge of the experimental biochemistry laboratory. See J. C. Todd and A. H. Sanford, *Clinical Diagnosis by Laboratory Methods* (Philadelphia: W. B. Saunders, 1931); and A. H. Sanford, "A Collective Review of Recent Books on Clinical Pathology," *Arch. Pathol.*, 1931, *12*: 857–867.

30. M. S. Henderson to W. J. Mayo, November 12, 1929, MCA. See also A. M. Harvey, "Clinical Science at the Mayo Clinic: The Concept of Team Research," in *Science at the Bedside: Clinical Research in American Medicine, 1905–1945* (Baltimore: Johns Hopkins University Press, 1981), 368–392; and J. L. Graner, "Leonard Rowntree and the Birth of the Mayo Clinic Research Tradition," *Mayo Clin. Proc.*, 2005, *80*: 920–922.

31. W. J. Mayo to M. S. Henderson, November 21, 1929, MCA.

32. For the committees, see "Present Organization of the Mayo Clinic," in *Sketch of the History of the Mayo Clinic and the Mayo Foundation* (Philadelphia: W. B. Saunders, 1926), 117–132. See also "Development of Laboratories," in *History of the Mayo Clinic*, 71–91.

33. L. B. Wilson, "Twelve Years' Experience of the University of Minnesota in Graduate Medical Education," *Bull. Assoc. Am. Med. Coll.*, 1928, *3*: 210–219, quotation from 211. See also L. B. Wilson, "Coordinating the Relations of the Laboratory and Clinical Staffs," *Mod. Hosp.*, 1928, *31*: 49–56.

34. W. J. Mayo to C. H. Mayo, February 7, 1930, MCA.

35. Minutes, MC BOG, February 12, 1930, MCA.

36. L. G. Rowntree to W. J. Mayo, February 16, 1930, MCA.

37. Minutes, MC BOG, February 12, 1930, MCA.

38. L. G. Rowntree to W. H. Welch, September 17, 1930, box 46, folder 10, Welch Papers, the Alan Mason Chesney Archives of the Johns Hopkins Medical Institutions.

39. C. H. Mayo, "Remarks," *PSMMC*, 1931, *6*: 590.

40. Minutes, MC BOG, November 18, 1931, MCA.

41. L. G. Rowntree to W. J. Mayo, December 18, 1931, in Minutes, MC BOG, December 23, 1931, MCA.

42. L. G. Rowntree, *Amid Masters of Twentieth Century Medicine* (Springfield, IL: Charles C Thomas, 1958), 399–419.

43. R. M. Wilder, "Recollections and Reflections on Education, Diabetes, Other Metabolic Diseases, and Nutrition in the Mayo Clinic and Associated Hospitals, 1919–1950," *Perspect. Biol. Med.*, 1958, *1*: 237–277, quotation from 259.

44. W. C. Alvarez, *Incurable Physician: An Autobiography* (Englewood Cliffs, NJ: Prentice-Hall, 1963), 150–153, quotations from 151. For a discussion of the tensions between researchers and practitioners, see J. B. Herrick, "The Practitioner of the Future," *JAMA*, 1934, *103*: 881–885.

45. See N. W. Barker, "The History of the Medical Vascular Section of the Mayo Clinic," typescript ca. 1957, MCA; and J. A. Spittell Jr. and J. F. Fairbairn II, "Vascular Medicine at Mayo Clinic: Some Highlights of the Early History and Development as a Subspecialty," *Int. Angiology*, 1992, *11*: 2–7.

46. L. G. Rowntree, "Foreword," in G. E. Brown, E. V. Allen, and H. R. Mahorner, *Thrombo-angiitis Obliterans: Clinical, Physiologic and Pathologic Studies* (Philadelphia: W. B. Saunders, 1928), 11.

47. W. B. Fye, "Organizing the American Heart Association," in *American Cardiology: The History of a Specialty and Its College* (Baltimore: Johns Hopkins University Press, 1996), 51–84.

48. Irving S. Wright, interview by W. B. Fye, New York, NY, August 14, 1991.

49. Minutes, AHA EC, June 11, 1935, American Heart Association National Center Corporate Records, Dallas, TX (hereafter AHA archives). The Committee for the Study of the Peripheral Circulation would become the first of several "councils" formed

by the AHA. See *A History of the Scientific Councils of the American Heart Association* (New York: AHA, 1967).

50. L. A. Conner, "Retrospect and Prospect," *Am. Heart J.*, 1935, *10*: 830–831, quotation from 830.

51. Ibid.

52. W. S. Middleton, "Activities in Medical Organizations," in *George Elgie Brown, M.D., F.A.C.P., 1885–1935* (Rochester, MN: Whiting Press, 1937), 12–17, quotation from 16–17.

53. "Section of the American Heart Association for the Study of the Peripheral Circulation," *Bull. Am. Heart Assn.*, 1938, *13*: 1–2.

54. F. A. Willius, "The Prevention of Heart Disease," *Minn. Med.*, 1929, *12*: 355–359. See also P. D. White, "The Early Infancy of Preventive Cardiology," *Trans. Am. Clin. Climatol. Assoc.*, 1973, *84*: 17–21.

55. See Fye, *American Cardiology*, 62–67; and P. K. J. Han, "Historical Changes in the Objectives of the Periodic Health Examination," *Ann. Intern. Med.*, 1997, *127*: 910–917.

56. C. H. Mayo, "Prevention of Disease," typescript, 1930, MCA.

57. A. R. Barnes, "The Treatment of Some Common Types of Heart Disease," *Northwest Med.*, 1932, *31*: 363–368, quotation from 368.

58. P. D. White, *Heart Disease* (New York: Macmillan, 1931), 498 (aortic valve disease), 400 (hypertension), and 424 (coronary disease). See also J. B. Herrick, "Comments on the Treatment of Heart Disease," *Trans. Cong. Am. Phys. Surg.*, 1929, *14*: 76–90.

59. F. A. Willius, Cardiology Section Report to MC BOG for 1934, MCA. Willius spoke at nine meetings in Nebraska, North and South Dakota, Virginia, and Tennessee in 1934.

60. F. A. Willius, "A Series of Cardiac Clinics," *PSMMC*, 1934, *9*: 535. See also J. T. Priestley, "The First Fifty Years of *Mayo Clinic Proceedings*," *Mayo Clin. Proc.*, 1976, *51*: 794–795.

61. W. J. Mayo to F. A. Willius, April 12, 1936, in Fredrick Willius Scrapbook, original in the possession of David L. Holmes Jr., Rochester, MN, copy in the author's possession (hereafter Willius Scrapbook). Thomas Lewis's London-based journal *Heart* was renamed *Clinical Science* in 1933 to reflect its new expanded scope.

62. William H. Allen to F. A. Willius, June 14, 1936, Willius Scrapbook.

63. F. A. Willius, Cardiology Section Report to MC BOG for 1933, MCA.

64. Minutes, MC BOG, March 28, 1934, MCA. Robert Parker, who joined the staff in 1937, admired Willius, but he explained that some individuals perceived the senior cardiologist as being reluctant "to carry his own weight" in terms of seeing patients. Robert L. Parker, interview by W. B. Fye, Rochester, MN, September 18, 2000.

65. Minutes, MC BOG, May 1, 1935, MCA.

66. Ibid. See also Minutes, MC BOG, May 15, 1935, MCA.

67. W. L. Bierring, "Early Recognition of Myocardial Disease," *Ann. Intern. Med.*, 1934, *8*: 497–503, quotation from 498. Bierring was an influential member of the Board of Regents of the American College of Physicians in the 1930s. See W. S. Middleton, "Walter L. Bierring, M.D., and the American Board of Internal Medicine," *Journal-Lancet*, 1963, *83*: 466–470. See also G. Weisz, "Regulating Specialists the American Way," in *Divide and Conquer: A Comparative History of Medical Specialization* (New York: Oxford University Press, 2006), 127–146; and R. Stevens, "The Curious Career of Internal Medicine: Functional Ambivalence, Social Success," in *Grand Rounds: One Hundred Years of Internal Medicine*, ed. R. C. Maulitz and D. E. Long (Philadelphia: University of Pennsylvania Press, 1988), 339–364.

68. R. Stevens, *American Medicine and the Public Interest*, rev. ed. (Berkeley: University of California Press, 1998), 130. Except for Stevens, historians have not appreciated Wilson's major contributions to American medical education and postgraduate training.

69. J. S. Rodman to C. H. Mayo, February 9, 1923, MCA. See also J. P. Hubbard and E. J. Levit, *The National Board of Medical Examiners: The First Seventy Years* (Philadelphia: National Board of Medical Examiners, 1985).

70. L. B. Wilson, "The Distinctive Functions of Undergraduate and Graduate Medical Schools," *South. Med. J.*, 1924, *17*: 707–713, quotation from 710.

71. Ibid. The comments of Charles Minor of Asheville, NC, are on 711.

72. "Washington University School of Medicine," *Am. Heart J.*, 1925, *1*: advertising section, page 8.

73. L. B. Wilson, "Some Suggestions for the Improved Training of the Medical Specialist," *Trans. Med. Assoc. Alabama*, 1929, *62*: 121–132, quotation from 124–125.

74. L. B. Wilson, "The Function of the Graduate School in the Training of Specialists," *Fed. Bull.*, 1932, *18*: 304–311, quotation from 304.

75. L. B. Wilson. "Report of Special Representative," in Association of American Medical Colleges, Minutes of the Proceedings of the Forty-Fourth Annual Meeting Held in Rochester and Minneapolis, MN. October 30 and 31 and November 1, 1933, *J. Assoc. Am. Medical Colleges*, 1933, *8* (6 Suppl): 3–45, quotation from 26. See also M. D. Bowles and V. P. Dawson, *With One Voice: The Association of American Medical Colleges, 1876–2000* (Washington DC: AAMC, 2003). For a very comprehensive list of organizations, see J. B. Kirsner, *The Development of American Gastroenterology* (New York: Raven Press, 1990), 146–150.

76. R. L. Wilbur, "Order in the Specialties: The Relation of the [AMA] Council on Medical Education and Hospitals to the Special Practice of Medicine," *Fed. Bull.*, 1933, *19*: 241–244, quotation from 242. See also E. E. Robinson and P. C. Edwards, eds., *The Memoirs of Ray Lyman Wilbur, 1875–1949* (Stanford, CA: Stanford University Press, 1960).

77. W. L. Bierring, in "Discussion of Papers of Drs. Gifford, Bierring, Cutter, and Wilbur," *Fed. Bull.*, 1933, *19*: 244–255, quotation from 251.

78. L. B. Wilson, in "Discussion of Papers," 252.

79. Louis B. Wilson, interview by Helen Clapesattle, January 25, 1940, MCA.

80. Stevens, *American Medicine*, 216.

81. "Advisory Board for Medical Specialties," in *Directory of Medical Specialists Certified by American Boards*, ed. P. Titus (New York: Columbia University Press, 1939), 3–16, quotation from 10.

82. Ibid., 11. Because the Advisory Board recognized that it was setting very high training standards, it agreed that they would not be mandatory until 1942.

83. W. L. Bierring, "The American Board of Internal Medicine (Inc)," *Fed. Bull.*, 1936, *22*: 281–283. See also W. L. Bierring, "The American Board of Internal Medicine," in *The American College of Physicians: Its First Quarter Century*, ed. W. G. Morgan (Philadelphia: American College of Physicians, 1940), 87–102.

84. For negotiations regarding the creation of a subspecialty board in cardiology, see Fye, *American Cardiology*, 86–93.

85. W. L. Bierring to L. B. Wilson, February 24, 1936, MCA.

86. L. B. Wilson to W. L. Bierring, March 8, 1937, MCA.

87. "Index According to the University or College by Which the Degree of Doctor of Medicine Was Conferred," in *Physicians of the Mayo Clinic and the Mayo Foundation* (Minneapolis: University of Minnesota Press, 1937), 1543–1557.

88. J. H. Musser, "Opportunities for the Training of Future Internists," *JAMA*, 1938, *110*: 1328–1331, quotation from 1330.

89. W. J. Mayo, "The Establishment of 'The Mayo Foundation House' and Its Purpose," *PSMMC*, 1938, *13*: 553–554.

90. G. W. Crile to W. J. Mayo, June 24, 1939, MCA. See also Amy Rowland, *Cleveland Clinic Foundation* (Cleveland, OH: William Feather, 1938).

91. H. Cushing, "The Mayo Brothers and Their Clinic," *Science*, 1939, *90*: 225–226. See also A. A. Cohen-Gadol, J. M. Homan, E. R. Laws, J. L. D. Atkinson, and R. H. Miller, "The Mayo Brothers and Harvey Cushing: A Review of Their 39-Year Friendship Through Their Personal Letters," *J. Neurosurg.*, 2005, *102*: 396. See also "Dr. Charles H. Mayo Dies,"

Rochester Post-Bulletin, May 26, 1939, MHA; and "Dr. William J. Mayo Dies," *Rochester Post-Bulletin*, July 28, 1939, MHA.

92. H. M. Zimmerman, "The Last Days of Harvey Cushing," *Neurology India*, 1969, *17*: 151–163, quotation from 154. For Cushing's illness and death, see also J. F. Fulton, *Harvey Cushing, A Biography* (Springfield, IL: Charles C Thomas, 1946), 640, 669, 713–714; and M. Bliss, *Harvey Cushing: A Life in Surgery* (New York: Oxford University Press, 2005), 515–516.

93. Zimmerman, "Last Days of Harvey Cushing," 161. Samuel Levine, Cushing's former colleague at Boston's Peter Bent Brigham Hospital, was a leading authority on acute myocardial infarction. See S. A. Levine, *Coronary Thrombosis: Its Various Clinical Features* (Baltimore: Williams & Wilkins, 1929).

94. See D. Y. Solandt and C. H. Best, "Heparin and Coronary Thrombosis in Experimental Animals," *Lancet*, 1938, *232*: 130–132; and D. Y. Solandt, R. Nassim, and C. H. Best, "Production and Prevention of Cardiac Mural Thrombosis in Dogs," *Lancet*, 1939, *234*: 592–595.

95. A. R. Barnes, "Pulmonary Embolism," *JAMA*, 1937, *109*: 1347–1353. See also L. B. Wilson, "Fatal Postoperative Embolism," *Ann. Surg.*, 1912, *56*: 809–817.

96. Barnes, "Pulmonary Embolism," 1347.

97. C. H. Best, "Preparation of Heparin and Its Use in the First Clinical Cases," *Circulation*, 1959, *19*: 79–86. See also S. McKellar, *Surgical Limits: The Life of Gordon Murray* (Toronto: University of Toronto Press, 2003), 38–51; W. B. Fye, "Heparin: The Contributions of William Henry Howell," *Circulation*, 1984, *69*: 1198–1203; and J. A. Marcum, "The Development of Heparin in Toronto," *J. Hist. Med. Allied Sci.*, 1997, *52*: 310–337.

98. H. E. Essex to C. H. Best, June 21, 1937, and C. H. Best to H. E. Essex, June 24, 1937, MCA. See also C. A. Owen Jr., *A History of Blood Coagulation* (Rochester, MN: Mayo Foundation, 2001); and E. J. W. Bowie and G. S. Gilchrist, *Bleeding and Thrombosis at Mayo Clinic: A Brief History* (Rochester, MN: Mayo Scientific Press, 2008).

99. D. W. G. Murray, L. B. Jaques, T. S. Perrett, and C. H. Best, "Heparin and Thrombosis of Veins Following Injury," *Surgery*, 1937, *2*: 163–187.

100. H. E. Essex to C. H. Best, November 11, 1937, MCA. New York City vascular specialist Irving Wright claimed to have been the first American physician to treat a patient with heparin, but he first got a sample of heparin thirteen months after Priestley had administered it to his postoperative patient. See I. S. Wright, "Experience with Anticoagulants," *Circulation*, 1959, *19*: 110–113. For Best's clarification of the priority, see "Preparation of Heparin."

101. C. H. Best to H. E. Essex, November 23, 1937, MCA.

102. Priestley's comments in Minutes, MC BOG, December 29, 1937, MCA.

103. A. R. Barnes, "Diagnostic Electrocardiographic Changes Observed Following Acute Pulmonary Embolism," *PSMMC*, 1936, *11*: 11–13, quotation from 11.

104. C. H. Best, "Heparin and Thrombosis," *PSMMC*, 1939, *14*: 81–84, quotation from 84, paper presented on October 31, 1938.

105. J. T. Priestley, H. E. Essex, and N. W. Barker, "The Use of Heparin in the Prevention and Treatment of Postoperative Thrombosis and Embolism: A Preliminary Report," *PSMMC*, 1941, *16*: 60–64. The title of a book that a pioneering Canadian surgeon published a half-century later reveals how heparin played a critical role in the surgical treatment of millions of patients with heart disease: W. G. Bigelow, *Mysterious Heparin: The Key to Open Heart Surgery* (Toronto: McGraw-Hill Ryerson, 1990).

106. H. R. Butt, E. V. Allen, and J. L. Bollman, "A Preparation from Spoiled Sweet Clover [3,3'-methylene-bis-(4-hydroxycoumarin)] Which Prolongs Coagulation and Prothrombin Time of the Blood: Preliminary Report of Experimental and Clinical Studies," *PSMMC*, 1941, *16*: 388–395.

107. "Heparin and a Rival," *Lancet* 1941, *238*: 314.

108. K. P. Link, "The Discovery of Dicumarol and Its Sequels," *Circulation*, 1959, *19*: 97–107.

109. H. R. Butt, A. M. Snell, and A. E. Osterberg, "Further Observations on the Use of Vitamin K in the Prevention and Control of the Hemorrhagic Diathesis in Cases of Jaundice," *PSMMC*, 1938, *13*: 753–764, quotation from 762.

110. E. V. Allen, "My Early Experience with Bishydroxycoumarin (Dicumarol)," *Circulation*, 1959, *19*: 118–121. Allen explains that Karl Link had already given a sample to a hematologist at the Wisconsin General Hospital, but that the Mayo researchers published their findings first. See also Link, "Discovery of Dicumarol," 103.

111. Butt, Allen, and Bollman, "A Preparation from Spoiled Sweet Clover." Link's group studied several compounds related to dicumarol and concluded that one was superior. It was marketed as warfarin in 1954. See R. L. Mueller and S. Scheidt, "History of Drugs for Thrombotic Disease: Discovery, Development, and Directions for the Future," *Circulation*, 1994, *89*: 432–449.

112. "Sigma Xi Lecture," *Clinic Bulletin*, February 21, 1942, MCA.

113. "Sigma Xi Lecture Postponed," *Clinic Bulletin*, February 25, 1942, MCA.

114. "Sigma Xi Lecture," *Clinic Bulletin*, March 7, 1942, MCA. See also R. Buderi, *The Invention That Changed the World: How a Small Group of Radar Pioneers Won the Second World War and Launched a Technological Revolution* (New York: Simon and Schuster, 1996).

115. A. R. Barnes Section Report to MC BOG for 1941, MCA. See also O. H. Beahrs, "Contributions of the Mayo Clinic in World Wars I and II," *Ann. Surg.*, 1995, *221*: 196–201; and D. Kenney, *Minnesota Goes to War: The Home Front during World War II* (St. Paul: Minnesota Historical Society Press, 2005).

Chapter 7

1. Significant studies of Franklin Roosevelt's health, listed in date order, include K. R. Crispell and C. F. Gomez, "Franklin D. Roosevelt: The Diagnosis of an 'Unexpected' Death," in *Hidden Illness in the White House* (Durham, NC: Duke University Press, 1988), 75–120; R. H. Ferrell, *The Dying President: Franklin D. Roosevelt, 1944–1945* (Columbia: University of Missouri Press, 1998); H. E. Evans, *The Hidden Campaign: FDR's Health and the 1944 Election* (Armonk, NY: Sharpe, 2002); M. B. Wills, *A Diminished President: FDR in 1944* (Raleigh, NC: Ivy House, 2003); H. S. Goldsmith, *A Conspiracy of Silence: The Health and Death of Franklin D. Roosevelt* (New York: iUniverse, 2007); and S. Lomazov and E. Fettmann, *FDR's Deadly Secret* (New York: Public Affairs, 2009). I focus on Roosevelt's cardiovascular disease and do not discuss non-cardiac conditions that Roosevelt had or may have had. See A. Karenberg, "Retrospective Diagnosis: Use and Abuse in Medical Historiography," *Prague Med. Rep.*, 2009, *110*: 140–145. A brief overview of Roosevelt's life with a list of biographies is A. Brinkley, "Franklin Delano Roosevelt," in *American National Biography*, ed. J. A. Garraty and M. C. Carnes (New York: Oxford University Press, 1999), 18: 816–826. Political historian James Burns corresponded with Roosevelt's cardiologist, Howard Bruenn, and Roosevelt's daughter Anna. His biography is a valuable source for the war years. J. M. Burns, *Roosevelt: The Soldier of Freedom* (New York: Harcourt Brace Jovanovich, 1970). General studies of the health of American and world leaders include R. H. Ferrell, *Ill-Advised: Presidential Health and the Public Trust* (Columbia: University of Missouri Press, 1992); B. E. Park, *The Impact of Illness on World Leaders* (Philadelphia: University of Pennsylvania Press, 1986); and R. McDermott, *Presidential Leadership, Illness, and Decision Making* (New York: Cambridge University Press, 2008).

2. See, for example, A. R. Barnes and M. B. Whitten, "Study of the R-T Interval in Myocardial Infarction," *Am. Heart J.*, 1929, *5*: 142–171; and A. R. Barnes, "Electrocardiogram

in Myocardial Infarction," *Arch. Int. Med.* 1935, *55*: 457–483. See also R. D. Pruitt, "Arlie Ray Barnes, 1892–1970," *Trans. Assoc. Am. Phys.* 1970; *83*: 12–13.

3. A. R. Barnes, *Electrocardiographic Patterns: Their Diagnostic and Clinical Significance* (Springfield, IL: Charles C Thomas, 1940), 4. See also C. C. Wolferth and F. C. Wood, "The Electrocardiographic Diagnosis of Coronary Occlusion by the Use of Chest Leads," *Am. J. Med. Sci.*, 1932, *183*: 30–35; W. B. Fye, "A History of the Origin, Evolution, and Impact of Electrocardiography," *Am. J. Cardiol.*, 1994, *73*: 937–949; and G. E. Burch and N. P. DePasquale, *A History of Electrocardiography*, with a new introduction by J. D. Howell (San Francisco: Jeremy Norman, 1990).

4. A. R. Barnes, H. E. B. Pardee, P. D. White, F. N. Wilson, and C. C. Wolferth, "Standardization of Precordial Leads: Supplementary Report," *Am. Heart J.*, 1938, *15*: 235–239.

5. C. C. Wolferth, Review of Barnes, *Electrocardiographic Patterns*, in *Am. J. Med. Sci.* 1940, *199*: 406–407.

6. S. A. Levine, "Electrocardiography and the General Practitioner," *Med. Clin. North Am.*, 1940, *24*: 1325–1345, quotation from 1340.

7. See W. B. Fye, *American Cardiology: The History of a Specialty and Its College* (Baltimore: Johns Hopkins University Press, 1996), 86–93; "Specialties and Sub-Specialties among Members of the American College of Physicians," *Ann. Intern. Med.*, 1942, *17*: 1042–1043; and B. R. Kirklin, "Summary of Eligibility Requirements of Certifying Boards," *JAMA*, 1941, *116*: 2626–2628.

8. Alex to Jack in Virginia, July 13, 1944, postcard in the author's possession. See also O. H. Beahrs, "Contributions of the Mayo Clinic in World Wars I and II," *Ann. Surg.*, 1995, *221*: 196–201.

9. A. R. Barnes Section Report to MC BOG for 1944, Mayo Clinic Archives, Mayo Historical Unit, Rochester, MN (hereafter MCA). During Barnes's first year as editor of the monthly publication, Mayo authors wrote one-half of the articles.

10. H. M. Marvin to P. D. White, May 5, 1944, Paul Dudley White Papers, Harvard Medical Library in the Francis A. Countway Library of Medicine, Boston, MA (hereafter White Papers).

11. P. D. White to H. M. Marvin, May 12, 1944, White Papers.

12. F. D. Roosevelt, "Statement of the President on Signing the Public Health Service Act. July 1, 1944," in *The Public Papers and Addresses of Franklin D. Roosevelt...1944–45 volume*, ed. S. I. Rosenman (New York: Harper, 1950), 191–193. See also S. P. Strickland, *Politics, Science, and Dread Disease: A Short History of United States Medical Research Policy* (Cambridge, MA: Harvard University Press, 1972), 15–31.

13. A. R. Barnes to H. S. Diehl, August 14, 1944, box 6, Maurice B. Visscher Papers, University of Minnesota Archives, Minneapolis, MN (hereafter Visscher Papers).

14. M. B. Visscher to A. R. Barnes, August 15, 1944, box 6, Visscher Papers.

15. Barnes Section Report for 1944.

16. See D. M. Jordan, *FDR, Dewey, and the Election of 1944* (Bloomington: Indiana University Press, 2011); and S. Weintraub, *Final Victory: FDR's Extraordinary World War II Presidential Campaign* (Boston: Da Capo, 2012).

17. J. E. Hoover to S. Early, November 1, 1944 [cover letter with] "Memorandum Re: Circulation of Story Alleging the President has a Serious Heart Affliction," October 29, 1944, FDR corres. and White House Matters, McIntire Collection, Franklin D. Roosevelt Library, Hyde Park, NY (herafter FDRL).

18. Dwight J. Dalbey to H. S. Goldsmith, June 27, 1983, published in Goldsmith, *Conspiracy of Silence*, 81–82.

19. L. L. Levin, *The Making of FDR: The Story of Stephen T. Early, America's First Modern Press Secretary* (Amherst, NY: Prometheus, 2008), 74–79. For an account of Harding's death by a physician who was caring for him at the time, see E. E. Robinson and P. C. Edwards, eds., *The Memoirs of Ray Lyman Wilbur, 1875–1949* (Stanford, CA: Stanford University Press, 1960), 377–385.

20. Steve Early, Confidential Memorandum for Dr. McIntire, August 23, 1937, quotation from B. H. Winfield, *FDR and the News Media* (Urbana: University of Illinois Press, 1990), 114. See also R. J. Ruben, "Dr Ross McIntire, Otolaryngologist, and His Care of President Franklin D. Roosevelt," *Otolaryngol. Head Neck Surg.*, 2009, *141*: 4–6. The definitive study of the interplay of Roosevelt's polio, the public, and his political career is J. Tobin, *The Man He Became: How FDR Defied Polio to Win the Presidency* (New York: Simon & Schuster, 2013). See also H. G. Gallagher, *FDR's Splendid Deception* (New York: Dodd, Mead, 1985); D. W. Houck and A. Kiewe, *FDR's Body Politics: The Rhetoric of Disability* (College Station: Texas A&M University, 2003); and M. Pressman, "Ambivalent Accomplices: How the Press Handled FDR's Disability and How FDR Handled the Press," *J. Historical Soc.*, 2013, *13*: 325–359. Although Roosevelt downplayed his disability from polio, he was very open about having had the disease. See R. H. Berg, *The Challenge of Polio: The Crusade Against Infantile Paralysis* (New York: Dial Press, 1946); and D. M. Oshinsky, *Polio: An American Story* (New York: Oxford University Press, 2005), 43–60.

21. "Have You Heard? The Story of Wartime Rumors," *Life*, July 13, 1942, 68–73.

22. "Text of Roosevelt Speech," *New York Times*, August 9, 1934. The local newspaper covered the visit extensively. See *Rochester Post-Bulletin*, August 8, 1934, MCA.

23. C. T. Grayson to W. J. and C. H. Mayo, October 6, 1934, MCA. Grayson had undergone surgery at Mayo for a kidney tumor nine months earlier. See "Grayson Has Operation," *New York Times*, January 9, 1934.

24. H. Cushing to Roosevelt, September 8, 1938, published in R. L. Rovit and W. T. Couldwell, "No Ordinary Time, No Ordinary Men: The Relationship Between Harvey Cushing and Franklin D. Roosevelt, 1928–1939," *J. Neurosurg.* 2001, *95*: 354–368, quotation from 364. Mayo gastroenterologist George Eusterman coordinated James Roosevelt's visit to Mayo Clinic in the spring of 1938. See G. B. Eusterman to J. Roosevelt, May 27, 1938, James Roosevelt Collection, box 47, folder Mayo Clinic, FDRL. Several high-ranking government officials had sought (or would seek) care at Mayo. See *Mayo Clinic and the White House*, DVD (Rochester, MN: Mayo Foundation, 2006).

25. "President Reaches City; Son James Operated On," *Rochester Post-Bulletin*, September 11, 1938, MCA.

26. "The Presidency," *Time*, September 19, 1938, 11. See also H. N. Dorris, "James Roosevelt Is Operated on When President Gets to Hospital," *New York Times*, September 12, 1938.

27. H. C. Habein to Whom It May Concern, June 21, 1939, published in B. H. Lerner, "The First Modern Patient: The Public Death of Lou Gehrig," in *When Illness Goes Public: Celebrity Patients and How We Look at Medicine* (Baltimore: Johns Hopkins University Press, 2006), 19–40. See also J. Eig, *Luckiest Man: The Life and Death of Lou Gehrig* (New York: Simon & Schuster, 2005), 295–311.

28. Roosevelt, "Address Broadcast from a Naval Base on the Pacific Coast to the Democratic National Convention in Chicago, July 20, 1944," in *Public Papers*, 201–206, quotation from 201–202. For a video of the convention that includes Roosevelt delivering portions of his speech, see http://www.criticalpast.com/video/65675023163_Franklin-Delano-Roosevelt_renominated-President_lasting-peace_Democratic-Convention.

29. S. I. Rosenman, *Working with Roosevelt* (New York: Harper & Brothers, 1952), 453.

30. S. Early to G. Tully, July 28, 1944, box 24, Tully folder, Early Collection, FDRL. An article in *Time* magazine reproduced two photographs of Roosevelt taken moments apart in October 1944. One showed him smiling broadly, but the other one showed him looking very tired. The writer explained: "Pictures of him smiling or tired were taken by all newspapers, and they made their selections according to their political sympathies." "The Campaign," *Time*, October 30, 1944, 11–14, quotation from 12.

31. G. Skadding to S. Early, August 2, 1944, box 33, folder: Pictures of the President, Good and Bad, Early Collection, FDRL. Skadding's photograph was published in "Roosevelt Nominated for Term IV," *Life*, July 31, 1944, 13.

32. "Roosevelt Nominated." The caption lists all but two individuals in the picture, one of whom was cardiologist Howard Bruenn. James Roosevelt's second wife, the former Romelle Schneider, was seated between him and the president. He had met her in 1938, when he was hospitalized at St. Mary's Hospital, where she worked as a nurse. They had been married in 1941 after the president's son and Betsey Cushing were divorced. See "Princely Prize for the Cinderella Nurse," [2 page newspaper article] *King Features Syndicate*, ca. March 1941, MCA. For a detailed summary of Roosevelt's trip to San Diego and the Pacific, see W. M. Rigdon, *Log of the President's Inspection Trip to the Pacific, July–August 1944* (Washington DC: White House, 1945). The document was restricted when it was issued on March 16, 1945, copy in the author's possession.

33. W. Trohan, "Disclose Heart Specialist Is with Roosevelt," *Chicago Tribune*, August 6, 1944. See also W. Trohan, *Political Animals: Memoirs of a Sentimental Cynic* (Garden City, NY: Doubleday, 1975); and L. Wendt, *Chicago Tribune: The Rise of a Great American Newspaper* (Chicago: Rand McNally, 1979). Trohan and Early were friends, which may help to explain why the Chicago reporter did not follow up his August 6 story. When Trohan thanked Early for his 1943 Christmas card, he told the president's press secretary: "I shall always treasure your friendship and stand ready to do you any service I can." W. Trohan to S. Early, December 29, 1943, box 20, Trohan folder, Early Collection, FDRL.

34. An overview of the war, arranged by topic, is I. C. B. Dear and M. R. D. Foot, eds., *The Oxford Companion to the Second World War* (New York: Oxford University Press, 1995). See also D. K. Goodwin, *No Ordinary Time: Franklin and Eleanor Roosevelt, The Home Front in World War II* (New York: Simon & Schuster, 1994), 401–410.

35. Margaret "Daisy" Suckley, Diary entry for January 11, 1943, published in G. C. Ward, *Closest Companion: The Unknown Story of the Intimate Friendship Between Franklin Roosevelt and Margaret Suckley* (Boston: Houghton Mifflin, 1995), 196 (hereafter Ward, *Closest Companion*).

36. Harry Hopkins, Diary entry for January 11, 1943, quotation from R. E. Sherwood, *Roosevelt and Hopkins: An Intimate History* (New York: Harper, 1948), 671.

37. Hopkins, Diary entry for January 12, 1943, Sherwood, *Roosevelt and Hopkins*, 672.

38. R. L. Levy, A. L. Barach, and H. G. Bruenn, "Effects of Induced Oxygen Want in Patients with Cardiac Pain," *Am. Heart J.*, 1938, *15*: 187–200, quotation from 198. An editorial, citing Mayo Clinic research, included a more general warning: "Passengers who are suffering from certain cardio-respiratory difficulties…can experience serious, sometimes even dangerous, symptoms from flying at altitudes of 5000 feet or even less, unless they are protected by efficient administration of oxygen." Anon., "Recent Developments in Use and Administration of Oxygen in Aviation and Therapeutics," *Ann. Intern. Med.* 1939, *12*: 560–563.

39. Roosevelt to Suckley, January 14, 1943, Ward, *Closest Companion*, 198.

40. Roosevelt to Laura Delano, Washington, January 14, 1944, in *F.D.R.: His Personal Letters. 1928–1945*, ed. Elliott Roosevelt (New York: Duell, Sloan and Pearce, 1950), 1483. For Suckley's firsthand observations of his flu, see Ward, *Closest Companion*, 265–273. Steve Early discussed Roosevelt's flu and the restrictions that White House physician Ross McIntire placed on him at several of his press conferences in January 1944. See Early Press Conferences, January–June 1944, Early Collection, FDRL.

41. For Suckley's description of the trip to the hospital, see Ward, *Closest Companion*, 275–276. Anna Roosevelt Boettiger's son wrote a biography of his parents: J. R. Boettiger, *A Love in Shadow* (New York: W. W. Norton, 1978).

42. Roosevelt, "Press Conference of 4 February 1944," in *Complete Presidential Press Conferences of Franklin D. Roosevelt*, vols. 23, 24, and 25 [in one], (New York: Da Capo, 1972), 17–22.

43. John William Pender, Video Interview by Elliott V. Miller, September 22, 1983, *Living History of Anesthesia*, part 1 (Park Ridge, IL: Wood Library-Museum of Anesthesiology, 1983), DVD.

44. W. M. Craig, "History of the Development of the Section of Neurologic Surgery at the Mayo Clinic. Appendix C. Some Wartime Experiences With Famous Patients: President F. D. Roosevelt," August 1958, typescript, MCA. For plastic surgeon George Webster's recollections of the operation, see Goldsmith, *Conspiracy of Silence*, 50–54.

45. W. M. Craig, "Essential Hypertension: The Selection of Cases and Results Obtained by Subdiaphragmatic Sympathectomy," *Surgery*, 1938, *13*: 502–509, quotation from 502.

46. Suckley, Diary entry for February 2, 1944, Ward, *Closest Companion*, 275–276.

47. For correspondence between Suckley and Anna Roosevelt Boettiger about the president's health at this time, see Ward, *Closest Companion*, 284–289.

48. Roosevelt, "Press Conference of 24 March 1944," in *Press Conferences*, 109–118. Three days earlier, Steve Early had informed the press that McIntire was treating Roosevelt for a "head cold" and that the president was "sneezing through the night [and] not resting too well." Early Press Conference, March 21, 1944, Early Collection, FDRL.

49. Roosevelt, "Press Conference of 28 March 1944," in *Press Conferences*, 119–120.

50. H. G. Bruenn, "Clinical Notes on the Illness and Death of President Franklin D. Roosevelt," *Ann. Intern. Med.*, 1970, *72*: 579–591, esp. 579–581. For an analysis of the dynamics leading to Bruenn's publication, see B. H. Lerner, "Crafting Medical History: Revisiting the 'Definitive' Account of Franklin D. Roosevelt's Terminal Illness," *Bull. Hist. Med.*, 2007, *81*: 386–406. Lerner discusses former Mayo cardiologist Howard Burchell's 1970 editorial on Bruenn's article, but he does not mention that Burchell was a protégé of Arlie Barnes. Burchell, who was a member of Barnes's medical section, was stationed in England in 1944 and 1945. See H. B. Burchell, "Minuscule Review: H. G. Bruenn: Clinical Notes on the Illness and Death of President Franklin D. Roosevelt," *Circulation*, 1970, *41*: 966; and W. C. Roberts, "Howard Bertram Burchell, MD: A Conversation with the Editor," *Am. J. Cardiol.*, 1998, *81*: 1187–1195.

51. H. E. B. Pardee, *Clinical Aspects of the Electrocardiogram*, 4th ed. (New York: Paul B. Hoeber, 1941), 171.

52. Bruenn, "Clinical Notes," 580–582. For contemporary perspectives on the disorders that Bruenn diagnosed, see W. Goldring and H. Chasis, *Hypertension and Hypertensive Disease* (New York: Commonwealth Fund, 1944); and A. M. Fishberg, *Heart Failure*, 2nd ed. (Philadelphia: Lea & Febiger, 1940). See also M. Moser, *Myths, Misconceptions, and Heroics: The Story of the Treatment of Hypertension from the 1930s* (Greenwich, CT: Le Jacq, 1997). William Hassett, Roosevelt's personal secretary, noted in his diary that the president had bronchitis and a fever. See W. D. Hassett, *Off the Record with F.D.R., 1942–1945* (New Brunswick, NJ: Rutgers University Press, 1958), 239–241.

53. Suckley, Diary entry for March 28, 1944, Ward, *Closest Companion*, 288–289.

54. Suckley, Diary entry for April 4, 1944, Ward, *Closest Companion*, 290–291.

55. Bruenn, "Clinical Notes," 581–582. See also M. E. Silverman and J. W. Hurst, "James Edgar Paullin: Internist to Franklin Delano Roosevelt, Oslerian, and Forgotten Leader of American Medicine," *Ann. Intern. Med.*, 2001, *134*: 428–431. See also a handwritten digitalis dosing schedule on White House Stationery, March 31, 1944, container 66, FDR medical treatment 1944, Anna Halsted Collection, FDRL; and D. Luten, *The Clinical Use of Digitalis* (Springfield, IL: Charles C Thomas, 1936). The day after Paullin and Lahey examined Roosevelt at the White House, Early told the press that the president was "doing nicely. He is working right along over at the [White] House." Early Press Conference, March 21, 1944, Early Collection, FDRL.

56. Ross McIntire, participating in Early Press Conference, April 4, 1944, Early Collection, FDRL.

57. T. J. Dry, "Congestive Heart Failure: Factors Influencing the Ultimate Prognosis," *JAMA*, 1942, *118*: 263–266, quotation from 266.

58. Ibid.

59. Early Press Conference, March 21, 1944, Early Collection, FDRL. See also C. B. Swisher, Joseph B. Eastman: Public Servant," *Public Admin. Rev.*, 1945, *5*: 34–54.

60. Early read Roosevelt's letter to Eastman to the press. Early Press Conference, March 21, 1944, Early Collection, FDRL.

61. E. V. Allen, "Medical Aspects of Arterial Hypertension," *Bull. N. Y. Acad. Med.*, 1941, *17*: 174–186, quotations from 177 and 175. The definition and significance of hypertension was debated, however, as explained by Allen's protégé Ray Gifford. See R. W. Gifford Jr., "Three Decades of Antihypertensive Therapy," *Clin. Pharmacol. Ther.*, 1980, *28*: 1–5. See also R. W. Piepho and J. Beal, "An Overview of Antihypertensive Therapy in the 20th Century," *J. Clin. Pharmacol.*, 2000, *40*: 967–977.

62. Ferrell, "President Roosevelt's Blood Pressures," in *Dying President*, 153–156.

63. E. A. Hines Jr., "The Background and Treatment of Hypertensive Disease," *J. South. Med. Surg.*, 1941, *103*: 301–306, quotation from 305.

64. P. D. White, *Heart Disease*, 3rd ed. (New York: Macmillan, 1944), 429. Henry Christian, a prominent Boston internist-cardiologist, warned that "a diastolic pressure maintained above 100 mm. Hg. is apt to soon cause important damage to heart and arteries." H. A. Christian, *The Principles and Practice of Medicine*, 14th ed. (New York: Appleton-Century, 1942), 1128.

65. Allen, "Arterial Hypertension," 182.

66. Early Press Conference, April 10, 1944, Early Collection, FDRL.

67. S. Early to R. McIntire, April 15, 1944, telegram, box 15, Eleanor Roosevelt, Early Collection, FDRL. For Baruch's relationship with Roosevelt, see B. M. Baruch, *Baruch: The Public Years* (New York: Holt, Rinehart and Winston, 1960). See also L. G. Brockington, *Plantation Between the Waters: A Brief History of Hobcaw Barony* (Charleston, SC: History Press, 2006).

68. Roosevelt, "Press Conference of 28 April 1944," in *Press Conferences*, 137–138.

69. S. Shalett, "Final Tribute Paid to Secretary Knox," *New York Times*, May 2, 1944.

70. M. Smith, *Thank You, Mr. President: A White House Notebook* (New York: Harper & Brothers, 1946), 141.

71. Bruenn, "Clinical Notes," 583.

72. Roosevelt to Suckley, ca. April 25, 1944, published in Ward, *Closest Companion*, 295.

73. Suckley, Diary entry for May 5, 1944, Ward, *Closest Companion*, 296–297, emphasis in the original.

74. Roosevelt to M. Quezon, Washington, July 16, 1943, in *F.D.R. Personal Letters*, 1435. See also T. Dormandy, *The White Death: A History of Tuberculosis* (New York: New York University Press, 2000), 173–186.

75. Roosevelt, "Statement and Messages Hailing the Landing of American Troops in the Philippines. October 20, 1944," in *Public Papers*, 337–341, quotation from 338.

76. Roosevelt to H. Hopkins, May 18, 1944, published in Sherwood, *Roosevelt and Hopkins*, 6–8. For Hopkins's illness and its treatment at the Mayo Clinic, see J. A. Halsted, "Severe Malnutrition in a Public Servant of the World War II Era: The Medical History of Harry Hopkins," *Trans. Am. Clin. Climatol. Assoc.*, 1975, *86*: 23–32. Halsted, a physician, was Anna Roosevelt's third husband. See also Sherwood, *Roosevelt and Hopkins*, 92–93, 119–122, 804, 874–876.

77. R. Wilson and W. Mylander, "The President's Job—Biggest in the World," *Look*, July 25, 1944, 21–27.

78. Roosevelt, "The 954th Press Conference: D-Day (Excerpts) June 6, 1944," in *Public Papers*, 154–160, quotation from 160. See also S. E. Ambrose, *D-Day June 6, 1944: The Climactic Battle of World War II* (New York: Simon & Schuster, 1995).

79. Ross McIntire, participating in Early Press Conference, June 8, 1944, Early Collection, FDRL.

80. Ibid.

81. C. Hurd, "President's Health 'Excellent,' Admiral McIntire Reports," *New York Times*, June 9 1944.

82. The average blood pressure was calculated from a complete listing of measurements published in Ferrell, "President Roosevelt's Blood Pressures."

83. Frank H. Lahey, Typewritten memo, July 10, 1944, reproduced in Weintraub, *Final Victory*, 51. Lahey explained that the memo was placed in safe keeping, "to be opened and utilized only in the event that there might be criticism of me should this later eventuate [i.e., should Roosevelt die in office] and the criticism be directed toward me for not having made this public." For details of the memo's long-delayed release, see Goldsmith, *Conspiracy of Silence*, 118–173. Lahey had also seen Roosevelt in May 1944, after the president developed symptoms of gall bladder disease. An X-ray text revealed cholesterol gallstones, and the president was placed on a low-fat diet. See Bruenn, "Clinical Notes," 584. For McIntire's account, see R. T. McIntire, *White House Physician* (New York: G. P. Putnam's Sons, 1946), 186–188.

84. See Dry, "Congestive Heart Failure;" and N. M. Keith, H. P. Wagener, and N. W. Barker, "Some Different Types of Essential Hypertension: Their Course and Prognosis," *Am. J. Med. Sci.*, 1939, *197*: 332–343.

85. Roosevelt, "Radio Address at Puget Sound Navy Yard, Bremerton, Washington, August 12, 1944," in *Public Papers*, 216–228.

86. G. Tully, *F.D.R. My Boss* (New York: Charles Scribner's Sons, 1949), 278. Samuel Rosenman described the speech as a "dismal failure." Rosenman, *Working with Roosevelt*, 462.

87. Bruenn, "Clinical Notes," 586, 591.

88. J. K. Herman, "The President's Cardiologist," *Navy Med.*, March–April 1990, 6–13, quotation from 9. This article is based on an interview of Bruenn ca. 1989.

89. Rigdon, *Log of the President's Inspection Trip*, 44. See also W. M. Rigdon and J. Derieux, *White House Sailor* (Garden City, NY: Doubleday, 1962), 129–132.

90. R. L. Levy, H. G. Bruenn, and D. Kurtz, "Facts on Coronary Artery Disease, Based on a Survey of the Clinical and Pathological Records of 762 Cases," *Trans. Am. Clin. Climatol. Assoc.*, 1933, *49*: 67–76, quotation from 67.

91. H. W. Baldwin, "Theodore Roosevelt, 56, Dies on Normandy Battlefield," *New York Times*, July 13, 1944. See also H. P. Jeffers, *Theodore Roosevelt Jr.: The Life of a War Hero* (Novato, CA: Presidio Press, 2002), 261–264.

92. Bruenn, "Clinical Notes," 587.

93. Suckley, Diary entry for September 17, 1944, Ward, *Closest Companion*, 326–327, emphasis in the original.

94. Roosevelt, "Joint Press Conference of the President, Prime Minister Churchill, and Prime Minister Mackenzie (Excerpts). Quebec, Canada. September 16, 1944," in *Public Papers*, 260–270, quotation from 261.

95. Suckley, Diary entry for September 20, 1944, Ward, *Closest Companion*, 327–328.

96. Jordan, *Election of 1944*, 268. See also G. J. White, *FDR and the Press* (Chicago: University of Chicago Press, 1979), 69–91.

97. "The Election III: Why Dewey Deserves the Independent Vote," *Life*, October 16, 1944, 34.

98. "Nation Mourns Death of Wendell Willkie," *Sarasota Herald-Tribune*, October 9, 1944. For Willkie and the 1940 election, see S. Dunn, *1940: FDR, Willkie, Lindbergh, Hitler—the Election amid the Storm* (New Haven, CT: Yale University Press, 2013); and R. Moe, *Roosevelt's Second Act: The Election of 1940 and the Politics of War* (New York: Oxford University Press, 2013). For a study of the 1940 campaign by Columbia University social scientists, see P. F. Lazarsfeld, B. Berelson, and H. Gaudet, *The People's Choice: How the Voter Makes Up His Mind in a Presidential Campaign* (New York: Duell, Sloan and Pearce, 1944).

99. W. Willkie to Mary Sleeth, September 1944, quotation from E. Barnard, *Wendell Willkie: Fighter for Freedom* (Marquette: Northern Michigan University Press, 1966), 494.

100. Barnard, *Wendell Willkie*, 494. For his heart disease and and death, see 494–499.

101. "Mr. Roosevelt's Health," *Chicago Tribune*, October 17, 1944.

102. "Both Parties Woo Key Cities in Final Drives of Campaign," *Newsweek*, October 23, 1944, 40–45, quotations from 40 and 45.

103. "He's Perfectly O.K.," *Time*, October 23, 1944, 17–18.

104. Winfield, *FDR and the News Media*, 216–229.

105. W. Mylander, "F.D.R. Hopes Trip Will End Health Tales," *Des Moines Register*, October 21, 1944, emphasis in the original, clipping in S. Early Scrapbook, August 1, 1944, to January 20, 1945, Early Collection, FDRL.

106. "Roosevelt: He Makes a Personal Tour of New York in Blustering Rain," *Life*, October 30, 1944, 23.

107. Sinclair Lewis, CBS Radio Address, November 1, 1944, quotation from Jordan, *Election of 1944*, 307–308.

108. Roosevelt, "Campaign Radio Address from the White House, November 2, 1944," in *Public Papers*, 383–388.

109. "Stephen Early's Sister in City: Widow of Newsman Undergoes Surgery," *Rochester Post-Bulletin*, October 21, 1944, clipping in S. Early Scrapbook, August 1, 1944, to January 20, 1945, Early Collection, FDRL.

110. Roosevelt to Breckinridge Long, February 22, 1936, in *F.D.R. Personal Letters*, 560.

111. Long, Diary entry for July 25, 1944, published in F. L. Israel, ed., *The War Diary of Breckinridge Long: Selections from the Years 1939–1944* (Lincoln: University of Nebraska Press, 1966), 367–370. Long had surgery at Mayo in 1936. Ibid., xxiii, 145, 314.

112. Long, Diary entry for November 3, 1940, Israel, ed., *War Diary*, 145.

113. Long, Diary entry for July 13, 1944, Israel, ed., *War Diary*, 364–366.

114. Long, Diary entry for July 25, 1944, Israel, ed., *War Diary*, 367–370. See also R. H. Ferrell, *Choosing Truman: The Democratic Convention of 1944* (Columbia: University of Missouri Press, 1994).

115. Long, Diary entry for July 25, 1944, Israel, ed., *War Diary*, 367–370.

116. "Memorandum Re: Circulation of Story Alleging the President Has a Serious Heart Affliction," October 29, 1944, with J. E. Hoover to S. Early, November 1, 1944, FDR corres. and White House Matters, McIntire Collection, FDRL. See also H. M. Weber, "Byrl Raymond Kirklin, M.D., 1888–1957," *Am. J. Roentgenol. Radium Ther. Nucl. Med.*, 1957, *78*: 906–910; and H. Harwick, *Forty-four Years with the Mayo Clinic* (Rochester, MN: Whiting Press, 1957).

117. Roosevelt, "Peace, Like War, Can Succeed Only Where There Is a Will to Enforce It, and Where There Is Available Power to Enforce It—Radio Address at Dinner of Foreign Policy Association, New York, N.Y. October 21, 1944 in *Public Papers*, 342–354. In this speech, Roosevelt reiterated his commitment to the creation of the United Nations.

118. "President Has a Serious Heart Affliction." Authors who have described the FBI investigation include Crispell and Gomez, *Hidden Illness*, 110–113; Ferrell, *Dying President*, 86–88; Goldsmith, *Conspiracy of Silence*, 45–46, 75–86; and Lomazov and Fettmann, *FDR's Deadly Secret*, 135–139.

119. "President Has a Serious Heart Affliction." For recollections of the FBI agents who interviewed Barnes and Kirklin, see Goldsmith, *Conspiracy of Silence*, 75–86.

120. "President Has a Serious Heart Affliction." See also B. Stuhler, "A Minnesota Footnote to the 1944 Presidential Election, Summer 1990," *Minn. Hist.*, 1990, 27–34. This article focuses on Harold Knutson, a Republican member of the House of Representatives, who started the rumor that Roosevelt's Scottish terrier Fala had been left behind when he visited the Aleutian Islands and that a naval destroyer had been sent to retrieve the dog. The president used this story in his speech to the Teamster's Union on September 23, 1944. In contrast to Roosevelt's Bremerton, Washington, speech (during which he got severe chest pain), he delivered the Teamster's speech flawlessly. Suckley, who had given Fala to Roosevelt, wrote in her diary: "He never spoke with more 'pep' and humor—A few speeches like that and we won't worry about the results of the election on Nov. 7th." Suckley, Diary entry for September 25, 1944, Ward, *Closest Companion*,

328–329. Daisy, like Steve Early and other White House insiders, knew that public perceptions mattered and influenced how individuals voted.

121. "President Has a Serious Heart Affliction."

122. Ibid.

123. Ibid. Howard Odel, a recognized heart expert in his own right, lectured on coronary artery disease and its complications to members of the Medical Society of the District of Columbia on October 4, 1944 (less than a month before the FBI interrogated him). H. M. Odel, "The Future of Our Coronaries," *Med. Ann. DC*, 1945, *14*: 57–62.

124. Hoover to Early, November 1, 1944.

125. See C. Gentry, *J. Edgar Hoover: The Man and His Secrets* (New York: W. W. Norton, 1991), 181, 225–238.

126. "Dewey Will Restore Responsible Rule," *Saturday Evening Post*, November 4, 1944, 112.

127. Jordan, *Election of 1944*, 321.

128. "Postelection: The Scoreboard, Studying Figures Shows How Election was Won and Playing Game with Them Shows How Results Could Be Reversed," *Life*, November 20, 1944, 24–25.

129. Jordan, *Election of 1944*, 329.

130. Bruenn, "Clinical Notes," 587.

131. Suckley, Diary entry for November 29, 1944, Ward, *Closest Companion*, 347–349.

132. Suckley, Diary entry for December 15, 1944, Ward, *Closest Companion*, 361–364.

133. Suckley, Diary entry for December 19, 1944, Ward, *Closest Companion*, 366–367, emphasis in the original.

134. Anna R. Boettiger to John Boettiger, February 4, 1945, quotation from Lomazow and Fettmann, *FDR's Deadly Secret*, 164. See also S. M. Plokhy, *Yalta: The Price of Peace* (New York: Viking, 2010). For Bruenn's concerns at Yalta, see his "Clinical Notes," 588–589.

135. Roosevelt to F. Murphy, Washington, April 9, 1945, in *F.D.R. Personal Letters*, 1581.

136. "Here's Ailment Which Killed the President," *Chicago Tribune*, April 13, 1945.

137. White, *Heart Disease*, 444.

138. For a photocopy of Roosevelt's death certificate, see Evans, *Hidden Campaign*, 135. See also W. S. Fields and N. A. Lemak, *A History of Stroke: Its Recognition and Treatment* (New York: Oxford University Press, 1989).

139. "Everybody Knew It but the People," *Saturday Evening Post*, May 19, 1945, 108. See also Ferrell, *Choosing Truman*; and D. McCullough, *Truman* (New York: Simon & Schuster, 1992), 292–324.

140. "Everybody Knew It but the People."

141. McIntire, *White House Physician*, 239.

142. Keith, Wagener, and Barker, "Essential Hypertension." See also H. Chasis, "Appreciation of the Keith, Wagener, and Barker Classification of Hypertensive Disease," *Am. J. Med. Sci.*, 1974, *268*: 347–351; and R. B. Singer, F.D.R.'s Fatal Stroke, Mortality in Severe Hypertension, 1944–45," *J. Insurance Med.* 1996, *27*: 294–304.

143. E. Roosevelt, *This I Remember* (New York: Harper & Brothers, 1949), 328–329. Eight days after her husband died, Eleanor wrote to Steve Early: "You and I have been 'fellow-travellers' since 1920, and you've always been loyal and kind. Franklin loved you, and I am deeply grateful to you and have a deep and abiding trust and affection for you." E. Roosevelt to S. Early, April 20, 1945, box 15, folder Eleanor Roosevelt, Early Collection, FDRL.

144. McIntire, *White House Physician*, 58, 67. McIntire wrote to Bruenn when the cardiologist left the Navy to resume his practice in New York City: "I have nothing but the highest praise for the manner in which you conducted yourself and for the meticulous care that you gave to his case. It is a pity that there is not some way that we would know when the cerebral arteries are going to go bad, for it is my belief that without that disaster we could have carried him on over a long period of time." R. McIntire to H. Bruenn, February 18, 1946, box 2,

corres. A-B, 1939–1946, McIntire Collection, FDRL. McIntire did not mention cancer, and he knew that Bruenn was aware of all of Roosevelt's health problems. Surgeon Frank Lahey, in his secret memorandum of August 1944, expressed concern about the president's hypertension and his episode of heart failure, but he did not mention cancer. See note 83. In 1949 the president's daughter Anna and son Elliott published separate articles refuting various claims about Roosevelt's health made by Minneapolis doctor Karl Wold (who never cared for the president and had no affiliation with the Mayo Clinic). See K. C. Wold, *Mr. President: How Is Your Health?* (St. Paul, MN: 1948); K. C. Wold, "The Truth about F.D.R.'s Health," *Look*, February 15, 1949, 23–29; A. Roosevelt, "My Life with F.D.R.: Part 1, The Real Truth about My Father's Health," *The Woman*, May 1949, 6–16, 112–113; and E. Roosevelt, "They're Lying about F.D.R.'s Health," *Liberty*, May 1949, 18, 73–76. See also Lerner, "Crafting Medical History," 389–391.

Chapter 8

1. The definitive summary is E. C. Andrus, D. W. Bronk, G. A. Carden Jr., C. S. Keefer, J. S. Lockwood, J. T. Wearn et al., eds., *Advances in Military Medicine Made by American Investigators Working under the Sponsorship of the Committee on Medical Research*, 2 vols. (Boston: Little, Brown, 1948). See also M. Fishbein, ed., *Doctors at War* (New York: E. P. Dutton, 1945).

2. P. Neushul, "Fighting Research: Army Participation in the Clinical Testing and Mass Production of Penicillin during the Second World War," in *War, Medicine and Modernity*, ed. R. Cooter, M. Harrison, and S. Sturdy (Phoenix Mill, England: Sutton, 1998), 203–224. Wallace Herrell and his colleagues at Mayo were among the first to study the use of penicillin in patients. See W. B. Herrell, *Penicillin and Other Antibiotic Agents* (Philadelphia: W. B. Saunders, 1945). See also D. Greenwood, *Antimicrobial Drugs: Chronicle of a Twentieth-Century Medical Triumph* (New York: Oxford University Press, 2008), 85–113; and P. C. English, *Rheumatic Fever in America and Britain: A Biological, Epidemiological, and Medical History* (New Brunswick, NJ: Rutgers University Press, 2004).

3. F. D. Roosevelt to V. Bush, November 17, 1944, published in V. Bush, *Science: The Endless Frontier* (Washington, DC: Government Printing Office, 1945), vii–viii. See also G. P. Zachary, *Endless Frontier: Vannevar Bush, Engineer of the American Century* (New York: Free Press, 2007).

4. Roosevelt to Bush, November 17, 1944.

5. Bush, *Science: The Endless Frontier*.

6. W. W. Palmer, Appendix 2. "Report of the Medical Advisory Committee," in Bush, *Science: The Endless Frontier*, 40–64, quotation from 43–44. For background on federal research funding, see V. A. Harden, *Inventing the NIH: Federal Biomedical Research Policy, 1887–1937* (Baltimore: Johns Hopkins University Press, 1986); S. P. Strickland, *Politics, Science, and Dread Disease: A Short History of United States Medical Research Policy* (Cambridge, MA: Harvard University Press, 1972); D. M. Fox, "The Politics of the NIH Extramural Program, 1937–1950," *J. Hist. Med. Allied Sci.*, 1987, *42*: 447–466; T. A. Appel, *Shaping Biology: The National Science Foundation and American Biological Research, 1945–1975* (Baltimore: Johns Hopkins University Press, 2000), 9–37; and G. B. Mider, "The Federal Impact on Biomedical Research," in *Advances in American Medicine: Essays at the Bicentennial*, ed. J. Z. Bowers and E. F. Purcell (New York: Josiah H. Macy Jr. Foundation, 1976), 806–871.

7. For changes in the philosophy, structure, and activities of the AHA in the late 1930s and 1940s, see W. B. Fye, *American Cardiology: The History of a Specialty and Its College* (Baltimore: Johns Hopkins University Press, 1996), 85–111.

8. S. M. Gunn and P. S. Platt, *Voluntary Health Agencies: An Interpretive Study* (New York: Ronald Press, 1945), 218–219.

9. For Roosevelt and polio, see H. G. Gallagher, *FDR's Splendid Deception* (New York: Dodd, Mead, 1985). See also R. H. Berg, *The Challenge of Polio: The Crusade Against Infantile Paralysis*

(New York: Dial Press, 1946); and D. M. Oshinsky, *Polio: An American Story* (New York: Oxford University Press, 2005), 43–60.

10. See J. T. Patterson, *The Dread Disease: Cancer and Modern American Culture* (Cambridge, MA: Harvard University Press, 1987), 114–136; D. Cantor, ed., *Cancer in the Twentieth Century* (Baltimore: Johns Hopkins University Press, 2008); and S. Mukherjee, *The Emperor of All Maladies: A Biography of Cancer* (New York: Scribner, 2010); 107–122.

11. H. B. Sprague, "A General Program for the American Heart Association Prepared by the Committee on Activities," [ca. March 1941], Howard Sprague Papers, Boston Medical Library in the Francis A. Countway Library of Medicine, Boston, MA.

12. H. M. Marvin to AHA EC, July 22, 1942, AHA History 1940s, American Heart Association National Center Corporate Records (hereafter AHA Archives).

13. H. M. Marvin, "Memorandum to the American Heart Association Board of Directors," September 26, 1945, Paul Dudley White Papers, Harvard Medical Library in the Francis A. Countway Library of Medicine, Boston, MA.

14. Minutes, AHA Board of Directors, June 28, 1946, AHA Archives.

15. "Mayo Clinic Official Named to Head Heart Association," *New York Times*, June 7, 1947.

16. W. L. Laurence, "Doctors Advocate U.S. Heart Institute," *New York Times*, June 9, 1947. The testimony provides insight into the Javits Bill and the context. *US Congress, Senate, National Heart Institute. Hearings on S. 720 and S. 2215 before a Subcommittee of the Committee on Labor and Public Welfare, 80th Cong., 2d sess. April 8–9, 1948.* (Washington, DC: Government Printing Office, 1948).

17. M. Ford, "Happy to Pay Taxes, Says $22,500 Winner," March 8, 1948. Newspaper clipping. Record group 450 C661-U, box 14, file 30, Cohn Papers, Rockefeller Archive Center.

18. M. Frederick Arkus to Arlie Barnes, November 4, 1957 [with script of Ralph Edwards's remarks at an AHA dinner], Barnes Papers, Mayo Clinic Archives, Mayo Historical Unit, Rochester, MN (hereafter MCA).

19. A.R. Barnes to Dear Doctor, May 19, 1948, AHA History 1940s, folder 2, AHA Archives. See also *Scientific Council of the American Heart Association* [May 1948], Pamphlet, AHA Archives; and *A History of the Scientific Councils of the American Heart Association* (New York: American Heart Association, 1965). For tensions surrounding the creation of the Scientific Council, see Fye, *American Cardiology*, 118–121.

20. Charles A. R. Connor to John J. Sampson, June 1, 1948 [with two attached lists]: "Cardiovascular Disease: Candidates Certified in Cardiovascular Disease to September 8, 1947" and "American Heart Association, Inc. Names Proposed for the Scientific Council." AHA History 1940s, folder 2, AHA Archives. For individuals who presented papers at the 1948 annual meeting, see *Am. Heart J.*, 1948, *35*: 687–688.

21. Congress passed a bill in 1930 that renamed the Hygienic Laboratory of the Public Health Service the National Institute of Health. Seven years later it passed another bill that created the National Cancer Institute. When Congress created the National Heart Institute in 1948, the National Institute of Health became the National Institutes of Health. See Harden, *Inventing the NIH*, 138–175; and Strickland, *Politics, Science, and Dread Disease*, 32–54. For Van Slyke's illness and appointment, see S. P. Strickland, *The Story of the NIH Grants Program* (Lanham, MD: University Press of America, 1989), 21–27. See also R. Mandel, "Mandate for Biomedical Research: The Awards Experience, 1945–1950," in *A Half Century of Peer Review, 1946–1996* (Bethesda, MD: Division of Research Grants, NIH, 1996), 15–49.

22. C. J. Van Slyke, "New Horizons in Medical Research," *Science*, 1946, *104*: 559–567, quotation from 561.

23. Minutes, MC BOG, October 8, 1947, MCA. See also H. E. Essex, "Heart," *Ann. Rev. Physiol.*, 1945, *7*: 405–426.

24. Thomas Parran to Hiram Essex, November 3, 1947, Essex collection, MCA. Parran, a 1915 Georgetown University medical graduate, recalled looking for an opportunity to do

research after his internship: "In those days there were only about three places in the country where a young physician could do proper research. One was Mayo Clinic which was quite new, another was the Rockefeller Institute, and the third was the Hygienic Laboratory of the Public Health Service, which was the antecedent of the present National Institutes of Health." Thomas Parran, interview by Harlan B. Phillips, July 16–18, 1962. George Rosen Public Health Oral History Collection, History of Medicine Division, National Library of Medicine, Bethesda, MD.

25. See J. P. Swann, *Academic Scientists and the Pharmaceutical Industry: Cooperative Research in Twentieth Century America* (Baltimore: Johns Hopkins University Press, 1988); and H. M. Marks, *The Progress of Experiment: Science and Therapeutic Reform in the United States, 1900–1990* (New York: Cambridge University Press, 1997).

26. "Basic Questions" [for the Survey of Cardiovascular Research, March 1948]. For an example of the letter Essex sent to medical school deans, see H. E. Essex to Maxwell Lapham, March 23, 1948. See also "Survey by Cardiovascular Study Section—NIH," May 28, 1948. Both in box 46, PHS-NIH CV Study Section 1948, George E. Burch Papers, MS C376, Modern Manuscripts Collection, History of Medicine Division, National Library of Medicine, Bethesda, MD.

27. *Senate, National Heart Institute Hearings*.

28. F. Donnell in *Senate. National Heart Institute Hearings*, quotations from 74–75.

29. A. R. Barnes in *Senate. National Heart Institute Hearings*, quotations from 74–75.

30. D. Rutstein in *Senate, National Heart Institute Hearings*, quotations from 83, 81, 79. See also "O. Zimmerman, 67, Long in Congress," *New York Times*, April 8, 1948.

31. *National Heart Institute Awards $11,000,000 in Grants to Aid Large-Scale Attack Against Heart Disease,* National Heart Institute Circular, No. 2, November 1949. Copy in the Rutstein Papers in the Francis A. Countway Library of Medicine, Boston, MA. This total does not include the support of intramural programs (at the NIH). See F. W. Reynolds and D. E. Price, "Federal Support of Medical Research Through the Public Health Service," *Am. Scientist*, 1949, *37*: 578–586; and E. T. Lanahan, *A Salute to the Past: A History of the National Heart, Lung, and Blood Institute Based on Personal Recollections* (Bethesda, MD: National Heart, Lung, and Blood Institute, 1987).

32. I. S. Wright, "Proposed Establishment of a Cardio-Vascular Institute or Division at Cornell University Medical College and the New York Hospital," [June 1948], box 2, misc. corres., Irving S. Wright Papers, Medical Center Archives, New York Presbyterian/Weill Cornell, New York.

33. S. F. Haines, "Report of the Research Administrative Committee of the Board of Governors to the Staff of the Mayo Clinic," November 21, 1949, MCA.

34. Ibid.

35. E. V. Allen, N. W. Barker, and E. A. Hines Jr., *Peripheral Vascular Diseases* (Philadelphia: W. B. Saunders, 1946).

36. Minutes, AHA EC, February 18, 1947, AHA Archives.

37. Minutes, AHA Board of Directors, June 8, 1947, AHA Archives.

38. Irvine Page of the Cleveland Clinic had founded the American Foundation for High Blood Pressure in 1945. Four years later it was incorporated into the AHA as the Council on High Blood Pressure Research. See *History of the Scientific Councils*, 15–20; and I. H. Page, *Hypertension Research: A Memoir, 1920–1960* (New York: Permagon, 1988).

39. H. M. Marvin, "Foreword," *Circulation*, 1950, *1*: 1.

40. B. W. Zweifach, "Peripheral Circulatory Changes as Criteria for Hemorrhagic Shock Therapy," *Circulation*, 1950, *1*: 433–444. See also C. J. Wiggers, *Physiology of Shock* (New York: Commonwealth Fund, 1950); P. C. English, *Shock, Physiological Surgery, and George Washington Crile: Medical Innovation in the Progessive Era* (Westport, CT: Greenwood, 1980); and R. A. Manji, K. E. Wood, and A. Kumar, "The History and Evolution of Circulatory Shock," *Crit. Care Med.*, 2009, *25*: 1–29.

41. W. T. Porter, *Shock at the Front* (Boston: Atlantic Monthly Press, 1918), 5. See also W. B. Fye, "William Townsend Porter," *Clin. Cardiol.* 1990, *13*: 585–587.

42. S. Benison, A. C. Barger, and E. L. Wolfe, "Walter B. Cannon and the Mystery of Shock: A Study of Anglo-American Co-operation in World War I," *Med. Hist.*, 1991, *35*: 217–249. See also W. B. Cannon, *Traumatic Shock* (New York: D. Appleton, 1923).

43. F. C. Mann and H. E. Essex, "The Present Status of the Problem of Traumatic Shock," *Am. J. Surg.*, 1935, *28*: 160–162, quotation from 160.

44. F. C. Mann, "Report of a European Trip," 1938, MCA. See also W. O. Fenn, ed., *History of the International Congresses of Physiological Sciences, 1889–1968* (Bethesda, MD: American Physiological Society, 1968).

45. R. A. Kilduffe and M. E. DeBakey, *The Blood Bank and the Technique and Therapeutics of Transfusions* (St. Louis: C. V. Mosby, 1942), 126–129.

46. E. A. Graham to A. Blalock, June 26, 1940, folder National Research Council, Blalock Papers, the Alan Mason Chesney Archives of the Johns Hopkins Medical Institutions (hereafter Blalock Papers). See also A. Blalock, *Principles of Surgical Care: Shock and Other Problems* (St. Louis: C. V. Mosby, 1940); and N. K. Chambers and T. G. Buchman, "Shock at the Millennium: 1. Walter B. Cannon and Alfred Blalock," *Shock*, 2000, *13*: 497–504.

47. A. Cournand and H. A. Ranges, "Catheterization of the Right Auricle in Man," *Proc. Soc. Exp. Biol. Med.*, 1941, *46*: 462–466. See also W. Forssmann, *Experiments on Myself: Memoirs of a Surgeon in Germany* (New York: Saint Martin's Press, 1974); A. Cournand, "Cardiac Catheterization: Development of the Technique, Its Contributions to Experimental Medicine, and Its Initial Applications in Man," *Acta. Med. Scand.*, 1975, *Suppl. 579*: 3–32; M. E. Bertrand, ed., *The Evolution of Cardiac Catheterization and Interventional Cardiology* (St. Albans, UK: Iatric Press and European Society of Cardiology, 2006); and T. Seed, "The Introduction of Cardiac Catheterization," in *Nobel Prizes That Changed Medicine*, ed. G. Thompson (London: Imperial College Press, 2012), 69–87. Several early papers on cardiac catheterization are reprinted in J. V. Warren, ed., *Cardiovascular Physiology* (Stroudsburg, PA: Dowden, Hutchinson & Ross, 1975).

48. A. Grollman, *The Cardiac Output of Man in Health and Disease* (Springfield, IL: Charles C Thomas, 1932), 10–11.

49. W. F. Hamilton and D. W. Richards, "The Output of the Heart," in *Circulation of the Blood: Men and Ideas*, ed. A. P. Fishman and D. W. Richards (New York: Oxford University Press, 1964), 71–126.

50. Cournand and Ranges, "Catheterization of the Right Auricle in Man."

51. A. Blalock to D. W. Richards, November 12, 1941, folder National Research Council, Blalock Papers.

52. D. W. Richards to A. Blalock, November 24, 1941, folder National Research Council, Blalock Papers.

53. H. W. Smith to A. Blalock, November 14, 1941, folder National Research Council, Blalock Papers.

54. D. W. Richards, "The Contributions of Right Heart Catheterization to Physiology and Medicine, with Some Observations on the Physiopathology of Pulmonary Heart Disease," in *Les Prix Nobel en 1956* (Stockholm: Norstedt & Söner, 1957), 182–195, quotation from 185.

55. "Aviation Medicine Laboratory Opened at Mayo Clinic," *Science News Letter*, May 6, 1939, 279. See also M. P. Mackowski, *Testing the Limits: Aviation Medicine and the Origins of Manned Space Flight* (College Station: Texas A&M University Press, 2006).

56. W. R. Lovelace II, "Oxygen for Therapy and Aviation: An Apparatus for the Administration of Oxygen or Oxygen and Helium by Inhalation," *Proceedings of the Staff Meetings of the Mayo Clinic* (hereafter *PSMMC*), 1938, *13*: 646–654. See also W. M. Boothby, "Oxygen Administration: The Value of High Concentration of Oxygen for Therapy," *PSMMC*, 1938, *13*: 641–646; L. D. Vandam, "Walter M. Boothby, MD: The Wellspring of Anesthesiology,"

N. Engl. J. Med., 1967, *276*: 558–563; R. G. Elliott, "'On a Comet, Always': A Biography of Dr. W. Randolph Lovelace II," *New Mexico Quart.*, 1966, *35*: 351–388; and J. Stepanek, "Aviation Medicine at Mayo," *Minn. Med.*, 2003, *86*: 44–46.

57. W. M. Boothby, E. J. Baldes, and C. F. Code, "The Mayo Aero Medical Unit, Rochester, Minnesota: Final Report Including a Brief History…and Complete Bibliography for Both the High Altitude and Acceleration Laboratories," June 15, 1946, MCA.

58. "Rochester Scientists Awarded Collier Trophy, Aviation's Highest Honor," *Rochester Post-Bulletin*, November 15, 1940, MCA. See also W. M. Boothby, A. H. Bulbulian, and W. R. Lovelace II, "B-L-B Oxygen Masks: Stages in Its Development," ca. 1940, MCA.

59. Minutes, MC BOG, April 16, 1941, MCA. See also W. J. Boyne, *Beyond the Horizons: The Lockheed Story* (New York: St. Martin's Press, 1998), 88–129.

60. See E. H. Wood, "Charlie Code: Reminiscences," *Mayo Clin. Proc.*, 1975, *50*: 476–506; C. Kopp, "Interview with Charles F. Code," *Cure News*, June 1980, *2*: 1–3, MCA; and C. F. Code, "Critical Issues in the Development of Research at Mayo," September 15, 1995, MCA.

61. I. C. B. Dear, and M. R. D. Foot, eds., *The Oxford Companion to the Second World War* (New York: Oxford University Press, 1995).

62. F. D. Roosevelt, "'December 7, 1941—A Date Which Will Live in Infamy'—Address to the Congress Asking That a State of War Be Declared Between the United States and Japan. December 8, 1941," in *The Public Papers and Addresses of Franklin D. Roosevelt…1941 volume*, ed. S. I. Rosenman (New York: Harper, 1950), 514–516.

63. Code's report in MC BOG, 10 December 1941, MCA.

64. Ibid.

65. See W. C. Roberts, "Howard Bertram Burchell, MD: A Conversation with the Editor," *Am. J. Cardiol.*, 1998, *81*: 1187–1195.

66. The number of officers in the Medical Army Corps tripled to almost 36,000 during 1942. See table 1 in J. H. McGinn and M. Levin, *Medical Department, United States Army: Personnel in World War II* (Washington, DC: Office of the Surgeon General, 1963), 10.

67. M. B. Visscher to C. F. Code, May 19, 1942, box 8, Maurice B. Visscher Papers, University of Minnesota Archives, Minneapolis, MN (hereafter Visscher Papers). See also H. B. Burchell, "Earl H. Wood: Outstanding Twentieth Century Investigator of the Heart and Circulation," *Clin. Cardiology*, 1987, *10*: 372–374.

68. C. F. Code to M. B. Visscher, May 20, 1942, box 8, Visscher Papers. See also E. H. Wood, "Reminiscences and Thoughts concerning the Relationship and Evolution of Cardiovascular Physiology, Cardiology and Cardiac Surgery at Mayo from the 1940s to the Present," December 15, 1978, MCA.

69. See C. A. Lindbergh, *The Wartime Journals of Charles A. Lindbergh* (New York, 1970), 718–731; and Boothby, Baldes, and Code, "Mayo Aero Medical Unit."

70 See E. M. Landis, "The Effects of Acceleration and Their Amelioration," in *Advances in Military Medicine*, *1*: 232–260; E. Engle and A. S. Lott, *Man in Flight: Biomedical Achievements in Aerospace* (Annapolis, MD: Leeward, 1979), 217–230; and D. R. Jenkins, *Dressing for Altitude: U.S. Aviation Pressure Suits—Wiley Post to Space Shuttle* (Washington, DC: NASA, 2012), 71–119, 425–435.

71. C. F. Code, Report of the Section on Clinical Physiology to the MC BOG for 1943, MCA.

72. J. F. Fulton, "Effects of Acceleration: Dim-Out and Black-Out; Protective Measures," in *Aviation Medicine in Its Preventive Aspects* (New York: Oxford University Press, 1948), 119–150, quotation from 148.

73. Minutes, MC Laboratory and Research Committee, August 21, 1945, MCA. See also E. H. Wood, "Evolution of Instrumentation and Techniques for the Study of Cardiovascular Dynamics from the Thirties to 1980," *Ann. Biomed. Eng.*, 1978, *6*: 250–309; and Earl H. Wood, interview by W. B. Fye, Rochester, MN, February 5, 2001.

74. G. M. Roth, H. E. Essex, E. H. Wood, C. F. Code, E. H. Lambert, and F. C. Mann, [Proposal to Establish a Section on Physiology] with Minutes, MC BOG, September 26, 1945, MCA.

75. C. F. Code to M. B. Visscher, September 27, 1945, box 8, Visscher Papers. For Mayo's physiologists and their activities, see Code, Report of the Section of Physiology to the MC BOG for 1945, MCA.

76. G. L. Geison, "International Relations and Domestic Elites in American Physiology, 1900–1940," in *Physiology in the American Context, 1850–1940* (Bethesda, MD: American Physiological Society, 1987), 115–154, esp. tables 5 and 9. See also M. B. Visscher, "Frank Charles Mann," *Biogr. Mem. Nat. Acad. Sci.*, 1965, *38*: 161–204.

77. E. H. Wood, Untitled typescript beginning "At Dr. Balfour's request," February 5, 1946, MCA.

78. J. McMichael and E. P. Sharpey-Schafer, "Cardiac Output in Man by a Direct Fick Method: Effects of Posture, Venous Pressure Change, Atropine, and Adrenaline," *Br. Heart J.*, 1944, *6*: 33–40. See also J. McMichael, "Foreword," in *Cardiac Catheterization and Angiography*, ed. D. Verel and R. G. Grainger (Edinburgh: E. & S. Livingstone, 1969), v–viii; and M. E. Silverman, P. R. Fleming, A. Hollman, D. G. Julian, and D. M. Krikler, *British Cardiology in the 20th Century* (London: Springer, 2000), 103–110.

79. This summary of the patient's care is based mainly on the published article. See B. E. Taylor, J. E. Geraci, A. A. Pollack, H. B. Burchell, and E. H. Wood, "Interatrial Mixing of Blood and Pulmonary Circulatory Dynamics in Atrial Septal Defects," *PSMMC*, 1948, *23*: 500–505. Additional details came from a review of the patient's medical record and H. B. Burchell, "History of Cardiac Catheterization," 1976, MCA.

80. Details and quotations from the patient's medical record.

81. E. S. Brannon, H. S. Weens, and J. V. Warren, "Atrial Septal Defect: Study of Hemodynamics by the Technique of Right Heart Catheterization," *Am. J. Med. Sci.*, 1945, *210*: 480–491, quotation from 491. See also C. F. Wooley, "The Warren Interview," in *Academic Heritage, The Transmission of Excellence: Cardiology at the Ohio State University* (Mount Kisco, NY: Futura, 1992), 117–145. The definitive contemporary review of congenital heart disease is H. B. Taussig, *Congenital Malformations of the Heart* (New York: Commonwealth Fund, 1947).

82. Details from the patient's medical record. See also H. B. Shumacker Jr., "Atrial Septal Defects," in *The Evolution of Cardiac Surgery* (Bloomington: Indiana University Press, 1992), 143–149.

83. E. H. Wood to L. Dexter, December 5, 1946, MCA. See also L. Dexter, C. S. Burwell, F. W. Haynes, and R. E. Seibel, "Venous Catheterization for the Diagnosis of Congenital Heart Disease," *Bull. N. Engl. Med. Ctr.*, 1946, *8*: 113–121; C. S. Burwell and L. Dexter, "Venous Catheterization in Congenital Heart Disease," *Mod. Concepts Cardiovasc. Dis.*, 1947, *16*: 1–2; and R. C. Schlant, "Lewis Dexter," *Clin. Cardiol.*, 1990, *13*: 232–235.

84. Wood interview. Burchell made the same point. Howard B. Burchell, interviews by W. B. Fye, St. Paul, MN, June 17–18, 2000.

85. E. H. Wood, Annual Report for 1947, MCA.

86. "Tube into the Heart," *Life*, August 18, 1947, 81–82. See also B. Hansen, "*Life* Looks at Medicine: Magazine Photography and the American Public," in *Picturing Medical Progress from Pasteur to Polio: A History of Mass Media Images and Popular Attitudes in America* (New Brunswick, NJ: Rutgers University Press, 2009), 207–255.

87. A. R. Barnes, MC BOG Annual Report to the Staff, November 17, 1947, with Minutes, MC BOG, November 11, 1947, MCA.

88. "Symposium on Cardiac Catheterization," *PSMMC*, 1948, *23*: 481–520.

89. H. B. Burchell, R. L. Parker, T. J. Dry, E. H. Wood, J. W. Pender, and D. G. Pugh, "Cardiac Catheterization in the Diagnosis of Various Cardiac Malformations and Diseases,"

PSMMC, 1948, *23*: 481–487, quotation from 482. See also E. H. Wood, J. E. Geraci, A. A. Pollack, D. Groom, B. E. Taylor, J. W. Pender et al., "General and Special Technics in Cardiac Catheterization," *PSMMC*, 1948, *23*: 494–500.

90. Minutes, MC BOG, October 27, 1948, MCA.

91. Lewis Dexter to E. H. Wood, November 24, 1948, MCA.

92. John McMichael to E. H. Wood, January 18, 1949, MCA.

93. André Cournand to E. H. Wood, November 16, 1948, MCA.

94. E. H. Wood to André Cournand, December 3, 1948, MCA.

95. A. Cournand, J. S. Baldwin, and A. Himmelstein, *Cardiac Catheterization in Congenital Heart Disease* (New York: Commonwealth Fund, 1949), 107–108.

96. "Engineer Role in Medicine Grows in Technological Era," *Mayovox*, April 15, 1961.

97. Minutes, MC Laboratory and Research Committee, October 9, 1945, MCA.

98. C. Sheard, E. J. Baldes, and M. M. D. Williams, Memo to the MC BOG, January 30, 1946, MCA.

99. H. B. Burchell and E. H. Wood, "Remarks on the Technic and Diagnostic Applications of Cardiac Catheterization," *PSMMC*, 1950, *25*: 41–48.

100. Lewis Dexter to E. H. Wood, May 4, 1951, MCA.

101. A. R. Barnes Section Report to MC BOG for 1951, MCA.

102. E. H. Wood to A. R. Barnes, May 15, 1950, MCA.

103. Minutes, MC Sciences Committee, January 26, 1951, MCA.

104. See J. W. Hurst, "H. J. C. Swan," *Clin. Cardiol.*, 1988, *11*: 727–728; I. C. Roddie and J. T. Shepherd, "Recollections of Professor Henry Barcroft, F.R.S.," *Clin. Autonomic Res.*, 1998, *8*: 317–327; and Harold J. C. Swan, interview by W. B. Fye, San Diego, CA, October 7, 2000.

105. H. J. C. Swan, "Early Development of the Pulmonary Artery Catheter: A Personal Perspective," *Proc. Bayl. Univ. Med. Cent.*, 1996, *9*: 3–7, quotation from 4.

106. C. F. Code, Report of the Section of Physiology to the MC BOG for 1949, MCA. See also "Medical Sciences Building, Old and New," *Mayovox*, May 12, 1951.

107. "Dedication of Frank C. Mann Hall, Medical Sciences Building," *PSMMC*, 1952, *27*: 529–530. For the research programs, floor plans, and dedication day addresses, see *Medical Sciences Building of the Mayo Clinic and the Mayo Foundation for Medical Education and Research* (Rochester, MN: Mayo Clinic, 1952). See also O. H. Wangensteen, "The Impact of Physiology on Progress in Surgery," *PSMMC*, 1952, *27*: 532–545.

108. H. E. Essex to Drs. Code, Wood, Helmholz, Lambert, Wakim, Bickford, and Fowler, November 7, 1952, MCA.

109. James Callaway to Hiram Essex, November 20, 1952, MCA. See also B. S. Park, "Disease Categories and Scientific Disciplines: Reorganizing the NIH Intramural Program, 1945–1960," in *Biomedicine in the Twentieth Century: Practices, Policies, and Politics*, ed. C. Hannaway (Amsterdam: IOS Press, 2008), 27–58.

110. C. F. Code, Report of the Section of Physiology to the MC BOG for 1952, MCA.

Chapter 9

1. S. Paget, *The Surgery of the Chest* (Bristol, England: John Wright, 1896), quotation from 121. For the history of thoracic and cardiac surgery, see L. A. Hochberg, *Thoracic Surgery before the 20th Century* (New York: Vantage, 1960); R. H. Meade, *A History of Thoracic Surgery* (Springfield, IL: Charles C Thomas, 1961); H. B. Shumacker Jr., *The Evolution of Cardiac Surgery* (Bloomington: Indiana University Press, 1992); and S. Westaby and C. Bosher, *Landmarks in Cardiac Surgery* (Oxford: Isis Medical Media, 1997).

2. L. Rehn, "Penetrating Cardiac Wounds and Cardiac Suture [1897]," trans. R. E. Asnis, in J. A. Callahan, T. E. Keys, and J. D. Key, eds., *Classics of Cardiology: A Collection of*

Classic Works on the Heart and Circulation with Comprehensive Biographic Accounts of the Authors. 4 vols. in 5 (Malabar, FL: Krieger, 1983), 3: 34–44, quotation from 44. See also K. B. Absolon and M. A. Naficy, *First Successful Cardiac Operation in a Human, 1896, A Documentation: The Life, the Times and the Work of Ludwig Rehn, 1849–1930* (Rockville, MD: Kabel Publishers, 2002).

3. See L. L. Hill, "A Report of a Case of Successful Suturing of the Heart, and Table of Thirty-seven Other Cases of Suturing by Different Operators with Various Terminations, and the Conclusions Drawn," *Med. Rec.*, 1902, *62*: 846–848; and V. Alexi-Meskishvili and W. Böttcher, "Suturing of Penetrating Wounds to the Heart in the Nineteenth Century: The Beginnings of Heart Surgery," *Ann. Thorac. Surg.*, 2011, *92*: 1926–1931.

4. B. M. Ricketts, *The Surgery of the Heart and Lungs* (New York: Grafton, 1904), 3.

5. See J. Mead, "Mechanics of Lung and Chest Wall," in *Respiratory Physiology: People and Ideas*, ed. J. B. West (New York: Oxford University Press, 1996), 173–207.

6. E. Rixford, "Excision of Portions of the Chest Wall for Malignant Tumors," *Ann. Surg.*, 1906, *43*: 35–47, quotation from 37.

7. J. G. Scannell, "Samuel Robinson, Pioneer Thoracic Surgeon (1875–1947)," *Ann. Thorac. Surg.*, 1986, *41*: 692–699. The maintenance of respiration was critical, and competing approaches involved placing a patient inside a negative or a positive pressure chamber to keep the lungs from collapsing. See S. Robinson, "Progress in Surgery: Thoracic Surgery," *Boston Med. Surg. J.*, 1910, *163*: 875–877, 914–918.

8. F. Sauerbruch, *A Surgeon's Life* (London: Andre Deutsch, 1953), 84. See also J. Moerchel, "Sauerbruch und die Mayos," *Dtsch. Med. Wochenschr.*, 1980, *105*: 697–699.

9. F. Sauerbruch and S. Robinson, "Investigations Concerning the Technic of Lung Resection with the Application of Both Forms of Differential Pressure," *Ann. Surg.*, 1910, *51*: 320–339.

10. S. Robinson, "Surgery of the Heart, Pericardium and Diaphragm," *Clifton Med. Bull.*, 1914, *2*: 120–126, quotations from 120.

11. For innovations in transfusion and anesthesia, see S. E. Lederer, *Flesh and Blood: Organ Transplantation and Blood Transfusion in Twentieth-Century America* (New York: Oxford University Press, 2008); and W. W. Mushin, *The Origins of Thoracic Anaesthesia* (Park Ridge, IL: Wood Library-Museum of Anesthesiology, 1991).

12. S. Robinson, "The Surgical Aspects of Bronchiectasis," *Clifton Med. Bull.* 1914, *3*: 31–35. Will Mayo was president of the organization. For a summary of the 1914 meeting, see M. M. Ravitch, *A Century of Surgery: The History of the American Surgical Association* (Philadelphia: J. B. Lippincott, 1981), 481–500.

13. S. Robinson to W. J. Mayo, December 8, 1914, Mayo Clinic Archives, Mayo Historical Unit, Rochester, MN (hereafter MCA).

14. W. J. Mayo to S. Robinson, December 11, 1914, MCA.

15. *Twenty-fourth Annual Report of St. Mary's Hospital* [for 1913] (Rochester, MN: St. Mary's Hospital, 1914), 22, 29.

16. S. Robinson to W. J. Mayo, December 15, 1914, MCA. See also S. Robinson, "Intratrachial Ether Anesthesia; 1400 Cases from 15 Surgical Clinics," *Clifton Med. Bull.*, 1913, *1*: 3–8.

17. S. Robinson, "Thoracic Diseases: The Status of Surgical Therapy," *JAMA*, 1916, *67*: 556–559, quotation from 556.

18. S. Robinson, "The Present and Future of Thoracic Surgery," *Arch. Surg.*, 1923, *6*: 247–255.

19. Samuel Robinson in "Harvard College, Class of 1898. IV Report, 1923," quotation from Scannell, "Samuel Robinson," 692.

20. Churchill quotation in J. G. Scannell, ed., *Wanderjahr: The Education of a Surgeon, Edward D. Churchill* (Boston: Francis A. Countway Library of Medicine, 1990), 202.

21. C. A. Hedblom, "The Treatment of Pericarditis with Effusion," *Minn. Med.*, 1922, *5*: 40–51. See also E. A. Graham, "Carl Arthur Hedblom," *J. Thorac. Surg.*, 1934, *3*: 552–558; and J.

M. Barry, *The Great Influenza: The Epic Story of the Deadliest Plague in History* (New York: Viking Penguin, 2004).

22. C. A. Hedblom, "The Evolution of Thoracic Surgery as a Specialty," *Arch. Surg.*, 1924, *10*: 267–277. See also D. S. Allen and E. A. Graham, "Intracardiac Surgery: A New Method," *JAMA*, 1922, *79*: 1028–1030.

23. S. W. Harrington, "Early Thoracic Surgery," Mayo Foundation Lecture, February 27, 1959, MCA. See also P. E. Bernatz, "Historical Perspectives of the American Association for Thoracic Surgery: Stuart Harrington, MD (1889–1975)," *J. Thorac. Cardiovasc. Surg.*, 2005, *129*: 670–671.

24. Harrington, "Early Thoracic Surgery." See also H. Lilienthal, *Thoracic Surgery: The Surgical Treatment of Thoracic Disease*, 2 vols. (Philadelphia: W. B. Saunders, 1925).

25. W. J. Mayo, "The Future of the Clinic," *Trans. Assoc. Resident and Ex-resident Phys. Mayo Clinic*, 1925, *5*: 121–124, quotation from 124.

26. S. W. Harrington, "Report of a European Trip," *Proceedings of the Staff Meetings of the Mayo Clinic* (hereafter *PSMMC*), 1927, *2*: 42–46.

27. C. A. Hedblom, "Thoracic Surgery with Special Reference to Postgraduate Treatment," *Trans. Assoc. Resident and Ex-resident Phys. Mayo Clinic*, 1927, *7*: 281–291, quotation from 281.

28. E. C. Cutler and C. S. Beck, "Surgery of the Heart and Pericardium," in *Nelson's Loose Leaf Surgery*, ed. A. O. Whipple (New York: T. Nelson & Sons, 1927), 4: 233–386, quotation from 233. See also R. M. Zollinger, *Elliott Carr Cutler and the Cloning of Surgeons* (Mount Kisco, NY: Futura, 1988); and E. C. Cutler, "The Origins of Thoracic Surgery," *N. Engl. J. Med. Surg.*, 1933, *208*: 1233–1243.

29. H. Cushing to E. Cutler [1928], original in author's possession. Cushing had been interested in heart valve surgery early in his career. See H. Cushing and J. R. B. Branch, "Experimental and Clinical Notes on Chronic Valvular Lesions in the Dog and Their Possible Relation to a Future Surgery of the Cardiac Valves," *J. Med. Res.*, 1908, n.s., *12*: 471–486; N. L. Tilney, "Cushing, Cutler and the Mitral Valve," *Surg. Gynecol. Obstet.*, 1981, *152*: 91–96; and S. P. Kiefer and M. L. Hlavin, "Harvey Cushing and Claude Beck: A Surgical Legacy," *Neurosurgery*, 1996, *38*: 1223–1231.

30. C. F. Coombs, *Rheumatic Heart Disease* (Bristol, England: John Wright & Sons, 1924), 143.

31. F. A. Willius, "Life Expectancy with Mitral Stenosis," *Ann. Clin. Med.*, 1923, *1*: 326–330.

32. E. C. Cutler and C. S. Beck, "The Present Status of the Surgical Procedures in Chronic Valvular Disease of the Heart," *Arch. Surg.*, 1929, *18*: 403–416, quotation from 416.

33. E. A. Graham, J. J. Singer, and H. C. Ballon, *Surgical Diseases of the Chest* (Philadelphia: Lea & Febiger, 1935), 335.

34. J. P. Swazey and R. C. Fox, "The Clinical Moratorium: A Case Study of Mitral Valve Surgery," in *Experimentation with Human Subjects*, ed. P. A. Freund (New York: George Braziller, 1970), 315–357.

35. E. A. Graham, "Diseases of the Heart and Pericardium," in Graham, Singer, and Ballon, *Surgical Diseases of the Chest*, 270–366.

36. E. A. Graham, "A Brief Account of the Development of Thoracic Surgery and Some of Its Consequences," in *From the Surgeon's Library*, ed. L. Davis (Chicago: Franklin H. Martin Memorial Foundation, 1959), 114–122, quotation from 116.

37. Graham, Singer, and Ballon, *Surgical Diseases of the Chest*, 3.

38. E. A. Graham, "Training of the Thoracic Surgeon from the Standpoint of the General Surgeon," *J. Thorac. Surg.*, 1936, *5*: 575–578, quotation from 576.

39. E. F. Butler, "Discussion of Symposium on the Training of the Thoracic Surgeon," *J. Thorac. Surg.*, 1936, *5*: 587.

40. B. Bates, *Bargaining for Life: A Social History of Tuberculosis, 1876–1938* (Philadelphia: University of Pennsylvania Press, 1992).

41. "Feels Heart Beat Again: Melbourne Man Has Stone Casing Cut Away at Mayo Clinic," *New York Times*, July 17, 1938.

42. Harrington reported his first patient's case with others six years later. S. W. Harrington, "Chronic Constrictive Pericarditis: Partial Pericardiectomy and Epicardiolysis in Twenty-four Cases," *Ann. Surg.*, 1944, *120*: 468–487.

43. A. R. Barnes and S. W. Harrington, "Calcified Constricting Pericardium," *PSMMC*, 1938, *13*: 673–678, quotation from 678.

44. M. E. Abbott, *Atlas of Congenital Cardiac Disease* (New York: American Heart Association, 1936). See also R. Fraser, "Maude Abbott and the 'Atlas of Congenital Heart Disease,'" *Cardiovasc. Path.*, 2006, *15*: 233–235.

45. T. J. Dry, "An Approach to the Diagnosis of Congenital Heart Disease," *Am. Heart J.*, 1937, *14*: 135–154. Although Fredrick Willius and a few other Mayo doctors published short articles on congenital heart disease in the 1920s and 1930s, Thomas Dry was the first physician at the clinic to focus on this area.

46. R. E. Gross and J. P. Hubbard, "Surgical Ligation of a Patent Ductus Arteriosus: Report of First Successful Case," *JAMA*, 1939, *112*: 729–731. See also F. D. Moore and J. Folkman, "Robert Edward Gross," *Biogr. Mem. Nat. Acad. Sci.*, 1988, *66*: 131–148; and V. V. Alexi-Meskishvili and W. Böttcher, "The First Closure of the Persistent Ductus Arteriosus," *Ann. Thorac. Surg.*, 2010, *90*: 349–356.

47. "The Heart of Innovation—Lorraine Sweeney Nicoli—Boston Children's Hospital. Video interview 'published' May 25, 2012," www.youtube.com/watch?v=JOq_-L24WBs.

48. P. D. White, "Foreword," in Abbott, *Atlas of Congenital Heart Disease*, v.

49. M. E. Abbott, "Congenital Cardiac Abnormalities," in *The Diagnosis and Treatment of Cardiovascular Disease*, ed. W. D. Stroud (Philadelphia: F. A. Davis, 1940), 14–41, quotation from 37, emphasis in the original.

50. Ibid., 38.

51. Elliott Cutler, Discussion of R. E. Gross, "Surgical Management of the Patent Ductus Arteriosus, With Summary of Four Surgically Treated Cases," *Ann. Surg.*, 1939, *110*: 321–356, quotation from 354.

52. Harrington, "Chronic Constrictive Pericarditis."

53. The attendees are listed in *American Surgical Association: Registration Book* [1881–1961] (Philadelphia: J. B. Lippincott, 1963).

54. H. B. Taussig, *Congenital Malformations of the Heart* (New York: Commonwealth Fund, 1947), 109–149.

55. H. B. Taussig, "The Development of the Blalock-Taussig Operation and Its Results Twenty-five Years Later," *Proc. Amer. Phil. Soc.*, 1976, *120*: 13–20. See also W. N. Evans, "The Blalock-Taussig Shunt: The Social History of an Eponym," *Cardiol. Young*, 2009, *19*: 119–128.

56. See V. T. Thomas, *Pioneering Research in Surgical Shock and Cardiovascular Surgery: Vivien Thomas and his Work with Alfred Blalock, An Autobiography* (Philadelphia: University of Pennsylvania Press, 1985), 80–104. Thomas and Blalock's relationship was the subject of the award–winning television movie *Something the Lord Made* (HBO, 2004). See also S. Timmermans, "A Black Technician and Blue Babies," *Soc. Stud. Sci.*, 2003, *33*: 197–229.

57. A. Blalock and H. B. Taussig, "The Surgical Treatment of Malformations of the Heart in Which There Is Pulmonary Stenosis or Pulmonary Atresia," *JAMA*, 1945, *128*: 189–202. See also D. G. McNamara, "The Blalock-Taussig Operation and Subsequent Progress in Surgical Treatment of Cardiovascular Diseases," *JAMA*, 1984, *251*: 2139–2141.

58. W. H. B[arker], "Brighter Blood for Blue Babies," *Ann. Int. Med.*, 1946, *24*: 285–288, quotations from 285, 287.

59. "Blue Baby Research," *Life*, March 14, 1949, 105–109, quotation from 105.

60. J. I. E. Hoffman and S. Kaplan, "The Incidence of Congenital Heart Disease," *J. Am. Coll. Cardiol.*, 2002, *39*: 1890–1900.

61. O. T. Clagett to A. Blalock, October 21, 1946, box 47, number 12, folder corres. MAX-MEA, Blalock Papers, the Alan Mason Chesney Archives of the Johns Hopkins Medical Institutions (hereafter Blalock Papers). See also O. T. Clagett, *Reflections of O. T. "Jim" Clagett* (Rochester, MN: privately printed, 1979).

62. A. Blalock to O. T. Clagett, October 28, 1946, Blalock Papers. See also A. Blalock, "The Surgical Treatment of Congenital Pulmonic Stenosis," *Ann. Surg.*, 1946, *124*: 879–887.

63. O. T. Clagett to A. Blalock, November 1, 1946, Blalock Papers.

64. T. J. Dry, "Introduction [to] Symposium on Tetralogy of Fallot," *PSMMC*, 1947, *22*: 161–162, quotation from 162.

65. O. T. Clagett, "Surgical Considerations in Tetralogy of Fallot," *PSMMC*, 1947, *22*: 180–182, quotations froms 180.

66. Ibid., 182. See also O. T. Clagett, "Advances in Cardio-Vascular Surgery," *Aust. N. Z. J. Surg.*, 1951, *20*: 201–214.

67. R. P. Glover, "The J. William White Travelling Scholarship," July 1, 1947, [with O. T. Clagett to A. Blalock, July 31, 1947], Blalock Papers. See also O. T. Clagett to A. Blalock, March 26, 1947, Blalock Papers; and J. R. Kitchell, "Memoir of Robert P. Glover (1913–1961)," *Trans. Coll. Phys. Phila.*, 1962, *4th ser. 29*: 191–192. Will Mayo had operated on Philadelphia surgeon J. William White in 1906. When White died a decade later, he endowed a prize that was awarded every five years to an exceptional surgical fellow. See A. Repplier, *J. William White, M.D., A Biography* (Boston: Houghton Mifflin, 1919), 139–143.

68. O. T. Clagett to A. Blalock, July 31, 1947, Blalock Papers.

69. Glover, "White Travelling Scholarship."

70. J. Parkinson, "Enlargement of the Heart," *Lancet*, 1936, *1*: 1337–1345, 1391–1399, quotation from 1338.

71. Howard B. Burchell, interviews by W. B. Fye, St. Paul, MN, June 17–18, 2000.

72. See, for example, D. G. Pugh, "Roentgenologic Diagnosis of Tetralogy of Fallot," *PSMMC*, 1947, *22*: 174–177. See also G. D. Davis and O. W. Kincaid, "Development of Cardiovascular Radiology at the Mayo Clinic," chap. 10 in "Diagnostic Radiology at the Mayo Clinic: Personal Recollections of People and Practice from the 1940s to 1970s," 1990, typescript, MCA.

73. D. E. Harken and E. M. Glidden, "Experiments in Intracardiac Surgery. II. Intracardiac Visualization," *J. Thorac. Surg.*, 1943, *12*: 566–572, quotation from 566. See also F. D. Moore, "Dwight Emory Harken, MD," *Circulation*, 1993, *88*: 2985–2986.

74. D. E. Harken, "A Review of the Activities of the Thoracic Center for the III and IV Hospital Groups, 160th General Hospital European Theater of Operations, June 10, 1944, to Jan. 1, 1945," *J. Thorac. Surg.*, 1946, *15*: 31–43. See also D. E. Harken, "Administrative and Basic Clinical Considerations in the European Theater of Operations," in *Thoracic Surgery*. Vol. 1. *Medical Department, United States Army, Surgery in World War II*, ed. F. B. Berry (Washington, DC: Office of the Surgeon General, Dept. of the Army, 1963), 113–160. A valuable perspective on the European Theater by a pioneer of thoracic surgery is E. D. Churchill, *Surgeon to Soldiers: Diary and Records of the Surgical Consultant, Allied Force Headquarters, World War II* (Philadelphia: J. B. Lippincott, 1972).

75. D. E. Harken and P. M. Zoll, "Foreign Bodies in and in Relation to the Thoracic Blood Vessels and Heart. III. Indications for the Removal of Intracardiac Foreign Bodies and the Behavior of the Heart during Manipulation," *Am. Heart J.*, 1946, *32*: 1–19, quotations from 7, 9. See also D. E. Harken, "Foreign Bodies in, and in Relation to, the Thoracic Blood Vessels and Heart: I. Techniques for Approaching and Removing Foreign Bodies from the Chambers of the Heart," *Surg. Gynecol. Obstet.*, 1946, *83*: 117–125.

76. Glover, "White Travelling Scholarship."

77. Ibid.

78. D. E. Harken, "The Surgical Treatment of Mitral Stenosis. I. Valvuloplasty," *N. Engl. J. Med.*, 1948, *239*: 801–809.

79. Glover, "White Travelling Scholarship."

80. O. T. Clagett to A. Blalock, 31 July 1947, Blalock Papers.

81. A. B. Weisse, "Charles P. Bailey, M.D., Sc.D., J.D.," in *Conversations in Medicine: The Story of Twentieth-Century American Medicine in the Words of Those Who Created It* (New York: New York University Press, 1984), 132–156, quotation from 142.

82. L. W. Kinsell, ed., *The Medic: Hahnemann Medical College* (Philadelphia: Hahnemann Medical College, 1932), 107. This yearbook entry was written before the existence of any sustained research program on an artificial heart or cardiac transplantation. See G. B. Griffenhagen and C. H. Hughes, "The History of the Mechanical Heart," *Ann. Rept. Smithsonian Inst. for 1955*, 1956, 339–356.

83. C. P. Bailey, "The Surgical Treatment of Mitral Stenosis (Mitral Commissurotomy)," *Dis. Chest*, 1949, *15*: 377–397. For a summary of the patients, see Swazey and Fox, "Clinical Moratorium," 325–326.

84. C. P. Bailey, "The Surgical Treatment of Mitral Stenosis (Mitral Commissurotomy): A Review after Forty Years," typescript received by the journal *Chest* on September 18, 1959, but not published, copy sent to the author by Bailey. See also J. C. Davila, "The Birth of Intracardiac Surgery: A Semicentennial Tribute (June 10, 1948–1998)," *Ann. Thorac. Surg.*, 1998, *65*: 1809–1820.

85. E. A. Graham, Discussion of Bailey, "The Surgical Treatment of Mitral Stenosis," *Dis. Chest*, 1949, *15*: 377–397, quotation from 393. Bailey delivered his lecture on June 20, 1948.

86. H. G. Smithy, Discussion of Bailey, "Surgical Treatment of Mitral Stenosis," 393–395.

87. S. M. Spencer, "Can We Rebuild Damaged Hearts?" *Saturday Evening Post* November 6, 1948, 34–35, 120–124.

88. Ibid., 123.

89. B. L. Woolridge to H. G. Smithy, December 6, 1947, quotation from F. A. Crawford Jr., "Horace Smithy: Pioneer Heart Surgeon," *Ann. Thorac. Surg.*, 2010, *89*: 2067–2071. Several contemporary newspaper reports of Smithy's operation on Woolridge are reprinted in J. C. Kiley, *The Heart of a Surgeon: The Life and Writings of Horace Gilbert Smithy, M.D., Heart Surgeon (1914–1948)* (Berryville, VA: privately printed, 1984). Smithy's experience with valve surgery was summarized in a posthumous article: H. G. Smithy, J. A. Boone, and J. M. Stallworth, "Surgical Treatment of Constrictive Valvular Disease of the Heart," *Surg. Gynecol. Obstet.*, 1950, *90*: 175–192.

90. For the photograph, see Crawford, "Horace Smithy."

91. Minutes, MC BOG, September 1, 1948, MCA.

92. Ibid.

93. W. C. Roberts, "John Webster Kirklin, MD: A Conversation with the Editor," *Am. J. Cardiol.*, 1998, *81*: 1027–1044.

94. J. W. Kirklin, "The Middle 1950s and C. Walton Lillehei," *J. Thorac. Cardiovasc. Surg.*, 1989, *98*: 822–824, quotation from 822.

95. R. E. Gross, "Introduction of Caldwell Lecturer, 1967," *Am. J. Roentgenol. Radium Ther. Nucl. Med.*, 1968, *102*: 251–252, quotation from 251.

96. Minutes, MC BOG, November 12, 1947, MCA.

97. Minutes, MC BOG, October 18, 1950. MCA.

98. See, for example, D. E. Harken, L. Dexter, L. B. Ellis, R. F. Farrand, and J. F. Dickson III, "The Surgery of Mitral Stenosis. III. Finger-Fracture Valvuloplasty," *Ann. Surg.*, 1951, *134*: 722–742; C. P. Bailey, R. P. Glover, and T. J. E. O'Neill, "The Surgery of Valvular Heart Disease," *Dis. Chest*, 1951, *20*: 453–468; and E. C. Andrus, A. Blalock, and R. J. Bing, "The Surgical Treatment of Mitral Stenosis and Its Physiological Consequences," *Bull. Johns Hopkins Hosp.*, 1952, *90*: 175–178.

99. J. W. Pender, "Care of the Patient during Operation on the Mitral Valve for Stenosis," *PSMMC*, 1952, *27*: 310–316. See also E. A. Hessel II, "Evolution of Cardiac Anesthesia and

Surgery," in *Kaplan's Cardiac Anesthesia*, ed. J. A. Kaplan, 5th ed. (Philadelphia: Saunders Elsevier, 2006), 3–32.

100. Roberts, "John Webster Kirklin," 1032–1033.

101. J. W. Kirklin, "Surgical Treatment of Diseases of the Heart and Great Vessels," *Minn. Med.*, 1951, *34*: 865–870.

102. C. Baker, R. C. Brock, and M. Campbell, "Valvulotomy for Mitral Stenosis: Report of Six Successful Cases," *Brit. Med. J.*, 1950, *1*: 1283–1293, quotation from 1285.

103. Chapter 10 is devoted to the development of open-heart surgery. See also D. K. C. Cooper, *Open Heart: The Radical Surgeons Who Revolutionized Medicine* (New York: Kaplan, 2010).

104. Richard J. Bing to W. B. Fye, August 20, 1996. See also D. G. McNamara, "Contributions of Richard Bing to the Field of Congenital Heart Disease," *J. Applied Cardiol.*, 1989, *4*: 351–356.

105. Blalock, "Surgical Treatment of Congenital Pulmonic Stenosis."

106. Longmire, *Alfred Blalock*, 109.

107. Harken, "Surgical Treatment of Mitral Stenosis," 801.

108. L. Dexter, Untitled lecture on the history of cardiac catheterization presented to the Harvard Club ca. 1980, typescript, copy sent to the author by Dexter. See also L. Dexter, R. Gorlin, B. M. Lewis, F. W. Haynes, and D. E. Harken, "Physiologic Evaluation of Patients with Mitral Stenosis before and after Mitral Valvuloplasty," *Trans. Am. Clin. Climatol. Assoc.*, 1950, *62*: 170–180.

109. A. R. Barnes, "Fear Banished, Hunger for Facts Satisfied," *The American Heart*, 1950, *1*: 7. This is a review of H. M. Marvin, T. D. Jones, I. H. Page, I. S. Wright, and D. D. Rutstein, *You and Your Heart* (New York: Random House, 1950).

110. D. S. Fleming and B. Wolcyn, "Minnesota Reports Heart Disease," *Minn. Med.*, 1951, *34*: 218–220.

111. Barnes, "Fear Banished."

112. J. D. Ratcliff, "Surgery's New Frontier: The Human Heart," *Reader's Digest*, May 1952, 45–48, quotations from 45, 48.

113. The first article reporting the administration of cortisone to patients with rheumatoid arthritis is P. S. Hench, E. C. Kendall, C. H. Slocumb, and H. F. Polley, "The Effect of a Hormone of the Adrenal Cortex (17-hydroxy-11-dehydrocorticosterone: Compound E) and of Pituitary Adrenocorticotropic Hormone on Rheumatoid Arthritis; Preliminary Report," *PSMMC*, 1949, *24*: 181–197. See also E. C. Kendall, "The Development of Cortisone as a Therapeutic Agent. Nobel Lecture, December 11, 1950," in *Nobel Lectures Including Presentation Speeches and Laureates' Biographies. Physiology or Medicine, 1942–1962* (Amsterdam: Elsevier, 1964), 270–290; G. Hetenyi Jr. and J. Karsh, "Cortisone Therapy: A Challenge to Academic Medicine in 1949 to 1952," *Perspect. Biol. Med.*, 1977, *40*: 426–439; C. E. Gastineau, "Remembrance of Things Adrenal: A Historical Perspective," *Endocr. Practice*, 2004, *10*: 376–380; and T. Rooke, *The Quest for Cortisone* (East Lansing: Michigan State University Press, 2012).

114. "Arthritis: Mayo Clinic Finds a Treatment for Man's Most Crippling Disease," *Life*, June 6, 1949, 106–113.

115. L. A. Scheele, "A New Era in Medical Research and Practice," *Am. J. Med.*, 1950, *9*: 1–2, quotation from 1.

116. P. S. Hench, C. H. Slocumb, A. R. Barnes, H. L. Smith, H. F. Polley, and E. C. Kendall, "The Effects of the Adrenal Cortical Hormone 17-hydroxy-11-dehydrocorticosterone (Compound E) on the Acute Phase of Rheumatic Fever: Preliminary Report," *PSMMC*, 1949, *24*: 277–297, quotation from 296. See also P. D. White, "Rheumatic Heart Disease" in *Heart Disease*, 4th ed. (New York: Macmillan, 1951), 352–384.

117. L. Thomas, ed., *Rheumatic Fever: A Symposium* (Minneapolis: University of Minnesota Press, 1952).

118. P. C. English, *Rheumatic Fever in America and Britain: A Biological, Epidemiological, and Medical History* (New Brunswick, NJ: Rutgers University Press, 2004), 147–150. See also D. M. Dunlop, "Cortisone in Practice," *Br. Med. J.*, 1955, *2*: 1263–1266.

119. J. W. Kirklin, "Surgical Intrathoracic Cardiovascular Lesions," *Postgrad. Med.*, 1952, *12*: 118–123, quotation from 118.

Chapter 10

1. For the history of cardiac surgery, see H. B. Shumacker Jr., *The Evolution of Cardiac Surgery* (Bloomington: Indiana University Press, 1992); S. Westaby and C. Bosher, *Landmarks in Cardiac Surgery* (Oxford: Isis Medical Media, 1997); and D. K. C. Cooper, *Open Heart: The Radical Surgeons Who Revolutionized Medicine* (New York: Kaplan, 2010). A collection of oral histories is W. S. Stoney, ed., *Pioneers of Cardiac Surgery* (Nashville, TN: Vanderbilt University Press, 2008). For reprints of important articles with commentaries by Mayo staff members, see J. A. Callahan, D. C. McGoon, and J. D. Key, *Classics of Cardiology: A Collection of Classic Works on the Heart and Circulation*, 4 vols. in 5 (Malabar, FL: Robert E. Krieger, 1989).

2. Various heart-lung machines and issues associated with their use are detailed in P. M. Galletti and G. A. Brecher, *Heart-Lung Bypass: Principles and Techniques of Extracorporeal Circulation* (New York: Grune & Stratton, 1962).

3. J. H. Gibbon Jr., "The Maintenance of Life during Experimental Occlusion of the Pulmonary Artery Followed by Survival," *Surg. Gynecol. Obstet.*, 1939, *69*: 602–614, quotation from 602. See also A. Romaine-Davis, *John Gibbon and His Heart-Lung Machine* (Philadelphia: University of Pennsylvania Press, 1991); and H. B. Shumacker Jr., *A Dream of the Heart: The Life of John H. Gibbon Jr., Father of the Heart-Lung Machine* (Santa Barbara, CA: Fithian Press, 1999).

4. "Artificial Heart: Mechanical Device Substitutes for Living Organ," *Life*, May 8, 1950, 90–92. For *Life* magazine's role in popularizing developments in medicine, see B. Hansen, *Picturing Medical Progress from Pasteur to Polio: A History of Mass Media Images and Popular Attitudes in America* (New Brunswick NJ: Rutgers University Press, 2009), 207–255.

5. O. T. Clagett, "Advances in Cardio-Vascular Surgery," *Aust. N. Z. J. Surg.*, 1951, *20*: 201–214, quotation from 213–214.

6. The Mayo surgeons who attended each meeting are listed in *American Surgical Association: Registration Book* [1881–1961] (Philadelphia: J. B. Lippincott, 1963).

7. B. J. Miller, J. H. Gibbon Jr., and M. H. Gibbon, "Recent Advances in the Development of a Mechanical Heart and Lung Apparatus," *Ann. Surg.*, 1951, *134*: 694–708, quotation from 707. Miller, Gibbon's research assistant, did not attend the meeting. See B. J. Miller, "Laboratory Work Preceding the First Clinical Application of Cardiopulmonary Bypass," *Ann. Thorac. Surg.*, 2003, *76*: S2203–S2209. Using animals, especially dogs, in experiments designed to develop operations that might benefit humans has a long history. See W. W. Keen, *Animal Experimentation and Medical Progress* (Boston: Houghton Mifflin, 1914); A. Guerrini, *Experimenting with Humans and Animals: From Galen to Animal Rights* (Baltimore: Johns Hopkins University Press, 2003); and F. B. Orlans, *In the Name of Science: Issues in Responsible Animal Experimentation* (New York: Oxford University Press, 1993).

8. C. Dennis, D. S. Spreng Jr., G. E. Nelson, K. E. Karlson, R. M. Nelson, J. V. Thomas et al., "Development of a Pump-Oxygenator to Replace the Heart and Lungs; An Apparatus Applicable to Human Patients, and Application to One Case," *Ann. Surg.*, 1951, *134*: 709–721, emphasis added.

9. Ibid., 719. See also V. V. Alexi-Meskishvili and I. E. Konstantinov, "Surgery for Atrial Septal Defect: From the First Experiments to Clinical Practice," *Ann. Thorac. Surg.*, 2003, *76*: 322–327.

566 _Notes to Pages 207–211_

10. Dennis et al., "Development of a Pump-Oxygenator," 718.

11. L. Engel, "The Automatic Heart," _Harper's Magazine_, June 1952, 90–92, quotation from 92.

12. F. D. Moore, "Therapeutic Innovation: Ethical Boundaries in the Initial Clinical Trials of New Drugs and Surgical Procedures," _Daedalus_, 1969, 502–522. General reviews include P. A. Freund, ed., _Experimentation with Human Subjects_ (New York: George Braziller, 1970); R. R. Faden and T. L. Beauchamp, _A History and Theory of Informed Consent_ (New York: Oxford University Press, 1986); D. J. Rothman, _Strangers at the Bedside: A History of How Law and Bioethics Transformed Medical Decision Making_ (New York: Basic Books, 1991); and L. Stark, _Behind Closed Doors: IRBs and the Making of Ethical Research_ (Chicago: University of Chicago Press, 2012).

13. Dennis et al., "Development of a Pump-Oxygenator."

14. A. Blalock [Discussion of three papers], _Ann. Surg._, 1951, _134_: 741–742.

15. L. G. Wilson, "The Development of Cardiac Surgery at Minnesota, 1940–1960," in _Medical Revolution in Minnesota: A History of the University of Minnesota Medical School_ (St. Paul, MN: Midewiwin Press, 1989), 481–528, quotation from 487.

16. J. H. Gibbon Jr., "Application of a Mechanical Heart and Lung Apparatus to Cardiac Surgery," _Minn. Med._, 1954, _37_: 171–180, delivered in Minneapolis on September 16, 1953.

17. A. Cournand, R. J. Bing, L. Dexter, C. T. Dotter, L. N. Katz, J. V. Warren, and E. Wood, "Report of Committee on Cardiac Catheterization and Angiocardiography of the American Heart Association," _Circulation_, 1953, _7_: 769–773. Cournand chaired the committee; the other members' names were listed alphabetically. The participating institutions included the University of Alabama; Columbia University, Bellevue Hospital Service; Columbia University, Presbyterian Hospital; Emory University; Johns Hopkins Hospital; Mayo Clinic, Michael Reese Hospital; New York Hospital; and Peter Bent Brigham Hospital.

18. Minutes, MC Sciences Committee, August 29, 1952, Mayo Clinic Archives, Mayo Historical Unit, Rochester, MN (hereafter MCA).

19. D. E. Donald, "Talk at [Sigma Xi] Honorary Society," Rochester, MN, November 9, 1989, MCA.

20. F. J. Lewis and M. Taufic, "Closure of Atrial Septal Defects with the Aid of Hypothermia: Experimental Accomplishments and the Report of One Successful Case," _Surgery_, 1953, _33_: 52–59. See also W. G. Bigelow, _Cold Hearts: The Story of Hypothermia and the Pacemaker in Heart Surgery_ (Toronto: McClelland and Stewart, 1984).

21. J. W. Kirklin to G. S. Shuster, September 17, 1952, MCA.

22. E. H. Wood, "Report of Meeting Concerning Project to Develop Equipment for By-pass of the Right Heart," October 22, 1952, MCA.

23. C. Dennis to E. H. Wood, November 17, 1952, MCA.

24. E. H. Wood to J. H. Gibbon Jr., January 13, 1953, MCA.

25. J. H. McPherson to Secretary, Mayo BOG, January 29, 1953, MCA.

26. E. H. Wood to J. H. McPherson, February 11, 1953, MCA.

27. J. W. Kirklin to E. H. Wood, February 9, 1953, MCA.

28. E. H. Wood to J. W. Kirklin, February 11, 1953, MCA.

29. Minutes, MC BOG, April 1, 1953, MCA.

30. J. W. Kirklin to J. W. Harwick [for the MC BOG], June 17, 1953, MCA.

31. L. H. Cohn, "Fifty Years of Open-Heart Surgery," _Circulation_, 2003, _107_: 2168–2170, quotation from 2169.

32. "Recent Advances in Cardiovascular Physiology and Surgery: A Symposium Presented by the Minnesota Heart Association and the University of Minnesota. September 14, 15 and 16, 1953. University of Minnesota, Minneapolis." Reprinted from _Minn. Med._, January, February, and March 1954, _37_, copy in the author's possession. Mayo physiologist Grace Roth,

the Minnesota Heart Association's immediate past president, chaired the planning committee. They invited North American and European investigators who had made important contributions to cardiovascular physiology, diagnosis, and surgery.

33. Gibbon, "Application of a Mechanical Heart and Lung Apparatus," 112.

34. J. H. Gibbon Jr. to E. H. Wood, September 23, 1953, MCA.

35. A. Blalock to O. T. Clagett, November 24, 1953, box 18 F7, folder Clagett, Blalock Papers, the Alan Mason Chesney Archives of the Johns Hopkins Medical Institutions (hereafter Blalock Papers). Vivien Thomas, Blalock's laboratory assistant, recalled that when the surgeon returned to Baltimore, "He couldn't wait to send a team to Mayo to study the design, construction, and operation of their animal-care and research facilities." Thomas describes his own visit to Rochester, where surgical research director John Grindley hosted him, an architect, and an engineer. V. T. Thomas, *Pioneering Research in Surgical Shock and Cardiovascular Surgery: Vivien Thomas and his Work with Alfred Blalock, An Autobiography* (Philadelphia: University of Pennsylvania Press, 1985), 186.

36. J. W. Kirklin, "Report on Pump Project," January 28, 1954, MCA. Kirklin explained that during the previous twelve months he had personally done 143 cardiovascular operations, his mentor Jim Clagett had done "a large number" of cases, and his junior associate Henry Ellis was "doing more and more."

37. O. H. Wangensteen to A. Blalock, September 23, 1948, folder Lillehei, Blalock Papers. See also G. W. Miller, *King of Hearts: The True Story of the Maverick Who Pioneered Open Heart Surgery* (New York: Random House, 2000). An annotated summary of Lillehei's many publications is R. W. M. Frater, ed., *The Key to the Door: A Cardiac Surgical Anthology, C. Walton Lillehei* (London: ICR Publishers, 1998). See also C. Walton Lillehei, MD, PhD [Oral history, May 4, 1998], in Stoney, ed., *Pioneers of Cardiac Surgery*, 83–99.

38. For Lillehei's tumor and its treatment, see Miller, *King of Hearts*, 35–35. Vincent L. Gott, interview by W. B. Fye, Minneapolis, MN, December 13, 2007.

39. H. E. Warden, M. Cohen, R. C. Read, and C. W. Lillehei, "Controlled Cross Circulation for Open Intracardiac Surgery: Physiologic Studies and Results of Creation and Closure of Ventricular Septal Defects," *J. Thorac. Surg.*, 1954, *28*: 331–343.

40. C. W. Lillehei to O. H. Wangensteen, January 22, 1954, box 18, University of Minnesota Department of Surgery Papers, University of Minnesota Archives, Minneapolis, MN (hereafter UMN Surgery Papers).

41. Ibid. See also Miller, *King of Hearts*, 99–139.

42. O. H. Wangensteen to C. W. Lillehei, January 23, 1954, box 18, UMN Surgery Papers.

43. J. E. Edwards, T. J. Dry, R. L. Parker, H. B. Burchell, E. H. Wood, and A. H. Bulbulian, *An Atlas of Congenital Anomalies of the Heart and Great Vessels* (Springfield, IL: Charles C Thomas, 1954). See also B. S. Edwards and J. H. Moller, eds., *Jesse E. Edwards: His Legacy to Cardiovascular Medicine* (Stamford, CT: Science International, 2011).

44. For Cecil Watson's attempt to block the operation, see Miller, *King of Hearts*, 119–123.

45. C. W. Lillehei, "Historical Development of Cardiopulmonary Bypass," in *Cardiopulmonary Bypass: Principles and Practice*, ed. G. P. Gravlee, R. F. Davis, and J. R. Utley (Baltimore: Williams and Wilkins, 1993), 1–26. The patient and the donor (who was always a parent or a close blood relative) had to have compatible blood types.

46. O. H. Wangensteen to A. Blalock, April 1, 1954, box 18, UMN Surgery Papers.

47. Warden, Cohen, Read, and Lillehei, "Controlled Cross Circulation," 342–343. For additional details on the eight patients, see C. W. Lillehei, M. Cohen, H. E. Warden, N. R. Ziegler, and R. L. Varco, "The Results of Direct Vision Closure of Ventricular Septal Defects in Eight Patients by Means of Controlled Cross Circulation," *Surg. Gynecol. Obstet.*, 1955, *101*: 446–466.

48. J. H. Gibbon Jr., comments on Warden et al., "Controlled Cross Circulation," quotation from 343.

49. J. H. Gibbon Jr., B. J. Miller, A. R. Dobell, H. C. Engell, and G. B. Voigt, "The Closure of Interventricular Septal Defects in Dogs during Open Cardiotomy with the Maintenance of the Cardiorespiratory Functions by a Pump-Oxygenator," *J. Thorac. Surg.*, 1954, *28*: 235–240.

50. R. H. Berg, "New Miracles to Save Your Heart," *Look*, September 7, 1954. 50–57.

51. Ibid., 52.

52. J. W. Kirklin, "The Middle 1950s and C. Walton Lillehei," *J. Thorac. Cardiovasc. Surg.*, 1989, *98*: 822–824, quotation from 823.

53. S. F. Haines, Untitled 7-page memo beginning "It is Tradition," with Minutes, MC BOG, April 21, 1954, MCA.

54. Ibid. For the cultural context, see D. Halberstam, *The Fifties* (New York: Villard Books, 1993).

55. Table 14-1. "NIH Obligations of Appropriations, 1939–1988," in W. Shonick, *Government and Health Services: Government's Role in the Development of U.S. Health Services, 1930–1980* (New York: Oxford University Press, 1995), 416.

56. Minutes, National Advisory Heart Council, June 14–16, 1954, copy in the author's possession obtained from bound minute books located outside Claude Lenfant's office at the NIH in May 2000.

57. O. H. Wangensteen to J. F. Yeager, July 9, 1954, box 18, UMN Surgery Papers.

58. A. Blalock to C. W. Lillehei, September 24, 1954, box 18, UMN Surgery Papers. For Blalock's assessment of cardiac surgery at this time, see A. Blalock, "The Expanding Scope of Cardiovascular Surgery," in *The Papers of Alfred Blalock*, ed. M. M. Ravitch (Baltimore: Johns Hopkins Press, 1966), 1757–1765, paper presented on May 14, 1954.

59. D. C. Balfour to J. W. Kirklin, October 4, 1954, MCA.

60. C. W. Lillehei, "Controlled Cross Circulation for Direct-Vision Surgery: Correction of Ventricular Septal Defects, Atrioventricularis Communis, and Tetralogy of Fallot," *Postgrad. Med.*, 1955, *17*: 388–396, quotation from 396, paper presented in November 1954.

61. "A Baby's Heart Is Mended," *Life*, November 1, 1954. 43–46.

62. James Watt commenting on "Management of Congenital Cardiac Anomalies by Direct Vision Intracardiac Surgery. Dr. Lillehei," Minutes, National Advisory Heart Council, November 4–6, 1954, copy in the author's possession.

63. H. B. Shumacker Jr., "Heart and Great Vessels: Introduction," *Surg. Forum*, 1955, *5*: 1–2. See also Harris B. Shumacker Jr., MD [Oral history, December 3, 1996], in Stoney, ed., *Pioneers of Cardiac Surgery*, 125–137.

64. C. P. Bailey to A. Blalock, October 12, 1954, box 10 F3, folder Bailey, Blalock Papers.

65. H. B. Taussig to A. Blalock [December 1954], folder Taussig, Blalock Papers. For the perspectives of two individuals involved in the development and performance of the Blalock-Taussig operation, see Thomas, *Pioneering Research in Surgical Shock*; and W. P. Longmire Jr., *Alfred Blalock: His Life and Times* (Los Angeles: privately printed, 1991).

66. M. M. Ravitch, "Alfred Blalock, 1899–1964," in *Papers of Alfred Blalock*, xiii–lvii, quotation from lv. Henry Bahnson and Frank Spencer performed the first open-heart operation at Johns Hopkins in March 1956. See Henry T. Bahnson, MD [Oral history, August 3, 1999], in Stoney, ed., *Pioneers of Cardiac Surgery*, 185–193.

67. "Excerpt from Minutes of Sciences Committee," January 7, 1955, MCA.

68. J. W. Kirklin to J. W. Harwick [for the MC BOG], February 14, 1955, MCA.

69. Ibid. Priestley's note is on the copy of the minutes circulated among board members.

70. Minutes, Administrative Committee of MC BOG, March 2, 1955, MCA.

71. C. W. Lillehei, M. Cohen, H. E. Warden, R. C. Read, R. A. DeWall, J. B. Aust et al., "Direct Vision Intracardiac Surgery by Means of Controlled Cross Circulation or Continuous Arterial Reservoir Perfusion for Correction of Ventricular Septal Defects, Atrioventricularis Communis, Isolated Infundibular Pulmonic Stenosis and Tetralogy of Fallot," in *Henry Ford Hospital International Symposium on Cardiovascular Surgery*, ed. C. R. Lam (Philadelphia: W. B. Saunders, 1955), 371–393.

72. R. C. Brock, "Foreword," in *Ford Symposium on Cardiovascular Surgery*, xv–xxiii, quotation from xvii.

73. R. E. Jones, D. E. Donald, H. J. C. Swan, H. G. Harshbarger, J. W. Kirklin, and E. H. Wood, "Apparatus of the Gibbon Type for Mechanical Bypass of the Heart and Lungs: Preliminary Report," *Proceedings of the Staff Meetings of the Mayo Clinic* (hereafter *PSMMC*), 1955, *30*: 105–113. For a description of the Mayo-Gibbon machine, see J. W. Kirklin, D. E. Donald, H. G. Harshbarger, P. S. Hetzel, R. T. Patrick, H. J. C. Swan et al., "Studies in Extracorporeal Circulation. I. Applicability of Gibbon-Type Pump-Oxygenator to Human Intracardiac Surgery: 40 Cases," *Ann. Surg.*, 1956, *144*: 2–8. Colonial Hospital, one block from the Mayo Clinic, was renamed Methodist Hospital in 1954. See W. Holmes, *Dedicated to Excellence: The Rochester Methodist Hospital Story* (Rochester, MN: RMH Foundation, 1984).

74. J. R. Eckman, "Memorandum: Inquiry of Victor Cohn, of the *Minneapolis Morning Tribune* and Others, concerning the First Application of the Extracorporeal Heart-Lung Bypass Apparatus in Operation for Ventricular Septal Defect on Linda Stout, 6, of Bismarck, North Dakota," March 23, 1955, MCA. See also D. L. Breo, "Meet Vic Cohn: Dean of American Science Writers," *JAMA*, 1989, *262*: 968–970.

75. Linda Stout returned to Rochester in 2005 to participate in the fiftieth anniversary celebration. See *The Development of Cardiopulmonary Bypass at Mayo Clinic: Presentations, Interviews and Photographs from May 12, 2005* (Rochester, MN: Mayo Foundation, 2005), 8 DVD set.

76. Eckman, "Memorandum."

77. "First 'Bypass' Operation: Girl Doing Well after Surgery," *Rochester Post-Bulletin*, March 23, 1955, MCA.

78. Jones et al., "Apparatus of the Gibbon Type." See also D. E. Donald, H. G. Harshbarger, P. S. Hetzel, R. T. Patrick, E. H. Wood, and J. W. Kirklin, "Experiences with a Heart-Lung Bypass (Gibbon Type) in the Experimental Laboratory," *PSMMC*, 1955, *30*: 113–115.

79. Kirklin, "Middle 1950s," 824. See also J. W. Kirklin, J. W. DuShane, R. T. Patrick, D. E. Donald, P. S. Hetzel, H. G. Harshbarger et al., "Intracardiac Surgery with the Aid of a Mechanical Pump-Oxygenator System (Gibbon Type): Report of Eight Cases," *PSMMC*, 1955, *30*: 201–206.

80. A. Blalock, Discussion of C. W. Lillehei, M. Cohen, H. E. Warden, R. C. Read, J. B. Aust, R. A. DeWall et al., "Direct Vision Intracardiac Surgical Correction of the Tetralogy of Fallot, Pentalogy of Fallot, and Pulmonary Atresia Defects: Report of First Ten Cases," *Ann. Surg.*, 1955, *142*: 418–445, quotation from 442.

81. J. W. Kirklin to E. H. Wood, April 22, 1955, MCA.

82. Ibid.

83. Ibid.

84. Kirklin, "Intracardiac Surgery ... Eight Cases," 202.

85. D. McRae, *Every Second Counts: The Race to Transplant the First Human Heart* (New York: G. P. Putnam's Sons, 2006), 330.

86. "'Proceedings of the Staff Meetings' Provides Information and Record on Clinic, Foundation," *Mayovox*, July 19, 1952. See also fig. 2, "Circulation of *Proceedings of the Staff Meetings of the Mayo Clinic* in various years [1929–1954]," in Report of the Section of Publications for the Year ending December 31, 1954, MCA.

87. Shumacker, *Dream of the Heart*, 197.

88. Donald N. Ross, MD [Oral history, August 13, 1997], in Stoney, ed., *Pioneers of Cardiac Surgery*, 285–296, quotations from 292–293.

89. Norman E. Shumway, MD, PhD [Oral history, October 16, 1997], in Stoney, ed., *Pioneers of Cardiac Surgery*, 427–439, quotation from 431.

90. M. F. and her mother, interview by W. B. Fye, Rochester, MN, February 19, 2008. The adult patient and her mother gave the author written permission to publish details of her case. For a description of the atrial well technique, see J. W. Kirklin, W. H. Weidman, J. T. Burroughs,

H. B. Burchell, and E. H. Wood, "The Hemodynamic Results of Surgical Correction of Atrial Septal Defects: A Report of Thirty-three Cases," *Circulation*, 1956, *13*: 825–833.

91. "Medical Horizons. No. 1, September 12, 1955," typescript, MCA. Mayo Clinic Media Support Services has a video of the original program. See also "Clinic on National TV Monday," *Mayovox*, September 10, 1955; D. J. Cook, "Cardiothoracic Anesthesia," in *Art to Science: Department of Anesthesiology, Mayo Clinic*, ed. K. Rehder, P. Southorn, and A. Sessler (Rochester, MN: Mayo Clinic, 2000), 45–50; and D. Selkin, *Imagining Illness: Public Health and Visual Culture* (Minneapolis: University of Minnesota Press, 2010), 223–244.

92. "Medical Horizons" typescript.

93. E. H. Wood to W. H. Weidman, October 4, 1955, MCA.

94. Minutes, MC Sciences Committee, February 3, 1956, MCA.

95. E. H. Wood to J. T. Shepherd, April 9, 1956, MCA. See also J. T. Shepherd, *Inside the Mayo Clinic: A Memoir* (Afton, MN: Afton Historical Society Press, 2003).

96. "Second Heart-Lung Bypass is 'Valentine,'" *Mayovox*, February 25, 1956.

Chapter 11

1. Minutes, MC Sciences Committee, February 3, 1956, Mayo Clinic Archives, Mayo Historical Unit, Rochester, MN (hereafter MCA).

2. Ibid. Of the first 440 open-heart operations performed at Mayo (between March 1955 and June 1958), all but eight were done on patients with congenital heart disease. See F. H. Ellis Jr. and J. W. Kirklin, "The Use of Extracorporeal Circulation in Cardiac Surgery," *Dis. Chest*, 1959, *36*: 173–178.

3. W. S. Stoney, "A Short History of Cardiac Surgery," in *Pioneers of Cardiac Surgery* (Nashville, TN: Vanderbilt University Press, 2008), 1–60, quotation from 30.

4. The base price was $19,725. See *Mayo-Gibbon Pump-Oxygenator, Model 10*, March 1, 1963, Price List (St. Louis: Med-Science Electronics), John H. Gibbon Papers, MS C313, Modern Manuscripts Collection, National Library of Medicine, Bethesda, MD. A typed description of the machine and accessories accompanied this printed price list. For Gibbon's perspective on the rapidly changing field that he had helped to invent less than five years earlier, see J. H. Gibbon Jr. and J. Y. Templeton III, "Current Status of Pump Oxygenators in Cardiac Surgery and Persistent Problems in Their Use," *Prog. Cardiovasc. Dis.*, 1958, *1*: 56–65; A. Romaine-Davis, *John Gibbon and His Heart-Lung Machine* (Philadelphia: University of Pennsylvania Press, 1991), 138–154; and P. M. Galletti and G. A. Brecher, *Heart-Lung Bypass: Principles and Techniques of Extracorporeal Circulation* (New York: Grune & Stratton, 1962), 61–78.

5. "Clinic's Blood Bank Seeking New Donors from Staffs, Area," *Mayovox*, February 22, 1958.

6. C. W. Lillehei, R. A. DeWall, R. C. Read, H. E. Warden, and R. L. Varco, "Direct Vision Intracardiac Surgery in Man Using a Simple, Disposable Artificial Oxygenator," *Dis. Chest*, 1956, *29*: 1–8. See also R. A. DeWall, "The Evolution of the Helical Reservoir Pump-Oxygenator System at the University of Minnesota," *Ann. Thorac. Surg.*, 2003, *76*: S2210–S2215. Lillehei had used the cross-circulation technique in forty-five patients before abandoning it in favor of using a pump-oxygenator that he and DeWall had developed. See J. H. Moller, S. Shumway, and V. L. Gott, "The First Open-Heart Repairs Using Extracorporeal Circulation by Cross-Circulation: A 53-Year Follow-up," *Ann. Thorac. Surg.*, 2009, *88*: 1044–1046.

7. R. C. Brock, "The Present Position of Cardiac Surgery," *Ann. R. Coll. Surg. Engl.*, 1958, *23*: 213–237, quotation from 235, paper presented in London, December 11, 1957.

8. C. W. Lillehei to O. H. Wangensteen, October 4, 1956, box 18, University of Minnesota Department of Surgery Papers, University of Minnesota Archives, Minneapolis, MN.

9. See J. D. Clough, ed., *To Act as a Unit: The Story of the Cleveland Clinic*, 4th ed. (Cleveland, OH: Cleveland Clinic Press, 2004); W. C. Sheldon, *Pathfinders of the Heart: The History of Cardiology at the Cleveland Clinic* (n.p.: Xlibris Corporation, 2008); W. C. Sheldon, "F. Mason Sones, Jr.: Stormy Petrel of Cardiology," *Clin. Cardiol.*, 1994, *17*: 405–407; W. L. Proudfit, "F. Mason Sones, Jr., M.D. (1918–1985): The Man and His Work," *Cleve. Clin. Q.*, 1986, *53*: 121–124; P. Heiney, *The Nuts and Bolts of Life: Willem Kolff and the Invention of the Kidney Machine* (Stroud, England: Sutton, 2002).

10. Willem J. Kolff to E. H. Wood, May 4, 1955, MCA. Kolff was referring to D. E. Donald, H. G. Harshbarger, P. S. Hetzel, R. T. Patrick, E. H. Wood, and J. W. Kirklin, "Experiences with a Heart-Lung Bypass (Gibbon Type) in the Experimental Laboratory," *Proceedings of the Staff Meetings of the Mayo Clinic*, (hereafter *PSMMC*), 1955, *30*: 113–115.

11. Kolff to Wood, May 4, 1955, MCA.

12. E. H. Wood to Willem J. Kolff, May 16, 1955, MCA. For insight into how requests for blueprints of the Gibbon-IBM machine were handled, see Romaine-Davis, *John Gibbon*, 147–152.

13. "Sequence of Events and Time Table for Operation in Open Heart," [February 17, 1956], 7-page typewritten memo, Cleveland Clinic Archives.

14. "Surgery in the Heart," *Time*, April 30, 1956, 61. The Cleveland group pioneered "stopped-heart surgery," using a solution that caused cardiac arrest. See D. B. Effler, L. K. Groves, and F. M. Sones Jr., "Elective Cardiac Arrest in Open-Heart Surgery," *Cleveland Clin. Q.*, 1956, *23*: 105–114; J. D. Ratcliff, "The 'Stopped Heart' Operation: New Era in Surgery?" *Reader's Digest*, August 1956, 29–33; and M. S. Shirorishi, "Myocardial Protection: The Rebirth of Potassium-Based Cardioplegia," *Texas Heart Inst. J.*, 1999, *26*: 71–86.

15. Interview of Donald Effler, 1974. "Oral History of Twenty-five Years of American Cardiology.…Celebrating the 25th Anniversary of the American College of Cardiology, 1949–1974," transcript in the author's possession. For a Mayo perspective on patient selection and surgical outcomes, see H. B. Burchell and E. H. Wood, "The Interdependence of the Medical, Surgical and Laboratory Disciplines in the Selection of Cases for Cardiac Surgery," *Surg. Clin. North Am.*, August 1955, 919–936. British pioneers of open-heart surgery Denis Melrose and William Cleland, who worked at Hammersmith Hospital in London, spent three months in Minnesota in 1955 to learn why Walt Lillehei and John Kirklin's patients had much better survival rates than theirs' did. See Cleland's recollections in M. E. Silverman, P. R. Fleming, A. Hollman, D. G. Julian, and D. M. Krikler, *British Cardiology in the 20th Century* (London: Springer, 2000), 107–108.

16. J. D. Clough ed., *To Act as a Unit: The Story of the Cleveland Clinic*, 3rd ed. (Cleveland, OH: Cleveland Clinic Foundation, 1996), 102.

17. William L. Proudfit, interview by W. B. Fye, Cleveland, OH, July 21, 2005.

18. J. W. Kirklin to J. W. Harwick [for the MC BOG], February 15, 1956, MCA.

19. W. C. Roberts, "John Webster Kirklin, MD: A Conversation with the Editor," *Am. J. Cardiol.*, 1998, *81*: 1027–1044.

20. See O. T. Clagett, *General Surgery at the Mayo Clinic 1900–1970* (Rochester, MN: privately printed, 1980).

21. The author thanks Mayo cardiologist Michael McGoon for sharing copies of his father's correspondence and granting permission to incorporate quotations from these letters in this book. See also S. H. McKellar and S. D. Cassivi, "Historical Perspectives of the American Association for Thoracic Surgery: Dwight C. McGoon (1925–1999)," *J. Thorac. Cardiovasc. Surg.*, 2012, *144*: 759–761.

22. Paul Doege had recently resigned from the Marshfield Clinic after the institution adopted an equal salary plan (for all doctors regardless of specialty) that would have dramatically reduced his income when it was phased in over five years. See D. J. McCarty, D. L. Schiedermayer, G. S. Custer, R. F. Lewis, and G. Magnin, "Equity in Physician Compensation: The Marshfield

Experiment," *Perspect. Biol. Med.*, 1992, *35*: 261–270. For a description of the Marshfield Clinic and the group practice model, see S. M. Spencer, "Is the Clinic Your Best Bet?" *Saturday Evening Post*, March 22, 1947, 30–31, 121–122, 124, 126. See also *The Marshfield Story, 1872–1997: Piecing Together Our Past* (Marshfield WI: Marshfield History Project, 1997).

23. P. Doege to A. Blalock, October 18, 1955, box 45, folder 6, McGoon, Blalock Papers, the Alan Mason Chesney Archives of the Johns Hopkins Medical Institutions (hereafter Blalock Papers).

24. A. Blalock to P. Doege, October 22, 1955, box 45, folder 6, McGoon, Blalock Papers.

25. D. C. McGoon to P. Doege, October 24, 1955, Dwight C. McGoon correspondence, copy in the author's possession thanks to the generosity of Michael D. McGoon (hereafter McGoon Papers).

26. I. R. Trimble to D. C. McGoon, October 21, 1955, McGoon Papers.

27. D. C. McGoon to I. R. Trimble, October 31, 1955, McGoon Papers.

28. J. T. Priestley to I. R. Trimble, November 29, 1955, McGoon Papers.

29. D. C. McGoon to John Farrell, January 2, 1956, McGoon Papers. For a recent perspective on medical student debt and career choices, see R. Steinbrook, "Medical Student Debt—Is There a Limit?" *N. Engl. J. Med.*, 2009, *359*: 2629–2632.

30. J. T. Priestley to I. R. Trimble, February 3, 1956, McGoon Papers.

31. I. R. Trimble to D. C. McGoon, February 14, 1956, McGoon Papers.

32. D. C. McGoon to I. R. Trimble, February 22, 1956. McGoon Papers.

33. D. C. McGoon to P. Doege, February 23, 1956. McGoon Papers.

34. P. Doege to D. C. McGoon, March 4, 1956, McGoon Papers.

35. Erville Doege to D. C. McGoon, March 21, 1956, McGoon Papers.

36. V. Cohn, "The Marvelous Mayos. Part Two: How the Clinic Works," *Saturday Evening Post*, December 3, 1960. 24–25, 98–100, 102, quotation from 99.

37. Erville Doege to D. C. McGoon, March 21, 1956. For contemporary perspectives on practice alternatives, see J. Garland, *The Physician and His Practice* (Boston: Little, Brown, 1954); and J. H. Means, "Choice of Opportunities in Medicine," *N. Engl. J. Med.*, 1954, *250*: 766–770. For the group practice model, see C. R. Rorem, "Pattern and Problems of Group Medical Practice," *Am. J. Public Health*, 1950, *40*: 1521–1528.

38. A. Blalock to D. C. McGoon, April 3, 1956, McGoon Papers.

39. J. T. Priestley to D. C. McGoon, April 18, 1956, McGoon Papers.

40. A. Blalock to D. C. McGoon, April 30, 1956, McGoon Papers.

41. Erville Doege to D. C. McGoon, Sunday [1956], McGoon Papers.

42. D. C. McGoon to A. Blalock, August 24, 1956, box 45, folder 6, McGoon, Blalock Papers.

43. J. W. Kirklin to A. Blalock, January 16, 1957, folder Kirklin, Blalock Papers.

44. L. Engel, "Heart Surgery: A New Attack on Our Number 1 Killer," *Harper's Magazine*, April 1957, 38–43, quotation from 38. Engel also published a book about heart surgery at the University of Minnesota. See L. Engel, *The Operation: A Minute-by-Minute Account of a Heart Operation, and the Story of Medicine and Surgery That Led Up to It* (New York: McGraw-Hill, 1958).

45. Engel, "Heart Surgery," 38. See also H. E. Mozen, "Impact of Heart Surgery on Hospitals," *Mod. Hosp.*, 1957, *89*: 67–70, 144.

46. C. W. Lillehei, "Contributions of Open Cardiotomy to the Correction of Congenital and Acquired Cardiac Disease," *N. Engl. J. Med.*, 1958, *258*: 1044–1049, 1090–1095, quotation from 1044.

47. J. P. Swazey and R. C. Fox, "The Clinical Moratorium: A Case Study of Mitral Valve Surgery," in *Experimentation with Human Subjects*, ed. P. A. Freund (New York: George Braziller, 1970), 315–357.

48. H. G. Smithy, H. W. Pratt-Thomas, and H. P. Deyerle, "Aortic Valvulotomy: Experimental Methods and Early Results," *Surg. Gynecol. Obstet.*, 1948, *86*: 513–523, quotation

from 522. For the history of the surgical treatment of aortic valve disease, see W. H. Muller Jr., "The Evolution and Current Status of Surgery of the Aortic Valve," *Bull. Am. Coll. Surg.*, 1977, *62*: 20–31; and S. Westaby and C. Bosher, "Development of Surgery for Valvular Heart Disease," in *Landmarks in Cardiac Surgery* (Oxford: Isis Medical Media, 1997), 139–185. See also C. P. Bailey, ed., *Surgery of the Heart* (Philadelphia: Lea & Febiger, 1955), 738–806.

49. F. A. Crawford Jr., "Horace Smithy: Pioneer Heart Surgeon," *Ann. Thorac. Surg.*, 2010, *89*: 2067–2071, Cooley quotation from 2070.

50. S. M. Spencer, "Can We Rebuild Damaged Hearts?" *Saturday Evening Post*, November 6, 1948, 34–35, 120–124.

51. R. P. Glover, C. P. Bailey, and T. J. E. O'Neill, "Surgery of Stenotic Valvular Disease of the Heart," *JAMA*, 1950, *144*: 1049–1057.

52. G. Lawton, *Straight to the Heart: A Personal Account of Thoughts and Feelings While Undergoing Heart Surgery* (New York: International Universities Press, 1956), 10.

53. Ibid., 219.

54. Ibid., 249.

55. Ibid., 253, 254–255.

56. F. H. Ellis Jr. and J. W. Kirklin, "Aortic Stenosis," *Surg. Clin. North Am.*, August 1955, 1029–1034, quotation from 1033.

57. Ibid., 1033–1034. See also F. H. Ellis Jr. and M. W. Anderson, "Surgical Treatment of Aortic Stenosis: Results of Closed Technics and of Direct Operation Using Hypothermia," *PSMMC*, 1961, *36*: 451–456.

58. Lillehei reported his results in a series of articles published in 1956 and 1957 that are summarized in R. W. M. Frater, ed., *The Key to the Door: A Cardiac Surgical Anthology, C. Walton Lillehei* (London: ICR Publishers, 1998), 123–166.

59. C. W. Lillehei, R. A. DeWall, V. L. Gott, and R. L. Varco, "The Direct Vision Correction of Calcific Aortic Stenosis by Means of a Pump-Oxygenator and Retrograde Coronary Perfusion," *Dis. Chest*, 1956, *30*: 123–140, quotation from 127.

60. J. W. Kirklin and H. T. Mankin, "Open Operation in the Treatment of Aortic Stenosis," *Circulation*, 1960, *21*: 578–586.

61. C. A. Hufnagel, "Basic Concepts in the Development of Cardiovascular Prostheses," *Am. J. Surg.*, 1979, *137*: 285–300.

62. B. Pearse, "Spare Parts for Defective Hearts," *Saturday Evening Post*, August 30, 1958, 18–19, 45–47, quotation from 18. Pearse had watched Hufnagel operate.

63. F. H. Ellis Jr. and J. W. Kirklin, "Aortic Insufficiency," *Surg. Clin. North Am.*, August 1955, 1035–1039, quotation from 1038.

64. E. H. Wood to C. Dennis, February 15, 1956, MCA.

65. E. H. Wood to S. Sarnoff, May 31, 1956, MCA. See also S. Sarnoff to E. H. Wood, May 29, 1956, MCA.

66. J. E. Edwards, T. J. Dry, R. L. Parker, H. B. Burchell, E. H. Wood, and A. H. Bulbulian, *An Atlas of Congenital Anomalies of the Heart and Great Vessels* (Springfield, IL: Charles C Thomas, 1954).

67. F. H. Ellis Jr. and A. H. Bulbulian, "Prosthetic Replacement of the Mitral Valve. I. Preliminary Experimental Observations," *PSMMC*, 1958, *33*: 532–534a.

68. F. H. Ellis Jr., R. O. Brandenburg, J. A. Callahan, and H. W. Marshall, "Open Heart Surgery for Acquired Mitral Insufficiency," *Arch. Surg.*, 1959, *79*: 222–236, quotation from 222.

69. D. B. Effler, Discussion of Ellis et al., "Acquired Mitral Insufficiency," 236.

70. D. C. McGoon, "Repair of Mitral Insufficiency Due to Ruptured Chordae Tendineae," *J. Thorac. Cardiovasc. Surg.*, 1960, *39*: 357–362, quotation from 361. See also D. C. McGoon, "An Early Approach to the Repair of Ruptured Mitral Chordae," *Ann. Thorac. Surg.*, 1989, *47*: 628–629.

71. F. H. Ellis Jr., J. A. Callahan, D. C. McGoon, and J. W. Kirklin, "Results of Open Operation for Acquired Mitral Valve Disease," *N. Engl. J. Med.*, 1965, *272*: 869–874, quotation from 873.

72. See A. B. Weisse, "Mitral Valve Prolapse: Now You See It; Now You Don't: Recalling the Discovery, Rise and Decline of a Diagnosis," *Am. J. Cardiol.*, 2007, *99*: 129–133; and H. Boudoulas and C. F. Wooley, eds., *Mitral Valve Prolapse and the Mitral Valve Prolapse Syndrome* (Mount Kisco, NY: Futura, 1988).

73. French surgeon Alain Carpentier, a major innovator and promoter of mitral valve repair, cited four Americans who had a major influence on him: Walt Lillehei, John Kirklin, Dwight McGoon and Albert Starr. Alain F. Carpentier, MD, PhD [Oral history, September 16, 2000], in Stoney, ed., *Pioneers of Cardiac Surgery*, 322–331. See also T. A. Orszulak, H. V. Schaff, G. K. Danielson, J. M. Piehler, J. R. Pluth, R. L. Frye et al., "Mitral Regurgitation Due to Ruptured Chordae Tendineae: Early and Late Results of Valve Repair," *J. Thorac. Cardiovasc. Surg.*, 1985, *89*: 491–498; and W. R. Chitwood Jr., "Mitral Valve Repair: An Odyssey to Save the Valves!" *J. Heart Valve Dis.*, 1998, *7*: 255–261.

74. H. K. Hellems, F. W. Haynes, and L. Dexter, "Pulmonary 'Capillary' Pressure in Man," *J. Applied Physiol.*, 1949, *2*: 24–29. See also D. C. Connolly, J. W. Kirklin, and E. H. Wood, "The Relationship Between Pulmonary Artery Wedge Pressure and Left Atrial Pressure in Man," *Circ. Res.*, 1954, *2*: 434–440. James Warren, a catheterization pioneer who chronicled the procedure's history, cited Connolly's 1954 article and three earlier papers by others as evidence that they had "fully explored the right side of the heart." See J. V. Warren, ed., *Cardiovascular Physiology* (Stroudsburg, PA: Dowden, Hutchinson & Ross, 1975), 115.

75. H. K. Hellems, F. W. Haynes, L. Dexter, and T. D. Kinney, "Pulmonary Capillary Pressure in Animals Estimated by Venous and Arterial Catheterization," *Am. J. Physiol.*, 1948, *155*: 98–105, quotation from 104.

76. H. A. Zimmerman, R. W. Scott, and N. O. Becker, "Catheterization of the Left Side of the Heart in Man," *Circulation*, 1950, *1*: 357–359.

77. For a description of the various techniques for left heart catheterization, see D. L. Fisher, "Catheterization of the Left Heart," in *Intra Vascular Catheterization*, ed. H. A. Zimmerman (Springfield, IL: Charles C Thomas, 1959), 34–79.

78. H. B. Burchell to E. H. Wood, May 5, 1955, MCA. See also A. G. Morrow, E. Braunwald, J. A. Haller Jr., and E. H. Sharp, "Left Heart Catheterization by the Transbronchial Route," *Circulation*, 1957, *16*: 1033–1039.

79. Burchell to Wood, May 5, 1955. Fisher's technique was a modification of a procedure developed by Swedish surgeon Viking Björk. See D. L. Fisher, "The Use of Pressure Recordings Obtained at Transthoracic Left Heart Catheterization in the Diagnosis of Valvular Heart Disease," *J. Thorac. Surg.*, 1955, *30*: 379–396.

80. E. H. Wood to H. B. Burchell, May 6, 1955, MCA.

81. E. H. Wood, W. Sutterer, H. J. C. Swan, and H. F. Helmholz Jr., "The Technic and Special Instrumentation Problems Associated with Catheterization of the Left Side of the Heart," *PSMMC*, 1956, *31*: 108–115, quotation from 115.

82. E. H. Wood, "Evolution of Instrumentation and Techniques for the Study of Cardiovascular Dynamics from the Thirties to 1980." *Ann. Biomed. Eng.*, 1978, *6*: 250–309, quotation from 268.

83. H. B. Burchell, "The Selection of Patients for Catheterization of the Left Side of the Heart," *PSMMC*, 1956, *31*: 105–108. See also "Symposium on the Diagnostic Value of Simultaneous Catheterization of the Aorta and the Right and Left Sides of the Heart," *PSMMC*, 1956, *31*: 105–145.

84. J. W. Kirklin and F. H. Ellis Jr., "Surgical Implications of Catheterization of the Left Side of the Heart," *PSMMC*, 1956, *31*: 144–145.

85. See G. P. Robb, *An Atlas of Angiocardiography* (Washington, DC: American Registry of Pathology, 1951); and H. L. Abrams, "Angiocardiography and Thoracic Aortography,"

in *Classic Descriptions in Diagnostic Radiography*, ed. A. J. Bruwer (Springfield, IL: Charles C Thomas, 1964), 492–652.

86. A. Cournand, R. J. Bing, L. Dexter, C. T. Dotter, L. N. Katz, J. V. Warren, and E. H. Wood, "Report of Committee on Cardiac Catheterization and Angiocardiography of the American Heart Association," *Circulation*, 1953, *7*: 769–773, quotation from 773.

87. R. H. Morgan and R. E. Sturm, "The Johns Hopkins Fluoroscopic Screen Intensifier," *Radiology*, 1951, *57*: 556–560. See also R. H. Morgan, "Screen Intensification: A Review of Past and Present Research with an Analysis of Future Development," *Am. J. Roentgenol. Radium Ther. Nucl. Med.*, 1956, *75*: 69–76.

88. E. H. Wood to R. E. Sturm, September 25, 1954, MCA.

89. E. H. Wood to J. T. Shepherd, October 26, 1955, MCA.

90. E. H. Wood to H. R. Butt and M. W. Comfort, July 16, 1956, MCA.

91. E. H. Wood to H. R. Butt and M. W. Comfort, July 21, 1956, MCA.

92. "Just What You've Asked For…Dynamic Fluoroscopic Records.…Westinghouse Electric Corporation," Advertisement in *Radiology*, February 1966, *66*, [iii].

93. Wood to Butt and Comfort, July 21, 1956.

94. C. T. Dotter, "New Horizons in Cardiovascular Roentgenology," *Am. J. Roentgenol. Radium Ther. Nucl. Med.*, 1956, *76*: 817–818, quotations from 818.

95. H. M. Weber, Radiology Section Report to MC BOG for 1956, MCA.

96. Ibid.

97. See T. Yipintsoi and E. H. Wood, "The History of Circulatory Indicator Dilution," in *Dye Curves: The Theory and Practice of Indicator Dilution*, ed. D. A. Bloomfield (Baltimore: University Park Press, 1974), 1–19; and I. J. Fox, "History and Developmental Aspects of the Indicator-Dilution Technics," *Circ. Res.*, 1962, *10*: 381–392.

98. "Symposium on Diagnostic Applications of Indicator-Dilution Technics," *PSMMC*, 1957, *32*: 463–553.

99. J. W. Kirklin, "Introduction" [to Symposium on Indicator-Dilution], 463–464.

100. H. B. Burchell, "Assessment of Clinical Value," *PSMMC*, 1957, *32*: 551–553, quotation from 553. See also I. J. Fox and E. H. Wood, "Indocyanine Green: Physical and Physiological Properties," *PSMMC*, 1960, *35*: 732–744.

101. H. B. Burchell, "Relative Roles of Various Technics in Diagnosis and Selection of Cases for Surgical Treatment," in *Congenital Heart Disease: A Symposium*, ed. A. D. Bass and G. K. Moe (Washington, DC: American Association for the Advancement of Science, 1960), 289–308, quotation from 295, symposium held in December 1958. Indicator-dilution techniques fell out of favor as newer and simpler technologies replaced them. In 1995, two North Carolina cardiologists claimed that finding a catheterization laboratory "that performs green dye curves is like finding a doctor who still makes house calls." G. J. Dehmer and W. A. Rutala, "Current Use of Green Dye Curves," *Am. J. Cardiol.*, 1995, *75*: 170–171, quotation from 171.

102. Benjamin D. McCallister, interview by W. B. Fye, Atlanta, GA, March 13, 2006. Two individuals who worked closely with Wood made the same point: his colleague Jeremy Swan and laboratory technician James Fellows. Harold J. C. (Jeremy) Swan, interview by W. B. Fye, San Diego, CA, October 7, 2000. James Fellows, interview by W. B. Fye, Rochester, MN, December 7, 2011.

103. E. H. Wood and H. J. C. Swan to H. M. Odel, R. L. Parker, J. W. Kirklin, F. H. Ellis Jr., J. W. DuShane, November 5, 1956, MCA.

104. Ibid. Emphasis in the original.

105. For additional perspective on Wood's philosophy, see E. H. Wood, "Graduate Training in Cardiovascular Physiology at a Clinical Center: An Analysis of 15 Years' Experience," *PSMMC*, 1961, *36*: 567–580; and E. H. Wood, "Four Decades of Physiology, Musing, and What Now," *Physiologist*, 1982, *25*: 19–32.

106. J. T. Priestley, "The Head, the Heart, and the Hand," *Arch. Surg.*, 1954, *69*: 135–139, quotation from 137.

107. For contemporary perspectives on these themes, see J. E. Deitrick and R. C. Berson, *Medical Schools in the United States at Mid-Century* (New York: McGraw-Hill, 1953); and E. E. Lape, *Medical Research: A Midcentury Survey*, Volume I. *American Medical Research in Principle and Practice* (Boston: Little, Brown, 1955).

108. Minutes, MC Sciences Committee, March 14, 1958, MCA.

109. Minutes, MC BOG, August 28, 1958, MCA.

110. Ibid.

111. For a history of angiography that emphasizes Swedish contributions, see E. Boijsen, "Heart and Blood Vessels: Evolution of Angiography," in *Radiology in Medical Diagnosis: Evolution of X-Ray Applications, 1895–1995*, ed. G. Rosenbusch, M. Oudkerk, and E. Ammann (Cambridge, MA: Blackwell Science, 1995), 176–199.

112. "New Clinic Laboratory to Begin Operations at St. Marys Hospital," *Mayovox*, February 20, 1960.

113. H. J. C. Swan, "Cardiac Catheterization at the St. Marys Laboratory," [Typescript prepared for John Callahan in 1997], MCA.

114. O. W. Kincaid, "Development and Early Years in the Saint Marys Clinical Cardiovascular Laboratory." July 12, 1993, MCA. An anesthesiologist participated in the catheterization of infants and children, who were anesthetized prior to the procedure.

115. D. E. Harken, H. S. Soroff, W. J. Taylor, A. A. Lefemine, S. K. Gupta, and S. Lunzer, "Partial and Complete Prostheses in Aortic Insufficiency," *J. Thorac. Cardiovasc. Surg.*, 1960, *40*: 744–762, 799–812, quotation from 760.

116. J. Watt, "Address of Welcome," in *Prosthetic Valves for Cardiac Surgery*, ed. K. A. Merendino, A. G. Morrow, C. W. Lillehei, and W. H. Muller Jr. (Springfield, IL: Charles C Thomas, 1961), xvii–xviii, quotation from xvii. The papers presented at the September 1957 symposium were published; see J. G. Allen, ed., *Extracorporeal Circulation* (Springfield, IL: Charles C Thomas, 1958).

117. N. S. Braunwald, "It Will Work: The First Successful Mitral Valve Replacement," *Ann. Thorac. Surg.*, 1989, *48*: S1–S3. See also T. H. Lee, *Eugene Braunwald and the Rise of Modern Medicine* (Cambridge, MA: Harvard University Press, 2013), 114–177.

118. For example, University of Oregon surgeon Albert Starr told the audience that the Bethesda group's presentation was "quite exciting" despite the 80 percent mortality rate. See A. Starr, "Discussion," in Merendino et al., eds., *Prosthetic Valves*, 319–328, quotation from 319.

119. F. H. Ellis Jr., Discussion of Frater and Ellis, "Problems in the Development of a Mitral Valve Prosthesis," in Merendino et al., eds., *Prosthetic Valves*, 281–284. For the date of the first procedure, see F. H. Ellis Jr., D. C. McGoon, R. O. Brandenburg, and J. W. Kirklin, "Clinical Experience with Total Mitral Valve Replacement with Prosthetic Valves," *J. Thorac. Cardiovasc. Surg.*, 1963, *46*: 482–497.

120. F. H. Ellis Jr. and J. A. Callahan, "Clinical Application of a Flexible Monocusp Prosthesis: Report of a Case," *PSMMC*, 1961, *36*: 605–609, quotation from 605.

121. Starr, "Discussion," in Merendino et al., eds., *Prosthetic Valves*. See also A. Starr, "The Artificial Heart Valve," *Nature Medicine*, 2007, *13*: 1160–1164. For the link between the Starr-Edwards and Ellis-Bulbulian valves, see A. M. Matthews, "The Development of the Starr-Edwards Heart Valve," *Texas Heart Inst. J.*, 1998, *25*: 282–293.

122. A. Starr to A. Blalock, March 27, 1963, Blalock Papers. This letter includes a detailed description of the development of the Starr-Edwards valve. See also A. Starr and M. L. Edwards, "Mitral Replacement: Clinical Experience with a Ball-Valve Prosthesis," *Ann. Surg.*, 1961, *154*: 740.

123. T. A. Wilson, "Miracle for Amanda," *McCall's*, June 1964, 52, 54, 56.

124. F. H. Ellis Jr., "Development of Mitral Valve Surgery," in *Surgery for Acquired Mitral Valve Disease* (Philadelphia: W. B. Saunders, 1967), 3–45, quotation from 29.

125. H. B. Shumacker Jr., *The Evolution of Cardiac Surgery* (Bloomington: Indiana University Press, 1992), 308.

126. D. C. McGoon, C. Pestana, and E. A. Moffitt, "Decreased Risk of Aortic Valve Surgery," *Arch. Surg.*, 1965, *91*: 779–786. See also S. H. Rahimtoola, "The Twenty-fifth Anniversary of Valve Replacement: A Time for Reflection," *Circulation*, 1985, *71*: 1–3.

127. D. C. McGoon, F. H. Ellis Jr., and J. W. Kirklin, "Late Results of Operation for Acquired Aortic Valvular Disease," *Circulation*, 1965, suppl. 1 to vols. *31* and *32*: I-108–I-116, quotation from I-108.

128. B. Barratt-Boyes, "Homograft Aortic Valve Replacement in Aortic Incompetence and Stenosis," *Thorax*, 1964, *19*: 131–150.

129. R. B. Wallace, E. R. Giuliani, and J. L. Titus, "Use of Aortic Valve Homografts for Aortic Valve Replacement," *Circulation*, 1971, *43*: 365–373. For insights gained by a decade of experience implanting tissue valves at the Mayo Clinic, see R. B. Wallace, "Tissue Valves," *Am. J. Cardiol.*, 1975, *35*: 866–871.

130. A. Starr, "Commentary" on J. R. Pluth, "The Starr Valve Revisited," *Ann. Thorac. Surg.*, 1991, *51*: 333–334. Dwight McGoon wrote in 1982: "Literally hundreds of differing types, models, and concepts of valves have been promoted, tried in patients, and often heralded as the best, only to be discovered in practice to have certain flaws and limitations." D. C. McGoon, "Changing Trends in Cardiac Disease and Cardiac Surgery," *Can. Anaesth. Soc. J.*, 1982, *29*: 330–335, quotation from 332–333.

131. "Ten Years since First Open-Heart Operation," *Mayovox*, March 26, 1965.

132. A. F. Crocetti, "Cardiac Diagnostic and Surgical Facilities in the United States," *Public Health Rep.*, 1965, *80*: 1035–1053, esp. 1039–1040, survey completed in 1961.

133. C. W. Lillehei, "Should YOUR Hospital Have an Open-Heart Surgery Team?" *Hospital Practice*, 1966, 21–27, quotations from 21 and 26. See also B. Eiseman and F. C. Spencer, "The Occasional Open-Heart Surgeon," *Circulation*, 1965, *31*: 161–162.

134. F. D. Moore, "Foreword," in *Cardiac Surgery*, ed. J. C. Norman (New York : Appleton-Century-Crofts, 1967), xv–xviii, quotation from xv.

135. Ibid., xvii. See also F. D. Moore, "Opening Its Valves and Then the Heart Itself," in *A Miracle and a Privilege: Recounting a Half Century of Surgical Advance* (Washington DC: Joseph Henry Press, 1995), 213–231.

Chapter 12

1. "New Mayo Clinic Construction Program Announced: Set to Begin Next Summer," *Mayovox*, January 7, 1950. See also R. C. Roesler, "The Ecology of the Physical Mayo," *Mayo Clin. Proc.*, 1968, *43*: 393–419.

2. "Barnes, Harwick Statements [about the Mayo Clinic's construction program]," *Mayovox*, January 7, 1950.

3. "Same Architects, Same Client, Same Problem: Ellerbee and Company, Mayo Clinic, Diagnostic Center," *Architectural Forum*, 1954, *100*: 136–145. The main "problem" was designing a building that would enhance the efficiency of the outpatient practice, something that had been emphasized in the development of the 1914 and 1928 buildings.

4. Ibid., 137. In 1956 formal names were attached to the clinic's outpatient buildings. What had been called the 1914 and 1928 buildings were renamed "Mayo Clinic-Plummer Building," and the new one was named "Mayo Clinic-Mayo Building." See "Mayo, Plummer Honored in Choice of Building Names," *Mayovox*, July 28, 1956. Three decades later, a writer in a Twin Cities newspaper characterized the Mayo Building as a marble monolith that was a "misbegotten bow to modernism." W. Parker, "Famous Clinic Faces Future as It Remains True to Tradition," *St. Paul Pioneer Press Dispatch*, July 13, 1986, Mayo Clinic Archives, Mayo Historical Unit, Rochester, MN (hereafter MCA).

5. A. Deutsch, "Group Medicine…The Mayo Clinic," *Consumer Reports*, January 1957, 37–40, quotation from 39.

6. Ibid., 39.

7. Ibid., 40.

8. "Same Architects," 140.

9. "Guiding Principles of the Mayo Clinic Group Practice of Medicine," January 16, 1958, MCA.

10. D. L. Wilbur, "The Future of the Practice of Internal Medicine," *Ann. Intern. Med.*, 1959, *51*: 185–195, quotation from 194. See also L. Rantz, "The Image of an Internist," *Clin. Res.*, 1961, *9*: 218–220.

11. D. L. Wilbur, "You as a Specialist in Internal Medicine," in *Listen to Leaders in Medicine*, ed. A. Love and J. S. Childers (New York: Holt, Rinehart and Winston, 1963), 95–114, quotation from 98.

12. Robert L. Parker, interview by John T. Shepherd, Rochester, MN, October 14, 1994, MCA.

13. J. A. Shannon, "Federal Support of Biomedical Sciences: Development and Academic Impact," *J. Med. Educ.*, 1976, *51*. *Suppl to July 1976, part 2*: 1–98. See table 5, "NIH Appropriations for Selected Years, 1950–1975," 87. See also S. P. Strickland, *The Story of the NIH Grants Program* (Lanham, MD: University Press of America, 1989); and W. B. Fye, "Cardiology and the Federal Funding of Academic Medicine," in *American Cardiology: The History of a Specialty and Its College* (Baltimore: Johns Hopkins University Press, 1996), 150–181.

14. Paul Dudley White, who cared for President Dwight Eisenhower, recalled that some politicians "became especially interested in our work when they themselves developed heart disease (as many of them did) and became our patients." P. D. White, *My Life and Medicine: An Autobiographical Memoir* (Boston: Gambit, 1971), 58.

15. Lyndon Johnson characterized James Cain as "my family physician…[and] a longtime personal friend." See L. B. Johnson, "My Heart Attack Taught Me How to Live," *American Magazine*, July 1956, 15–17, 85–87, quotation from 87. See also R. Dallek, *Lone Star Rising: Lyndon Johnson and His Times, 1908–1960* (New York: Oxford University Press, 1991), 469, 483–492; and R. A. Caro, *The Years of Lyndon Johnson: Master of the Senate* (New York: Alfred A. Knopf, 2002), 618–658.

16. J. W. Hurst, "Coronary Events in World Leaders," *Ann. Intern. Med.*, 2001, *134*: 338–339. See also J. W. Hurst and J. C. Cain, *LBJ: To Know Him Better*, ed. R. L. Hardesty and T. Gittinger (Austin, TX: LBJ Foundation, 1995); and H. B. Burchell, "Acute Myocardial Infarction: A Discussion of Certain Controversial Issues," *Calif. Med.*, 1954, *80*: 281–287.

17. D. D. Eisenhower to L. B. Johnson, September 23, 1955, quotation from C. G. Lasby, *Eisenhower's Heart Attack: How Ike Beat Heart Disease and Held on to the Presidency* (Lawrence: University of Kansas Press, 1997), 70–71.

18. Lasby, *Eisenhower's Heart Attack*. See also P. D. White, "President Eisenhower's Heart Attack," in *My Life and Medicine*, 175–194; and R. E. Gilbert, "Eisenhower's Heart Attack: Medical Treatment, Political Effect, and the 'Behind the Scenes' Leadership Style," *Politics and Life Sciences*, 2008, *27*: 2–21.

19. F. H. Messerli, A. W. Messerli, and T. F. Lüscher, "Eisenhower's Billion-Dollar Heart Attack—50 Years Later," *N. Engl. J. Med.*, 2005, *353*: 1205–1207, quotation from 1205.

20. "Heart Attack: The President's Ailment, Coronary Thrombosis, Is the Worst U.S. Killer, Deadlier than Cancer," *Life*, October 10, 1955, 150–159.

21. Their conclusion was based on a poll that revealed 60 percent of 234 heart specialists thought the president was "physically able to serve a second term." See "3 out of 5 Heart Specialists Say Ike Could Serve a Second Term," *U.S. News & World Report*, January 13, 1956, 19–29.

22. AP Wirephoto caption accompanying image of Lyndon Johnson, Lady Bird Johnson, and James Cain at the Mayo Clinic, December 29, 1955, original in the author's possession.

23. J. Willis Hurst to W. B. Fye, June 13, 2007, e-mail. For a similar perspective, see Philip R. Lee quoted in D. Blumenthal and J. A. Morone, *The Heart of Power: Health and Politics in the Oval Office* (Berkeley: University of California Press, 2009), 170.

24. E. V. Allen, "The American Heart Association: Its Aims and Accomplishments," *Circulation*, 1957, *16*: 323–331, quotation from 323–324. See also E. V. Allen, "The American Heart Association in 1956–1957" [address as outgoing president to AHA Assembly], October 1957, American Heart Association National Center Corporate Records, Dallas, TX (hereafter AHA Archives).

25. "Summary of Currently Active (as of Nov. 1, 1956) National Heart Institute Research Grants," attachment B to NAHC Minutes, November 26–28, 1956, box 32, University of Minnesota Department of Surgery Papers, University of Minnesota Archives, Minneapolis, MN (hereafter UMN Dept. Surgery Papers).

26. O. H. Wangensteen to Edward J. Thye, February 17, 1956, box 23, UMN Dept. Surgery Papers.

27. O. H. Wangensteen to E. V. Allen, February 13, 1957, box 4, UMN Dept. Surgery Papers. At the time, Mayo did not solicit research funds from the AHA or the NIH; see R. L. Parker, "Minnesota Heart Association," *Minn. Med.*, 1957, *40*: 47–49.

28. Minutes, MC BOG, November 14, 1956, MCA.

29. S. F. Haines, "Confidential Report to the Staff," November 24, 1956, MCA.

30. Ibid. See also W. W. Moore, *Fighting for Life: The Story of the American Heart Association, 1911–1975* (Dallas: American Heart Association, 1983); R. Carter, *The Gentle Legions: A Probing Study of the National Voluntary Health Organizations* (Garden City, NY: Doubleday, 1961); and J. T. Patterson, *The Dread Disease: Cancer and Modern American Culture* (Cambridge, MA: Harvard University Press, 1987).

31. K. J. Ladner, "Mayo Association Extramural Funds," June 1964, MCA. Physiologist Earl Wood was among those who received a grant. See E. H. Wood, "Four Decades of Physiology, Musing, and What Now," *Physiologist*, 1982, *25*: 19–32.

32. "Dr. Rowntree," *Clinic Bulletin*, October 15, 1920, MCA. See also L. G. Rowntree and R. Fitz, "Studies of Renal Function in Renal, Cardiorenal and Cardiac Diseases," *Arch. Int. Med.*, 1913, *11*: 258–287.

33. S. J. Peitzman, *Dropsy, Dialysis, Transplant: A Short History of Failing Kidneys* (Baltimore: Johns Hopkins University Press, 2007).

34. James C. Broadbent, interview by W. B. Fye, Rochester, MN, January 29, 2008.

35. J. T. McCarthy, "The Division of Nephrology," in *History of the Department of Internal Medicine at the Mayo Clinic*, ed. J. L. Graner (Rochester, MN: Mayo Foundation, 2002), 187–204.

36. "Nephrology Subspecialty Develops Varied Roles," *Mayovox*, January 14, 1966.

37. L. T. Coggeshall, *Planning for Medical Progress Through Education* (Washington, DC: Association of American Medical Colleges, 1965), 97–104. See also R. A. Stevens, "Health Care in the Early 1960s," *Health Care Manage Rev.*, 1996, *18*: 11–22; and E. Freidson, *Profession of Medicine: A Study of the Sociology of Applied Knowledge* (New York: Dodd, Mead, 1970).

38. Cancer and Stroke. The President's Commission on Heart Disease, *Report to the President: A National Program to Conquer Heart Disease, Cancer and Stroke,* 2 vols. (Washington, DC: Government Printing Office, 1965), quotation from 1: 88. In 1956, one year after Johnson had his heart attack, he had written, "I joined a huge throng when I became, unwillingly like all the others, a member of the Coronary Club. Last year about 810,000 deaths in the United States were attributed to heart disease." Johnson, "My Heart Attack," 87. The definitive study of the Commission on Heart Disease, Cancer and Stroke is S. P. Strickland, *The History of Regional Medical Programs* (Lanham, MD: University Press of America, 2000).

39. I. S. Wright, S. Bellet, J. W. Hurst, P. Sanger, and H. B. Taussig, "Report of the Subcommittee on Heart Disease," in *Report to the President*, 2: 1–102, quotation from 1.

40. Ibid., 7. See also R. Fein, *The Doctor Shortage: An Economic Diagnosis* (Washington, DC: Brookings Institution, 1967).

41. "Next Week Is Apex of Centennial Year," *Mayovox*, September 11, 1964.

42. "Mayo Stamp Issued Today," *Mayovox*, September 11, 1964.

43. "Long-Term Planning Essential to Insure Future: Dr. Priestley," *Mayovox*, November 23, 1963.

44. "A Prospectus: Adult Clinical Cardiology at the Mayo Clinic," January 13, 1964, MCA. For the cultural context, see D. Farber and B. Bailey, eds., *The Columbia Guide to America in the 1960s* (New York: Columbia University Press, 2001); and A. Toffler, *Future Shock* (New York: Random House, 1970).

45. M. W. Anderson, G. W. Daugherty, R. O. Brandenburg and 13 additional cardiologists to J. William Harwick, January 20, 1964, MCA. The cardiologists are listed in Table 12.2 of this chapter.

46. "Adult Clinical Cardiology at the Mayo Clinic."

47. Ibid.

48. Ibid. The Mayo cardiologists' publications were found by searching for 1963 articles at http://www.ncbi.nlm.nih.gov/pubmed. See also W. B. Fye, "Medical Authorship: Traditions, Trends, and Tribulations," *Ann. Intern. Med.*, 1990, *113*: 317–325.

49. Minutes, Joint Meeting of the MC BOG and Officers and Councilors of the Voting Staff, July 11, 1962, MCA. For a national comparison, see H. N. Beaty, D. Babbott, E. J. Higgins, P. Jolly, and G. S. Levey, "Research Activities of Faculty in Academic Departments of Medicine," *Ann. Int. Med.*, 1986, *104*: 90–97.

50. "Adult Clinical Cardiology at the Mayo Clinic."

51. R. O. Brandenburg Section Report to MC BOG for 1964, MCA.

52. G. W. Thorn, "A Department of Medicine in 1963–1973," *N. Engl. J. Med.*, 1964, *270*: 281–286, quotation from 281–282.

53. "Mayo's Magic: The Human Touch," *Business Week*, December 1965, 107.

54. See B. Hansen, *Picturing Medical Progress from Pasteur to Polio: A History of Mass Media Images and Popular Attitudes in America* (New Brunswick, NJ: Rutgers University Press, 2009); P. E. Dans, *Doctors in the Movies: Boil the Water and Just Say Aah* (Bloomington, IL: Medi-Ed Press, 2000); and K. Ostherr, *Medical Visions: Producing the Patient Through Film, Television, and Imaging Technologies* (New York: Oxford University Press, 2013).

55. Deutsch, "Group Medicine," 37

56. W. R. Young, "Rx for Modern Medicine: Some Sympathy Added to Science," *Life*, October 12, 1959, 144–160, quotation from 148.

57. For a summary of changes in postgraduate training during the 1950s and 1960s, see R. Stevens, "Graduate Medical Education," in *American Medicine and the Public Interest*, 2nd ed. (Berkeley: University of California Press, 1998), 378–414; and K. M. Ludmerer, "The Maturation of Graduate Medical Education," in *Time to Heal: American Medical Education from the Turn of the Century to the Era of Managed Care* (New York: Oxford University Press, 1999), 180–195. Contemporary perspectives include S. E. Bradley, "Medical Education and Medical Research: An Interaction," *N. Engl. J. Med.*, 1963, *269*: 1292–1296; and J. A. Shannon, "The Place of the National Institutes of Health in American Medicine," *N. Engl. J. Med.*, 1963, *269*: 1352–1357. Because Mayo did not offer internships until 1969 or open a medical school until 1972, each Mayo medical fellow (resident) had trained somewhere else before he or she moved to Rochester. See "Mayo Graduate School Plans Internship Program," *Mayovox*, February 23, 1968. Mayo had already launched advanced fellowships in pediatric cardiology, dermatology, and gastroenterology. See "New Advanced Fellowship Training 'Meets Demand,'" *Mayovox*, March 30, 1963.

58. V. Johnson, "Memorandum: Proposed Training Program in Advanced Cardiology (Doctors Parker, Broadbent, Connolly)," February 14, 1963, MCA.

59. M. W. Anderson Section Report to MC BOG for 1962, MCA.

60. For Corne, see H. N. Segall, *Pioneers of Cardiology in Canada 1820–1970: The Genesis of Canadian Cardiology* (Willowdale, Ontario: Hounslow Press, 1988), 321–322. The terminology of postgraduate training at Mayo was unusual because the institution continued to use the term "fellowship" to describe the post-internship experience that almost every other institution described as a "residency."

61. "Adult Clinical Cardiology at the Mayo Clinic."

62. M. W. Anderson, "An Application for Grant Support for Cardiology Research and Education" with letter from Anderson to H. Mankin, G. W. Daugherty, D. C. Connolly, and R. O. Brandenburg, September 23, 1964, MCA. See also M. W. Anderson, *A Sojourn with Family, Career, and Time* (Rochester, MN: privately printed, 1983), 117–122.

63. K. B. Corbin, "The Mayo Foundation Fellowship Program," *PSMMC*, 1961, *36*: 562–566.

64. "Recent Events of Major Significance to Medical Education," *JAMA*, 1966, *198*: 848–850.

65. *The Graduate Education of Physicians: The Report of the Citizens Commission on Graduate Medical Education* (Chicago: American Medical Association, 1966), 112. This document, known as the Millis Report, was named for the commission's chair, Western Reserve University President John Millis. See also R. Stevens, "Graduate Medical Education: A Continuing History," *J. Med. Educ.*, 1978, *53*: 1–18.

66. For background on the Residency Review Committee for Internal Medicine, see E. C. Rosenow Jr., *History of the American College of Physicians: Executive Perspectives, 1959–1977* (Philadelphia: American College of Physicians, 1984), 9, 157–159.

67. Table 8. "Activity of Residency Review Committees, July 1, 1965 to June 30, 1966," in: "Graduate Medical Education," *JAMA*, 1966, *198*: 874–892, table on 880. See also C. H. Kohrman, R. M. Andersen, and M. M. Clements, *Training Physicians: The Case of Internal Medicine* (San Francisco: Jossey-Bass, 1994).

68. J. Star, "My Checkup at Mayos," *Look*, March 24, 1964, 66–69, quotation from 66.

69. "Hypertension Clinic Proves Worth in Services to Patients and Staff," *Mayovox*, October 12, 1963. See also A. Schirger, "The Division of Hypertension," in Graner, ed., *Department of Internal Medicine*, 243–247; J. E. Estes, "Hypertension in 1958: A Tale of Pills, Philosophy, and Perplexity," *Med. Clin. North Am.*, July 1958, 899–915; R. W. Gifford Jr., "The Use of Diuretics in Hypertension," *JAMA*, 1961, *177*: 140–141; and N. Postel-Vinay, *A Century of Arterial Hypertension, 1896–1996* (New York: John Wiley & Sons, 1996).

70. Star, "My Checkup at Mayos," 69.

71. Ibid., 68.

72. Hugh Butt, interview by Carolyn S. Beck, June 23, 1997, MCA.

73. George Mixter Jr. to Victor Johnson and R. Drew Miller, May 12, 1966, excerpts in Graner, ed., *Department of Internal Medicine*, 28.

74. J. V. Warren, "The Training of the Internist: Today and Tomorrow," *JAMA*, 1966, *195*: 935–938, quotation from 938.

75. T. B. Turner, *Fundamentals of Medical Education* (Springfield, IL: Charles C Thomas, 1963), 58.

76. Ibid., 23–24. Robert Howard, who had become dean of University of Minnesota Medical School in 1958, made a similar point. See R. B. Howard, "The Academic Health Center: On the Rocks with a Twist of Dilemma," *J. Med. Educ.*, 1970, *45*: 839–846. See also Ludmerer, *Time to Heal*, 173–179. In 1966, one-half of the 462 hospitals that offered internal medicine residencies were not affiliated with a medical school. See table 11, "Number of Residencies, by Specialty, in [Medical School] Affiliated and Nonaffiliated Hospitals," in "Graduate Medical Education," *JAMA*, 1966, *198*: 874–892, table on 882.

77. Turner, *Medical Education*, 58. Expanding health insurance coverage was the main reason for a decline in the number of so-called service or ward patients.

78. See P. A. Tumulty, "House Staff Education on a Private Medical Service," *JAMA*, 1963, *185*: 943–948; and A. M. Harvey, V. A. McKusick, and J. D. Stobo, *Osler's Legacy: The Department of Medicine at Johns Hopkins, 1889–1989* (Baltimore: Johns Hopkins University Department of Medicine, 1990).

79. "Definition of Terms Used in Mayo Foundation and Mayo Graduate School of Medicine: Categories of Temporary Professional Appointments," MCA. For a summary of the changes in Mayo's internal medicine residency, see Richard J. Reitemeier to Members of Sections of Internal Medicine, January 29, 1968, MCA.

80. For John Spittell's important role in reforming Mayo's residency program, see Graner, ed., *Department of Internal Medicine*, 43–45.

81. C. F. Code, "Report to Mayo Foundation Board of Trustees upon Completion of Directorship for Medical Education and Research," MCA.

82. R. J. Reitemeier, "History of the Department of Medicine," July 6, 1987, MCA.

83. G. Weisz, "The Rise of American Specialties," in *Divide and Conquer: A Comparative History of Medical Specialization* (New York: Oxford University Press, 2006), 63–83.

84. R. Stevens, *In Sickness and in Wealth: American Hospitals in the Twentieth Century*, reprint with new preface (Baltimore: Johns Hopkins University Press, 1999), 245.

85. V. Cohn, "The Marvelous Mayos, Part Two: How the Clinic Works," *Saturday Evening Post*, December 3, 1960, 24–25, 98–100, 102, quotation from 100.

86. Reitemeier, "History of the Department of Medicine."

87. Minutes, MC BOG, November 4, 1965, MCA. For a summary of the creation of the Department of Medicine and the transformation of Mayo's horizontal leadership structure (autonomous sections) into a pyramidal model (empowered departments) common to medical schools, see Graner, ed., *Department of Internal Medicine*, 25–35.

88. "Chairman of Sections of Internal Medicine" [Job Description] with Minutes, MC BOG, November 17, 1966, MCA.

89. R. O. Brandenburg Section Report to MC BOG for 1965, MCA. See also D. W. Mulder, *Neurology at Mayo: The Formative Years* (Rochester, MN, privately printed, 1989).

90. Brandenburg Section Report to MC BOG for 1965, MCA. Ward's comments are in the margin. For a national perspective on balancing general medical and subspecialty practice, see W. Adams, "Internal Medicine under Stress," *JAMA*, 1963, *186*: 934–937.

91. Shortly after I joined the Marshfield Clinic in Wisconsin in 1978, the Cardiology Division (which was part of the Department of Medicine) lobbied successfully to become a separate department in order to focus on patients with heart disease and not participate in general medical on-call responsibilities. This move frustrated many other medical subspecialists (such as hematologists, nephrologists, and rheumatologists) because they also wanted to focus on their fields of interest. For an overview of tensions surrounding cardiology's success as a specialty, see W. B. Fye, "Fueling the Growth of Cardiology: Patients, Procedures, and Profits," in *American Cardiology*, 249–294.

92. N. W. Barker, R. J. Kennedy, L. M. Eaton, H. M., Odel, L. M. Randall, E. A. Hines Jr. et al., "Recommendations of the Executive Committee for the Diagnostic and Medical Care of Adult Rochester Residents," January 27, 1947, MCA.

93. G. R. Geier Jr., *Shadows: A History of the Olmsted Medical Center* (Rochester, MN: Olmsted Medical Center, 2010).

94. K. G. Berge, G. W. Morrow Jr., M. I. Lindsay, and R. D. Hurt, *A History of Community Internal Medicine, Mayo Clinic, Rochester* (Rochester, MN, 1996).

95. "To the Board of Governors" [Majority Report of the Heck Committee to Review Problems Concerned with Local Practice], 1959, MCA.

96. Meeting of L. A. Smith Section with the Administrative Committee of the Board of Governors regarding Future Policies regarding Local Practice, October 29, 1959, Community Medicine Collection, MCA.

97. R. O. Brandenburg Report to MC BOG for 1967, May 8, 1968, MCA.

98. M. W. Anderson Section Report to MC BOG for 1968, February 24, 1969, MCA.

99. "Instructions for Fellows on Cardiology Hospital Services," [Mayo Clinic, ca. 1968], MCA.

100. [Fifteen cardiologists] to MC BOG with two-page memo "Proposed Change in Mode of Practice," August 26, 1969, with Minutes, MC BOG, August 28, 1969, MCA.

101. Minutes, MC BOG, August 28, 1969, MCA.

102. R. O. Brandenburg to R. J. Reitemeier, May 26, 1970, MCA.

103. For background on the role of the general internist in the context of increasing subspecialization within internal medicine, see R. H. Williams, "Departments of Medicine in 1970, I. Staff Policies," *Ann. Int. Med.*, 1959, *50*: 1252–1276.

104. "Consultation-Only Plan Provided Area Physicians," *Mayovox*, July 24, 1970.

105. E. J. Levit, M. Sabshin, and C. B. Mueller, "Trends in Graduate Medical Education and Specialty Certification," *N. Engl. J. Med.*, 1974, *290*: 545–549, quotations from 548–549. See also F. H. Adams and R. C. Mendenhall, "Profile of the Cardiologist: Training and Manpower Requirements for the Specialist in Adult Cardiovascular Disease," *Am. J. Cardiol.*, 1974, *34*: 389–456.

106. "Specialty Board Certification and Appointment to the Mayo Clinic Staff" with Minutes, MC BOG, August 23, 1967, MCA. Two Mayo staff members served as secretary-treasurers of the Advisory Board for Medical Specialties for a quarter century: radiologist Byrl Kirklin (1944–1957) and surgeon Louis Buie (1957–1970). See B. R. Kirklin, "The Specialty Boards," *JAMA*, 1956, *160*: 1327–1329; and L. A. Buie, "Specialty Certifying Boards in American Medicine," *Br. Med. J.*, 1965, *1*: 543–547.

107. J. F. Fairbairn II, J. L. Juergens, and J. A. Spittell Jr., *Peripheral Vascular Diseases* 4th ed. (Philadelphia: W. B. Saunders, 1972), 2.

108. "Quarterly Directory. Mayo Clinic, Mayo Foundation…[for the Quarter Beginning] Summer 1968," 39, MCA.

109. J. A. Spittell Section Report to MC BOG for 1968, MCA.

110. J. F. Fairbairn Section Report to MC BOG for 1968, MCA, emphasis in the original.

111. R. O. Brandenburg to R. J. Reitemeier, May 5, 1971, MCA. See also R. O. Brandenburg to J. C. Hunt, June 24, 1974, MCA.

112. D. L. Wilbur, W. E. Burger, H. R. Butt, G. S. Schuster, G. S. and J. W. Harwick, "Report of Special Committee Mayo Association," December 1962, MCA. The "Wilbur Report" explains the histories of (and relationships among) the Mayo Clinic, the Mayo Foundation, and the Mayo Association. Wilbur was one of the original public trustees appointed to the Mayo Association in 1951. See R. C. Roesler, "The Origin and Evolution of the Mayo Foundation Board of Trustees," February 1981, MCA.

113. See "LBJ to Serve on Mayo Board," *Rochester Post Bulletin*, February 13, 1969; and "Lyndon Johnson Accepts Mayo Foundation Trusteeship," *Mayovox*, February 21, 1969. Johnson did not serve on any other institutional or corporate boards.

114. *Trusteeship of Health* (Rochester, MN: Mayo Foundation, 1969), 1.

115. Ibid., 23. See also H. M. Somers and A. R. Somers, *Medicare and the Hospitals: Issues and Prospects* (Washington, DC: Brookings Institution, 1967); and E. Witkin, *The Impact of Medicare* (Springfield, IL: Charles C Thomas, 1971).

116. *Trusteeship of Health*, 26. See also A. S. Bridwell, "The Mayo Development Program: Laying the Foundation, 1965–1985," ca. 1990, MCA.

117. *Trusteeship of Health*, 15–16.

118. Ibid., 17. The first Mayo Medical School class entered in the fall of 1972. Addresses marking the occasion are contained in *The Unending Adventure* (Rochester, MN: Mayo Clinic, 1972). Cardiologist Raymond Pruitt was the first dean of the medical school. See R. D. Pruitt, "Mayo Medical School," in *New Medical Schools at Home and Abroad*, ed. J. Z. Bowers and E. F. Purcell (New York: Josiah Macy Jr. Foundation, 1978), 147–177; and V. Johnson, "Mayo Medical School," in *Mayo Clinic: Its Growth and Progress* (Bloomington, MN: Voyageur Press, 1984), 195–218.

119. C. F. Code, "Procurement of Medical Manpower in the Mayo Setting, Report to the Annual Staff Meeting," November 21, 1966, MCA.

120. See W. Shonick, *Government and Health Services: Government's Role in the Development of U.S. Health Services, 1930–1980* (New York: Oxford University Press, 1995), 367–412; and J. R. Schofield, *New and Expanded Medical Schools: Mid-Century to the 1980s* (San Francisco: Jossey-Bass, 1984).

121. *Trusteeship of Health*, 25.

122. Fye, "Fueling the Growth of Cardiology."

Chapter 13

1. Dwight Eisenhower to Clark Gable, November 7, 1960, published in C. G. Lasby, *Eisenhower's Heart Attack* (Lawrence: University Press of Kansas, 1997), 281–282.

2. L. Tornabene, *Long Live the King: A Biography of Clark Gable* (New York: G. P. Putnam's Sons, 1976), 391–398. See also E. Corday and D. W. Irving, *Disturbances of Heart Rate, Rhythm and Conduction* (Philadelphia: W. B. Saunders, 1961); and H. E. Stephenson Jr., *Cardiac Arrest and Resuscitation* (St. Louis: C.V. Mosby, 1958).

3. T. B. Morgan, "The Heart," *Look*, January 15, 1963, 62–69, quotation from 62.

4. C. A. Imboden Jr., "Coronary Care Units," *Med. Ann. D. C.*, 1964, *33*: 442–444, quotation from 442.

5. L. Poole, *I Am a Chronic Cardiac* (New York: Dodd, Mead, 1964), 20.

6. "Stevenson of Illinois," *Life*, July 23, 1965, 22–29, quotation from 28.

7. R. E. Spiekerman, J. T. Brandenburg, R. W. P. Achor, and J. E. Edwards, "The Spectrum of Coronary Heart Disease in a Community of 30,000: A Clinicopathologic Study," *Circulation*, 1962, *25*: 57–65. See also L. Kuller, A. M. Lilienfeld, and R. Fisher, "An Epidemiological Study of Sudden and Unexpected Deaths in Adults," *Medicine*, 1967, *46*: 341–361.

8. W. B. Fye, "Resuscitating a *Circulation* Abstract to Celebrate the 50th Anniversary of the Coronary Care Unit Concept," *Circulation*, 2011, *124*: 1886–1893. See also T. H. Lee and L. Goldman, "The Coronary Care Unit Turns 25: Historical Trends and Future Directions," *Ann. Intern. Med.*, 1988, *108*: 887–894; and K. K. Khush, E. Rapaport, and D. Waters, "The History of the Coronary Care Unit," *Can. J. Cardiol.*, 2005, *21*: 1041–1045.

9. J. S. Lundy and R. P. Gage, "'P.A.R.' Spells Better Care for Postanesthesia Patients," *Mod. Hosp.*, 1944, *63*: 63–64. More than 4,000 postoperative patients were admitted to the Mayo unit during its first year of operation. See R. T. Patrick and J. S. Lundy, "The Postanesthesia Room: A Life Saver," *Hosp. Prog.*, 1953, *34*: 58–60.

10. J. S. Lundy, E. B. Tuohy, R. C. Adams, L. H. Mousel, and T. H. Seldon, "Annual Report for 1942 of the Section on Anesthesia," *Proceedings of the Staff Meetings of the Mayo Clinic*, 1943, *18*: 129–140, quotation from 130–131. The name of St. Mary's Hospital changed gradually to Saint Marys Hospital beginning around 1940. In general, I use the older version up to that date and the newer version thereafter.

11. H. G. A. Charbon and H. M. Livingstone, "Planning a Postoperative Recovery Room for Adequate Postoperative Care," *Hospitals*, 1949, *23*: 35–38, quotation from 35. See also A. C. Bachmeyer and G. Hartman, eds., *Hospital Trends and Developments, 1940–1946* (New York: New York Commonwealth Fund, 1948).

12. M. S. Sadove, J. Cross, H. G. Higgins, and M. J. Segall, "The Recovery Room Expands Its Service," *Mod. Hosp.*, 1954, *83*: 65–70, quotation from 65. Other factors that contributed to the acceptance of the ICU model included experiences with specialized "shock units" for critically injured soldiers during World War II and the Korean War. A notable non-surgical example of the special care concept was the clustering of patients who needed mechanical respiration (with so-called iron lungs) following polio epidemics in the early 1950s. See D. J. Rothman, "The Iron Lung and Democratic Medicine," in *Beginnings Count: The Technological Imperative in American Health Care* (New York: Oxford University Press, 1997), 41–66.

13. R. Stevens, *In Sickness and in Wealth: American Hospitals in the Twentieth Century*, reprint with new preface (Baltimore: Johns Hopkins University Press, 1999), 228.

14. M. R. Taufic, "Nursing Care of the Cardiovascular Surgery Patient," *Nursing World*, February 1956, 10–13, quotations from 10, 12. See also L. G. Wilson, "The Development of Cardiac Surgery at Minnesota, 1940–1960," in *Medical Revolution in Minnesota: A History of the University of Minnesota Medical School* (St. Paul, MN: Midewiwin Press, 1989), 481–528.

15. J. W. Kirklin, D. E. Donald, H. G. Harshbarger, P. S. Hetzel, R. T. Patrick, H. J. C. Swan et al., "Studies in Extracorporeal Circulation. I. Applicability of Gibbon-Type Pump-Oxygenator to Human Intracardiac Surgery: 40 Cases," *Ann. Surg.*, 1956, *144*: 2–8.

16. E. H. Wood to J. W. Kirklin, July 24, 1956, Mayo Clinic Archives, Mayo Historical Unit, Rochester, MN (hereafter MCA).

17. Ibid.

18. Ibid, emphasis in the original. DuShane's handwritten notes are in the margin of a copy that Wood circulated to him, Howard Burchell, and Robert Brandenburg.

19. "Saint Marys Hospital Annals," 1956, MCA. See also W. S. Lyons, J. W. DuShane, and J. W. Kirklin, "Postoperative Care after Whole-Body Perfusion and Open Intracardiac Operations," *JAMA*, 1960, *173*: 625–630. The neurology-neurosurgery unit opened two years later. See E. F. M. Wijdicks, W. R. Worden, A. G. Miers, and D. G. Piepgras, "The Early Days of the Neurosciences Intensive Care Unit," *Mayo Clin. Proc.*, 2011, *86*: 903–906.

20. Sister Elizabeth Gillis, interview by Sister Ellen Whelan, September 11, 2005, in E. Whelan, *The Sisters' Story, Part Two: Saint Marys Hospital—Mayo Clinic, 1939 to 1980* (Rochester, MN: Mayo Foundation, 2007), 163–165. The University of Minnesota did not have an ICU for open-heart surgery patients until the 1960s. Prior to its opening, patients were cared for in the recovery room until they were moved to a standard room. See C. N. Barnard, R. A. DeWall, R. L. Varco, and C. W. Lillehei, "Pre and Postoperative Care for Patients Undergoing Open Cardiac Surgery," *Dis. Chest*, 1959, *35*: 194–211.

21. M. Brigh and M. Amadeus, "Intensive Care: Effective Care," *Hosp. Prog.*, 1958, *39*: 64–66, 131–132, quotations from 66 and 132. See also R. A. Klein, "A Vocation Is a Call from God: An Interview with Sister Mary Brigh," *Mayo Alumnus*, January 1981, 8–12.

22. M. Brigh, "Is Intensive Care the Answer?" typescript, paper presented at St. Louis University, April 14, 1959, MCA.

23. Ibid. See also F. G. Abdellah and E. J. Strachan, "Progressive Patient Care," *Am. J. Nursing*, 1959, *59*: 649–655. See also P. Southorn, "Intensive Care," in *Art to Science: Department of Anesthesiology, Mayo Clinic*, ed. K. Rehder, P. Southorn, and A. Sessler (Rochester, MN: Mayo Clinic, 2000), 55–71; M. Hilberman, "The Evolution of Intensive Care Units," *Crit. Care Med.*, 1975, *3*: 159–165; S. J. Reiser, "The Intensive Care Unit: The Unfolding and Ambiguities of Survival Therapy," *Int. J. Technol. Asses. Health Care*, 1992, *8*: 382–394; and A. Kumar and J. E. Parrillo, eds., *Historical Aspects of Critical Illness and Critical Care Medicine* (Philadelphia: W. B. Saunders, 2009).

24. M. Brigh, "Is Intensive Care the Answer?"

25. M. Brigh, "Intensive Care Unit at Saint Marys." Typescript, paper presented at the Idaho State Hospital Convention, Boise, ID, October 19, 1959, MCA.

26. W. T. Mosenthal and D. D. Boyd, "Special Unit Saves Lives, Nurses and Money," *Mod. Hosp.*, 1957, *89*: 83–86.

27. M. E. Fordham, *Cardiovascular Surgical Nursing* (New York: Macmillan, 1962). Fordham, describing the Saint Marys Hospital unit three decades later, exclaimed: "It was the best care I have ever seen anywhere. . . . There was a fantastic setup there, and they had fantastic surgeons." She spoke from experience, having worked at hospitals in London, Johannesburg, Capetown, and New York City. Mary E. Fordham interviews by Jacqueline Wilkie, August 31, 1994, and November 25, 1994, MCA. For the artificial pacemaker, see P. M. Zoll, A. J. Linenthal, L. R. Norman, M. H. Paul, and W. Gibson, "Treatment of Unexpected Cardiac Arrest by External Electrical Stimulation of the Heart," *N. Engl. J. Med.*, 1956, *254*: 541–546; D. C. Schechter, *Exploring the Origins of Electrical Cardiac Stimulation* (Minneapolis: Medtronic, 1983); and K. Jeffrey, *Machines in Our Hearts: The Cardiac Pacemaker, the Implantable Defibrillator, and American Health Care* (Baltimore: Johns Hopkins University Press, 2001).

28. J. A. M[a]cWilliam, "Cardiac Failure and Sudden Death," *Brit. Med. J.*, 1889, *1*: 6–8, quotations from 6, 8. See also W. B. Fye, "Ventricular Fibrillation and Defibrillation: Historical Perspectives with Emphasis on the Contributions of John MacWilliam, Carl Wiggers, and William Kouwenhoven," *Circulation*, 1985, *71*: 858–865.

29. C. S. Beck, W. H. Pritchard, and H. S. Feil, "Ventricular Fibrillation of Long Duration Abolished by Electric Shock," *JAMA*, 1947, *135*: 985–986, quotation from 985.

30. Ibid. See also R. M. Hosler, *A Manual on Cardiac Resuscitation* (Springfield, IL: Charles C Thomas, 1954); H. E. Natof and M. S. Sadove, *Cardiovascular Collapse in the Operating Room* (Philadelphia: J. B. Lippincott, 1958); and C. S. Beck, "Reminiscences of Cardiac Resuscitation," *Rev. Surg.*, 1970, *27*: 77–86.

31. K. K. Keown, M. L. Buckley, and H. S. Ruth, "Cardiac Resuscitation," in *Surgery of the Heart*, ed. C. P. Bailey (Philadelphia: Lea & Febiger, 1955), 38–48, quotation from 41.

32. S. L. Cole and E. Corday, "Four-Minute Limit for Cardiac Resuscitation," *JAMA*, 1956, *161*: 1454–1458, quotation from 1457.

33. C. S. Beck, E. C. Weckesser, and F. M. Barry, "Fatal Heart Attack and Successful Defibrillation: New Concepts in Coronary Artery Disease," *JAMA*, 1956, *161*: 434–436, quotation from 435.

34. J. S. Butterworth, J. V. Warren, A. Friedlich, and L. Dexter, "Prevention and Treatment of Cardiac Emergencies: A Panel Discussion," *Rhode Island Med. J.*, 1958, *41*: 677–683, 700–709. Dexter quotation from 705. Two decades later, Dexter was in a CCU when he had a cardiac arrest. For his description of the heroic treatment he received, see L. Dexter, "Cardiac Arrest," in *When Doctors Get Sick*, ed. H. Mandell and H. Spiro (New York: Plenum, 1987), 39–43.

35. H. L. Russek, "Evaluation of Status and Results of Management in Coronary Heart Disease," *Minn. Med.*, 1955, *38*: 891–900, quotation from 898. Contemporary articles on heart attack treatment by Mayo cardiologists include H. B. Burchell, "Acute Myocardial Infarction: A Discussion of Certain Controversial Issues," *Calif. Med.*, 1954, *80*: 281–287; and M. W. Anderson, "The Management of Acute Myocardial Infarction," *Med. Clin. North Am.*, 1958, 849–858.

36. Russek, "Coronary Heart Disease," 898.

37. H. B. Burchell, Discussion of Russek, "Coronary Heart Disease," 917.

38. P. M. Zoll, A. J. Linenthal, W. Gibson, M. H. Paul, and L. R. Norman, "Termination of Ventricular Fibrillation in Man by Externally Applied Electric Countershock," *N. Engl. J. Med.*, 1956, *254*: 727–732.

39. W. B. Kouwenhoven, J. R. Jude, and G. G. Knickerbocker, "Closed-Chest Cardiac Massage," *JAMA*, 1960, *173*: 1064–1067, quotation from 1064. See also P. Safar, "History of Cardiopulmonary-Cerebral Resuscitation," in *Cardiopulmonary Resuscitation*, ed. W. Kaye and N. G. Bircher (New York: Churchill Livingstone, 1989), 1–53; and M. S. Eisenberg, *Life in the Balance: Emergency Medicine and the Quest to Reverse Sudden Death* (New York: Oxford University Press, 1997).

40. Kouwenhoven, Jude, and Knickerbocker, "Closed-Chest Cardiac Massage," 1067.

41. C. S. Beck, Discussion of J. S. Jude, W. B. Kouwenhoven, and G. G. Knickerbocker. "A New Approach to Cardiac Resuscitation," *Ann. Surg.*, 1961, *154*: 311–319, quotation from 318.

42. Minutes, Saint Marys Hospital Joint Conference Committee, December 13, 1960, MCA.

43. Ibid. See also T. Hale, "Why the Nursing Shortage Persists," *N. Engl. J. Med.*, 1964, *270*: 1092–1097.

44. See J. Zalumas, *Caring in Crisis: An Oral History of Critical Care Nursing* (Philadelphia: University of Pennsylvania Press, 1995). For the cultural context, see D. Halberstam, *The Fifties* (New York: Villard Books, 1993); and T. Brokaw, *Boom! Voices of the Sixties* (New York: Random House, 2007).

45. M. Brigh, "Emerging Hospital Problems," typescript, paper presented to the South Dakota Conference of Catholic Hospitals, Aberdeen, SD, October 15, 1962, MCA.

46. S. J. Reiser and M. Anbar, eds., *The Machine at the Bedside: Strategies for Using Technology in Patient Care* (New York: Cambridge University Press, 1984).

47. John A. Hartford Foundation. Board Book entry summarizing Bethany Hospital application of May 15, 1961. Grant approved on July 26, 1961. Copy provided to the author by the Hartford Foundation, New York. See also J. S. Jacobson, *The Greatest Good: A History of the John A. Hartford Foundation* (New York: John A. Hartford Foundation, 1984), 84–86.

48. H. W. Day, "An Intensive Coronary Care Area," *Dis. Chest*, 1963, *44*: 423–427. For a description and depiction of the equipment and nurses in the Bethany Hospital unit, see R. M. Harris, "Laying the Right Lines for Electronic Monitoring," *Nursing Outlook*, 1963, *11*: 573–576. I thank Arlene Keeling for providing an unpublished manuscript: A. W. Keeling, "Scene I Stage Left: Hughes Day and the Concept of Coronary Care, Kansas City," November 16, 2005.

49. Fye, "Resuscitating a *Circulation* Abstract." British cardiologist Desmond Julian published a substantial article on the CCU model that year. D. G. Julian, "Treatment of Cardiac Arrest in Acute Myocardial Ischaemia and Infarction," *Lancet*, 1961, *2*: 840–844.

50. M. Wilburne and J. Fields, "Cardiac Resuscitation in Coronary Artery Disease: A Central Coronary Care Unit," *JAMA*, 1963, *184*: 453–457, quotation from 455.

51. M. I. Lindsay and R. E. Spiekerman, "Re-evaluation of Therapy of Acute Myocardial Infarction," *Am. Heart J.*, 1964, *67*: 559–564. See also Ralph Spiekerman and Malcolm Lindsay Jr., joint interview by W. B. Fye, Rochester, MN, February 2, 2011.

52. Lindsay and Spiekerman, "Acute Myocardial Infarction," 562. For a summary of the early phase of the CCU movement, see R. L. Flynn and S. M. Fox III, "Coronary Care Programs in the United States," *Isr. J. Med. Sci.*, 1967, *3*: 279–286. See also B. Lown, A. M. Fakhro, W. B. Hood Jr., and G. W. Thorn, "The Coronary Care Unit: New Perspectives and Directions," *JAMA*, 1967, *199*: 188–198.

53. "Medical Intensive Care Unit Opened on Monday," *Saint Marys Hospital News Bulletin*, December 1964, MCA.

54. J. A. Callahan, J. C. Broadbent, R. E. Spiekerman, E. R. Giuliani, and M. Henry, "St. Marys Hospital-Mayo Clinic Medical Intensive-Care Unit. II. Patient Population," *Mayo Clin. Proc.*, 1967, *42*: 332–338, quotation from 332. See also "Saint Marys' New Medical Unit to Serve Critically Ill Adults," *Mayovox*, December 4, 1964; and "Engineers Install Monitor System in St. Mary's Unit," *Mayovox*, June 4, 1965.

55. M. B. Cassidy, "A Plan for the Organization and Construction of a Medical Intensive Care Unit," April 10, 1965, 24-page typescript, MCA.

56. R. O. Brandenburg Section Report to MC BOG for 1964, MCA. See also P. N. Yu, C. A. Imboden, S. M. Fox, and T. Killip, "Coronary Care Unit: A Specialized Intensive Care Unit for Acute Myocardial Infarction," *Mod. Concepts Cardiovasc. Dis.*, 1965, *34*: 23–30.

57. E. C. Andrus and C. H. Maxwell, eds., *The Heart and Circulation: Second National Conference on Cardiovascular Diseases*, Vol. 1, *Research* (Bethesda, MD: Federation of American Societies for Experimental Biology, 1965). Fogarty's comments are on 7–10.

58. E. B. Drew, "The Health Syndicate: Washington's Noble Conspirators," *Atlantic Monthly*, December 1967, 75–82, quotation from 78. Houston cardiovascular surgeon Michael DeBakey was an influential member of the health lobby. See also J. Robinson, *Noble Conspirator: Florence Mahoney and the Rise of the National Institutes of Health* (Washington, DC: Francis Press, 2001); S. P. Strickland, *Politics, Science, and Dread Disease: A Short History of United States Medical Research Policy* (Cambridge, MA: Harvard University Press, 1972); J. A. Shannon, "The Advancement of Medical Research: A Twenty-Year View of the Role of the National Institutes of Health," *J. Med. Educ.*, 1967, *42*: 97–108; and W. Shonick, *Government and Health Services: Government's Role in the Development of U.S. Health Services, 1939–1980* (New York: Oxford University Press, 1995).

59. Fogarty had his first heart attack in 1953. See J. P. Crowley, "Health for Peace: John E. Fogarty's Vision of American Leadership in Health Care and International Biomedical Research," *Rhode Island Med.*, 1992, *75*: 561–582.

60. See W. B. Fye, "Washington, Medicine, and the American College of Cardiology," in *American Cardiology: The History of a Specialty and Its College*, (Baltimore: Johns Hopkins University Press, 1996), 215–248; and "American College of Cardiology Committees for 1966–1967," *Am. J. Cardiol.*, 1966, *17*: 594–595.

61. Public Law 89-239. 89th Cong. S. 596. An Act to Amend the Public Health Service Act to Assist in Combating Heart Disease, Cancer, Stroke, and Related Diseases. October 6, 1965 (Washington, DC: Government Printing Office, 1965). See also S. P. Strickland, *The History of Regional Medical Programs* (Lanham, MD: University Press of America, 2000).

62. "Training Technics for the Coronary Care Unit.," *Am. J. Cardiol.*, 1966, *17*: 736–747, quotation from 737. See also E. E. Corday to H. W. Day, September 20, 1965, American College of Cardiology Archives, MS C599, Modern Manuscripts Collection, History of Medicine Division, National Library of Medicine, Bethesda, MD.

63. See B. Bates, "Doctor and Nurse: Changing Roles and Relations," *N. Engl. J. Med.*, 1970, *283*: 129–134; J. Fairman and J. E. Lynaugh, *Critical Care Nursing: A History* (Philadelphia: University of Pennsylvania Press, 1998); and Zalumas, *Caring in Crisis*.

64. E. Corday, "The Coronary Care Area: A Tiger by the Tail," *Am. J. Cardiol.*, 1965, *16*: 466–468, quotation from 466.

65. See G. Church and R. O. Biern, "Intensive Coronary Care: A Practical System for a Small Hospital Without House Staff," *N. Engl. J. Med.*, 1968, *281*: 1155–1159.

66. Fordham, *Cardiovascular Surgical Nursing*.

67. Fordham interviews by Jacqueline Wilkie, quotation from 82–83.

68. Thomas Killip, interview by W. B. Fye, Dallas, TX, November 13, 1994.

69. S. Scheidt, "Thirty Years of Cardiology Research at the New York Hospital-Cornell Medical Center," *Cardiovasc. Rev. Rep.*, 1991, *12*: 7–8, 11–12, quotation from 7. See also A. W. Keeling, "Blurring the Boundaries Between Medicine and Nursing: Coronary Care Nursing, Circa the 1960s," *Nursing Hist. Rev.*, 2004, *12*: 139–164. A contemporary text, coauthored by two cardiologists and a nurse, was based on the principle of empowering nurses in the CCU context. See L. E. Meltzer, R. Pinneo, and J. R. Kitchell, *Intensive Coronary Care: A Manual for Nurses* (Philadelphia: Presbyterian Hospital, 1965).

70. J. A. Callahan, J. C. Broadbent, R. E. Spiekerman, and E. R. Giuliani, "St. Marys Hospital-Mayo Clinic Medical Intensive-Care Unit. I. Organization," *Mayo Clin. Proc.*, 1967, *42*: 326–331.

71. Callahan, Spiekerman, Broadbent, M. Henry, and Giuliani, "St. Marys Hospital-Mayo Clinic Medical Intensive-Care Unit. II," quotation from 336. In addition to Sister Henry, the unit was staffed by four assistant head nurses, eight registered nurses, two licensed practical nurses, and four nurse aides.

72. "Policy regarding Defibrillation" and "Policy regarding Cardiopulmonary Resuscitation," Nursing Service, Saint Marys Hospital, March 1, 1968, MCA.

73. M. Henry, "Coronary Care: Expanded Directions for Nursing," *Hosp. Prog.*, 1968, *49*: 104–119, quotation from 106.

74. O. Paul, C. G. Leigh, and G. A. Smyth, "The Patient with a Major Acute Coronary Attack and the Role of a Coronary Care Unit," *Illinois Med. J.*, 1967, *132*: 721–731, 738, quotation from 722–723.

75. J. R. Jude, W. B. Kouwenhoven, and G. G. Knickerbocker, "External Cardiac Resuscitation," *Monographs Surg. Sci.*, 1964, *1*: 59–117, quotation from 85.

76. H. W. Day, "A Cardiac Resuscitation Program," *Journal-Lancet*, 1962, *82*: 153–156. See also I. Greenfield, "Emergency Red: A Plan for Hospital Personnel in the Treatment of Cardiac and Respiratory Emergencies," *Minn. Med.*, 1964, *47*: 745–747.

77. "When a Man's Heart Stops and His Life Flickers 'Code 99!' Calls a Hospital to Battle Against Death," *Life*, February 28, 1964, 52B-61, quotation from 53–54.

78. Ibid., 60.

79. Minutes, MC Executive Committee, May 24, 1965, MCA.

80. E. P. Didier to K. J. Ladner, November 4, 1965, MCA.

81. For some of the issues surrounding resuscitation, see V. J. Collins, "Limits of Medical Responsibility in Prolonging Life," *JAMA*, 1968, *206*: 389–392; and J. R. Benfield and R. C. Hickey, "Cardiopulmonary Resuscitation at University of Wisconsin," *Arch. Surg.*, 1968, *96*: 664–670.

82. H. B. Burchell, "Coronary Care Units: Panel Discussion," *Isr. J. Med. Sci.*, 1967, *3*: 319–325, quotation from 320.

83. "'Dial 45' Mobilizes Hospital Resuscitation Team," *Mayovox*, August 25, 1967. The name for the code team was derived from nursing station 45 at Methodist Hospital, where an ICU directed by anesthesiologist Paul Didier had opened in January 1966.

84. Minutes, Saint Marys Hospital Joint Conference Committee, January 10, 1968, MCA. Other institutions reported similar results. At the University of Pennsylvania Hospital, for example, only 5 of 103 patients in whom resuscitation was attempted in a one-year period survived. See E. J. Stemmler, "Cardiac Resuscitation: A One-Year Study of Patients within a University Hospital," *Ann. Intern. Med.*, 1965, *63*: 613–618.

85. E. Corday, "Impact of Recent Legislation on Cardiology," *Am. J. Cardiol.*, 1966, *17*: 144–148, quotation from 148.

86. "Faculties Leave on Circuit Courses 8 and 9," *Am. J. Cardiol.*, 1964, *13*: 717. See also E. G. Dimond, "Medicine, a Universal Language: The International Circuit Courses of the American College of Cardiology," *Medical Times*, 1967, *95*: 1058–1071.

87. "Dr. Swan Will Leave Clinic Staff," *Rochester Post-Bulletin*, May 4, 1965, MCA.

88. Robert O. Brandenburg, interview by W. B. Fye, Orlando, FL, March 18, 2001. H. J. C. (Jeremy) Swan, interview by W. B. Fye, San Diego, CA, October 7, 2000.

89. H. J. C. Swan, "Cardiac Catheterization at the St. Mary's Laboratory," typescript prepared for John Callahan, July 30, 1993, MCA. See also J. W. Hurst, "H. J. C. Swan," *Clin. Cardiol.*, 1988, *11*: 727–728.

90. Swan interview by Fye.

91. H. J. C. Swan, "Early Development of the Pulmonary Artery Catheter: A Personal Perspective," *Proc. Bayl. Univ. Med. Cent.*, 1996, *9*: 3–7, quotation from 5. See also E. Corday and H. J. C. Swan, eds., *Myocardial Infarction: New Perspectives in Diagnosis and Management* (Baltimore: Williams & Wilkins, 1973).

92. E. Braunwald and H. J. C. Swan, eds., "Cooperative Study on Cardiac Catheterization," *Circulation*, 1968, *37*: III-1-113.

93. R. P. Grant, "The Coronary Spectrum: The Public Health Service Contribution," *J. Rehabil.*, 1966, *32*: 86–88, quotation from 86.

94. P. L. Frommer, "The Myocardial Infarction Research Program of the National Heart Institute," *Am. J. Cardiol.*, 1968, *22*: 108–110.

95. E. Braunwald, "Robert P. Grant, M.D., 1915–1966," *Am. J. Cardiol.*, 1966, *18*: 803.

96. "Deaths," *JAMA*, 1966, 603–604.

97. See L. E. Meltzer and J. R. Kitchell, "The Development and Current Status of Coronary Care," in *Textbook of Coronary Care*, ed. L. E. Meltzer and A. J. Dunning (Amsterdam: Excerpta Medica, 1972), 3–25; and R. M. Gunnar and H. Loeb, "Shock in Acute Myocardial Infarction: Evolution of Physiologic Therapy," *J. Am. Coll. Cardiol.*, 1983, *1*: 154–163.

98. M. W. Anderson Section Report to MC BOG for 1968, February 24, 1969, MCA.

99. See H. J. C. Swan, W. Ganz, J. S. Forrester, H. Marcus, G. Diamond, and D. Chonette, "Catheterization of the Heart in Man with Use of a Flow-Directed Balloon-Tipped Catheter," *N. Engl. J. Med.*, 1970, *283*: 447–451; J. S. Forrester, G. Diamond, K. Chatterjee, and H. J. C. Swan, "Medical Therapy of Acute Myocardial Infarction by Application of Hemodynamic Subsets," *N. Engl. J. Med.*, 1976, *295*: 1356–1362, 1404–1413; and K. Chatterjee, "The Swan-Ganz Catheters: Past, Present, and Future. A Viewpoint," *Circulation*, 2009, *119*: 147–152.

100. P. N. Yu, M. T. Bielski, A. Edwards, C. K. Friedberg, W. J. Grace, L. E. January et al., "Resources for the Optimal Care of Patients with Acute Myocardial Infarction," *Circulation*, 1971, *43*: A171–183, quotation from A-178.

101. Meltzer and Dunning, eds., *Coronary Care*, xiii.

102. R. O. Brandenburg, "Cardiovascular Division History," typescript, May 8, 1993, MCA. A new Methodist Hospital opened in 1966, and it contained an MICU where some patients with acute cardiac problems were admitted. See "Research Made This Hospital Go Round—and Square," *Mod. Hosp.*, 1967, *109*: 98–101. For the perspective of the unit's first head nurse, see Maureen Hardtke, interview by W. B. Fye, Rochester, MN, 8 July 2005.

103. Minutes of the Meeting of the Intensive Cardiac Care Service Director with Representatives from Nursing Service, July 7, 1970, MCA, emphasis in the original.

104. Spiekerman interview by Fye, February 2, 2011. See also G. W. Morrow Jr., "The Formative Years (1970–1979)," in *A History of Community Internal Medicine, Mayo Clinic Rochester*, ed. K. G. Berge, G. W. Morrow Jr., M. I. Lindsay, and R. D. Hurt (Rochester: Mayo Clinic, 1996), 9–25.

105. See F. H. Adams and R. C. Mendenhall, "Profile of the Cardiologist: Training and Manpower Requirements for the Specialist in Adult Cardiovascular Disease," *Am. J. Cardiol.*, 1974, *34*: 389–456; and W. B. Fye, "Cardiology Training Programs and Cardiology Fellows (1941–1995)," in *American Cardiology*, table A9, 346.

106. T. P. B. O'Donovan, J. Thierer, H. T. Mankin, and J. P. Stokes, "Training Physicians and Nurses for Intensive Coronary Care Units," *Minn. Med.*, 1972, *55*, *suppl. 3*: 56–60, quotation from 56.

107. Ibid., 58.

108. J. A. Callahan and R. C. Bahn, "Cardiac Care Unit," in *Medical Engineering*, ed. C. D. Ray (Chicago: Year Book Medical Publishers, 1974), 636–644, quotation from 636.

109. Ibid., 641. For a discussion of dynamics of new nurse-physician interaction by two nurses who directed the Coronary Care Training Program at a hospital in St. Paul, see C. A. Baden and J. A. Huebsch, "Staffing and Staff Relations in Coronary Care Units," *Nurs. Clin. North Am.*, 1969, *4*: 573–583.

110. "Medical Science 'Big Wheel' to Whirl for U.S. Air Force," *Mayovox*, February 7, 1959.

111. E. H. Wood, "Evolution of Instrumentation and Techniques for the Study of Cardiovascular Dynamics from the Thirties to 1980," *Ann. Biomed. Eng.*, 1978, *6*: 250–309. See also "New Electronic Device will Speed Data Analysis," *Mayovox*, May 27, 1961.

112. "Computer-Linked Monitor System Studied in Relation to Patient Care," *Mayovox*, June 14, 1968.

113. H. R. Warner, "Experiences with Computer-Based Patient Monitoring," *Anesth. Analg.*, 1968, *47*: 453–462, quotation from 461. For Warner's pioneering role in medical computing and

monitoring, see M. L. Millenson, *Demanding Medical Excellence: Doctors and Accountability in the Information Age* (Chicago: University of Chicago Press, 1997), 80–89.

114. "Collaborative Study Seeks Computer Role in Cardiac Care," *Mayovox*, December 8, 1972. For the coronary care group, see Minutes, MC Clinical Practice Committee, December 3, 1973, MCA. For later developments in the organization and computerization of Mayo's CCUs, see "Major Upgrading Project Begun in Coronary Care Units," *Mayovox*, February 1983.

115. "Computerized Medicine at Mayo," *Mayovox*, October 1978.

116. Byron Olney and Jean Lee quoted in "Computerized Medicine at Mayo."

117. See J. B. Herrick, "The Relation of the Clinical Laboratory to the Practitioner of Medicine," *JAMA*, 1907, *48*: 1915–1919. For a Mayo surgeon's expression of concern about the need to focus on the patient rather than his or her test results, see J. T. Priestley, "The Head, the Heart, and the Hand," *Arch. Surg.*, 1954, *69*: 135–139.

118. "Heart Attack: Curbing the Killers," *Newsweek*, May 1, 1972, 73–82, quotation from 73.

119. See T. Clavin and D. Peary, *Gil Hodges* (New York: New American Library, 2012), 316–319, 358–360; and "Jackie Robinson, First Black in Major Leagues, Dies," *New York Times*, October 25, 1972.

120. "Heart Attack: Curbing the Killers," 76.

121. Ibid. The world's first mobile CCU service was launched in Belfast, Ireland, in 1967. See J. F. Pantridge and J. S. Geddes, "A Mobile Intensive Care Unit in the Management of Myocardial Infarction," *Lancet*, 1967, *2*: 271–273; and J. F. Pantridge and C. Wilson, "A History of Prehospital Coronary Care," *Ulster Med. J.*, 1996, *65*: 68–73. The first mobile CCU service in America was inaugurated at St. Vincent's Hospital in New York City in 1968. See W. J. Grace and J. A. Chadbourne, "The Mobile Coronary Care Unit," *Dis. Chest*, 1969, *55*: 452–455. See also A. T. Simpson, "Transporting Lazarus: Physicians, the State, and the Creation of the Modern Paramedic and Ambulance, 1955–1973," *J. Hist. Med. Allied Sci.*, 2013, *68*: 163–197.

122. L. Janos, "The Last Days of the President," *Atlantic Monthly*, July 1973, 35–41. The author thanks Arlene Keeling for sharing her unpublished manuscript "Lyndon Johnson and the University of Virginia CCU," 2005.

123. "Mayo Mourns LBJ: He Served with Distinction," *Mayovox*, February 1973.

124. "Ambulance-Hospital ECG Telemetry System will be Operational by April 1," *Mayovox*, February 1973.

125. Ibid. See also E. L. Nagel, J. C. Hirschman, S. R. Nussenfeld, D. Rankin, and E. Lundblad, "Telemetry-Medical Command in Coronary and Other Mobile Emergency Care Systems," *JAMA*, 1970, *214*: 332–338.

126. R. D. White and T. P. B. O'Donovan, "Prehospital Life-Support Systems in Traumatic and Cardiac Emergencies," *Anesth. Analg.*, 1974, *53*: 734–743, quotations from 742.

127. L. Thomas, "Notes of a Biology Watcher: The Technology of Medicine," *N. Engl. J. Med.*, 1971, *285*: 1366–1368, quotation from 1366–1367.

128. Ibid., 1367–1368.

129. Ibid., 1368. See also A. J. Angyal, *Lewis Thomas* (Boston: Twayne, 1989).

130. See B. S. Bloom and O. L. Peterson, "Patient Needs and Medical-Care Planning: The Coronary-Care Unit as a Model," *N. Engl. J. Med.*, 1974, *290*: 1171–1177. The definitive work that traces the basic research origins of a series of clinical breakthroughs in cardiovascular disease is J. H. Comroe Jr. and R. D. Dripps, *The Top Ten Clinical Advances in Cardiovascular-Pulmonary Medicine and Surgery 1945–1975*, 2 vols. (Washington, DC: Government Printing Office, 1978).

Chapter 14

1. For a description of angina written for the general public, see B. J. Gersh, ed., *Mayo Clinic Heart Book*, 2nd ed. (New York: William Morrow, 2000), 29–31, 88–91. See also M. B. Matthews,

"Historical Background," in *Angina Pectoris*, ed. D. G. Julian (New York: Churchill Livingstone, 1977), 1–13; and J. O. Leibowitz, *The History of Coronary Heart Disease* (London: Wellcome Institute of the History of Medicine, 1970).

2. See W. B. Fye, "Coronary Arteriography: It Took a Long Time," *Circulation*, 1984, *70*: 781–787; M. E. Bertrand and M. G. Bourassa, "Coronary Angiography," in M. E. Bertrand, ed., *The Evolution of Cardiac Catheterization and Interventional Cardiology* (St Albans, UK: Iatric Press and European Society of Cardiology, 2006), 47–60; and D. A. Killen, "Angiographic Contrast Media: A Historical Résumé," *Surgery*, 1973, *73*: 333–346.

3. See W. L. Proudfit, "F. Mason Sones, Jr., M.D. (1918–1985): The Man and His Work," *Cleveland Clin. Q.*, 1986, *53*: 121–124; and A. V. G. Bruschke, W. C. Sheldon, E. K. Shirey, and W. L. Proudfit, "A Half Century of Selective Coronary Arteriography," *J. Am. Coll. Cardiol.*, 2009, *54*: 2139–2144.

4. F. Jamin and H. Merkel, *Die Koronararterien des Menschlichen Herzens Unter Normalen und Pathologischen Verhältnissen* (Jena: Gustav Fischer, 1907).

5. E. D. Osborne, C. G. Sutherland, A. J. Scholl Jr., and L. G. Rowntree, "Roentgenography of Urinary Tract during Excretion of Sodium Iodid[e]," *JAMA*, 1923, *80*: 368–373, quotation from 372. Historians of radiology have described this Mayo article as a classic contribution that helped lay the foundations for angiography. See R. Brecher and E. Brecher, *The Rays: A History of Radiology in the United States and Canada* (Baltimore: Williams and Wilkins, 1959), 231; and R. L. Tondreau, "Roentgenography of the Urinary Tract," in *Classic Descriptions in Diagnostic Roentgenology*, ed. A. J. Bruwer (Springfield: Charles C Thomas, 1964), 1605–1728, esp. 1688–1701. German investigators also pioneered the use of intravascular contrast. See J. Berberich and S. Hirsch, "Die Röntgenographische Darstellung der Arterien und Venen am Lebenden Menschen," *Klin. Wschr.*, 1923, *2*: 2226–2228; and U. Speck, "Development of Intravascular Contrast Media," in *Radiology in Medical Diagnostics: Evolution of X-Ray Applications 1895–1995*, ed. G. Rosenbusch, M. Oudkerk, and E. Ammann; trans. P. F. Winter (Oxford: Blackwell Scientific, 1995), 121–130.

6. See B. Brooks and F. A. Jostes, "A Clinical Study of Diseases of the Circulation of the Extremities; A Description of a New Method of Examination," *Arch. Surg.*, 1924, *9*: 485–503; B. Brooks, "Intra-Arterial Injection of Sodium Iodid[e]: Preliminary Report," *JAMA*, 1924, *82*: 1016–1019; J. H. Foster, "Arteriography: Cornerstone of Vascular Surgery," *Arch. Surg.*, 1974, *109*: 605–611; and M. A. Meyers, *Happy Accidents: Serendipity in Modern Medical Breakthroughs* (New York: Arcade, 2007).

7. G. E. Brown and M. S. Henderson, "The Diagnosis and Treatment of Arterial Vascular Disease of the Extremities," *J. Bone Joint Surg.*, 1927, *9*: 613–626.

8. E. V. Allen and J. D. Camp, "Roentgenography of the Arteries of the Extremities," *Proceedings of the Staff Meetings of the Mayo Clinic* (hereafter *PSMMC*), 1932, *7*: 657–662.

9. E. V. Allen and J. D. Camp, "Arteriography: A Roentgenographic Study of the Peripheral Arteries of the Living Subject Following Their Injection with a Radiopaque Substance," *JAMA*, 1935, *104*: 618–623, paper presented in Cleveland on June 14, 1934. Irving Wright's comments are on 623. See also E. V. Allen, "How Arteries Compensate for Occlusion: An Arteriographic Study of Collateral Circulation," *Arch. Int. Med.*, 1936, *57*: 601–609. For contributions from investigators outside of the United States, see T. Doby, *Development of Angiography and Cardiovascular Catheterization* (Littleton, MA: Publishing Sciences Group, 1976).

10. See D. C. Elkin and M. E. DeBakey, eds., *Vascular Surgery in World War II* (Washington, DC: Government Printing Office, 1955); and M. E. DeBakey, "The Development of Vascular Surgery," *Am. J. Surg.*, 1979, *137*: 697–738.

11. See "Symposium on Recent Advances in the Surgical Treatment of Aneurysms," *PSMMC*, 1953, *28*: 705–728; and F. H. Ellis Jr., O. T. Clagett, and J. W. Kirklin, "Aneurysms of the Aorta," *Surg. Clin. North Am.*, August 1955, 953–963.

12. See J. M. Janes, "Arteriography," *Am. Practice Digest Treat*, 1951, *2*: 569–573; O. W. Kincaid and G. D. Davis, "Abdominal Aortography," *N. Engl. J. Med.*, 1958, *259*: 1017–1024, 1067–1073; and G. D. Davis, J. R. Hodgson, and O. W. Kincaid, "Diagnostic Radiology at the Mayo Clinic: Personal Recollections of People and Practice from the 1940s to 1970s, Including Reflections on the Beginning Years," 1990, Mayo Clinic Archives, Mayo Historical Unit, Rochester, MN (hereafter MCA).

13. J. H. Kotte, Discussion of J. A. Helmsworth J. McGuire, and B. Felson, "Arteriography of the Aorta and Its Branches by Means of the Polyethylene Catheter," *Am. J. Roentgenol. Radium Ther.*, 1950, *64*: 196–213, quotation from 213. See also L. Di Guglielmo and M. Guttadauro, "A Roentgenologic Study of the Coronary Arteries in the Living," *Acta Radiologica*, 1952, *Suppl. 97*, 1–82, esp. 11.

14. See R. C. Cabot, "The Historical Development and Relative Value of Laboratory and Clinical Methods of Diagnosis," *Boston Med. Surg. J.*, 1907, *157*: 150–153; J. C. Todd and A. H. Sanford, *Clinical Diagnosis by Laboratory Methods* (Philadelphia: W. B. Saunders, 1931); and Rosenbusch, Oudkerk, and Ammann, eds., *Radiology in Medical Diagnostics*.

15. C. K. Friedberg, *Diseases of the Heart* (Philadelphia: W. B. Saunders, 1956), 481. See also W. B. Fye, "Nitroglycerin: A Homeopathic Remedy," *Circulation*, 1986, *73*: 21–29.

16. Friedberg, *Diseases of the Heart*, 477.

17. H. B. Burchell, "The Management of the Patient with Anginal Pain," in *Conference on Atherosclerosis and Coronary Heart Disease* (New York: New York Heart Association, 1957), 33–45, quotation from 43.

18. J. W. Kirklin, "Surgical Treatment of Coronary Arterial Disease," *Minn. Med.*, 1955, *38*: 570. For a contromporary review of the operations for coronary heart disease, see C. P. Bailey, ed., *Surgery of the Heart* (Philadelphia: Lea & Febiger, 1955), 915–1005.

19. The papers presented at the symposium were published in several issues of the 1955 volume of *Minnesota Medicine*. For the history and definitions of arteriosclerosis and atherosclerosis, see A. M. Gotto Jr., "Some Reflections on Arteriosclerosis: Past, Present, and Future," *Circulation*, 1985, *72*: 8–17; and W. B. Fye, "A Historical Perspective on Atherosclerosis and Coronary Artery Disease," in *Atherosclerosis and Coronary Artery Disease*, ed. V. Fuster, R. Ross, and E. J. Topol (Philadelphia: Lippincott-Raven, 1996), 1–12.

20. C. W. Lillehei, Discussion of E. J. Wylie, "Occlusive Arterial Disease: Management by Thromboendarterectomy," *Minn. Med.*, 1955, *38*: 910–911. See also E. V. Allen, N. W. Barker, E. A. Hines Jr., J. A. Spittell Jr., J. F. Fairbairn II, and J. L. Juergens, *Peripheral Vascular Diseases*, 3rd ed. (Philadelphia: W. B. Saunders, 1962), 259–341. For historical perspective, see W. F. Barker, "Direct Management of Arterial Occlusive Disease," in *Clio: The Arteries, The Development of Ideas in Arterial Surgery* (Austin, TX: Landes, 1992), 161–229.

21. Application for National Institutes of Health Research Grant H-2795: "Contrast Visualization of the Coronary Circulation," Principal Investigator: F. Mason Sones Jr., June 29, 1956, Cleveland Clinic Archives (CCA), (hereafter Sones grant application).

22. Ibid.

23. See E. Blacksher and J. D. Moreno, "A History of Informed Consent in Clinical Research," in *The Oxford Textbook of Clinical Research Ethics*, ed. E. J. Emanuel, C. Grady, R. A. Crouch, R. K. Lie, F. K. Miller, and D. Wendler (New York: Oxford University Press, 2008), 591–605; and R. R. Faden and T. L. Beauchamp, *A History and Theory of Informed Consent* (New York: Oxford University Press, 1986).

24. Sones grant application.

25. Sones to Thal, November 30, 1956, box 9, University of Minnesota Department of Surgery Papers, University of Minnesota Archives, Minneapolis, MN (hereafter UMN Dept. Surgery Papers). See also C. R. Hughes, H. Sartorius, and W. J. Kolff, "Angiography of the Coronary Arteries in the Live Dog," *Cleveland Clin. Q.*, 1956, *23*: 251–255. See also D. B. Effler,

L. K. Groves, and F. M. Sones Jr., "Elective Cardiac Arrest in Open-Heart Surgery," *Cleveland Clin. Q.*, 1956, *23*: 105–114. Effler adopted the elective cardiac arrest technique, which would be termed "cardioplegia," from British surgeon Denis Melrose, who had described it one year earlier. It caused the heart to stop beating so a surgeon could operate on an organ that did not move. See S. Westaby and C. Bosher, *Landmarks in Cardiac Surgery* (Oxford: Isis Medical Media, 1997) 79–80, 348–349; and M. S. Shiroishi, "Myocardial Protection: The Rebirth of Potassium-Based Cardioplegia," *Texas Heart Inst. J.*, 1999, *26*: 71–86.

26. Sones to Thal, November 30, 1956, box 9, UMN Dept. Surgery Papers.

27. A. Thal to F. M. Sones, December 10, 1956, box 9, UMN Dept. Surgery Papers. See also A. Thal, J. M. Perry Jr., F. A. Miller, and O. H. Wangensteen, "Direct Suture Anastomosis of the Coronary Arteries in the Dog," *Surgery*, 1956, *40*: 1023–1029; and A. Thal, R. G. Lester, L. S. Richards, and M. J. Murray, "Coronary Arteriography in Arteriosclerotic Disease of the Heart," *Surg. Gynecol. Obstet.*, 1957, *105*: 457–464.

28. J. Watt to F. M. Sones [regarding application for research grant, H-2795], 26 December 1956, CCA. See also J. Watt, "Role of the National Heart Institute in Meeting the Challenge of Arteriosclerosis," *Minn. Med.*, 1955, 38: 734–735, 742.

29. "New Look for Heart Lab," *Cleveland Clin. Newsletter*, October 1958, CCA.

30. F. M. Sones, "Retrograde Aortic Catheterization and Selective Cardiography Summary," October 30, 1958, typewritten copy of procedure note, CCA.

31. Ibid.

32. Ibid. Years later, Sones recalled being "horrified" because he was "certain that the patient would develop ventricular fibrillation." Sones to J. W. Hurst [August 9, 1982], published in Hurst, "History of Cardiac Catheterization," in S. B. King III and J. S. Douglas Jr., eds. *Coronary Arteriography and Angioplasty* (New York: McGraw Hill, 1985), 1–8, quotation from 5–6. For the date of the letter, see W. C. Sheldon, "F. Mason Sones, Jr.: Stormy Petrel of Cardiology," *Clin. Cardiol.*, 1994, *17*: 405–407. The original procedure note, which is much longer than the brief excerpt that I have included, reveals some inaccuracies in accounts by persons who did not have access to these manuscripts and who based their conclusions on recollections by Sones and others. See, for example, T. J. Ryan, "The Coronary Angiogram and Its Seminal Contributions to Cardiovascular Medicine over Five Decades," *Trans. Am. Clin. Climatol. Assoc.*, 2002, *113*: 261–271.

33. F. M. Sones Jr., "Cinecardioangiography," in *Clinical Cardiopulmonary Physiology*, 2nd ed., ed. B. L. Gordon (New York: Grune & Stratton, 1960), 130–144. The abstract of his lecture at the American Heart Association meeting does not mention inserting a catheter tip into a coronary artery. See F. M. Sones Jr., E. K. Shirey, W. L. Proudfit, and R. N. Westcott, "Cine-Coronary Arteriography," *Circulation* 1959, *20*: 773–774, abstract.

34. D. Dunham, "Clinic Team Scores Breakthrough in Heart Diagnosis," *Cleveland Press*, February 11, 1960, CCA.

35. E. C. Andrus, "Coronary Artery Disease," March 11, 1960, 28A-28D with Minutes, NAHC, March 10–12, 1960, copy in the author's possession, obtained from bound minute books located outside Claude Lenfant's office at the NIH in May 2000. See also E. C. Andrus, "Diagnosis of Angina Pectoris," *Circulation*, 1960, *22*: 979–985. Burchell had used coronary angiography in animal experiments in the late 1930s. See H. Burchell, "Adjustments in Coronary Circulation after Experimental Coronary Occlusion," *Arch. Int. Med.*, 1940, *65*: 240–262.

36. D. B. Effler to F. A. LeFevre, November 8, 1960, Effler Papers, CCA. See also C. P. Bailey, D. P. Morse, and W. M. Lemmon, "Thromboendarterectomy for Coronary Artery Disease," *Am. J. Cardiol.*, 1960, *5*: 3–13.

37. F. A. LeFevre to D. B. Effler, November 11, 1960, Effler Papers, CCA.

38. R. A. Gottron to F. M. Sones, April 14, 1961, Sones Papers, CCA.

39. R. A. Gottron, "Dr. Sones' Projects," July 18, 1961, Sones Papers, CCA. See also J. H. Nichols, Minutes of Meeting on Interesting Developments in the Field of Cineangiography and Cardiac Catheterization, July 18, 1961, CCA.

40. G. G. Gensini, S. Di Giorgi, and A. Black, "New Approaches to Coronary Arteriography," *Angiology*, 1961, *12*: 223–238, quotation from 237.

41. R. G. Petersdorf and P. B. Beeson, "Fever of Unexplained Origin: Report on 100 Cases," *Medicine*, 1961, *40*: 1–30, quotation from 27.

42. W. Sutton and E. Linn, *Where the Money Was* (New York: Viking Press, 1976), 120.

43. H. E. Klarman, "Socioeconomic Impact of Heart Disease," in *The Heart and Circulation: Second National Conference on Cardiovascular Diseases*, Vol. 2, *Community Services and Education*, ed. E. C. Andrus and C. H. Maxwell (Bethesda, MD: Federation of American Societies for Experimental Biology, 1965), 693–707.

44. F. M. Sones Jr. and E. K. Shirey, "Cine Coronary Arteriography," *Mod. Concepts Cardiovasc. Dis.*, 1962, *31*: 735–738, quotation from 738.

45. Ibid., 737.

46. E. M. Rogers, *Diffusion of Innovations* (New York: Free Press, 1962), 148–192. See also Rogers, *Diffusion of Innovations*, 5th ed. (New York: Free Press, 2003), 1–38, and J. B. McKinlay, "From 'Promising Report' to 'Standard Procedure': Seven Stages in the Career of a Medical Innovation," *Milbank Q.*, 1981, *59*: 374–411.

47. D. C. Sabiston Jr., "Observations on the Coronary Circulation with Tributes to My Teachers," *J. Thorac. Cardiovasc. Surg.*, 1985, *90*: 321–340.

48. See E. K. Lang and D. C. Sabiston Jr., "Coronary Arteriography in the Selection of Patients for Surgery," *Radiology*, 1961, *76*: 32–38; and D. C. Sabiston Jr., "Direct Surgical Management of Congenital and Acquired Lesions of the Coronary Circulation," *Prog. Cardiovasc. Dis.*, 1963, *6*: 299–316.

49. G. C. Friesinger to W. B. Fye, February 20, 2011. See R. S. Ross, "Clinical Applications of Coronary Arteriography," *Circulation*, 1963, *27*: 107–112.

50. A. M. Harvey, V. A. McKusick, and J. D. Stobo, *Osler's Legacy: The Department of Medicine at Johns Hopkins, 1889–1989* (Baltimore: Johns Hopkins University Department of Medicine, 1990), 78–82.

51. D. C. Sabiston Jr. and A. Blalock, "Coronary Thromboendarterectomy for Angina Pectoris," *Postgrad. Med.*, 1961, *29*: 439–450, quotation from 439.

52. Ibid., 450.

53. D. B. Effler, L. K. Groves, F. M. Sones Jr., and E. K. Shirey, "Endarterectomy in the Treatment of Coronary Artery Disease," *J. Thorac. Cardiovasc. Surg.*, 1964, *47*: 98–108, Effler quotation from 108.

54. "Surgery: The Best Hope of All," *Time*, May 3, 1963, 44–60, quotation from 58.

55. D. B. Effler, F. M. Sones Jr., R. G. Favaloro, and L. K. Groves, "Coronary Endarterotomy with Patch-Graft Reconstruction: Clinical Experience with 34 Cases," *Ann. Surg.*, 1965, *162*: 590–601, Effler quotations from 590, 601, emphasis in the original.

56. Ibid., 601, emphasis in the original.

57. R. L. Parker, "An Internist's Evaluation of the Present Surgical Treatment of Acquired and Congenital Heart Disease," *Coll. Papers Mayo Clinic*, 1958, *50*: 84–93, quotation from 89.

58. J. W. Kirklin and D. C. McGoon, "Evaluation and Current Applications of Open Heart Surgery in Congenital and Acquired Heart Disease," *Prog. Cardiovasc. Dis.*, 1958, *1*: 66–79, quotation from 78–79.

59. Minutes, MC BOG, January 16, 1958, MCA.

60. For an overview of these operations, see R. H. Jones, "Development of Surgical Treatments for Coronary Artery Disease," *Ann. Surg.*, 2003, *238*: S121–S131.

61. See A. Vineberg, D. D. Munro, H. Cohen, and W. Buller, "Four Years' Clinical Experience with Internal Mammary Artery Implantation in the Treatment of Human Coronary Artery Insufficiency Including Additional Experimental Studies," *J. Thorac. Surg.*, 1955, *29*: 1–36; and J. B. Shrager, "The Vineberg Procedure: The Immediate Forerunner of Coronary Artery Bypass Grafting," *Ann. Thorac. Surg.*, 1994, *57*: 1354–1364.

Mayo experimental surgeon John Grindlay had mentored three fellows who performed the Vineberg operation in animals in 1957. Based on blood flow measurements and microscopic analysis, they concluded that the few collateral vessels that developed would "allow only relatively small blood flow." M. C. Fuquay, L. S. Carey, E. V. Dahl, and J. H. Grindlay, "Myocardial Revascularization: A Comparison of Internal Mammary and Subclavian Artery Implantation in the Laboratory," *Surgery*, 1958, *43*: 226–235, quotation from 235.

62. Thal, Perry, Miller, and Wangensteen, "Direct Suture Anastomosis."

63. N. H. Baker and J. H. Grindlay, "Technic of Experimental Systemic-to-Coronary-Artery Anastomosis," *PSMMC*, 1959, *34*: 497–501, quotation from 501. The first article describing the application of this anastamosis procedure in a patient is C. P. Bailey and T. Hirose, "Successful Internal Mammary-Coronary Arterial Anastomosis Using a 'Minivascular' Suturing Technic," *Int. Surg.*, 1968, *49*: 416–427.

64. J. H. Eusterman, R. W. P. Achor, O. W. Kincaid, and A. L. Brown Jr., "Atherosclerotic Disease of the Coronary Arteries: A Pathologic-Radiologic Correlative Study," *Circulation*, 1962, *26*: 1288–1295, quotations from 1294 and 1295, paper presented in Miami Beach on October 20, 1961.

65. N. R. Niles and C. T. Dotter, "Coronary Radiography and Endarterectomy: Postmortem Study of Feasibility of Surgery," *Circulation*, 1963, *28*: 190–202, quotation from 201, paper presented in Miami Beach on October 24, 1961.

66. C. T. Dotter and L. H. Frische, "An Approach to Coronary Arteriography," in *Angiography*, ed. H. L. Abrams (Boston: Little, Brown, 1961), 259–273, quotation from 259.

67. C. A. Good, Radiology Section Report to MC BOG for 1960, MCA.

68. Ibid.

69. Earl K. Shirey, interview by W. B. Fye, Cleveland, OH, July 21, 2005.

70. H. B. Burchell to the Mayo Foundation Office, November 9, 1959, MCA.

71. Minutes, MC BOG, October 3, 1963, MCA.

72. Ross, "Clinical Applications of Coronary Arteriography," 107.

73. W. G. Bigelow, H. Basian, and G. A. Trusler, "Internal Mammary Artery Implantation for Coronary Heart Disease," *J. Thorac. Cardiovasc. Surg.*, 1963, *45*: 67–79, quotation from 77.

74. Ross, "Coronary Arteriography," 108.

75. "Coronary Angiography," *Br. Med. J.*, 1961, *2*: 878–879, quotation from 879. London cardiologist Aubrey Leatham, who surely wrote this editorial, encouraged his group at St. George's Hospital to perform coronary angiography after he had visited Sones in 1960. See G. Hale, D. Dexter, K. Jefferson, and A. Leatham, "Value of Coronary Arteriography in the Investigation of Ischæmic Heart Disease," *Brit. Heart J.*, 1966, *28*: 40–54.

76. Frye interviews. See also T. H. Lee, *Eugene Braunwald and the Rise of Modern Medicine* (Cambridge, MA: Harvard University Press, 2013), 114–177.

77. Minutes, MC BOG, November 12, 1964, MCA. Frye interviews.

78. G. W. Daugherty Section Report to MC BOG for 1965, MCA; C. A. Good, Radiology Section Report to MC BOG for 1965, MCA.

79. Frye interviews; and Benjamin D. McCallister, interview by W. B. Fye, Atlanta, GA, March 13, 2006.

80. Minutes, MC BOG, April 1, 1965, MCA.

81. "Preliminary Report from the Committee on the Cardiac Laboratory at St. Marys Hospital," with Minutes, MC BOG, April 21, 1965, MCA. See also Davis, Hodgson, and Kincaid, "Diagnostic Radiology at the Mayo Clinic."

82. D. B. Effler, F. M. Sones Jr., L. K. Groves, and E. L. Suarez, "Myocardial Revascularization by Vineberg's Internal Mammary Implant: Evaluation of Postoperative Results," *J. Thorac. Cardiovasc. Surg.*, 1965, *50*: 527–533.

83. Ibid. Bigelow and Sones's quotations are from the discussion on 532.

84. W. L. Proudfit, "Surgical Treatment of Coronary Artery Disease," *J. Iowa Med. Soc.*, 1966, *56*: 661–662.

85. Ibid., 662.

86. "Coronary Angiography," *Lancet*, 1966, *1*: 1084–1085, quotation from 1084.

87. D. B. Effler, "Coronary Angiography," *Lancet*, 1966, *2*: 169–170, quotation from 169.

88. "Healing the Heart: New Operations Hold Promise of Normal Life for Numerous Patients," *Wall Street Journal*, May 17, 1966.

89. D. C. Sabiston Jr., "Role of Surgery in the Management of Myocardial Ischemia," *Mod. Concepts Cardiovasc. Dis.*, 1966, *35*: 123–127, quotation from 127.

90. E. Braunwald and H. J. C. Swan, eds., "Cooperative Study on Cardiac Catheterization," *Circulation*, 1968, *37*: III-1–III-113.

91. R. S. Ross and R. Gorlin, "Coronary Arteriography," *Circulation*, 1968, *37*: III-67–III-73.

92. R. O. Brandenburg Section Report to MC BOG for 1966, MCA.

93. Robert B. Wallace, MD [Oral history, May 5, 2003], in W. Stoney, *Pioneers of Cardiac Surgery* (Nashville, TN: Vanderbilt University Press, 2008), 308–315.

94. J. R. Hodgson, Radiology Section Report to MC BOG for 1969, MCA. See also R. G. Favaloro, D. B. Effler, L. K. Groves, F. M. Sones Jr., and D. J. G. Fergusson, "Myocardial Revascularization by Internal Mammary Artery Implant Procedures," *J. Thorac. Cardiovasc. Surg.*, 1967, *54*: 359–368.

95. R. G. Favaloro, "Saphenous Vein Graft in the Surgical Treatment of Coronary Artery Disease: Operative Technique," *J. Thorac. Cardiovasc. Surg.*, 1969, *58*: 178–185.

Chapter 15

1. D. C. McGoon, "Surgery of the Heart and Great Vessels," *N. Engl. J. Med.*, 1968, *278*: 143–148, 194–198, quotation from 197.

2. Ibid.

3. D. B. Effler, "A New Era of Surgery for Ischemic Heart Disease," *Dis. Chest*, 1968, *54*: 399–400, quotation from 399.

4. Ibid. See also D. B. Effler, L. K. Groves, F. M. Sones Jr., and E. K. Shirey, "Increased Myocardial Perfusion by Internal Mammary Artery Implant: Vineberg's Operation," *Ann. Surg.*, 1963 *158*: 526–536; J. B. Shrager, "The Vineberg Procedure: The Immediate Forerunner of Coronary Artery Bypass Grafting," *Ann. Thorac. Surg.*, 1994, *57*: 1354–1364; R. H. Jones, "Development of Surgical Treatments for Coronary Artery Disease," *Ann. Surg.*, 2003, *238*: S121-S131; and W. B. Fye, "Coronary Arteriography: It Took a Long Time," *Circulation*, 1984, *70*: 781–787.

5. R. G. Favaloro, "Saphenous Vein Graft in the Surgical Treatment of Coronary Artery Disease: Operative Technique," *J. Thorac. Cardiovasc. Surg.*, 1969, *58*: 178–185. For the development of the operation, see R. G. Favaloro, *Surgical Treatment of Coronary Arteriosclerosis* (Baltimore: Williams & Wilkins, 1970); R. G. Favaloro, "The Developmental Phase of Modern Coronary Artery Surgery," *Am. J. Cardiol.*, 1990, *66*: 1496–1503; and D. B. Effler, "Myocardial Revascularization Surgery since 1945 A.D.: Its Evolution and Impact," *J. Thorac. Cardiovasc. Surg.*, 1976, *72*: 823–828. See also R. G. Favaloro, *The Challenging Dream of Heart Surgery: From the Pampas to Cleveland* (Boston: Little, Brown, 1994); and G. Captur, "Memento for René Favaloro," *Texas Heart Inst. J.*, 2004, *31*: 47–60.

6. D. B. Effler, R. G. Favaloro, and L. K. Groves, "Coronary Artery Surgery Utilizing Saphenous Vein Graft Techniques: Clinical Experience with 224 Operations," *J. Thorac. Cardiovasc. Surg.*, 1970, *59*: 147–154, paper presented on April 2, 1969.

7. W. Kerth, Discussion of W. D. Johnson and D. Lepley Jr., "An Aggressive Surgical Approach to Coronary Disease," *J. Thorac. Cardiovasc. Surg.*, 1969, *59*: 128–138, quotation from 136–137. Kerth's percentages referred to patients who were thought to be candidates for coronary endarterectomy compared to those who might be candidates for bypass surgery.

8. J. W. Kirklin to D. C. McGoon, June 6, 1966, Dwight C. McGoon correspondence, copy in the author's possession thanks to the generosity of Michael D. McGoon (hereafter McGoon Papers). See also "Dr. Kirklin Will Take Alabama Post," *Mayovox*, June 17, 1966.

9. D. C. McGoon Section Report to MC BOG for 1966, Mayo Clinic Archives, Mayo Historical Unit, Rochester, MN (hereafter MCA). Kirklin's sudden departure upset Mayo's surgical residents. One of them explained, "No man is indispensable, but we feel that he comes pretty close.... His support of the surgical fellows in establishing a program for independent operating and exercise of surgical judgment has contributed much to the training of mature, capable surgeons. His insistence upon intellectual honesty and accuracy is an example to us all." H. Houston, "Fellows' News," *Mayovox*, September 9, 1966.

10. J. W. Kirklin to D. C. McGoon, September 9, 1967, McGoon Papers, emphasis in the original. See also J. W. Kirklin, "Lessons Learned from the Mayo Clinic," in M. G. McGuinn, ed., *The Reynolds Historical Lectures, 1980–1991* (Birmingham: University of Alabama at Birmingham, 1993), 118–154; W. C. Roberts, "John Webster Kirklin, MD: A Conversation with the Editor," *Am. J. Cardiol.*, 1998, *81*: 1027–1044; L. W. Stephenson, "John W. Kirklin: Reminiscences of a Surgical Resident," *J. Card. Surg.*, 2004, *19*: 367–374; P. Skates, "The Elegance of Efficiency: A Profile of John Kirklin," in *Architecture & Medicine: I. M. Pei Designs the Kirklin Clinic*, ed. A. Betsky (Lanham, MD: University Press of America, 1992), 11–31; and J. W. Kirklin, "A University Department of Surgery," *Ann. Surg.*, 1971, *37*: 706–712.

11. D. B. Effler to F. A. LeFevre, March 1, 1962, Effler Papers, CCA. Edwards confirmed that salary was the main factor in his decision to leave Mayo. Jesse E. Edwards, interview by W. B. Fye, Rochester, MN, December 20, 2005. See also N. J. Hall and M. B. Smith, *Traditions United: The History of St. Luke's and Charles T. Miller Hospitals and Their Service to St. Paul* (St. Paul, MN: United Hospital Foundation, 1987). Pruitt returned to Rochester in 1968. See R. O. Brandenburg, "Raymond Pruitt," *Clin. Cardiol.*, 1987, *10*: 683–684.

12. Effler to LeFevre, March 1, 1962.

13. M. M. Ravitch, *A Century of Surgery: The History of the American Surgical Association*, 2 vols. (Philadelphia: J. B. Lippincott, 1981), 2:1399.

14. James DuShane, Mayo's first pediatric cardiologist, had trained the other four staff members: William Weidman, Patrick Ongley, Donald Ritter, and Robert Feldt. Two second-generation pediatric cardiologists explained that DuShane played "a major role in defining the clinical specialty." See C. A. Neill and E. B. Clark, *The Developing Heart: A 'History' of Pediatric Cardiology* (Boston: Kluwer, 1995), 72. See also J. A. Noonan, "A History of Pediatric Specialties: The Development of Pediatric Cardiology," *Pediatr. Res.*, 2004, *56*: 298–306. For a list of board-certified pediatric cardiologists in the United States at the time, see *Directory of Medical Specialists Holding Certification by American Specialty Boards*, 14th ed. (Chicago: Marquis-Who's Who, 1970), 1305–1308.

15. See I. E. Konstantinov, F. Rosapepe, J. A. Dearani, V. V. Alexi-Meskishvili, and J. Li, "A Tribute to Giancarlo Rastelli," *Ann. Thorac. Surg.*, 2005, *79*: 1819–1823.

16. Robert B. Wallace, MD [Oral history, May 5, 2003], in W. Stoney, *Pioneers of Cardiac Surgery* (Nashville, TN: Vanderbilt University Press, 2008), 308–315.

17. B. D. McCallister, D. R. Richmond, A. Saltups, F. J. Hallermann, R. B. Wallace, and R. L. Frye, "Left Ventricular Hemodynamics before and One Year after Internal Mammary Artery Implantation in Patients with Coronary Artery Disease and Angina Pectoris," *Circulation*, 1970, *42*: 471–477.

18. D. B. Effler, "Myocardial Revascularization with Internal Mammary Artery Implants," *Minn. Med.*, 1968, *51*: 1039–1042, quotation from 1042.

19. H. A. Zimmerman, "The Dilemma of Surgery in the Treatment of Coronary Artery Disease," *Am. Heart J.*, 1969, *77*: 577–578.

20. D. B. Effler to H. A. Zimmerman, May 16, 1969, George E. Burch Papers, MS C376, Modern Manuscripts Collection, History of Medicine Division, National Library of Medicine, Bethesda, MD.

21. H. A. Zimmerman, "And Now—Vein Grafts," *Am. Heart J.*, 1970, *80*: 585.

22. D. C. McGoon, "Response of a Cardiovascular Surgeon to the Editorial of Henry A. Zimmerman, M.D.," *Am. Heart J.*, 1970, *80*: 586, emphasis in the original.

23. G. K. Danielson, G. T. Gau, and G. D. Davis, "Early Results of Vein Bypass Grafts for Coronary Artery Disease," *Circulation*, 1971, *44* suppl. 2: II-101, abstract. G. K. Danielson to W. B. Fye, October 30, 2007, e-mail.

24. D. C. McGoon Section Report to MC BOG for 1967, MCA.

25. Minutes, Saint Marys Hospital Joint Conference Committee, June 18, 1968, MCA. See also T. Hale, "Why the Nursing Shortage Persists," *N. Engl. J. Med.*, 1964, *270*: 1092–1097; "Growing Nurses' Shortage Poses Problems for Mayo, Others," *Mayovox*, March 1979; and V. S. Wentzel, *Sincere et Constanter, 1906–1970: The Story of Saint Marys School of Nursing* (Rochester, MN: Mayo Foundation, 2006), 65–75.

26. The statistics are from W. W. L. Glenn, "Some Reflections on the Coronary Bypass Operation," *Circulation*, 1972, *45*: 869–877. See also J. K. Roche and J. M. Stengle, "Facilities for Open Heart Surgery in the United States," *Am. J. Cardiol.*, 1973, *32*: 224–228. The number of procedures in Rochester is from D. C. McGoon, Section of Thoracic and Cardiovascular Surgery Report to MC BOG for 1970, MCA.

27. Benjamin D. McCallister, interview by W. B. Fye, Atlanta, GA, March 13, 2006.

28. B. D. McCallister, "Indications for Coronary Arteriography," *Med. Clin. North Am.*, 1970, *54*: 979–995, quotations from 980 and 994.

29. McCallister interview. Another cardiologist who performed coronary angiograms at Mayo confirmed this impression: Gerald T. Gau, interview by W. B. Fye, Rochester, MN, July 27, 2006. McCallister and Crockett formed the Mid America Heart Institute in conjunction with St. Luke's Hospital in Kansas City in 1975. Their practice flourished, and other Mayo cardiologists would join it. See B. D. McCallister and D. M. Steinhaus, "The Mid-America Heart Institute," *Am. Heart Hosp. J.*, 2003, *1*: 183–187, 241–245.

30. G. D. Davis, J. R. Hodgson, and O. W. Kincaid, "Diagnostic Radiology at the Mayo Clinic: Personal Recollections of People and Practice from the 1940s to 1970s, Including Reflections on the Beginning Years," typescript, 1990, MCA. Hodgson quotation from 55.

31. J. T. Shepherd to MC BOG, December 15, 1970, MCA.

32. J. R. Hodgson, Radiology Section Report to MC BOG for 1970, MCA.

33. C. W. Lillehei to O. H. Wangensteen, March 25, 1958, box 18, University of Minnesota Department of Surgery Papers, University of Minnesota Archives, Minneapolis, MN (hereafter UMN Surgery Papers). See also R. Schmid, "Cecil James Watson," *Biogr. Mem. Nat. Acad. Sci.*, 1994, *65*: 354–372; and G. W. Miller, *King of Hearts: The True Story of the Maverick who Pioneered Open Heart Surgery* (New York: Random House, 2000), 119–123.

34. C. W. Lillehei to O. H. Wangensteen, April 14, 1958, box 18, UMN Dept. Surgery Papers. See also C. W. Lillehei to H. M. Cavert, May 10, 1958, box 18, UMN Dept. Surgery Papers.

35. Kurt Amplatz, interview by Kirk Jeffrey, Golden Valley, MN, October 23, 2000, transcript from the Minnesota Historical Society, St. Paul, MN. See also K. Amplatz, "Technics of Coronary Arteriography," *Circulation*, 1963, *27*: 101–106.

36. Miller, *King of Hearts*, 200–202. For the perspective of Wangensteen's successor, see J. S. Najarian, *The Miracle of Transplantation: The Unique Odyssey of a Pioneer Transplant Surgeon* (Beverly Hills, CA: Medallion Publishing, 2009), 63–84.

37. Thomas Killip, interview by W. B. Fye, Dallas, TX, November 13, 1994.

38. H. A. Baltaxe, K. Amplatz, and D. C. Levin, *Coronary Angiography* (Springfield: Charles C Thomas, 1973).

39. Richard Gorlin, interview by W. B. Fye, Atlanta, GA, March 15, 1994. See also H. L. Abrams and D. F. Adams, "The Coronary Arteriogram: Structural and Functional Aspects," *N. Engl. J. Med.*, 1969, *281*: 1276–1285, 1336–1342.

40. O. W. Linton, *Radiology at the Brigham, 1913–2002* (Boston: Department of Radiology, Brigham and Women's Hospital, 2003), 128.

41. D. C. Levin and H. L. Abrams, "Participation by Radiologists in Coronary Angiography," *Radiology*, 1977, *125*: 543–545.

42. D. C. Levin, D. F. Adams, and H. L. Abrams, "The Role of the Radiologist in Coronary Angiography," *Radiology*, 1977, *125*: 313–315. During the next three decades, Levin would author or coauthor more than two dozen editorials and articles about tensions between cardiology and radiology with respect to cardiac imaging. See, for example, D. C. Levin, H. L. Abrams, W. R. Castaneda-Zuñiga, K. E. Fellows, J. Grollman Jr., W. A. Mitchell et al., "Lessons from History: Why Radiologists Lost Coronary Angiography and What Can Be Done to Prevent Future Similar Losses," *Invest. Radiol.*, 1994, *29*: 480–484; and D. C. Levin and V. M. Rao, "Turf Wars in Radiology: Should It Be Radiologists or Cardiologists Who Do Cardiac Imaging?" *J. Am. Coll. Radiol.*, 2005, *2*: 749–752.

43. H. A. Baltaxe, "The Current Uses of Coronary Angiography," *Radiol. Clin. North Am.*, 1971, *9*: 597–607, quotation from 607.

44. See F. H. Adams and R. C. Mendenhall, "Profile of the Cardiologist: Training and Manpower Requirements for the Specialist in Adult Cardiovascular Disease," *Am. J. Cardiol.*, 1974, *34*: 389–456; and H. A. Baltaxe, "Past, Present, and Future Status of Cardiovascular Radiology," *Cardiovasc. Radiol.*, 1979, *2*: 57–66.

45. Spittell quotation from "Report to the BOG of the Review by the Residency Review Committee of the Educational Programs of the Department of Internal Medicine," December 6, 1971, MCA.

46. D. B. Effler, "Introduction," in Favaloro, *Surgical Treatment of Coronary Arteriosclerosis*, xi-xvi, quotation from xi.

47. W. B. Fye, "Fueling the Growth of Cardiology: Patients, Procedures, and Profits," in *American Cardiology: The History of a Specialty and Its College* (Baltimore: Johns Hopkins University Press, 1996), 249–294.

48. J. V. Warren, "A Revolution in Coronary Artery Disease," *J. Chron. Dis.*, 1973, *26*: 547–551, quotation from 547.

49. The procedural volumes are from the Radiology Section Report to MC BOG for 1968; and Minutes, MC Clinical Practice Committee, June 4, 1971, MCA.

50. Gau interview. Gau had been trained to perform coronary angiography in London by Shahbudin Rahimtoola, who had gone to England in 1966 after serving as co-director of the catheterization laboratory at Saint Marys Hospital in Rochester. See G. T. Gau, C. M. Oakley, S. Rahimtoola, M. J. Raphael, and R. E. Steiner, "Selective Coronary Arteriography: A Review of 18 Months' Experience," *Clin. Radiol.*, 1970, *21*: 275–286.

51. See D. S. Jones, "Visions of a Cure: Visualization, Clinical Trials, and Controversies in Cardiac Therapeutics, 1968–1998," *Isis*, 2000, *91*: 504–541; and D. S. Jones, *Broken Hearts: The Tangled History of Cardiac Care* (Baltimore: Johns Hopkins University Press, 2013).

52. See A. Selzer and W. J. Kerth, "Surgical Treatment of Coronary Artery Disease: Too Fast, Too Soon?" *Am. J. Cardiol.*, 1971, *28*: 490–492; and E. Braunwald, "Direct Coronary Revascularization: A Plea Not to Let the Genie Escape from the Bottle," *Hospital Practice*, 1971, *6*: 9–10. For a surgeon's perspective, see D. C. Sabiston Jr., "Direct Revascularization Procedure in the Management of Myocardial Ischemia," *Circulation*, 1971, *43*: 175–178.

53. R. Gore, "Lifeline for a Man with a Dying Heart: New Surgery Saves Doomed Coronary Victims," *Life*, February 5, 1971, 51–56, quotation from 52.

54. The name of the National Heart Institute was changed to the National Heart and Lung Institute in 1969. See E. T. Lanahan, *A Salute to the Past: A History of the National Heart, Lung, and Blood Institute Based on Personal Recollections* (Bethesda, MD: NHLBI, 1987), 18.

55. Minutes, National Advisory Heart and Lung Council, June 17–18, 1971, emphasis in the original, copy in the author's possession obtained from bound minute books located outside Claude Lenfant's office at the NIH in May 2000.

56. L. B. Johnson, *The Vantage Point: Perspectives of the Presidency 1963–1969* (New York: Holt, Rinehart and Winston, 1971), 425–426. Johnson's wife sought the opinion of her longtime family friend James Cain, a Mayo internist who had helped to care for her family for more than three decades. See Lady Bird Johnson, *A White House Diary* (New York: Holt, Rinehart and Winston, 1970), 583–584. See also D. Kearns, *Lyndon Johnson and the American Dream* (New York: Harper & Row, 1976), 309–352; D. Farber and B. Bailey, eds., *The Columbia Guide to America in the 1960s* (New York: Columbia University Press, 2001); and T. Brokaw, *Boom! Voices of the Sixties* (New York: Random House, 2007).

57. "Industry is Invited to Become an Ally of Medicine," *Mayovox*, November 27, 1970.

58. "Excerpts from an Address by the Honorable Lyndon B. Johnson," *Mayo Alumnus*, January 1971, 13–14. This entire issue was devoted to "Industry Day at Mayo."

59. L. Janos, "The Last Days of the President," *Atlantic*, July 1973, 35–41. See also R. Dallek, *Flawed Giant: Lyndon Johnson and His Times, 1961–1973* (New York: Oxford University Press, 1998), 523–526, 619–623.

60. T. Cooper, "Foreword," in *Coronary Artery Medicine and Surgery: Concepts and Controversies*, ed. J. C. Norman (New York: Appleton-Century-Crofts, 1975), xxxv–xxxvii.

61. P. L. Frommer, "The Ad Hoc Policy Board on Coronary Artery Surgery of the NHLI. Coronary Artery By-pass Surgery: Recommendations for a Program of Research." August 31, 1972, copy in the author's possession obtained from bound minute books located outside Claude Lenfant's office at the NIH in May 2000.

62. Anon., "Coronary-Bypass Surgery," *Lancet*, 1973, *301*: 137–139.

63. Ibid. For British medicine and cardiology, see R. Stevens, *Medical Practice in Modern England: The Impact of Specialization and State Medicine* (New Haven, CT: Yale University Press, 1966); and M. E. Silverman, P. R. Fleming, A. Hollman, D. G. Julian, and D. M. Krikler, *British Cardiology in the 20th Century* (London: Springer, 2000).

64. J. G. Mearns, "Effler and Sones and the Boys at Cleveland Clinic Have Taken the You-Bet-Your-Life Out of Heart Surgery, So Don't Wait Around to Get Zapped by a Heart Attack, Head It Off at the Coronary Artery," *Cleveland Magazine*, November 1973, quotation from 3. Reprint of article in the author's possession.

65. I. H. Page, "F. Mason Sones: The Importance of a Person," *Mod. Med.*, 1986, *54*: 11–12. See also W. C. Sheldon, "F. Mason Sones, Jr.: Stormy Petrel of Cardiology," *Clin. Cardiol.*, 1994, *17*: 405–407.

66. Mearns, "Effler and Sones," 4, emphasis in the original.

67. Ibid., 9, 10.

68. Ibid., 10.

69. R. D. Sautter, "Reply," *J. Thorac. Cardiovasc. Surg.*, 1974, *68*: 977–978, quotation from 978.

70. D. B. Effler, "Revascularization Surgery," *J. Thorac. Cardiovasc. Surg.*, 1974, *68*: 977.

71. Principal Investigators of CASS and their Associates, "National Heart, Lung, and Blood Institute Coronary Artery Surgery Study," *Circulation*, 1981, *63*, part 2, suppl. 1: I-1–I-81. See also "Mayo Takes Part in NIH Study on Coronary Artery Disease," *Mayovox*, November 1976.

72. Jones, "Visions of a Cure," 522. Houston surgeon Michael DeBakey complained in 1978 that "the insistence on the use of prospective randomized studies for the evaluation of surgical…techniques reflects a naïve obsession with this research tool." M. E. DeBakey, "Aortocoronary-Artery Bypass: Assessment after 13 Years," *JAMA*, 1978, *239*: 837–839, quotation from 838.

73. D. E. Harken, G. E. Green, W. D. Johnson, E. Dong, and F. M. Sones Jr., "Panel Discussion: Comparative Effects of Medical and Surgical Therapy on Prognosis of the Patient with Coronary Disease," in *Cardiovascular Disease: New Concepts in Diagnosis and Therapy*, ed. H. L. Russek (Baltimore: University Park Press, 1974), 495–507, Sones's quotation from 495–496.

74. S. P. Griffiths, B. M. Zazula, D. Courtney, F. C. Spencer, and J. R. Malm, "Trends in Cardiovascular Surgery (1961 to 1977): Review of the New York City and State Experience,"

Am. J. Cardiol., 1979, *44*: 555–562. By 1977, CABG accounted for 63 percent of the operations performed for acquired heart disease in New York State despite the fact that the procedure was less than a decade old. See also T. A. Preston, *Coronary Artery Surgery: A Critical Review* (New York: Raven Press, 1977).

75. E. Braunwald, "Coronary-Artery Surgery at the Crossroads," *N. Engl. J. Med.*, 1977, *297*: 661–663, quotation from 663.

76. Ibid. Results from CASS were not expected for several years because long-term follow-up of the patients was considered important.

77. N. E. Shumway, "Foreword," in *The Treatment of Acute Myocardial Ischemia: An Integrated Medical/Surgical Approach*, ed. L. H. Cohn (Mount Kisco, NY: Futura, 1979), vii–viii.

78. F. D. Loop, W. L. Proudfit, and W. C. Sheldon, "Coronary Artery Surgery Weighed in the Balance," *Am. J. Cardiol.*, 1978, *42*: 154–156, quotation from 155.

79. For a Mayo cardiologist's perspective, see R. G. Tancredi, "Medical Management of Patients with Chronic Stable Angina Pectoris," *Cardiovasc. Clin.*, 1980, *10*: 89–102. See also W. H. Frishman, "Beta-Adrenergic Blockers: A 50-Year Historical Perspective," *Am. J. Ther.*, 2008, *15*: 565–576; and R. Vos, *Drugs Looking for Diseases: Innovative Drug Research and the Development of the Beta Blockers and the Calcium Antagonists* (Boston: Kluwer, 1991).

80. J. H. Comroe Jr. and R. D. Dripps, "Ben Franklin and Open Heart Surgery," *Circ. Res.*, 1974, *35*: 661–669, quotation from 662. See also J. H. Comroe Jr. and R. D. Dripps, *The Top Ten Clinical Advances in Cardiovascular-Pulmonary Medicine and Surgery, 1945–1975*, 2 vols. (Washington, DC: Government Printing Office, 1978). A useful chronological bibliography of developments in cardiology and cardiac surgery (with annotations in French) is R. Khouri, *Références des Grandes Étapes en Cardiologie et Chirurgie Cardiovasculaire* (Paris: Éditions Louis Pariente, 1993).

81. "Open-Heart Surgery Techs Honored," *Mayovox*, April 1973.

82. R. B. Wallace, Surgery Report to MC BOG for 1977. MCA.

83. W. C. Sheldon to C. E. Wasmuth, April 23, 1976, CCA. See "The First Decade of Bypass Graft Surgery for Coronary Artery Disease: An International Symposium, September 15–17, 1977, Cleveland, Ohio, Proceedings," *Cleveland Clin. Q.*, 1978, *45*: 1–196.

84. See M. E. Bertrand, ed., *The Evolution of Cardiac Catheterization and Interventional Cardiology* (St Albans, UK: Iatric Press and European Society of Cardiology, 2006); and M. Picichè, ed., *Dawn and Evolution of Cardiac Procedures: Research Avenues in Cardiac Surgery and Interventional Cardiology* (New York: Springer, 2013).

85. R. L. Frye and P. L. Frommer, eds., "Consensus Development Conference on Coronary Artery Bypass Surgery: Medical and Scientifific Aspects," *Circulation*, 1982, *65*, suppl. 2: II-1–129, quotation from 129. The word "Blood" had been added to the name of the National Heart and Lung Institute and its associated council in 1976. For an overview of CASS and other bypass surgery trials, see Jones, "Visions of a Cure."

86. G. B. Kolata, "Consensus on Bypass Surgery," *Science*, 1981, *211*: 42–43.

87. D. M. Cosgrove, F. D. Loop, and W. C. Sheldon, "Results of Myocardial Revascularization: A 12-Year Experience," *Circulation*, 1982, *65*, suppl. 2: II-37–43.

88. The ABC television quote is reproduced in "Standing Behind Bypass Surgery," *Challenge*, Spring/Summer 1984, 16–23, CCA.

89. Effler's discussion of papers presented at the Fortieth Annual Meeting of the American Association for Thoracic Surgery, May 11–13, 1960. See *J. Thorac. Cardiovasc. Surg.*, 1960, *40*: 799–812, quotation from 810. See also J. L. Thomas, "The Vineberg Legacy: Internal Mammary Artery Implantation from Inception to Obsolescence," *Texas Heart Inst. J.*, 1999, *26*: 107–113.

90. Delos M. Cosgrove, interview by W. B. Fye, Cleveland, OH, September 20, 2007. For a list of visiting medical students, see "Quarterly Directory. Mayo Clinic, Mayo Foundation...[for

the Quarter Beginning] July 3, 1965," *Clinic Bulletin*, 1965, *43*. For background on the program, see R. D. Miller and V. Johnson, "Traineeships for Medical Students at the Mayo Graduate School of Medicine," *Mayo Clin. Proc.*, 1965, *40*: 917–922.

91. Cosgrove interview.

92. F. D. Loop, "CASS Continued," *Circulation*, 1985, *72*, suppl. 2: II-1–6. See also CASS Principlal Investigators and Their Associates, "Coronary Artery Surgery Study (CASS): A Randomized Trial of Coronary Bypass Surgery, Survival Data," *Circulation*, 1983, *68*: 939–950. CASS generated controversy beginning with the investigators' first report. See, for example, J. W. Hurst, "CASS November 1983: Two Years Later," *Clin. Cardiol.*, 1985, *8*: 561–564; and G. S. Weinstein and B. Levin, "The Coronary Artery Surgery Study (CASS): A Critical Appraisal," *J. Thorac. Cardiovasc. Surg.*, 1985, *90*: 541–548.

93. R. L. Frye, L. Fisher, H. V. Schaff, B. J. Gersh, R. E. Vlietstra, and M. B. Mock, "Randomized Trials in Coronary Artery Bypass Surgery," *Prog. Cardiovasc. Dis.*, 1987, *30*: 1–22, quotation from 18.

94. G. S. Reeder, H. C. Smith, and R. L. Frye, "Coronary Arteriography," in *Cardiology: Fundamentals and Practice*, ed. R. O. Brandenburg, V. Fuster, E. R. Giuliani, and D. C. McGoon (Chicago: Year Book Medical Publishers, 1987), 451–470, quotations from 451 and 468.

Chapter 16

1. "Clearing an Artery," *Life*, August 14, 1964, 43–46, quotation from 43. A technical review of peripheral artery angioplasty is G. J. van Andel, *Percutaneous Transluminal Angioplasty: The Dotter Procedure* (Amsterdam: Excerpta Medica, 1976).

2. C. T. Dotter and M. P. Judkins, "Transluminal Treatment of Arteriosclerotic Obstruction: Description of a New Technic and a Preliminary Report of Its Application," *Circulation*, 1964, *30*: 654–670, quotation from 669. See also C. T. Dotter, "Two Decades of Transluminal Angioplasty: An Overview," *J. Mal. Vasc.*, 1982, *7*: 357–361.

3. See M. E. Bertrand, ed., *The Evolution of Cardiac Catheterization and Interventional Cardiology* (St Albans, UK: Iatric Press and European Society of Cardiology, 2006); and M. Picichè, ed., *Dawn and Evolution of Cardiac Procedures: Research Avenues in Cardiac Surgery and Interventional Cardiology* (New York: Springer, 2013). For a discussion of the steps between the concept of PTCA and its first use in a human, see B. Meier, "The First Coronary Angioplasties in Zurich," in Bertrand, ed., *Evolution of Cardiac Catheterization*, 61–74. See also S. B. King III, "Angioplasty from Bench to Bedside," *Circulation*, 1996, *93*: 1621–1629; R. F. J. Shepherd and R. E. Vlietstra, "The History of Interventional Cardiology," in *Interventional Cardiology*, ed. D. R. Holmes Jr. and R. E. Vlietstra (Philadelphia: F. A. Davis, 1989), 3–19; and C. Handler and M. Cleman, eds., *Classic Papers in Coronary Angioplasty* (London: Springer, 2006). For oral histories of some pioneers of PTCA, see www.ptca.org/nv/interviews.html.

4. A. Grüntzig, "Transluminal Dilatation of Coronary Artery Stenosis," *Lancet*, 1978, *1*: 263. For the status of CABG just before the advent of PTCA, see H. D. McIntosh and J. A. Garcia, "The First Decade of Aortocoronary Bypass Grafting, 1967–1977," *Circulation*, 1978, *57*: 405–431. Most pioneers of PTCA experimented on animals (mainly dogs) before attempting the procedure in humans. For a comprehensive review of the historical, social, political, and ethical aspects of using of animals in biomedical research, see F. Barbara Orlans, *In the Name of Science: Issues in Responsible Animal Experimentation* (New York: Oxford University Press, 1993).

5. A. Grüntzig, A. Senning, and W. E. Siegenthaler, "Nonoperative Dilatation of Coronary Artery Stenoses: Percutaneous Transluminal Angioplasty (PTA)," in *Coronary Heart Disease: 3rd*

International Symposium, Frankfurt, February 1978, ed. M. Kaltenbach, P. R. Lichtlen, R. Balcon, and W.-D. Bussman (Stuttgart: Georg Thieme, 1978), 325–343, quotations from 338 and 342.

6. R. E. Vlietstra to W. B. Fye, April 28, 2008, e-mail. Vlietstra coauthored the paper that Harrison presented in Frankfurt, Germany, in February 1978. See I. P. Clements, R. E. Vlietstra, J. D. Dewey, and C. E. Harrison Jr., "Protective Effect of Verapamil Infusion on Mitochondrial Respiratory Function in Ischemic Myocardium," in Kaltenbach, Lichtlen, Balcon, and Bussman, eds., *Coronary Heart Disease,* 284–297.

7. Ronald E. Vlietstra, interview by W. B. Fye, Orlando, FL, March 8, 2005. See also D. S. Jones, "Visions of a Cure: Visualization, Clinical Trials, and Controversies in Cardiac Therapeutics, 1968–1998," *Isis,* 2000, *91:* 504–541; and D. S. Jones, *Broken Hearts: The Tangled History of Cardiac Care* (Baltimore: Johns Hopkins University Press, 2013).

8. Grüntzig had performed four *intraoperative* coronary angioplasties in the spring of 1977 with cardiac surgeon Elias Hanna and cardiologist Richard Myler at St. Mary's Hospital in San Francisco. See Meier, "First Coronary Angioplasties," 66–67.

9. "Blowup in the Arteries," *Time,* July 3, 1978, 85.

10. Ibid. See also R. K. Myler and S. H. Stertzer, "Coronary and Peripheral Angioplasty: Historical Perspective," in *Textbook of Interventional Cardiology,* ed. E. J. Topol (Philadelphia: W. B. Saunders, 1990), 187–198.

11. Minutes, MC Cardiovascular Practice Committee, November 10, 1978, Mayo Clinic Archives, Mayo Historical Unit, Rochester, MN (hereafter MCA). See also R. C. Fox and J. P. Swazey, "The Experiment-Therapy Dilemma," in *The Courage to Fail: A Social View of Organ Transplants and Dialysis* (Chicago: University of Chicago Press, 1974), 60–83; J. B. McKinlay, "From 'Promising Report' to 'Standard Procedure': Seven Stages in the Career of a Medical Innovation," *Milbank Q.,* 1981, *59:* 374–411; and G. Gordon and G. L. Fisher, eds., *The Diffusion of Medical Technology: Policy and Planning Perspectives* (Cambridge, MA: Ballinger, 1975).

12. J. K. Kahn, "Geoffrey O. Hartzler," *Clin. Cardiol.,* 2004, *27:* 58–59.

13. Minutes, MC Cardiovascular Practice Committee, March 9, 1979, MCA. For a summary of heart tests used at this time, see A. M. Weissler, ed., *Reviews of Contemporary Laboratory Methods* (Dallas: American Heart Association, 1980).

14. Cardiovascular Practice Committee, March 9, 1979.

15. R. E. Vlietstra to W. B. Fye, April 28, 2008, e-mail.

16. R. I. Levy, M. J. Jesse, and M. B. Mock, "Position on Percutaneous Transluminal Coronary Angioplasty (PTCA)," *Circulation,* 1979, *59:* 613.

17. Ibid.

18. T. R. Engel and S. G. Meister, "Coronary Percutaneous Transluminal Angioplasty," *Ann. Intern. Med.,* 1979, *90:* 268–269. See also S. Klaidman, *Health in the Headlines: The Stories behind the Stories* (New York: Oxford University Press, 1991).

19. Engel and Meister, "Angioplasty."

20. *Proceedings of the Workshop on Percutaneous Transluminal Coronary Angioplasty, June 15–16, 1979* (Bethesda, MD: NIH, 1980). Sones's quotation from 143. See also S. M. Mullin, E. R. Passamani, and M. B. Mock, "Historical Background of the National Heart, Lung, and Blood Institute Registry for Percutaneous Transluminal Coronary Angioplasty," *Am. J. Cardiol.,* 1984, *53:* 3C–6C

21. Minutes, MC Cardiovascular Practice Committee, October 26, 1979, MCA.

22. Vlietstra to Fye, April 28, 2008.

23. Information derived or quoted from Harvey Grummitt's medical record is used with the written permission of his wife. Lila Grummitt to W. B. Fye, May 16, 2008. A review of the patient's record reveals that a published account of the first PTCA at Mayo, based on conversations and correspondence with Hartzler between 1986 and 2006, contains inaccuracies. See D. Monagan and D. O. Williams, *Journey into the Heart: A Tale of Pioneering Doctors and Their Race to Transform Cardiovascular Medicine* (New York: Gotham Books, 2007), 199–201.

24. Grummitt medical record. For a Mayo cardiologist's perspective on the medical treatment of angina, see R. G. Tancredi, "Medical Management of Patients with Chronic Stable Angina Pectoris," *Cardiovasc. Clin.*, 1980, *10*: 89–102.

25. Grummitt medical record, October 8, 1979.

26. Ibid., October 9, 1979. John Bresnahan, a cardiology fellow at the time, recalls that the catheterization laboratory "was packed" with observers who wanted to watch Mayo's first angioplasty. J. F. Bresnahan to W. B. Fye, October 2013, e-mail.

27. G. Hartzler to H. Grummitt, November 19, 1979, copy in Grummitt medical record.

28. Cardiovascular Practice Committee, October 26, 1979.

29. G. O. Hartzler, H. C. Smith, R. E. Vlietstra, D. A. Oberle, and D. A. Strelow, "Coronary Blood Flow Responses during Successful Percutaneous Transluminal Coronary Angioplasty," *Mayo Clin. Proc.*, 1980, *55*: 45–49.

30. S. B. King III, "Andreas Gruentzig in Atlanta," in Bertrrand, ed., *Evolution of Cardiac Catheterization*, 75–83, quotation from 75.

31. W. C. Sheldon, *Pathfinders of the Heart: The History of Cardiology at the Cleveland Clinic* (n.p.: Xlibris Corporation, 2008), 96–98.

32. W. C. Sheldon to R. F. Farmer, November 19, 1979, CCA.

33. Minutes, Cleveland Clinic BOG, January 9, 1980, CCA.

34. King, "Gruentzig in Atlanta," 75. See also J. W. Hurst, "Andreas Roland Gruentzig, M.D.: The Teaching Genius," *Clin. Cardiol.*, 1986, *9*: 35–37.

35. King, "Gruentzig in Atlanta," 80.

36. Kahn, "Hartzler," 58. Kahn trained with Hartzler in Kansas City, MO, in 1990.

37. Vlietstra interview. Vlietstra left Mayo in 1989, when he joined the Watson Clinic in Lakeland, Florida.

38. W. B. Fye, "The Price of Success: Tensions in and Around Cardiology," in *American Cardiology: The History of a Specialty and Its College* (Baltimore: Johns Hopkins University Press, 1996), 295–334, esp. 317–322.

39. R. L. Frye to R. E. Weeks, April 13, 1981, with CV Annual Report for 1980, MCA.

40. Ibid.

41. Science writer Gina Kolata reported Detre's comment, which she made during an NHLBI-sponsored workshop on PTCA. G. B. Kolata, "Coronary Treatment Assessed," *Science*, 1981, *213*: 195.

42. The Society for Cardiac Angiography, founded in 1978, developed training guidelines, but they were voluntary. See P. J. Scanlon, "The Training for and Practice of Percutaneous Transluminal Coronary Angioplasty: Results of Two Surveys," *Cathet. Cardiovasc. Diagn.*, 1985, *11*: 561–570. See also W. C. Sheldon, "A Short History of the Society for Cardiac Angiography: The First Decade," *Cathet. Cardiovasc. Diagn.*, 1989, *17*: 1–4.

43. "The Departments of Medicine (Cardiology) and Radiology of Emory University School of Medicine...Present Demonstrations in Percutaneous Transluminal Angioplasty (PTA) by Andreas Gruentzig. Atlanta. February 1–5, 1981," brochure in the author's possession.

44. A. R. Gruentzig and B. Meier, "Percutaneous Transluminal Coronary Angioplasty: The First Five Years and the Future," *Int. J. Cardiol.*, 1983, *2*: 319–323, quotation from 321.

45. David R. Holmes Jr., interview by W. B. Fye, Snowmass, CO, August 7, 2004.

46. Spencer B. King III, M.D., interview by Burt Cohen, part 1, January 8, 1997, www.ptca.org.archive/interviews/970204int.html.

47. A. R. Gruentzig, "Percutaneous Transluminal Coronary Angioplasty, April 8–12, 1984." 21-page typescript given to course attendees, copy in the author's possession.

48. The Emory charges are from Gruentzig, "Coronary Angioplasty, April 8–12, 1984." For cardiologists' incomes, see P. R. Kletke, W. D. Marder, and S. L. Thran, *Socioeconomic Characteristics of Cardiology Practice* (Chicago: American Medical Association, 1988), table 2-10.

49. Alfred A. Bove, interview by W. B. Fye, New Orleans, LA, November 9, 2004. For the development of regulations regarding animal experimentation, see C. W. McPherson, ed., *50 Years of Laboratory Animal Science* (Memphis, TN: AALAS, 1999).

50. G. B. Kolata, "New Treatment for Coronary Artery Disease," *Science*, 1979, n.s. *206*: 917–918.

51. S. B. King III, "Who are Interventionalists? What about Surgeons?" *JACC Cardiovasc. Intervent.*, 2008, *1*: 109–110.

52. E. L. Jones, J. M. Craver, A. R. Grüntzig, S. B. King III, J. S. Douglas, D. K. Bone et al., "Percutaneous Transluminal Coronary Angioplasty: Role of the Surgeon," *Ann. Thorac. Surg.*, 1982, *34*: 492–503, quotation from 501, paper presented by Jones in January 1982.

53. F. Robicsek, Discussion of Jones et al., "Coronary Angioplasty," quotation from 502–503.

54. Jones, responding to Robicsek, in Jones, "Coronary Angioplasty," 503.

55. R. E. Vlietstra to W. B. Fye, April 29, 2008, e-mail.

56. D. C. McGoon, *The Parkinson's Handbook* (New York: W. W. Norton, 1990). See also O. T. Clagett, *General Surgery at the Mayo Clinic 1900–1970* (Rochester, MN: privately printed, 1980).

57. J. R. Pluth, "Balloon Angioplasty in Multivessel Coronary Artery Disease," *Mayo Clin. Proc.*, 1983, *58*: 624–625. See also D. C. Levin and H. L. Abrams, "Participation by Radiologists in Coronary Angiography," *Radiology*, 1977, *125*: 543–545.

58. J. M. Piehler, "PTCA and the Cardiovascular Surgeon," in *PTCA: Percutaneous Transluminal Coronary Angioplasty*, ed. R. E. Vlietstra and D. R. Holmes Jr. (Philadelphia: F. A. Davis, 1987), 189–199, quotation from 189. For another Mayo surgeon's perspective, see H. V. Schaff, "Role of the Surgeon in Interventional Cardiology," in Holmes and Vlietstra, eds., *Interventional Cardiology*, 42–52.

59. R. E. Vlietstra, D. R. Holmes Jr., H. C. Smith, G. O. Hartzler, and T. A. Orszulak, "Percutaneous Transluminal Coronary Angioplasty: Initial Mayo Clinic Experience," *Mayo Clin. Proc.*, 1981, *56*: 287–293.

60. R. O. Brandenburg, "Challenges and Frustrations," *Am. J. Cardiol.*, 1980, *46*: 905–906.

61. Vlietstra et al., "Angioplasty: Initial Mayo Clinic Experience," 287.

62. D. H. Spodick, "Percutaneous Transluminal Coronary Angioplasty," *Mayo Clin. Proc.*, 1981, *56*: 526–527.

63. For Chalmers, see Jones, "Visions of a Cure," 537–541. See also J. Daly, *Evidence-Based Medicine and the Search for a Science of Clinical Care* (Berkeley: University of California Press, 2005).

64. R. E. Vlietstra, D. R. Holmes Jr., H. C. Smith, G. O. Hartzler, and T. A. Orszulak, "The Authors Repond," *Mayo Clin. Proc.*, 1981, *56*: 526–527.

65. R. H. Kennedy, M. A. Kennedy, R. L. Frye, E. R. Giuliani, J. R. Pluth, H. C. Smith et al., "Use of the Cardiac Catheterization Laboratory in a Defined Population," *N. Engl. J. Med.*, 1980, *303*: 1273–1277. See also L. J. Melton III, "History of the Rochester Epidemiology Project," *Mayo Clin. Proc.*, 1996, *71*: 266–274.

66. Kennedy et al., "Cardiac Catheterization Laboratory," 1275. See also L. B. Russell, *Technology in Hospitals: Medical Advances and Their Diffusion* (Washington, DC: Brookings Institution, 1979); S. H. Altman and R. Blendon, eds., *Medical Technology: The Culprit behind Health Care Costs?* (Washington, DC: US Dept. of Health, Education, and Welfare, 1979); Institute of Medicine, *Assessing Medical Technologies* (Washington, DC: National Academy Press, 1985); J. D. Bronzino, V. H. Smith, and M. L. Wade, *Medical Technology and Society: An Interdisciplinary Perspective* (Cambridge, MA: MIT Press, 1990); E. M. Rogers, *Diffusion of Innovations*, 5th ed. (New York: Free Press, 2003); A. B. Cohen and R. S. Hanft, eds., *Technology in American Health Care: Policy Directions for Effective Evaluation and Management* (Ann Arbor: University of Michigan Press, 2004); and S. J. Reiser, *Technological Medicine: The Changing World of Doctors and Patients* (New York: Cambridge University Press, 2009).

67. Kennedy et al., "Cardiac Catheterization Laboratory," 1276.

68. M. P. Judkins, H. L. Abrams, J. D. Bristow, E. Carlsson, J. M. Criley, L. P. Elliott et al., "Report of the Inter-Society Commission for Heart Disease Resources. Optimal Resources for Examination of the Chest and Cardiovascular System: A Hospital Planning and Resource Guideline," *Circulation*, 1976, *53*: A1–37.

69. A. S. Relman, "Determining How Much Medical Care We Need," *N. Engl. J. Med.*, 1980, *303*: 1292–1293.

70. M. G. Brataas, "Public Affairs and the Mayo Clinic," *Med. Group Manage.*, 1983, *30*: 30–32. See also W. Shonick, *Government and Health Services: Government's Role in the Development of U.S. Health Services, 1930–1980* (New York: Oxford University Press, 1995); and C. S. Weissert and W. G. Weissert, *Governing Health: The Politics of Health Policy* (Baltimore: Johns Hopkins University Press, 1996).

71. "1983 Approaches Most Successful Year Ever for Mayo," *Mayovox*, December 1983.

72. For Eli Ginsberg's speech, see "Fewer Dollars will Mean More Competition in Medicine," *Mayovox*, June 1983. See also R. Mayes and R. A. Berenson, *Medicare Prospective Payment and the Shaping of U.S. Health Care* (Baltimore: Johns Hopkins University Press, 2006).

73. R. Avery, "The Medicare Prospective Payment System: Overview and Impact on PTCA," February 24, 1984, copy in the author's possession.

74. E. Ginzberg, *American Medicine: The Power Shift* (Totowa, NJ: Rowman & Allanheld, 1985), 177.

75. G. C. Jang, P. C. Block, M. J. Cowley, A. R. Gruentzig, G. Dorros, D. R. Holmes Jr. et al., "Relative Cost of Coronary Angioplasty and Bypass Surgery in a One-Vessel Disease Model," *Am. J. Cardiol.*, 1984, *53*: 52C–55C.

76. Ibid. See also J. D. Talley and P. D. Mauldin, "Publications Concerning Costs of Various Cardiovascular Procedures and Drugs," *Am. J. Cardiol.*, 1997, *79*: 70–72.

77. Kolata, "Coronary Treatment Assessed," 195.

78. R. E. Vlietstra, D. R. Holmes Jr., G. S. Reeder, M. B. Mock, H. C. Smith, A. A. Bove et al., "Balloon Angioplasty in Multivessel Coronary Artery Disease," *Mayo Clin. Proc.*, 1983, *58*: 563–567, quotation from 567.

79. M. B. Mock, G. S. Reeder, H. V. Schaff, D. R. Holmes Jr., R. E. Vlietstra, H. C. Smith et al., "Percutaneous Transluminal Coronary Angioplasty versus Coronary Artery Bypass: Isn't It Time for a Randomized Trial?" *N. Engl. J. Med.*, 1985, *312*: 916–919, quotation from 917. See also R. L. Frye, L. Fisher, H. V. Schaff, B. J. Gersh, R. E. Vlietstra, and M. B. Mock, "Randomized Trials in Coronary Artery Bypass Surgery," *Prog. Cardiovasc. Dis.*, 1987, *30*: 1–22; and D. C. Harrison, "Cost Containment in Medicine: Why Cardiology?" *Am. J. Cardiol.*, 1985, *56*: 10C–15C. Frye and Gersh would play significant roles in randomized clinical trials of CABG and PTCA for several decades. See, for example, B. J. Gersh and R. L. Frye, "Methods of Coronary Revascularization: Things May Not Be as They Seem," *N. Engl. J. Med.*, 2005, *352*: 2235–2237.

80. A. S. Relman, "Assessment and Accountability: The Third Revolution in Medical Care," *N. Engl. J. Med.*, 1988, *319*: 1220–1222. See also A. M. Epstein, "The Outcomes Movement: Will It Get Us Where We Want to Go?" *N. Engl. J. Med.*, 1990, *323*: 266–270.

81. See W. B. Fye, "Acute Myocardial Infarction: A Historical Summary," in *Acute Myocardial Infarction*, ed. B. J. Gersh and S. H. Rahimtoola, 2nd ed. (New York: Chapman & Hall, 1997), 1–15; and E. G. Nabel and E. Braunwald, "A Tale of Coronary Artery Disease and Myocardial Infarction," *N. Engl. J. Med.*, 2012, *366*: 54–63.

82. See A. Maroo and E. J. Topol, "The Early History and Development of Thrombolysis in Acute Myocardial Infarction," *J. Thromb. Haemost.*, 2004, *2*: 1867–1870; and R. L. Mueller and S. Scheidt, "History of Drugs for Thrombotic Disease: Discovery, Development, and Directions for the Future," *Circulation*, 1994, *89*: 432–449.

83. K. P. Rentrop, H. Blanke, K. R. Karsch, V. Wiegand, H. Köstering, H. Oster et al., "Acute Myocardial Infarction: Intracoronary Application of Nitroglycerin and Streptokinase,"

Clin. Cardiol., 1979, *2*: 354–363. A 1976 report on intracoronary streptokinase in acute myocardial infarction by Moscow cardiologist Evgeniĭ Chazov and his associates attracted almost no attention because it was published in Russian. See also K. P. Rentrop, "Development and Pathophysiological Basis of Thrombolytic Therapy in Acute Myocardial Infarction: Part I. 1912–1977," *J. Intervent. Cardiol.*, 1998, *11*: 255–263; and K. P. Rentrop, "Development and Pathophysiological Basis of Thrombolytic Therapy in Acute Myocardial Infarction: Part II. 1977–1980," *J. Intervent. Cardiol.*, 1998, *11*: 265–285.

84. E. Braunwald, "Personal Reflections on Efforts to Reduce Ischemic Myocardial Damage," *Cardiovasc. Res.*, 2002, *56*: 332–338.

85. A. B. Weisse, "The Elusive Clot: The Controversy over Coronary Thrombosis in Myocardial Infarction," *J. Hist. Med. Allied Sci.*, 2005, *61*: 66–78. See also E. Braunwald and D. A. Morrow, "Unstable Angina: Is It Time for a Requiem?" *Circulation*, 2013, *127*: 2452–2457.

86. Examples include E. Corday, ed., *Controversies in Cardiology* (Philadelphia: F.A. Davis, 1977); E. Corday and H. J. C. Swan, eds., *Clinical Strategies in Ischemic Heart Disease: New Concepts and Current Controversies* (Baltimore: Williams & Wilkins, 1979); E. Rapaport, ed., *Current Controversies in Cardiovascular Disease* (Philadelphia: W. B. Saunders, 1980); and S. H. Rahimtoola, ed., *Controversies in Coronary Artery Disease* (Philadelphia: F.A. Davis, 1983).

87. W. C. Roberts, "Valentin Fuster, MD, PhD: A Conversation with the Editor," *Am. J. Cardiol.*, 2000, *86*: 182–197, quotation from 188.

88. V. Fuster, R. L. Frye, D. C. Connolly, M. A. Danielson, L. R. Elveback, and L. T. Kurland, "Arteriographic Patterns Early in the Onset of the Coronary Syndromes," *Br. Heart J.*, 1975, *37*: 1250–1255, quotation from 1255.

89. D. R. Holmes Jr., G. O. Hartzler, H. C. Smith, and V. Fuster, "Coronary Artery Thrombosis in Patients with Unstable Angina," *Br. Heart J.*, 1981, *45*: 411–416, quotation from 411.

90. Ibid., 416.

91. M. A. DeWood, J. Spores, R. Notske, L. T. Mouser, R. Burroughs, M. S. Golden et al., "Prevalence of Total Coronary Occlusion during the Early Hours of Transmural Myocardial Infarction," *N. Engl. J. Med.*, 1980, *303*: 897–902.

92. E. R. González, "Intracoronary Thrombolysis to Abort Heart Attacks: Wave of the Future?" *JAMA*, 1981, *245*: 11–13. See also W. Ganz, N. Buchbinder, H. Marcus, A. Mondkar, J. Maddahi, Y. Charuzi et al., "Intracoronary Thrombolysis in Evolving Myocardial Infarction," *Am. Heart J.*, 1981, *101*: 4–13.

93. Minutes, MC Cardiovascular Practice Committee, January 9, 1981, MCA.

94. Details are from the author's review of the patient's medical record.

95. Ibid.

96. For Hartzler's role in pioneering emergency PTCA and for a general discussion of the strategy, see E. J. Topol, "Direct versus Sequential Percutaneous Transluminal Coronary Angioplasty," in *Acute Coronary Intervention* (New York: Alan R. Liss, 1988), 79–94.

97. G. O. Hartzler, B. D. Rutherford, D. R. McConahay, W. L. Johnson Jr., B. D. McCallister, R. C. Conn et al., "Percutaneous Transluminal Coronary Angioplasty with and without Thrombolytic Therapy for Treatment of Acute Myocardial Infarction," *Am. Heart J.*, 1983, *106*: 965–973. See also E. J. Topol, "Coronary Angioplasty for Acute Myocardial Infarction," *Ann. Intern. Med.*, 1988, *109*: 970–980. Emergency CABG was sometimes performed in patients with a heart attack or unstable angina. See L. H. Cohn, ed., *The Treatment of Acute Myocardial Ischemia: An Integrated Medical/Surgical Approach* (Mount Kisco, NY: Futura, 1979). For a Mayo surgeon's perspective, see J. R. Pluth, "What Is the Status of Coronary Revascularization for Acute Myocardial Infarction?" *Cardiovasc. Clin.*, 1983, *13*: 183–190.

98. B. D. McCallister and D. M. Steinhaus, "The Mid-America Heart Institute," 2 parts, *Am. Heart Hosp. J.*, 2003, *1*: 183–187, 241–245. During the final two decades of the twentieth

century, the single specialty group would become the most popular cardiology practice model in many parts of the United States. See Fye, *American Cardiology*, 317–334.

99. D. R. Holmes Jr., H. C. Smith, R. E. Vlietstra, R. A. Nishimura, G. S. Reeder, A. A. Bove et al., "Percutaneous Transluminal Coronary Angioplasty: Alone or in Combination with Strepokinase Therapy, during Acute Myocardial Infarction," *Mayo Clin. Proc.*, 1985, *60*: 449–456.

100. G. G. Gensini, "The Society for Cardiac Angiography: List of U.S. Cardiac Catheterization Laboratories," *Cathet. Cardiovasc. Diagn.*, 1984, *10*: 259–298.

101. E. Braunwald, "Happy Birthday, GISSI!" *Am. Heart J.*, 2004, *148*: 187. See also L. Tavazzi, A. P. Maggioni, and G. Tognoni, "Participation versus Education: The GISSI Story and Beyond," *Am. Heart J.*, 2004, *148*: 222–229.

102. D. Collen and H. R. Lijnen, "The Tissue-Type Plasminogen Activator Story," *Arterioscler. Thromb. Vasc. Biol.*, 2009, *29*: 1151–1155. See also S. S. Hughes, *Genentech: The Beginnings of Biotech* (Chicago: University of Chicago Press, 2011).

103. J. H. Chesebro, G. L. Knatterud, R. Roberts, J. S. Borer, L. S. Cohen, J. E. Dalen et al., "Thrombolysis in Myocardial Infarction (TIMI) Trial, Phase I: A Comparison between Intravenous Tissue Plasminogen Activator and Intravenous Streptokinase," *Circulation*, 1987, *76*: 142–154. See also E. Braunwald and M. S. Sabatine, "The Thrombolysis in Myocardial Infarction (TIMI) Study Group Experience," *J. Thorac. Cardiovasc. Surg.*, 2012, *144*: 762–770.

104. "Minimizing Heart Damage," *Mayovox*, August 1986.

105. W. C. Roberts, "Bernard John Gersh, MD: A Conversation with the Editor," *Am. J. Cardiol.*, 1998, *82*: 1087–1104, quotation from 1096.

106. N. Cousins, "The Healing Heart," *Int. J. Cardiol.*, 1983, *3*: 57–65, 219–229, quotation from 58.

107. The cover of a 1981 issue of *Time* magazine displayed a headline "Heart Attacks: New Insights, New Treatments" and featured an artist's image of a large heart with a door opening into it. The article described many recent developments in the diagnosis, treatment, and prevention of heart disease. See A.Toufexis, "Taming the No. 1 Killer: Doctors Attack Heart Disease with New Techniques and Potent Drugs," *Time*, June 1, 1981, 52–58.

108. Cousins, "Healing Heart," quotations from 58 and 64. See also N. Cousins, *The Healing Heart: Antidotes to Panic and Helplessness* (New York: W. W. Norton, 1983).

109. D. E. Rogers, "Some Observations on Having a Coronary," *Pharos*, Summer 1986, 12–14. See also H. Mandell and H. Spiro, eds., *When Doctors Get Sick* (New York: Plenum, 1987); and R. Klitzman, *When Doctors Become Patients* (New York: Oxford University Press, 2008).

110. Rogers, "Having a Coronary," 12–13.

111. D. E. Rogers, "Another Ode to High Technology—or Having Another Coronary Revisited," *Pharos*, Winter 1992, 13–14.

112. Ibid. See also D. E. Rogers, "Internists: More Specialists or More Generalists?" *Ann. Intern. Med.*, 1985, *102*: 702–703; and D. E. Rogers, *American Medicine: Challenge for the 1980s* (Cambridge, MA: Ballinger, 1978).

113. H. C. Smith, D. D. Mair, and P. R. Julsrud, Triennial Review, Cardiac Catheterization Laboratory, January 1983, MCA. Mayo doctors published the first report of using angioplasty to dilate arteries that carry blood to the brain. See T. M. Sundt Jr., H. C. Smith, J. K. Campbell, R. E. Vlietstra, R. F. Cucchiara, and A. W. Stanson, "Transluminal Angioplasty for Basilar Artery Stenosis," *Mayo Clin. Proc.*, 1980, *55*: 673–680.

114. "1983 Approaches Most Successful Year Ever for Mayo," *Mayovox*, December 1983. For the national context, see R. Blendon, C. J. Schramm, T. W. Moloney, and D. E. Rogers, "An Era of Stress for Health Institutions: The 1980s," *JAMA*, 1981, *245*: 1843–1845.

115. See H. Markel, "Patients, Profits, and the American People: The Bayh-Dole Act of 1980," *N. Engl. J. Med.*, 2013, *369*: 794–796.

116. G. Jacobson, "Ventures in Medicine and Plastics," *Management Rev.*, September 1989, 10–12, Colvin quotation from 11. The article describes several of Mayo Medical Venture's activities. It was also responsible for publishing the *Mayo Clinic Health Letter*, which had 300,000 paid subscribers by 1988. See "Mayo Medical Ventures Continues Its Treasure Hunt," *Mayovox*, March 1988; and K. Anderson, "Mayo Clinic Office of Intellectual Property: Exploring and Encouraging Invention and Innovation through Unique Mayo Clinic Funding Opportunities," *J. Cardiovasc. Trans. Res.*, 2008, *1*: 280.

117. See, for example, A. C. Gelijns and E. A. Halm, eds., *The Changing Economics of Medical Technology* (Washington, DC: National Academy Press, 1991); and N. Rosenberg, A. C. Gelijns, and H. Dawkins, eds., *Sources of Medical Technology: Universities and Industry* (Washington, DC: National Academy Press, 1995).

118. R. E. Vlietstra and R. L. Frye, "Topical Issues: A U.S. Viewpoint," *Int. J. Cardiol.*, 1989, *23*: 153–157.

119. Holmes and Vlietstra, eds., *Interventional Cardiology*, v.

120. M. E. Bertrand, "Atherectomy and Laser: 'New Devices,'" in *Evolution of Cardiac Catheterization*, 105–115.

121. "Tiny Cutting Tool Used to Remove Arterial Blockage," *Mayovox*, November 1988. See also J. Simpson, "How Atherectomy Began: A Personal Story," *Am. J. Cardiol.*, 1993, *72*: 3E–5E.

122. U. P. Kaufmann, K. N. Garratt, R. E. Vlietstra, K. K. Menke, and D. R. Holmes Jr., "Coronary Atherectomy: First 50 Patients at the Mayo Clinic," *Mayo Clin. Proc.*, 1989, *64*: 747–752, quotation from 750–751.

123. A. C. Clarke, *Profiles of the Future: An Inquiry into Limits of the Possible*, rev. ed., (New York: Harper & Row, 1973), 21.

124. D. R. Bresnahan, "Lasers in Cardiovascular Disease," in Holmes and Vlietstra, eds., *Interventional Cardiology*, 361–383, quotation from 372. For the early history of lasers, see J. L. Bromberg, *The Laser in America, 1950–1970* (Cambridge, MA: MIT Press, 1991)

125. R. A. White and W. S. Grundfest, eds., "Preface to the Second Edition," in *Lasers in Cardiovascular Disease: Clinical Applications, Alternative Angioplasty Devices, and Guidance Systems* (Chicago: Year Book Medical Publishers, 1989), xi.

126. See P. N. Ruygrok and P. W. Serruys, "Intracoronary Stenting: From Concept to Custom," *Circulation*, 1996, *94*: 882–890; and S. Xu, J. Avorn, and A. S. Kesselheim, "Origins of Medical Innovation: The Case of Coronary Artery Stents," *Circ. Cardiovasc. Qual. Outcomes*, 2012, *5*: 743–749. For a comparison of the adoption of heart care treatments (including PTCA and thrombolytic therapy) in the United States, Canada, and several European countries, see M. B. McClellan and D. P. Kessler, eds., *Technological Change in Health Care: A Global Analysis of Heart Attack* (Ann Arbor: University of Michigan Press, 2002). See also A. Sargentini and L. Mariani, "Regulations Governing Medical Devices," in *The Health Service Market in Europe*, ed. R. Rapparini (Brussels: Elsevier, 1984), 46–83; B. Stocking, ed., *Expensive Health Technologies: Regulatory and Administrative Mechanisms in Europe* (New York: Oxford University Press, 1988); and D. Banta, "The Development of Health Technology Assessment," *Health Policy*, 2003, *63*: 121–132.

127. A Mayo study revealed that the original estimates of the cost savings when PTCA was compared to CABG were exaggerated before the problem of restenosis at the site of dilatation was fully appreciated. See G. S. Reeder, I. Krishan, F. T. Nobrega, J. Naessens, M. Kelly, J. B. Christianson et al., "Is Percutaneous Coronary Angioplasty Less Expensive than Bypass Surgery?" *N. Engl. J. Med.*, 1984, *311*: 1157–1162.

128. This summary comes from the author's review of the patient's medical record. See also G. S. Roubin, "Trials and Tribulations in the Development of the Coronary Artery Stent: A Personal Perspective," *J. Invasive Cardiol.*, 1992, *4*: 69–74.

129. "Mayo Foundation Consent to Participation in Medical Research Study. Title: 'Gianturco-Roubin Coronary Stent.' Approved by IRB September 25, 1989," signed consent form in the patient's medical record, which was reviewed by the author.

130. L. Gustafson, "Interview with Kirk N. Garratt, MD," *J. Invasive Cardiol.*, 2001, *13*: 502–510, quotation from 508.

131. K. N. Garratt, D. R. Holmes Jr., and G. S. Roubin, "Early Outcome after Placement of a Metallic Intracoronary Stent: Initial Mayo Clinic Experience," *Mayo Clin. Proc.*, 1991, *66*: 268–275, quotation from 268.

132. Vlietstra and Frye, "Topical Issues," 153. See also S. B. Knoebel and S. Dack, eds., *An Era in Cardiovascular Medicine* (New York: Elsevier, 1991).

133. Vlietstra and Frye, "Topical Issues," 153.

134. R. L. Frye, "President's Page: Does It Really Make a Difference?" *J. Am. Coll. Cardiol.*, 1992, *19*: 468–470.

135. See L. H. Aiken and D. Mechanic, eds., *Applications of Social Science to Clinical Medicine and Health Policy* (New Brunswick, NJ: Rutgers University Press, 1986); and T. R. Marmor, *Understanding Health Care Reform* (New Haven, CT: Yale University Press, 1994).

136. E. J. Topol, "The Stentor and the Sea Change," *Am. J. Cardiol.*, 1995, *76*: 307–308.

137. W. B. Fye, "The Power of Clinical Trials and Guidelines, and the Challenge of Conflicts of Interest," *J. Am. Coll. Cardiol.*, 2003, *41*: 1237–1242; See also J. L. Ritchie, J. S. Forrester, and W. B. Fye, eds., "28th Bethesda Conference: Practice Guidelines and the Quality of Care," *J. Am. Coll. Cardiol.*, 1997, *29*: 1125–1179.

138. J. S. Kan, R. I. White Jr., S. E. Mitchell, and T. J. Gardner, "Percutaneous Balloon Valvuloplasty: A New Method for Treating Congenital Pulmonary Valve Stenosis," *N. Engl. J. Med.*, 1982, *307*: 540–542. William Rashkind had pioneered the use of a balloon catheter as an intracardiac therapeutic device. See W. J. Rashkind and W. W. Miller, "Creation of an Atrial Septal Defect Without Thoracotomy: A Palliative Approach to Complete Transposition of the Great Arteries," *JAMA*, 1966, *196*: 991–992; and T. O. Cheng, "The History of Balloon Valvuloplasty," *J. Intervent. Cardiol.*, 2000, *13*: 365–373.

139. D. J. Hagler, J. B. Seward, D. D. Mair, and P. R. Julsrud, "Valvuloplasty and Angioplasty in Congenital Heart Disease," in Holmes and Vlietstra, eds., *Interventional Cardiology*, 162–184.

140. K. Inoue, O. Takane, T. Nakamura, F. Kitamura, and N. Miyamoto, "Clinical Application of Transvenous Mitral Commisurotomy by a New Balloon Catheter," *J. Thorac. Cardiovasc. Surg.*, 1984, *87*: 394–402.

141. A. Cribier, N. Saoudi, J. Berland, T. Savin, P. Rocha, and B. Letac, "Percutaneous Transluminal Valvuloplasty of Acquired Aortic Stenosis in Elderly Patients: An Alternative to Valve Replacement?" *Lancet*, 1986, *327*: 63–67.

142. The author reviewed the patient's record.

143. Minutes, MC Cardiovascular Practice Committee, August 22, 1986, MCA.

144. The author reviewed the patient's record. For a Mayo perspective on the status of aortic and mitral balloon valvuloplasty at the end of the decade by Holmes, Nishimura, and Reeder, see Holmes and Vlietstra, eds., *Interventional Cardiology*, 120–147. See also T. M. Bashore and C. J. Davidson, eds., *Percutaneous Balloon Valvuloplasty and Related Techniques* (Baltimore: Williams & Wilkins, 1991).

145. D. R. Holmes Jr. and R. A. Nishimura, "Balloon Valvuloplasty," *Adv. Intern. Med.*, 1992, *37*: 363–389, quotation from 371.

146. Ibid., 382.

147. C. S. Rihal, R. A. Nishimura, and D. R. Holmes Jr., "Percutaneous Balloon Mitral Valvuloplasty: The Learning Curve," *Am. Heart J.*, 1991, *122*: 1750–1756, quotation from 1755.

148. The issue of individual (and institutional) volumes continued to be controversial. See, for example, T. J. Ryan, "The Critical Question of Procedure Volume Minimums for Coronary Angioplasty," *JAMA*, 1995, *274*: 1169–1170; S. E. Kimmel and D. M. Kolansky, "Operator Volume as a 'Risk Factor,'" *J. Am. Coll. Cardiol.*, 1997, *30*: 878–880; and K. A. Phillips and H. S. Luft, "The Policy Implications of Using Hospital and Physician Volumes as 'Indicators'

of Quality of Care in a Changing Health Care Environment," *Int. J. Qual. Health Care*, 1997, *9*: 341–348.

149. See Sheldon, "History of the Society for Cardiac Angiography;" and H. L. Page, "SCAI: 1977–1996," http://www.scai.org/About/History.aspx.

Chapter 17

1. R. S. Blacher and R. J. Cleveland, "Heart Surgery," *JAMA*, 1979, *242*: 2463–2464, quotation from 2463. See also F. Bound Alberti, *Matters of the Heart: History, Medicine, and Emotion* (New York: Oxford University Press, 2010).

2. J. C. Oates in Larry King, ed., *Taking on Heart Disease* (Emmaus, PA: Rodale, 2004), 226–233, quotation from 228.

3. See B. Lüderitz, *History of the Disorders of Cardiac Rhythm*, 3rd ed. (Armonk, NY: Futura, 2002); W. B. Fye, "The History of Cardiac Arrhythmias," in *Textbook of Cardiac Arrhythmias*, ed. J. A. Kastor (Philadelphia: W. B. Saunders, 1993), 1–24; and H. J. J. Wellens, "Cardiac Arrhythmias: The Quest for a Cure, A Historical Perspective," *J. Am. Coll. Cardiol.*, 2004, *44*: 1155–1163.

4. L. N. Katz and A. Pick, *Clinical Electrocardiography: Part 1. The Arrhythmias* (Philadelphia: Lea & Febiger, 1956), 15.

5. H. B. Burchell, "Important Events in Cardiology, 1940–1982," *JAMA*, 1983, *249*: 1197–1200, quotation from 1197.

6. R. L. Parker Section Report to MC BOG for 1957, Mayo Clinic Archives, Mayo Historical Unit, Rochester, MN (hereafter MCA). See also G. E. Burch and N. P. DePasquale, *A History of Electrocardiography*, with a new introduction by J. D. Howell (San Francisco: Jeremy Norman, 1990); and W. B. Fye, "A History of the Origin, Evolution, and Impact of Electrocardiography," *Am. J. Cardiol.*, 1994, *73*: 937–949.

7. "ECG Laboratory Changes Bring Major Savings in Time, Space," *Mayovox*, April 13, 1963.

8. A general overview is C. Pursell, *Technology in Postwar America: A History* (New York: Columbia University Press, 2007). For the history of technology and medicine, see J. D. Bronzino, V. H. Smith, and M. L. Wade, *Medical Technology and Society: An Interdisciplinary Perspective* (Cambridge, MA: MIT Press, 1990); S. S. Blume, *Insight and Industry: On the Dynamics of Technological Change in Medicine* (Cambridge, MA: MIT Press, 1992); and J. M. Edmondson, "Medicine and Technology," in *A Companion to American Technology*, ed. C. Pursell (Malden, MA: Blackwell, 2005), 156–176.

9. R. L. Parker Section Report to MC BOG for 1961, MCA. See also D. L. Morton Jr. and J. Gabriel, *Electronics: The Life Story of a Technology* (Baltimore: Johns Hopkins University Press, 2007); and P. W. Macfarlane, "A Brief History of Computer-Assisted Electrocardiography," *Meth. Inform. Med.*, 1990, *29*: 272–281.

10. "Computer Facility at Medical Sciences Now in Operation," *Mayovox*, August 4, 1962. See also "Clinic and IBM May Combine Efforts in Some Research Areas," *Mayovox*, March 21, 1959.

11. M. W. Anderson Section Report to MC BOG for 1962, MCA.

12. "ECG Laboratory Changes Bring Major Savings in Time, Space."

13. Earl Bakken, interview by W. B. Fye, Anaheim, CA, November 12, 1991.

14. C. A. Caceres, "The Use of Computers in Electrocardiography: The Present and the Future," in *Computers, Electrocardiography and Public Health: A Report of Recent Studies* (Washington, DC: US Public Health Service, 1966), 1-1–8, quotations from 1-1 and 1-7, paper presented in December 1964. See also R. S. Ledley, *Use of Computers in Biology and Medicine* (New York: McGraw-Hill, 1965); and J. A. November, *Biomedical Computing: Digitizing Life in the United States* (Baltimore: Johns Hopkins University Press, 2012).

15. "The Cybernated Generation," *Time*, April 2, 1965, 84–91, quotations from 86 and 84.

16. "Expanded Computer Use at Clinic Explored: Clinic and Lockheed Join in Year-Long Feasibility Study," *Mayovox*, September 23, 1966.

17. R. E. Smith and C. M. Hyde, "Computer Analysis of the Electrocardiogram in Clinical Practice," in *Electrical Activity of the Heart*, ed. G. W. Manning and S. P. Ahuja (Springfield, IL: Charles C Thomas, 1969), 305–315, paper presented in May 1967. See also "IBM Computer in Operation in ECG Laboratory," *Mayovox*, December 29, 1968. For interactions between Marquette Electronics and Mayo cardiologists Ralph Smith and Ralph Zitnik, see M. J. Cudahy, *Joyworks: The Story of Marquette Electronics and Two Lucky Entrepreneurs* (Milwaukee: Milwaukee County Historical Society, 2002), 73–80.

18. J. Wartak, *Computers in Electrocardiography* (Springfield, IL: Charles C Thomas, 1970), quotations from vii and viii.

19. E. G. Dimond and F. M. Berry, "Transmission of Electrocardiographic Signals over Telephone Circuits," *Am. Heart J.*, 1953, *46*: 906–910, quotation from 906. In fact, Willem Einthoven had transmitted the electrical impulses from the hearts of hospitalized patients over a telephone wire to the string galvanometer in his physiological laboratory one mile away before 1906. See Fye, "History of Electrocardiography," 939.

20. "ECG Telephonic Transmission Now Made Between Clinic and Hospital," *Mayovox*, June 2, 1967.

21. "Transoceanic ECG Demonstration Announced," *Mayovox*, August 6, 1971.

22. "Mayo ECG Service Links Clinic Facilities to Out-of-City Hospital," *Mayovox*, August 1973.

23. K-C. Hu, D. B. Francis, G. T. Gau, and R. E. Smith, "Development and Performance of Mayo-IBM Electronic Computer Analysis Programs (V70)," *Mayo Clin. Proc.*, 1973, *48*: 260–268, quotation from 268.

24. W. Einthoven, "Le télécardiogramme," *Arch. Int. Physiol.*, 1906, *4*: 132–164, plate 1 depicts complete heart block. For a translation, see W. Einthoven, "The Telecardiogram," trans. H. W. Blackburn Jr., *Am. Heart J.*, 1957, *53*: 602–615.

25. F. A. Willius, "A Study of Complete Heart Block," *Ann. Clin. Med.*, 1925, *3*: 129–135, quotations from 132 and 133.

26. See F. G. MacMurray, "Stokes-Adams Disease: A Historical Review," *N. Engl. J. Med.*, 1957, *256*: 643–650.

27. See K. Jeffrey, *Machines in Our Hearts: The Cardiac Pacemaker, the Implantable Defibrillator, and American Health Care* (Baltimore: Johns Hopkins University Press, 2001). Books written by pacemaker pioneers include W. G. Bigelow, *Cold Hearts: The Story of Hypothermia and the Pacemaker in Heart Surgery* (Toronto: McClelland and Stewart, 1984); J. A. Hopps, *Passing Pulses: The Pacemaker and Medical Engineering: A Canadian Story* (Gloucester, Ontario: John A. Hopps, 1995); E. Bakken, *One Man's Full Life* (Minneapolis: Medtronic, 1999); and W. Greatbatch, *The Making of the Pacemaker* (Amherst, NY: Prometheus Books, 2000). See also Å. Senning, "Cardiac Pacing in Retrospect," *Am. J. Surg.*, 1983, *145*: 733–739; D. C. Schechter, *Exploring the Origins of Electrical Cardiac Stimulation* (Minneapolis: Medtronic, 1983); and D. L. Hayes and S. Furman, "Cardiac Pacing: How It Started, Where We Are, Where We Are Going," *Pacing Clin. Electrophysiol.*, 2004, *27*: 693–704.

28. P. M. Zoll, A. J. Linenthal, L. R. Norman, and A. H. Belgard, "Treatment of Stokes-Adams Disease by External Electric Stimulation of the Heart," *Circulation*, 1954, *9*: 482–493, quotation from 488. Ten of the 25 patients survived for one to twenty-four months after they were resuscitated. For a contemporary summary of arrhythmias, see S. Bellet, *Clinical Disorders of the Heart Beat* (Philadelphia: Lea & Febiger, 1953).

29. P. M. Zoll, A. J. Linenthal, L. R. Norman, M. H. Paul, and W. Gibson, "External Electric Stimulation of the Heart in Cardiac Arrest," *Arch. Int. Med.*, 1955, *96*: 639–653.

30. D. E. Donald, J. E. Edwards, H. G. Harshbarger, and J. W. Kirklin, "Surgical Correction of Ventricular Septal Defect: Anatomic and Technical Considerations," *J. Thorac. Surg.*, 1957,

33: 45–59, paper presented by Kirklin in May 1956. Kirklin and Lillehei's comments on heart block as a result of surgery are on 57–59.

31. V. L. Gott, "Critical Role of Physiologist John A. Johnson in the Origins of Minnesota's Billion Dollar Pacemaker Industry," *Ann. Thorac. Surg.*, 2007, *83*: 349–353, quotation from 349–350.

32. W. L. Weirich, V. L. Gott, and C. W. Lillehei, "The Treatment of Complete Heart Block by the Combined Use of a Myocardial Electrode and an Artificial Pacemaker," *Surg. Forum*, 1958, *8*: 360–363, quotation from 363.

33. Senning, "Cardiac Pacing in Retrospect," 734.

34. D. Rhees and K. Jeffrey, "Earl Bakken's Little White Box: The Complex Meanings of the First Transistorized Pacemaker," in *Exposing Electronics*, ed. B. Finn, R. Bud, and H. Trischler (Amsterdam: Harwood, 2000), 75–113. David J. Rhees to W. B. Fye, July 17, 2013. Vincent L. Gott, interview by W. B. Fye, Minneapolis, MN, December 13, 2007.

35. Bakken, *One Man's Full Life*, 51. See also R. R. Munsey, "Trends and Events in FDA Regulation of Medical Devices Over the Last Fifty Years," *Food Drug Law J.*, 1995, *50*: 163–177.

36. Weirich, Gott, and Lillehei, "Artificial Pacemaker," 362.

37. R. M. Lauer, P. A. Ongley, J. W. DuShane, and J. W. Kirklin, "Heart Block after Repair of Ventricular Septal Defect in Children," *Circulation*, 1960, *22*: 526–534, paper presented on October 24, 1959.

38. C. W. Lillehei, V. L. Gott, P. C. Hodges Jr., D. M. Long, and E. Bakken, "Transistor Pacemaker for Treatment of Complete Atrioventriocular Dissociation," *JAMA*, 1960, *172*: 2006–2010, quotation from 2009. See also S. Furman and J. B. Schwedel, "An Intracardiac Pacemaker for Stokes-Adams Seizures," *N. Engl. J. Med.*, 1959, *261*: 943–948.

39. S. M. Spencer, "Making a Heartbeat Behave: An Amazing New Pocket-Size Ticker Sparks Hesitant Heartbeats and Provides Added Years of Near-Normal Life for Many Cardiac Patients," *Saturday Evening Post*, March 4, 1961, 13–14, 48, 50, quotation from 13.

40. Ibid., 13.

41. Ibid., 14–15. See also R. S. Blacher and R. H. Basch, "Psychological Aspects of Pacemaker Implantation," *Arch. Gen. Psychiat.*, 1970, *22*: 319–323; and W. M. Chardack, A. A. Gage, and W. Greatbatch, "A Transistorized, Self-Contained, Implantable Pacemaker for the Long-Term Correction of Complete Heart Block," *Surgery*, 1960, *48*: 643–654. Swedish surgeon Åke Senning implanted the first permanent pacemaker in the world in 1958. Chardack implanted the first permanent pacemaker in North America the following year. See Jeffrey, *Machines in Our Hearts*, 83–106.

42. D. C. McGoon, P. A. Ongley, and J. W. Kirklin, "Surgically Induced Heart Block," in "Cardiac Pacemakers," ed. W. W. L. Glenn, special issue, *Ann. NY Acad. Sci.*, 1964, *111 (art. 3)*: 830–834, symposium held September 27–28, 1963.

43. W. W. L. Glenn, "The Pacemaker Team," in "Cardiac Pacemakers," 815–816, quotation from 815. Several of the technologies and materials that made pacemakers possible were developed for military purposes during World War II and the early Cold War era. See Rhees and Jeffrey, "Bakken's Little White Box," 87; and D. C. Mowery and Nathan Rosenberg, "The Electronics Revolution," in *Paths of Innovation: Technological Change in 20th-Century America* (New York: Cambridge University Press, 1998), 123–166.

44. A. G. Morrow, W. M. Chardack, P. M. Zoll, A. Kantrowitz, D. A. Nathan, and J. W. Keller Jr., "Panel Discussion IV," in "Cardiac Pacemakers," 1105–1116, Chardack's comments are from 1105.

45. Ibid. Zoll's comments are from 1105. Medtronic licensed the Chardack-Greatbatch implantable pacemaker in 1960. At the time of the 1963 pacemaker symposium, they were selling about one hundred units a month. See Jeffrey, *Machines in Our Hearts*, 136–143. For insurance coverage, see W. B. Fye, *American Cardiology: The History of a Specialty and Its College* (Baltimore: Johns Hopkins University Press, 1996), 347.

46. F. H. Ellis Jr., P. C. Manning Jr., and D. C. Connolly, "Treatment of Stokes-Adams Disease," *Mayo Clin. Proc.*, 1964, *39*: 945–953, quotation from 951. See also H. B. Burchell, D. C. Connolly, and F. H. Ellis Jr., "Indications for and Results of Implanting Cardiac Pacemakers," *Am. J. Med.*, 1964, *37*: 764–777.

47. S. Furman, "Recollections of the Beginning of Transvenous Cardiac Pacing," *Pacing Clin. Electrophysiol.*, 1994, *17*: 1697–1705.

48. See R. G. Tancredi, B. D. McCallister, and H. T. Mankin, "Temporary Transvenous Catheter-Electrode Pacing of the Heart," *Circulation*, 1967, *36*: 598–608; and H. B. Burchell, "Experiences with Cardiac Pacemakers," in *Mechanisms and Therapy of Cardiac Arrhythmias*, ed. L. S. Dreifus and W. Likoff (New York: Grune & Stratton, 1966), 535–541.

49. R. J. Myers, *Medicare* (Bryn Mawr, PA: McCahn Foundation, 1970), 235. See also E. Witkin, *The Impact of Medicare* (Springfield IL: Charles C Thomas, 1971).

50. Bakken, *One Man's Full Life*, 92. For the interplay of insurance coverage and the development and diffusion of technology, see B. A. Weisbrod, "The Nature of Technological Change: Incentives Matter!" in *Adopting New Medical Technology*, ed. A. C. Gelijns and H. V. Dawkins (Washington, DC: National Academy Press, 1994), 8–48.

51. P. C. Hanley, R. E. Vlietstra, J. M. Merideth, D. R. Holmes Jr., J. C. Broadbent, M. J. Osborn et al., "Two Decades of Cardiac Pacing at the Mayo Clinic (1961 through 1981)," *Mayo Clin. Proc.*, 1984, *59*: 268–274.

52. John M. Merideth, interview by W. B. Fye, Rochester, MN, August 24, 2000.

53. S. Furman, V. Parsonnet, and S. Dack, "Complications of Pacemaker Therapy for Heart Block," *Am. J. Cardiol.*, 1966, *17*: 439–442, Parsonnet quotation from 440.

54. D. R. McConahay, B. D. McCallister, J. M. Merideth, and G. K. Danielson, "Clinical Experiences with Permanent Demand Pacemakers," *Mayo Clin. Proc.*, 1971, *46*: 44–51. A contemporary overview is S. Furman and D. J. W. Escher, *Principles and Techniques of Cardiac Pacing* (New York: Harper & Row, 1970).

55. See S. Furman, D. J. W. Escher, and B. Parker, "The Pacemaker Follow-up Clinic," *Prog. Cardiovasc. Dis.*, 1972, *14*: 515–530.

56. R. L. Frye to J. C. Hunt with CV Annual Report for 1974, June 16, 1975, MCA.

57. Jeffrey, *Machines in Our Hearts*, 186–205.

58. G. R. Ford, "Statement on Signing the Medical Device Amendments of 1976," May 28, 1976. Online by G. Peters and J. T. Woolley, *The American Presidency Project*. http://www. presidency.ucsb.edu/ws/index.php?pid=6069. See also S. H. Rahimtoola and G. A. Rahmoeller, "The Law on Cardiovascular Devices: The Role of the Food and Drug Administration and Physicians in Its Implementation," *Circulation*, 1980, *62*: 919–924; and S. B. Foote, *Managing the Medical Arms Race: Public Policy and Medical Device Innovation* (Berkeley: University of California Press, 1992).

59. James C. Broadbent, interview by W. B. Fye, Rochester, MN, January 29, 2008.

60. D. C. McGoon to R. B. Wallace, April 18, 1978, MCA.

61. R. L. Frye to J. C. Hunt, February 9, 1978, MCA. For the technique the Mayo cardiologists used, see F. A. Miller Jr., D. R. Holmes Jr., B. J. Gersh, and J. D. Maloney, "Permanent Transvenous Pacemaker Implantation via the Subclavian Vein," *Mayo Clin. Proc.*, 1980, *55*: 309–314. Mayo surgeons continued to implant pacemakers in the context of open-heart operations.

62. J. D. Maloney to R. L. Frye, Pacemaker-Electrophysiology Group Annual Report 1978, April 13, 1979. MCA. A contemporary review is M. E. Josephson and S. F. Seides, *Clinical Cardiac Electrophysiology: Techniques and Interpretations* (Philadelphia: Lea & Febiger, 1979).

63. R. L. Frye to J. C. Hunt, February 9, 1978, MCA.

64. J. M. Merideth, "Cardiac Pacemakers: Office Analysis of Common Problems," in *Office Cardiology*, ed. R. O. Brandenburg (Philadelphia: F. A. Davis, 1980), 241–246, quotation from 241. For the explosive growth in the number of articles after World War II, see D. T. Durack, "The Weight of Medical Knowledge," *N. Engl. J. Med.*, 1978, *298*: 773–775.

65. G. M. Lemole, "Foreword," in *A Guide to Cardiac Pacemakers*, ed. D. Morse, R. M. Steiner, and V. Parsonnet (Philadelphia: F. A. Davis, 1978), vii. This pacemaker atlas contained photographs and technical specifications of more than one hundred different models manufactured by twenty-one companies.

66. D. Morse and G. M. Lemole, "Programmable Pacemakers," in *A Guide to Cardiac Pacemakers*, ed. D. Morse, R. M. Steiner, and V. Parsonnet, 2nd ed. (Philadephia: F. A. Davis, 1983), 1–25.

67. V. Parsonnet, "The Proliferation of Cardiac Pacing: Medical, Technical, and Socioeconomic Dilemmas," *Circulation*, 1982, *65*: 841–845, quotation from 841. This situation contributed to the common practice of having an industry representative present when a doctor implanted a permanent pacemaker. See Jeffrey, *Machines in Our Hearts*, 184–185, 195–199; and V. Parsonnet, C. C. Crawford, and A. D. Bernstein, "The 1981 United States Survey of Cardiac Pacing Practices," *J. Am. Coll. Cardiol.*, 1984, *3*: 1321–1332.

68. For pacemaker sales, see Jeffrey, *Machines in Our Hearts*, 195.

69. See J. W. Hawthorne, M. Bilitch, S. Furman, B. S. Goldman, D. C. MacGregor, D. P. Morse et al., "North American Society of Pacing and Electrophysiology (NASPE)," *Pacing Clin. Electrophysiol.*, 1979, *2*: 521–522. Subspecialization in cardiology in this era was also evident with the formation of the American Society of Echocardiography in 1975 and the Society for Cardiac Angiography two years later. For these and other cardiology subspecialty societies, see Fye, *American Cardiology*, 341.

70. Hayes coauthored an article (based on his talk) with other Mayo cardiologists who implanted pacemakers. See D. L. Hayes, J. D. Maloney, J. M. Merideth, D. R. Holmes Jr., B. J. Gersh, J. C. Broadbent et al., "Initial and Early Follow-up Assessment of the Clinical Efficacy of a Multiparameter-Programmable Pulse Generator," *Pacing Clin. Electrophysiol.*, 1981, *4*: 417–431.

71. James D. Maloney, interview by W. B. Fye, Washington, DC, September 12, 2004. David L. Hayes, interview by W. B. Fye, Rochester, MN, October 14, 2005.

72. J. M. Merideth, Electrophysiology Group Annual Report, 1977, with R. L. Frye to J. C. Hunt, February 9, 1978, MCA.

73. "Pacemaker Testing by Telephone Brings Calls from Around the World," *Mayovox*, June 1982. See also S. Furman and D. J. W. Escher, "Transtelephone Pacemaker Clinic," *J. Thorac. Cardiovasc. Surg.*, 1971, *61*: 827–834.

74. V. Parsonnet and A. D. Bernstein, "Cardiac Pacing in the 1980s: Treatment and Techniques in Transition," *J. Am. Coll. Cardiol.*, 1983, *1*: 339–354, quotation from 339.

75. R. J. Blendon and D. E. Rogers, "Cutting Medical Care Costs: *Primum Non Nocere*," *JAMA*, 1983, *250*: 1880–1885, quotation from 1880. See also S. H. Altman and R. Blendon, eds., *Medical Technology: The Culprit behind Health Care Costs?* (Washington, DC: US Dept. of Health, Education, and Welfare, 1979). For a Mayo financial analyst's perspective, see J. H. Herrell, "Health Care Expenditures: The Approaching Crisis," *Mayo Clin. Proc.*, 1980, *55*: 705–710.

76. See G. Weisz, A. Cambrosio, P. Keating, L. Knaapen, T. Schlich, and V. J. Tournay, "The Emergence of Clinical Practice Guidelines," *Milbank Q.*, 2007, *85*: 691–727.

77. R. L. Frye, J. J. Collins, R. W. DeSanctis, H. T. Dodge, L. S. Dreifus, C. Fisch et al., "Guidelines for Permanent Cardiac Pacemaker Implantation, May 1984," *Circulation*, 1984, *70*: 331A–339A, quotation from 332A.

78. Ibid., Fisch quotation from 331A.

79. Ibid., 332A. See also R. J. Gibbons, S. Smith, and E. Antman, "American College of Cardiology/American Heart Association Clinical Practice Guidelines: Part I. Where Do They Come From?" *Circulation*, 2003, *107*: 2979–2986.

80. See P. Denes and M. D. Ezri, "Clinical Electrophysiology: A Decade of Progress," *J. Am. Coll. Cardiol.*, 1983, *1*: 292–305; Y. Grosgogeat and G. Fontaine, "From the First Endocardial

Electrocardiogram to the Ablative Techniques, Half a Century of Cardiac Electrophysiology," *Acta Cardiol.*, 1996, *51*: 203–234; and H. J. J. Wellens, "Forty Years of Invasive Clinical Electrophysiology, 1967–2007," *Circ. Arrhythmia Electrophysiol.*, 2008, *1*: 49–53. See also W. His Jr., "The Story of the Atrioventricular Bundle with Remarks Concerning Embryonic Heart Activity," *J. Hist. Med. Allied Sci.*, 1949, *4*: 319–333.

81. M. M. Scheinman, "History of Wolff-Parkinson-White Syndrome," *Pacing Clin. Electrophysiol.*, 2005, *28*: 152–156.

82. F. A. Willius and H. M. Carryer, "Electrocardiograms Displaying Short P-R Intervals with Prolonged QRS Complexes: An Analysis of Sixty-five Cases," *Proceedings of the Staff Meetings of the Mayo Clinic*, 1946, *21*: 438–444, quotation from 441.

83. H. B. Burchell, "Ventricular Preexcitation: Historical Overview," in *Cardiac Preexcitation Syndromes: Origins, Evaluation, and Treatment*, ed. D. G. Benditt and D. W. Benson Jr. (Boston: Martinus Nijhoff, 1986), 3–19.

84. H. B. Burchell, "Current Problems of Excitation," in "The Electrophysiology of the Heart," ed. H. H. Hecht, special issue, *Ann. NY Acad. Sci.*, 1957, *65 (art. 6)*: 741–742, symposium held February 15–16, 1956.

85. For the significance of the conference, see J. P. Boineau, "Electrocardiology: A 30-Year Perspective, Ah Serendipity, My Fulsome Friend," *J. Electrocardiology*, 1988, *21*, *suppl.*: S1–9.

86. H. B. Burchell, R. L. Frye, M. W. Anderson, and D. C. McGoon, "Atrioventricular and Ventriculoatrial Excitation in Wolff-Parkinson-White Syndrome (Type B)," *Circulation*, 1967, *36*: 663–672.

87. Quotations and other details are from the patient's medical record.

88. D. Durrer and J. P. Roos, "Epicardial Excitation of the Ventricles in a Patient with Wolff-Parkinson-White Syndrome (Type B)," *Circulation*, 1967, *35*: 15–21. See also H. B. Burchell, "Dirk Durrer: Thirty-five Years of Cardiology in Amsterdam," *Int. J. Cardiol.*, 1987, *14*: 239–254; and "'Circulation,' AHA Journal Now Has Clinic Editor," *Mayovox*, February 11, 1966.

89. H. B. Burchell's note in the patient's medical record, May 18, 1967.

90. Burchell, Frye, Anderson, and McGoon, "Wolff-Parkinson-White Syndrome," 667.

91. W. C. Sealy, "Reminiscences of the Beginning of Clinical Electrophysiology at Duke," *Pacing Clin. Electrophysiol.*, 1997, *20*: 382–387, quotation from 382.

92. Ibid., 385. For Frederick Cobb's description of the link between the operations at Mayo and Duke, see J. C. Greenfield Jr., *Duke Cardiology Fellows Training Program: Origin to the Present* (Durham, NC: Carolina Academic Press, 2004), 15. See also W. R. Chitwood Jr., "Will C. Sealy, MD: The Father of Arrhythmia Surgery, The Story of the Fisherman With a Fast Pulse," *Ann. Thorac. Surg.*, 1994, *58*: 1228–1239.

93. Boineau, "Electrocardiology," S4.

94. H. B. Burchell to G. K. Danielson, February 18, 1996, MCA.

95. See R. G. Petersdorf, "Departments of Medicine: Examples of Academic Hypertrophy," in *Academic Medicine: Present and Future*, ed. J. Z. Bowers and E. E. King (North Tarrytown, NY: Rockefeller Archive Center, 1983), 96–105; and H. N. Beaty, D. Babbott, E. J. Higgins, P. Jolly, and G. S. Levey, "Research Activities of Faculty in Academic Departments of Medicine," *Ann. Int. Med.*, 1986, *104*: 90–97.

96. For factors that accelerate or retard the adoption of innovations, see A. B. Cohen, "The Diffusion of New Medical Technology," in *Technology in American Health Care: Policy Directions for Effective Evaluation and Management*, ed. A. B. Cohen and R. S. Hanft (Ann Arbor: University of Michigan Press, 2004), 79–104.

97. T. N. James, "The Wolff-Parkinson-White Syndrome," *Ann. Intern. Med.*, 1969, *71*: 399–405, quotation from 399.

98. B. J. Scherlag, S. H. Lau, R. H. Helfant, W. D. Berkowitz, E. Stein, and A. N. Damato, "Catheter Technique for Recording His Bundle Activity in Man," *Circulation*, 1969, *39*: 13–18.

99. B. J. Scherlag, "The Development of the His Bundle Recording Technique," *Pacing Clin. Electrophysiol.*, 1979, *2*: 230–233, quotation from 231–232. See also M. R. Rosen, "The Links Between Basic and Clinical Cardiac Electrophysiology," *Circulation*, 1988, *77*: 251–263.

100. H. B. Burchell, "A Cardiologist's View of Modern Cardiovascular Surgery," *Dis. Chest*, 1969, *55*: 323–328, quotation from 327, paper presented on November 21, 1968. See also D. Crane, "The Gatekeepers of Science: Some Factors Affecting the Selection of Articles for Scientitfic Journals," *Am. Sociologist*, 1967, *2*: 195–201.

101. H. J. J. Wellens, *Electrical Stimulation of the Heart in the Study and Treatment of Tachycardias* (Baltimore: University Park Press, 1971), 10.

102. Maloney interview. See also J. D. Maloney, D. G. Ritter, D. C. McGoon, and G. K. Danielson, "Identification of the Conduction System in Corrected Transposition and Common Ventricle at Operation," *Mayo Clin. Proc.*, 1975, *50*: 387–394; and O. K. Narula, ed., *His Bundle Electrocardiography and Clinical Electrophysiology* (Philadelphia: F. A. Davis, 1975).

103. Merideth, Electrophysiology Group Annual Report, 1977.

104. G. O. Hartzler and J. D. Maloney, "Programmed Ventricular Stimulation in Management of Recurrent Ventricular Tachycardia," *Mayo Clin. Proc.*, 1977, *52*: 731–741, quotation from 732.

105. Ibid.

106. G. O. Hartzler, "Treatment of Recurrent Ventricular Tachycardia by Patient-Activated Radiofrequency Ventricular Stimulation," *Mayo Clin. Proc.*, 2012, *54*: 75–82, quotation from 75.

107. B. Surawicz, "Intracardiac Extrastimulation Studies: How To? Where? By Whom?" *Circulation*, 1982, *65*: 428–431. See also E. L. Michelson and L. S. Dreifus, "Present Status of Clinical Electrophysiologic Studies: Introduction—What Studies are Necessary?" *Pacing Clin. Electrophysiol.*, 1984, *7*: 421–431.

108. E. Rapaport, ed., *Current Controversies in Cardiovascular Disease* (Philadelphia: W. B. Saunders, 1980), 653. See also E. K. Chung, ed., *Artificial Cardiac Pacing: Practical Approach* (Baltimore, MD: Williams & Wilkins, 1978).

109. Maloney interview. Frye informed the chair of medicine: "It was felt necessary during the latter part of 1979 to change the administrative structure of the Clinical Electrophysiology Group which has been headed by Dr. James D. Maloney.... An administrative challenge during 1980 is to insure the appropriate relationships within this group to achieve the goal of an integrated electrophysiologic practice with provision of the best possible care of all the patients requiring these procedures and evaluations." R. L. Frye to R. E. Weeks, March 19, 1980, MCA.

110. Stephen C. Hammill, interview by W. B. Fye, Rochester, MN, July 11, 2005.

111. David Holmes became director of the catheterization laboratory in December 1984, when Hugh Smith succeeded Robert Frye as chief of the Cardiovascular Division. The following year, Holmes left the pacing-electrophysiology group to devote his time to catheterization techniques. D. R. Holmes Jr. to W. B. Fye, May 15, 2013, e-mail.

112. J. E. Osborn, "Progress Report, Cardiovascular Drug Assistant," with minutes, MC Cardiovascular Practice Committee, June 5, 1981, MCA. See also J. Federman and R. E. Vlietstra, "Series on Pharmacology in Practice: 2. Antiarrhythmic Drug Therapy," *Mayo Clin. Proc.*, 1979, *54*: 531–542; and B. Surawicz, "Pharmacologic Treatment of Cardiac Arrhythmias: 25 Years of Progress," *J. Am. Coll. Cardiol.*, 1983, *1*: 365–381. For the FDA, see E. L. C. Pritchett, "Evolution and Revolution in Drug Labeling: Regulation of Antiarrhythmic Drugs by the Food and Drug Administration 1962–1996," *Pacing Clin. Electrophysiol.*, 1998, *21*: 1457–1469; and D. Carpenter, *Reputation and Power: Organizational Image and Pharmaceutical Regulation at the FDA* (Princeton, NJ: Princeton University Press, 2010).

113. The Cardiac Arrhythmia Suppression Trial (CAST), reported in 1989, revealed that patients who received two drugs that had been thought to reduce the likelihood of sudden death after a heart attack were more likely to die than those who received a placebo. This trial had a major impact on the philosophy and practice of treating cardiac arrhythmias. For a journalist's

assessment of the situation, see T. J. Moore, *Deadly Medicine* (New York: Simon & Schuster, 1995). For a refutation of some of Moore's conclusions, see J. L. Anderson, C. M. Pratt, A. L. Waldo, and L. A. Karagounis, "Impact of the Food and Drug Administration Approval of *Flecainide and Encainide* on Coronary Artery Disease Mortality: Putting *Deadly Medicine* to the Test," *Am. J. Cardiol.*, 1997, *79*: 43–47.

114. J. J. Gallagher, R. H. Svenson, J. H. Kasell, L. D. German, G. H. Bardy, A. Broughton et al., "Catheter Technique for Closed-Chest Ablation of the Atrioventricular Conduction System," *N. Engl. J. Med.*, 1982, *306*: 194–200, quotation from 194.

115. See G. Fontaine and M. M. Scheinman, eds., *Ablation in Cardiac Arrhythmias* (Mount Kisco, NY: Futura, 1987).

116. W. C. Sealy, "The Obsolescence of Surgical Operations: Causes and Effects," *Bull. Am. Coll. Surg.*, 1995, *80*: 25–29, quotations from 25 and 29.

117. D. L. Wood, S. C. Hammill, D. R. Holmes Jr., M. J. Osborn, and B. J. Gersh, "Catheter Ablation of the Atrioventricular Conduction System in Patients with Supraventricular Tachycardia," *Mayo Clin. Proc.*, 1983, *58*: 791–796, quotation from 791.

118. M. M. Scheinman, "Interventional Electrophysiology," *Mayo Clin. Proc.*, 1983, *58*: 832–833.

119. Maloney interview.

120. Hammill interview. See also S. C. Hammill, D. D. Sugrue, B. J. Gersh, C-B. J. Porter, M. J. Osborn, D. L. Wood et al., "Clinical Intracardiac Electrophysiologic Testing: Technique, Diagnostic Indications, and Therapeutic Uses," *Mayo Clin. Proc.*, 1986, *61*: 478–503.

121. See W. B. Fye, "Resuscitating a *Circulation* Abstract to Celebrate the 50th Anniversary of the Coronary Care Unit Concept," *Circulation*, 2011, *124*: 1886–1893.

122. M. E. Josephson, ed., *Sudden Cardiac Death* (Philadelphia: F. A. Davis, 1985).

123. M. Mirowski, M. M. Mower, W. S. Staewen, B. Tabatznick, and A. I. Mendeloff, "Standby Automatic Defibrillator: An Approach to Prevention of Sudden Coronary Death," *Arch. Intern. Med.*, 1970, *126*: 158–161. For several perspectives on Mirowski and the development of the device, see "In Memoriam: Michel Mirowski, M.D.," special issue, *Pacing Clin. Electrophysiol.*, 1991, *14 (5, part 2)*: 865–966.

124. M. M. Mower and P. R. Reid, "Historical Development of the Automatic Implantable Cardioverter-Defibrillator," in *Implantable Cardioverter-Defibrillators*, ed. G. V. Naccarelli and E. P. Veltri (Boston: Blackwell Scientific, 1993), 15–25, quotation from 15.

125. M. Mirowski, P. R. Reid, M. M. Mower, L. Watkins, V. L. Gott, J. F. Schauble et al., "Termination of Ventricular Arrhythmias with an Implanted Automatic Defibrillator in Human Beings," *N. Engl. J. Med.*, 1980, *303*: 322–324. Eventually, the device would be referred to as an implantable cardiac defibrillator or ICD.

126. "Young Surgeon Brings New Hope to Heart Patients," *Ebony*, January 1982, 96–100, quotation from 100. Watkins had a special relationship with Vivien Thomas, another African-American who had moved from Vanderbilt to Hopkins four decades earlier. Alfred Blalock had brought Thomas to Baltimore, where he continued to work as the surgeon's research assistant. Thomas played a significant role in the development of the Blalock-Taussig "blue-baby" operation. See L. Watkins Jr., "Vivien T. Thomas, LL.D. (Hon.): Instructor in Surgery, Johns Hopkins University," in *A Century of Black Surgeons: The U.S.A. Experience*, ed. C. H. Organ and M. M. Kosiba (Norman, OK: Transcript Press, 1987), 2: 559–579. For segregation in Baltimore, see A. Pietila, *Not in My Neighborhood: How Bigotry Shaped a Great American City* (Chicago: Ivan R. Dee, 2010).

127. "Young Surgeon Brings New Hope to Heart Patients," 97.

128. Ibid., 98.

129. Details are from the patient's medical record. She signed a detailed consent form as required by Mayo's Institutional Review Board and the US FDA because implantable defibrillators had not been approved for clinical use. Minutes, MC Cardiovascular Practice Committee,

March 9, 1984, MCA. Schaff joined the Mayo staff in 1980 after having been a cardiac surgery chief resident at Johns Hopkins, where he had watched Levi Watkins implant the first automatic defibrillator. H. V. Schaff to W. B. Fye, October 11, 2012, e-mail.

130. W. Nehmer Jr., *Have a Heart: The Brighter Side of Recovery* (Cudahy, WI: Privately printed, 1985). The pages are not numbered.

131. Ibid. See also S. C. Hammill, "Antiarrhythmic Drugs," in *Cardiology: Fundamentals and Practice*, ed. R. O. Brandenburg, V. Fuster, E. R. Giuliani, and D. C. McGoon (Chicago: Year Book Medical Publishers, 1987), 566–593.

132. Nehmer, *Have a Heart.*

133. Ibid.

134. David L. Hayes, interview by W. B. Fye, Rochester, MN, October 14, 2005.

135. D. L. Packer to CV Division Clinical Practice and Quality Assurance Committee, March 16, 1990, MCA.

136. G. Gutfield and M. Sangiorgio, "Saved by AM Radio," *Prevention*, September 1991, 18–19. The date of the ablation is from Lisa Fanning to W. B. Fye, June 13, 2013, e-mail. See also J. J. Gallagher, "Wolff-Parkinson-White Syndrome: Surgery to Radiofrequency Catheter Ablation," *Pacing Clin. Electrophysiol.*, 1997, *20 (part 2)*: 512–533.

137. D. L. Packer, "Ablative Therapy for Cardiac Arrhythmias," in *Mayo Clinic Practice of Cardiology*, ed. E. R. Giuliani, B. J. Gersh, M. D. McGoon, D. L. Hayes, and H. V. Schaff (St. Louis: Mosby, 1996), 1020–1035, quotation from 1033.

Chapter 18

1. A contemporary summary is N. O. Fowler, ed., *Noninvasive Diagnostic Methods in Cardiology* (Philadelphia: F. A. Davis, 1983). The history and uses of medical imaging technologies are described for general readers in A. B. Wolbarst, *Looking Within: How X-Ray, CT, MRI, and Other Medical Images are Created and How They Help Physicians Save Lives* (Berkeley: University of California Press, 1999); B. Holtzmann Kevles, *Naked to the Bone: Medical Imaging in the Twentieth Century* (New Brunswick, NJ: Rutgers University Press, 1997); R. B. Gunderman, *X-Ray Vision: The Evolution of Medical Imaging and Its Human Significance* (New York: Oxford University Press, 2013); and B. J. Hillman and J. C. Goldsmith, *The Sorcerer's Apprentice: How Medical Imaging Is Changing Health Care* (New York: Oxford University Press, 2011).

2. E. Braunwald and H. J. C. Swan, eds., "Cooperative Study on Cardiac Catheterization," *Circulation*, 1968, *37*: III-1-113.

3. T. T. Schattenberg, "Echocardiographic Diagnosis of Left Atrial Myxoma," *Mayo Clin. Proc.*, 1968, *43*: 620–627.

4. See I. Edler and K. Lindström, "The History of Echocardiography," *Ultrasound Med. Biol.*, 2004, *30*: 1565–1644; and H. Feigenbaum, "Evolution of Echocardiography," *Circulation*, 1996, *93*: 1321–1327.

5. See I. Edler and C. H. Hertz, "The Use of Ultrasonic Reflectoscope for the Continuous Recording of the Movements of Heart Walls," *K. Fysiogr. Saellsk. Lund. Foerh.*, 1954, *24*: 1–19; and C. R. Joyner and J. M. Reid, "Applications of Ultrasound in Cardiology and Cardiovascular Physiology," *Prog. Cardiovasc. Dis.*, 1963, *5*: 482–497.

6. For brief biographies of several prominent figures in cardiology and cardiac surgery, see J. W. Hurst, C. R. Conti, and W. B. Fye, eds., *Profiles in Cardiology* (Mahwah, NJ: Foundation for Advances in Medicine and Science, 2003).

7. H. Feigenbaum, J. A. Waldhausen, and L. P. Hyde, "Ultrasonic Diagnosis of Pericardial Effusion," *JAMA*, 1965, *191*: 711–714. See also A. E. Weyman, "Harvey Feigenbaum: A Retrospective," *J. Am. Soc. Echocardiogr.*, 2008, *21*: 3–6.

8. Feigenbaum et al., "Ultrasound Diagnosis," 711 and 714.

9. "The Ekoline 20 Diagnostic Ultrasonoscope," (Philadelphia: Smith Kline Instrument Co., 1966), advertising brochure in the author's possession.

10. Thomas T. Schattenberg, interview by W. B. Fye, Rochester, MN, May 28, 2003.

11. R. A. Nichols, J. P. Whisnant, and H. L. Baker Jr., "A-Mode Echoencephalography: Its Value and Limitations and Report of 200 Verified Cases," *Mayo Clin. Proc.*, 1968, *43*: 36–53. The Ekoline 20 instrument that Schattenberg borrowed is pictured on 38.

12. M. W. Anderson Section Report to MC BOG for 1968, February 24, 1969, Mayo Clinic Archives, Mayo Historical Unit, Rochester, MN (hereafter MCA).

13. R. S. Zitnik to T. T. Schattenberg, June 25, 1969, MCA.

14. T. T. Schattenberg to R. S. Zitnik, July 1, 1969, MCA.

15. "About People: Vernon Weber," *Mayovox*, July 16, 1970. Vernon P. Weber, interview by W. B. Fye, Rochester, MN, February 13, 2008.

16. Gerald T. Gau, interview by W. B. Fye, Rochester, MN, July 27, 2006.

17. The standard phonocardiography text was M. E. Tavel, *Clinical Phonocardiography and External Pulse Tracing* (Chicago: Year Book Medical Publishers, 1972).

18. E. R. Giuliani to R. L. Frye, January 3, 1978, MCA.

19. Ibid.

20. Weber interview.

21. A. Jamil Tajik, interview by W. B. Fye, Scottsdale, AZ, January 4, 2007.

22. Titus C. Evans Jr., interview by W. B. Fye, Rochester, MN, October 26, 2004. George M. Gura, interview by W. B. Fye, Rochester, MN, December 26, 2005. In 1972 a one-room echocardiography laboratory opened at Saint Marys Hospital, where 220 inpatient studies were performed the following year. "Heart Station Workload Report for 1970 through 1977," series of tables, MCA.

23. A. S. Nadas, "Cardiovascular Disease in the Infant and Child," in *The Year Book of Cardiovascular Medicine and Surgery 1973*, ed. E. Braunwald, W. P. Harvey, W. M. Kirkendall, J. W. Kirklin, A. S. Nadas, O. Paul et al. (Chicago: Year Book Medical Publishers, 1973), 91–126, quotation from 117. One of the articles that Nadas reviewed was A. J. Tajik, G. T. Gau, D. G. Ritter, and T. T. Schattenberg, "Echocardiographic Pattern of Right Ventricular Diastolic Volume Overload in Children," *Circulation*, 1972, *46*: 36–43.

24. One of these articles was a pioneering study of the use of contrast echocardiography. See J. B. Seward, A. J. Tajik, J. G. Spangler, and D. G. Ritter, "Echocardiographic Contrast Studies: Initial Experience," *Mayo Clin. Proc.*, 1975, *50*: 163–192.

25. Edler and Lindström, "History of Echocardiography."

26. See A. E. Weyman, *Cross-Sectional Echocardiography* (Philadelphia: Lea & Febiger, 1982); and E. R. Giuliani, *Clinical Two-Dimensional Echocardiography* (Chicago: Year Book Medical Publishers, 1983).

27. Richard L. Popp, interview by W. B. Fye, Chicago, IL, March 29, 2008. See also H. Rakowski, R. P. Martin, J. W. French, and R. L. Popp, "The Clinical Utility of Two-Dimensional Echocardiography," *Acta Med. Scand.*, 1979, *627 suppl*: 68–78.

28. Tajik interview.

29. Minutes, MC BOG, February 3, 1977. Gura interview.

30. Minutes, MC BOG, September 8, 1977.

31. Ileen C. Marxhausen, interview by W. B. Fye, Rochester, MN, September 13, 2005.

32. A. J. Tajik, J. B. Seward, D. J. Hagler, D. D. Mair, and J. T. Lie, "Two-Dimensional Real-Time Ultrasonic Imaging of the Heart and Great Vessels: Technique, Image Orientation, Structure Identification, and Validation," *Mayo Clin. Proc.*, 1978, *53*: 271–303.

33. See, for example, J. A. Kisslo, O. T. von Ramm, and F. L. Thurstone, "Techniques for Real-Time, Two-Dimensional Echocardiography," in *Clinical Echocardiography*, ed. M. N. Kotler and B. L. Segal (Philadelphia: F. A. Davis, 1978), 21–38.

34. R. L. Frye and D. G. Ritter, "Ultrasonic Imaging of the Heart," *Mayo Clin. Proc.*, 1978, *53*: 339. For a perspective on how echocardiography contributed to the decline of older diagnostic technologies, see A. F. Parisi, "The Miracle of Echocardiography: A Clinician's Retrospective," *J. Am. Soc. Echocardiogr.*, 1997, *10*: 97–106.

35. S. H. Altman and R. Blendon, eds., *Medical Technology: The Culprit behind Health Care Costs?* (Washington, DC: US Dept. of HEW, 1979). For a Mayo financial analyst's perspective on cost containment, see J. H. Herrell, "Health Care Expenditures: The Approaching Crisis," *Mayo Clin. Proc.*, 1980, *55*: 705–710.

36. Frye and Ritter, "Ultrasonic Imaging of the Heart."

37. R. L. Frye to J. C. Hunt, February 9, 1978, MCA.

38. W. L. Henry, A. N. DeMaria, R. Gramiak, D. L. King, J. A. Kisslo, R. L. Popp et al., "Report of the American Society of Echocardiography Committee on Nomenclature and Standards in Two-Dimensional Echocardiography," *Circulation*, 1980, *62*: 212–217.

39. W. B. Fye, "You've Got to See It to Believe It!" lecture presented in Marshfield, WI, December 11, 1979. See also W. B. Fye, "Echocardiography 1980: Indications and Usefulness," *Wis. Med. J.*, 1980, *79*: 19–22.

40. J. V. Warren, "Medicine in the '80s: Cardiology," *Drug Therapy*, 1980, 26–32, quotation from 26.

41. E. R. Giuliani, "Role of Echocardiographic Studies in the Ambulatory Patient," in *Office Cardiology*, ed. R. O. Brandenburg (Philadelphia: F. A. Davis, 1980), 103–123, quotation from 122.

42. R. L. Frye to R. E. Weeks, May 29, 1979, MCA. Robert L. Frye, interviews by W. B. Fye, Rochester, MN, July 2, 2001, July 6, 2001, and July 20, 2001.

43. Minutes, MC BOG, February 21, 1979, MCA. See also J. B. Seward and A. J. Tajik, "Two-Dimensional Echocardiography," *Med. Clin. North Am.*, 1980, *64*: 177–203.

44. E. R. Giuliani to Robert Fleming, February 1, 1979, MCA.

45. A. J. Tajik to E. R. Giuliani, February 1, 1979, MCA.

46. Giuliani to Fleming, February 1, 1979.

47. R. L. Frye to R. E. Weeks, March 19, 1980, MCA.

48. Frye interviews, Tajik interviews, Gura interview, Gau interview.

49. Minutes, MC BOG, January 4, 1979, MCA.

50. Harvey Feigenbaum, interview by W. B. Fye, Chicago, IL, March 29, 2008.

51. "Learning Center Programs, January to July 1981," *Am. J. Cardiol.*, 1980, *46*: 1077.

52. Popp interview, Weber interview.

53. J. A. Kisslo, D. Adams, and D. B. Mark, eds., *Basic Doppler Echocardiography* (New York: Churchill Livingstone, 1986). For the development of Doppler echocardiography, see Edler and Lindström, "History of Echocardiography," 1626–1639.

54. Feigenbaum, "Evolution of Echocardiography," 1324. See also L. Hatle, E. A. Angelsen, and A. Tromsdal, "Non-invasive Assessment of Aortic Stenosis by Doppler Ultrasound," *Br. Heart J.*, 1980, *43*: 284–292. A contemporary review of valve disease is J. E. Dalen and J. S. Alpert, eds., *Valvular Heart Disease* (Boston: Little, Brown, 1981).

55. Hatle arrived in Rochester for a six-month sabbatical in October 1986. During the next five years, she coauthored ten articles on Doppler echocardiography with the Mayo group. Liv Hatle, interview by W. B. Fye, Rochester, MN, January 18, 2005.

56. R. L. Popp and P. G. Yock, "Noninvasive Intracardiac Measurement Using Doppler Ultrasound," *J. Am. Coll. Cardiol.*, 1985, *6*: 757–758.

57. Popp interview. Examples of Mayo contributions include P. J. Currie, J. B. Seward, G. S. Reeder, R. E. Vlietstra, D. R. Bresnahan, J. F. Bresnahan et al., "Continuous-Wave Doppler Echocardiographic Assessment of Calcific Aortic Stenosis: A Simultaneous Doppler-Catheter Correlative Study in 100 Adult Patients," *Circulation*, 1985, *71*: 1162–1169; and R. A. Nishimura, F. A. Miller Jr., M. J. Callahan, R. C. Benassi, J. B. Seward, and A. J. Tajik, "Doppler

Echocardiography: Theory, Instrumentation, Technique, and Application," *Mayo Clin. Proc.*, 1985, *60*: 321–343.

58. V. L. Roger, A. J. Tajik, G. S. Reeder, S. N. Hayes, C. J. Mullany, K. R. Bailey et al., "Effect of Doppler Echocardiography on Utilization of Hemodynamic Cardiac Catheterization in the Preoperative Evaluation of Aortic Stenosis," *Mayo Clin. Proc.*, 1996, *71*: 141–149. A Mayo article that emphasizes echocardiography's implications in terms of eliminating the need for invasive testing in some patients is R. A. Nishimura and A. J. Tajik, "Quantitative Hemodynamics by Doppler Echocardiography: A Noninvasive Alternative to Cardiac Catheterization," *Prog. Cardiovasc. Dis.*, 1994, *36*: 309–342.

59. J. A. Kisslo, D. B. Adams, and R. N. Belkin, *Doppler Color Flow Imaging* (New York: Churchill Livingstone, 1988).

60. A few individuals in Japan, Germany, and the United States pioneered TEE in the late 1970s, but it was not introduced into clinical practice for a decade. See J. B. Seward, "Transesophageal Echocardiography: Past, Present, and Future," in *Transesophageal Echocardiography*, ed. W. K. Freeman, J. B. Seward, B. K. Khandheria, and A. J. Tajik (Boston: Little, Brown, 1994), 1–8.

61. See B. I. Hirschowitz, "The Development and Application of Fiberoptic Endoscopy," *Cancer*, 1988, *61*: 1935–1941; and K. K. Djoa, N. De Jong, A. H. Cromme-Dukhuis, C. T. Lancée, and N. Bom, "Two Decades of Transesophageal Phased Array Probes," *Ultrasound Med. Biol.*, 1996, *22*: 1–9.

62. E. P. DiMagno, P. T. Regan, J. E. Clain, E. M. James, and J. L. Buxton, "Human Endoscopic Ultrasonography," *Gastroenterology*, 1982, *83*: 824–829, quotation from 826.

63. J. B. Seward, A. J. Tajik, and E. P. DiMagno, "Esophageal Phased-Array Sector Echocardiography: An Anatomic Study," in *Cardiovascular Diagnosis by Ultrasound: Transesophageal, Computerized, Contrast, Doppler Echocardiography*, ed. P. Hanrath, W. Bleifeld, and J. Souquet (The Hague: Martinus Nijhoff, 1982), 270–279.

64. See R. F. Cucchiara, M. Nugent, J. B. Seward, and J. M. Messick, "Air Embolism in Upright Neurosurgical Patients: Detection and Localization by Two-Dimensional Transesophageal Echocardiography," *Anesthesiology*, 1984, *60*: 353–355.

65. See M. D. Abel, R. A. Nishimura, M. J. Callahan, K. Rehder, D. M. Ilstrup, and A. J. Tajik, "Evaluation of Intraoperative Transesophageal Two-dimensional Echocardiography," *Anesthesiology*, 1987, *66*: 64–68; and Y. Oka, "The Evolution of Transesophageal Echocardiography," *Mt. Sinai J. Med.*, 2002, *69*: 18–20.

66. J. B. Seward to F. A. Miller, October 27, 1987, [with] "Proposal: Outpatient Transesophageal Echocardiography," MCA.

67. B. K. Khandheria, J. B. Seward, A. J. Tajik, and D. J. Ballard, "Implementation of Transesophageal Echocardiography: The Mayo Clinic Experience," *Advanced Hosp. Pract.*, September 1990, 27–30.

68. M. D. McGoon, ed., *Mayo Clinic Heart Book* (New York: William Morrow, 1993) 215.

69. J. B. Seward, B. K. Khandheria, J. K. Oh, M. D. Abel, C. R. Hughes, W. D. Edwards et al., "Transesophageal Echocardiography: Technique, Anatomic Correlations, Implementation, and Clinical Applications," *Mayo Clin. Proc.*, 1988, *63*: 649–680.

70. T. Ryan, "Transesophageal Echocardiography: Better Information at a Higher Price?" *J. Am. Soc. Echocardiogr.*, 1988, *1*: 311–312. For a comprehensive Mayo textbook on TEE, see Freeman, Seward, Khandheria and Tajik, eds., *Transesophageal Echocardiography.*

71. Feigenbaum interview.

72. N. O. Fowler, "Pericardial Disease," in *The Heart, Arteries and Veins*, ed. J. W. Hurst and R. B. Logue (New York: McGraw-Hill, 1966), 846–858, quotation from 853. See also D. H. Spodick, *Pericardial Diseases* (Philadelphia: F. A. Davis, 1976).

73. R. N. MacAlpin, "Percutaneous Catheter Pericardiocentesis," *Eur. Heart J.*, 1980, *1*: 287–291, quotation from 287.

74. L. K. Preis, G. J. Taylor, and R. P. Martin, "Traumatic Pericardiocentesis: Two-Dimensional Echocardiographic Visualization of an Unfortunate Event," *Arch. Int. Med.*, 1982, *142*: 2327–2329, quotations from 2329. See also R. P. Martin, H. Rakowski, J. French, and R. L. Popp, "Localization of Pericardial Effusion with Wide Angle Phased Array Echocardiography," *Am. J. Cardiol.*, 1978, *42*: 904–912.

75. J. A. Callahan, J. B. Seward, A. J. Tajik, D. R. Holmes Jr., H. C. Smith, G. S. Reeder et al., "Pericardiocentesis Assisted by Two-Dimensional Echocardiography," *J. Thorac. Cardiovasc. Surg.*, 1983, *85*: 877–879, quotation from 877.

76. For a two-decade summary of pericardiocentesis at Mayo, see T. S. M. Tsang, W. K. Freeman, L. J. Sinak, and J. B. Seward, "Echocardiographically Guided Pericardiocentesis: Evolution and State-of-the-Art Technique," *Mayo Clin. Proc.*, 1998, *73*: 647–652.

77. See L. S. Wann, J. V. Faris, R. H. Childress, J. C. Dillon, A. E. Weyman, and H. Feigenbaum, "Exercise Cross-Sectional Echocardiography in Ischemic Heart Disease," *Circulation*, 1979, *60*: 1300–1308; and W. F. Armstrong and T. Ryan, "Stress Echocardiography from 1979 to Present," *J. Am. Soc. Echocardiogr.*, 2008, *21*: 22–28.

78. V. L. Roger, P. A. Pellikka, J. K. Oh, F. A. Miller, J. B. Seward, and A. J. Tajik, "Stress Echocardiography: Part I. Exercise Echocardiography: Techniques, Implementation, Clinical Applications, and Correlations," *Mayo Clin. Proc.*, 1995, *70*: 5–15. Patricia A. Pellikka to W. B. Fye, 25 January 2013, e-mail.

79. By 1993, about one-third of the stress echocardiograms performed at Mayo involved the intravenous infusion of Dobutamine. See P. A. Pellikka, V. L. Roger, J. K. Oh, F. A. Miller, J. B. Seward, and A. J. Tajik, "Stress Echocardiography. Part II. Dobutamine Stress Echocardiography: Techniques, Implementation, Clinical Applications, and Correlations," *Mayo Clin. Proc.*, 1995, *70*: 16–27.

80. Roger et al., "Stress Echocardiography: Part I," 5.

81. Ibid., 13.

82. J. S. Alpert (chair), "Guidelines for Training in Adult Cardiovascular Medicine: Core Cardiology Training Symposium (COCATS)," *J. Am. Coll. Cardiol.*, 1995, *25*: 1–34.

83. In 1991 Mayo's cardiologists decided to make a four-year fellowship mandatory beginning in 1993. Minutes, MC CV Division Meeting, December 2, 1991, MCA. The first year included rotations through the diagnostic laboratories. The second year was spent on clinical rotations in the outpatient building and hospitals. The third year was devoted to research. The fourth year was devoted to elective clinical work. Most fellows spent that year in one cardiology subspecialty, such as echocardiography, electrophysiology, or interventional cardiology.

84. See, for example, R. A. Nishimura and G. S. Reeder, "Intravascular Ultrasound: Research Technique or Clinical Tool?" *Circulation*, 1992, *86*: 322–324; J. L. Orford, A. Lerman, and D. R. Holmes Jr., "Routine Intravascular Ultrasound Guidance of Percutaneous Coronary Intervention: A Critical Reappraisal," *J. Am. Coll. Cardiol.*, 2004, *43*: 1335–1342; and C. J. Bruce, D. L. Packer, and M. Belohlavek, "Intracardiac Echocardiography: Newest Technology," *J. Am. Soc. Echocardiogr.*, 2000, *13*: 788–795.

85. Radioisotopes were first used in cardiology in the 1920s to measure the time it took blood to circulate through the body. See H. N. Wagner Jr., "Nuclear Medicine: How It Began," *Hospital Practice*, 1974, *9*: 103–113. For overviews of nuclear medicine and nuclear cardiology written for the general reader, see Wolbarst, *Looking Within*, 111–127; and B. J. Gersh, ed., *Mayo Clinic Heart Book*, 2nd ed. (New York: William Morrow, 2000), 247–252.

86. R. L. Gibbons, "Nuclear Cardiology," in *Cardiology: Fundamentals and Practice*, ed. R. O. Brandenburg, V. Fuster, E. R. Giuliani, and D. C. McGoon (Chicago: Year Book Medical Publishers, 1987), 340–368, quotation from 340.

87. Minutes, MC BOG, August 28, 1946, MCA.

88. See G. E. Pfahler, "The Development of Roentgen Therapy during Fifty Years," *Radiology*, 1945, *45*: 503–521; and D. Cantor, "Radium and the Origins of the National Cancer Institute," in *Biomedicine in the Twentieth Century: Practices, Policies, and Politics*, ed. C. Hannaway (Amsterdam, IOS Press, 2008), 95–146.

89. C. A. Owen Jr., *Diagnostic Radioisotopes* (Springfield, IL: Charles C Thomas, 1959).

90. "Radioisotopes Prove Effective Diagnostic Tool," *Mayovox*, May 12, 1962.

91. "Scintigraphy: New Procedure in Radioisotope Laboratory," *Mayovox*, April 17, 1970. See also W. A. Wilcox and J. B. Marta, "Status of Nuclear Medicine in Minnesota: With Some Notes on Its History," *Minn. Med.*, 1975, *58*: 169–172.

92. See H. N. Wagner Jr., *A Personal History of Nuclear Medicine* (London: Springer-Verlag, 2006), 180–197; and F. J. Bonte, R. W. Parkey, and J. T. Willerson, "Past, Present, and Future of Nuclear Cardiology," in *Nuclear Cardiology*, ed. J. T. Willerson (Philadelphia: F. A. Davis, 1979), 1–7.

93. H. Wahner, Diagnostic Nuclear Medicine Section Report to MC BOG for 1971, MCA.

94. H. Wahner, Diagnostic Nuclear Medicine Section Report to MC BOG for 1975, MCA.

95. Ibid.

96. H. Wahner, Diagnostic Nuclear Medicine Section Report to MC BOG for 1977, MCA.

97. J. H. Chesebro, Consultant's Annual Report for 1976, MCA.

98. Minutes, Administrative Committee of MC BOG, April 20, 1977, MCA. See also Minutes, MC Clinical Practice Committee, April 4, 1977, MCA.

99. Minutes, MC Clinical Practice Committee, April 17, 1978, MCA. See also J. Federman, M. L. Brown, R. G. Tancredi, H. C. Smith, D. B. Wilson, and G. P. Becker, "Multiple-Gated Acquisition Cardiac Blood-Pool Isotope Imaging: Evaluation of Left Ventricular Function Correlated with Contrast Angiography," *Mayo Clin. Proc.*, 1978, *53*: 625–633.

100. H. Wahner to Michael O'Sullivan, March 8, 1979, MCA. See also J. S. Borer, P. Supino, D. Wencker, M. Aschermann, S. L. Bacharach, and M. V. Green, "Assessment of Coronary Artery Disease by Radionuclide Cineangiography: History, Current Applications, and New Directions," *Cardiol. Clin.*, 1994, *12*: 333–357.

101. I. P. Clements, A. R. Zinsmeister, R. J. Gibbons, M. L. Brown, and J. H. Chesebro, "Exercise Radionuclide Ventriculography in Evaluation of Coronary Artery Disease," *Am. Heart J.*, 1986, *112*: 582–588.

102. Raymond J. Gibbons, interview by W. B. Fye, Rochester, MN, April 3, 2002. See also M. W. Pozen, D. J. Lerner, R. B. D'Agostino, H. W. Strauss, and P. M. Gertman, "Cardiac Nuclear Imaging: Adoption of an Evolving Technology," *Med. Care*, 1984, *22*: 343–348; and R. J. Gibbons, "Nuclear Cardiology," in *Mayo Clinic Practice of Cardiology*, ed. E. R. Giuliani, B. J. Gersh, M. D. McGoon, D. L. Hayes, and H. V. Schaff (St. Louis: Mosby, 1996), 229–274.

103. J. Morganroth and G. M. Pohost, "Symposium: Two Dimensional Echocardiography versus Cardiac Nuclear Imaging Techniques," *Am. J. Cardiol.*, 1980, *46*: 1093–1283.

104. D. T. Mason, A. N. DeMaria, and D. S. Berman, *Principles of Noninvasive Cardiac Imaging: Echocardiography & Nuclear Cardiology* (n.p.: Le Jacq Publishing, 1980), xvii.

105. S. Webb, *From the Watching of Shadows: The Origins of Radiological Tomography* (Bristol, England: Adam Hilger, 1990).

106. Minutes, MC BOG, August 16, 1972, MCA. See also H. L. Baker Jr., "Historical Vignette: Introduction of Computed Tomography in North America," *Am. J. Neuroradiol.*, 1993, *14*: 283–287.

107. See E. L. Ritman, "Cardiac Computed Tomography Imaging: A History and Some Future Possibilities," *Cardiol. Clin.*, 2003, *21*: 491–513; and G. S. Hurlock, H. Higashino, and T. Mochizuki, "History of Cardiac Computed Tomography: Single to 320-Detector Row Multislice Computed Tomography," *Int. J. Cardiovasc. Imaging*, 2009, *25*: 31–42.

108. P. Skalka, "On the Inside Looking Out: The Body in 3-D," *Northwest Orient Magazine*, April 1983, 16, 18, 76, 78, quotation from 16.

109. Ibid., 78. For an example of human studies performed with the DSR, see L. J. Sinak, E. A. Hoffman, R. S. Schwartz, H. C. Smith, D. R. Holmes Jr., A. A. Bove et al., "Three-Dimensional Cardiac Anatomy and Function in Heart Disease in Adults: Initial Results with the Dynamic Spatial Reconstructor," *Mayo Clin. Proc.*, 1985, *60*: 383–392.

110. "NMR Scanner Begins Operation at Mayo," *Mayovox*, December 1982. See also K. A. Joyce, *Magnetic Appeal: MRI and the Myth of Transparency* (Ithaca, NY: Cornell University Press, 2008).

111. J. F. Breen and P. R. Julsrud, "Cardiac Magnetic Resonance Imaging," in *Mayo Clinic Practice of Cardiology*, 275–301, quotation from 275. For the development of another non-invasive diagnostic test, see D. J. Johnston, M. K. O'Connor, and L. A. Forstrom, "Positron-Emission Tomography," in *Mayo Clinic Practice of Cardiology*, 325–339.

112. J. J. Goodwin, "The Clinical Approach—Cui Bono?" *Eur. Heart J.*, 1991, *12*: 751–752, quotation from 751.

113. See S. J. Reiser, "The Medical Influence of the Stethoscope," *Scientific American*, February 1979, 148–156; and M. E. Tavel, "Cardiac Auscultation: A Glorious Past—But Does It Have a Future?" *Circulation*, 1996, *93*: 1250–1253.

114. E. J. Cassell, "The Sorcerer's Broom: Medicine's Rampant Technology," *Hastings Center Report*, 1993, *23, no. 2*: 32–39, quotation from 32, paper presented in Rochester, MN, on December 12, 1990. See also D. A. Grimes, "Technology Follies: The Uncritical Acceptance of Medical Innovation," *JAMA*, 1993, *269*: 3030–3033.

115. See, for example, Mayo Clinic Cardiovascular Working Group on Stress Testing, "Cardiovascular Stress Testing: A Description of the Various Types of Stress Tests and Indications for Their Use," *Mayo Clin. Proc.* 1996, *71*: 43–52.

Chapter 19

1. See A. M. Katz, "Overview, Definition, Historical Aspects," in *Heart Failure: Pathophysiology, Molecular Biology and Clinical Management* (Philadelphia: Lippincott Williams & Wilkins, 2000), 1–33; P. M. Edmonds, A. Rogers, J. M. Addington-Hall, A. McCoy, A. J. S. Coats, and S. R. Gibbs, "Patient Descriptions of Breathlessness in Heart Failure," *Int. J. Cardiol.*, 2004, *98*: 61–66; and J.-A. Costello and S. Boblin, "What Is the Experience of Men and Women with Congestive Heart Failure?" *Can. J. Cardiovasc. Nurs.*, 2004, *14*: 9–20.

2. P. D. White, *Heart Disease*, 4th ed. (New York: Macmillan, 1951), 808.

3. T. J. Dry, "Treatment of Congestive Heart Failure," *J. Tenn. Med. Assoc.*, 1950, *43*: 10–16. For a summary of available diuretics, see A. Grollman, *Pharmacology and Therapeutics* (Philadelphia: Lea & Febiger, 1951).

4. G. Eknoyan, "A History of Edema and Its Management," *Kidney Int.*, 1997, *51, suppl. 59*: S118–S126, quotation from S125. See also T. H. Maren, "Diuretics and Renal Drug Development," in *Renal Physiology: People and Ideas*, ed. C. W. Gottschalk, R. W. Berliner, and G. H. Giebisch (Bethesda, MD: American Physiological Society, 1987), 407–435; and J. A. Greene, *Prescribing by Numbers: Drugs and the Definition of Disease* (Baltimore: Johns Hopkins University Press, 2007). Contemporary perspectives include J. McMichael, "Cardiotonics and Diuretics in Human Heart Failure," *J. Chron. Dis.*, 1959, *9*: 602–616; and A. N. Brest and W. Likoff, "Hydrochlorothiazide in the Treatment of Congestive Heart Failure," *Am. J. Cardiol.*, 1959, *3*: 144–147.

5. V. Schrire and W. Beck, "Human Heart Transplantation: The Pre-Operative Assessment," *S. Afr. Med. J.*, 1967, *41*: 1263–1265, quotation from 1265.

6. Ibid. An insightful study of the pioneers of cardiac transplantation (Christiaan Barnard, Denton Cooley, Adrian Kantrowitz, Richard Lower, and Norman Shumway) is D. McRae,

Every Second Counts: The Race to Transplant the First Human Heart (New York: G. P. Putnam's Sons, 2006).

7. "Gift of a Heart," *Life*, December 15, 1967, 24–27, quotation from 27.

8. Ibid.

9. "Human Heart Transplantation," special issue, *S. Afr. Med. J.*, 1967, *41*: 1257–1278.

10. P. Blaiberg, *Looking at My Heart* (New York: Stein and Day, 1968), quotations from 56 and 15.

11. "The Future of Heart Transplantation," in *Experience with Human Heart Transplantation*, ed. H. A. Shapiro (Durban, South Africa: Butterworths, 1969), 235–261, Lillehei quotation from 235.

12. For the problem of organ rejection, see D. Hamilton, *A History of Organ Transplantation: Ancient Legends to Modern Practice* (Pittsburgh: University of Pittsburgh Press, 2012), 221–295; and A. De Vito Dabbs, J. H. Dauber, and L. A. Hoffman, "Rejection after Organ Transplantation: A Historical Review," *Am. J. Crit. Care*, 2000, *9*: 419–429.

13. J. F. Goodwin and C. M. Oakley, "Transplantation of the Heart," *Am. Heart J.*, 1969, *77*: 437–440, quotations from 438, 437. Complex social, economic, and ethical issues surrounding organ transplantation contributed to the development of the field of bioethics. See R. C. Fox and J. P. Swazey, *Spare Parts: Organ Replacement in American Society* (New York: Oxford University Press, 1992); A. R. Jonsen, *The Birth of Bioethics* (New York: Oxford University Press, 1998); and Margaret Lock, *Twice Dead: Organ Transplants and the Reinvention of Death* (Berkeley: University of California Press, 2002). See also N. L. Tilney, *Transplant: From Myth to Reality* (New Haven, CT: Yale University Press, 2003); and A. Nathoo, *Hearts Exposed: Transplants and the Media in 1960s Britain* (New York: Palgrave Macmillan, 2009).

14. Hamilton, *History of Organ Transplantation*, 350.

15. "Dr. Blaiberg Dies 19 Months after Historic Heart Transplant," *New York Times*, August 18, 1969.

16. T. Thompson, "The Year They Changed Hearts: A New and Disquieting Look at Transplants," *Life*, September 17, 1971, 56–70. The captions are on the magazine's cover.

17. Ibid., 66.

18. Ibid.

19. D. C. McGoon Section Report to MC BOG for 1967, Mayo Clinic Archives, Mayo Historical Unit, Rochester, MN (hereafter MCA).

20. Thompson, "The Year They Changed Hearts," 70.

21. A. K. Rider, J. G. Copeland, S. A. Hunt, J. Mason, M. J. Specter, R. A. Winkle et al., "The Status of Cardiac Transplantation, 1975," *Circulation*, 1975, *52*: 531–539.

22. N. E. Shumway, "The Experimental Basis for Heart Transplantation," *Bull. Am. Coll. Surg.*, 1981, *66*: 6–10.

23. F. C. Mann, J. T. Priestley, J. Markowitz, and W. M. Yater, "Transplantation of the Intact Mammalian Heart," *Arch. Surg.*, 1933, *26*: 219–224, quotations from 223 and 224.

24. Ibid., 219. See also F. C. Mann, "Transplantation of Organs," in *Contributions to the Medical Sciences in Honor of Dr. Emanuel Libman*, 3 vols. (New York: International Press, 1932), 2:757–771; and S. Sterioff and N. Rucker-Johnson, "Frank C. Mann and Transplantation at the Mayo Clinic," *Mayo Clin. Proc.*, 1987, *62*: 1051–1055.

25. Shumway, "Experimental Basis for Heart Transplantation," 7.

26. S. Westaby and C. Bosher, *Landmarks in Cardiac Surgery* (Oxford: Isis Medical Media, 1997), 255. See also D. K. C. Cooper, "Experimental Development of Cardiac Transplantation," *Brit. Med. J.*, 1968, *4*: 174–181.

27. L. M. Klainer, T. C. Gibson, and K. L. White, "The Epidemiology of Cardiac Failure," *J. Chron. Dis.*, 1965, *18*: 797–814.

28. D. Dempsey, "Transplants are Common: Now It's the Organs that Have Become Rare," *New York Times Magazine*, October 13, 1974, 56–68, quotation from 67. The esitmate was based on data from the American College of Cardiology. See also R. Fox, "Ethical and Existential

Developments of Contemporaneous American Medicine: Their Implications for Culture and Society," *Milbank Mem. Fund Q.*, 1974, *52*: 445–483.

29. E. Braunwald, "Introduction," in *The Myocardium: Failure and Infarction*, ed. E. Braunwald (New York: HP Publishing, 1974), xv–xviii, quotation from xviii. See also A. M. Katz, "Changing Strategies in the Management of Heart Failure," *J. Am. Coll. Cardiol.*, 1989, *13*: 513–523.

30. "Report of the WHO/ISFC Task Force on the Definition and Classification of Cardiomyopathies," *Br. Heart J.*, 1980, *44*: 672–673. Mayo cardiologist Robert Brandenburg (who was president of the American College of Cardiology at the time) represented the United States on the task force. See also J. F. Goodwin, "Prospects and Predictions for the Cardiomyopathies," *Circulation*, 1974, *50*: 210–219.

31. V. Fuster, B. J. Gersh, E. R. Giuliani, A. J. Tajik, R. O. Brandenburg, and R. L. Frye, "The Natural History of Idiopathic Dilated Cardiomyopathy," *Am. J. Cardiol.*, 1981, *47*: 525–531. See also J. B. Seward and A. J. Tajik, "Primary Cardiomyopathies: Classifica tion, Pathophysiology, Clinical Recognition and Management," in Brandenburg, ed., *Office Cardiology*, (Philadelphia: F. A. Davis, 1980), 199–230.

32. G. S. Francis, "Heart Failure," *J. Am. Coll. Cardiol.*, 1999, *33*: 291–294, quotation from 293.

33. W. C. Roberts, "Bernard John Gersh, MD: A Conversation with the Editor," *Am. J. Cardiol.*, 1998, *82*: 1087–1104. Bernard J. Gersh, interview by W. B. Fye, Rochester, MN, October 24, 2005.

34. Minutes, MC Clinical Practice Committee, January 29, 1980, MCA.

35. "Mayo Establishes Heart Transplant Program," *Mayovox*, November 1980.

36. Mayo record of the patient reviewed by the author. At the time of his admission to Saint Marys Hospital the patient was taking Aldactone, Amrinone, Coumadin, Isordil, Lanoxin, Lasix, Nitropaste, Tocainamide, and potassium. For a summary of these drugs, see B. J. Gersh, L. H. Opie, and N. M. Kaplan, "Which Drug for Which Disease?" *Drugs for the Heart*, ed. L. H. Opie (New York: Grune & Stratton, 1983), 153–191.

37. J. R. Pluth, "Cardiac Transplantation: Foolhardy or Farsighted?" *Mayo Clin. Proc.*, 1981, *56*: 202–203, quotation from 202.

38. A. Leaf, "The MGH Trustees Say No to Heart Transplants," *N. Engl. J. Med.*, 1980, *302*: 1087–1088, quotation from 1087. Leaf had spent two years at Mayo as a medical resident during World War II.

39. Pluth, "Cardiac Transplantation," 202. See also R. W. Evans, "The Economics of Heart Transplantation," *Circulation*, 1987, *75*: 63–76.

40. E. Braunwald, "Historical Overview and Pathophysiologic Considerations," in *Congestive Heart Failure: Current Research and Clinical Applications*, ed. E. Braunwald, M. B. Mock, and J. T. Watson (New York: Grune & Stratton, 1982), 3–9, quotation from 3.

41. Pluth, "Cardiac Transplantation," 203.

42. Minutes, MC Clinical Practice Committee, March 29, 1982, MCA. Two patients did not survive surgery, one died three months after surgery, and one died eleven months after surgery. See "Heart Transplant Program to Resume in Fall of 1986," *Mayovox*, January 1986.

43. The procedural volumes are from J. R. Pluth to D. C. McIlrath, March 5, 1982, MCA.

44. Minutes, MC Clinical Practice Committee, March 29, 1982, MCA.

45. Minutes, MC BOG, November 17, 1982, MCA.

46. M. B. Mock, "The Future of Clinical Investigation in Evaluating Treatment," in *Congestive Heart Failure: Current Research and Clinical Applications*, 337–340, quotation from 340. One diagnostic technique, endomyocardial biopsy, was a catheter-based procedure designed to obtain heart muscle for microscopic study. The Stanford group had pioneered the proceedure, which was first done at Mayo by Geoffrey Hartzler in December 1976. See T. B. Nippoldt, W. D. Edwards, D. R. Holmes Jr., G. S. Reeder, G. O. Hartzler, and H. C. Smith, "Right Ventricular Endomyocardial Biopsy: Clinicopathological Correlates in

100 Consecutive Patients," *Mayo Clin. Proc.*, 1982, *57*: 407–418; and K. R. Melvion and J. W. Mason, "Endomyocardial Biopsy: Its History, Techniques and Current Indications," *Can. Med. Assoc. J.*, 1982, *126*: 1381–1386.

47. J. R. Schneider, D. Alyono, J. R. Schwartz, T. B. Levine, J. N. Cohn, J. E. Molina et al., "Human Cardiac Transplantation at the University of Minnesota," *Minn. Med.*, 1984, *67*: 209–211, quotations from 210 and 211. See also J. N. Cohn, ed., *Drug Treatment of Heart Failure* (New York: Yorke Medical Books, 1983), 1–12. When the University of Minnesota began performing heart transplants, it was a world leader in pancreas, liver, and kidney transplants, due mainly to the influence of John Najarian, who had succeeded Owen Wangensteen as chief of surgery in 1967. See J. S. Najarian, *The Miracle of Transplantation: The Unique Odyssey of a Pioneer Transplant Surgeon* (Beverly Hills, CA: Medallion Publishing, 2009).

48. "The Heart: Miracle in Cape Town," *Newsweek*, December 18, 1967, 86–90, quotation from 90.

49. W. J. Kolff, "Artificial Heart inside the Chest," *Proc. Amer. Phil. Soc.*, 1965, *109*: 117–118, quotation from 117. See also P. Heiney, *The Nuts and Bolts of Life: Willem Kolff and the Invention of the Kidney Machine* (Stroud, England: Sutton, 2002).

50. S. McKellar, "Limitations Exposed: Willem J. Kolff and His Contentious Pursuit of a Mechanical Heart," in *Essays in Honour of Michael Bliss: Figuring the Social*, ed. E. A. Heaman, A. Li, and S. McKellar (Toronto: University of Toronto Press, 2008), 400–434.

51. R. J. Hegyeli, ed., *Proceedings: Artificial Heart Program Conference, National Heart Institute, Washington, DC, 9–13 June 1969* (Washington, DC: Government Printing Office, 1969). See 1110–1122 for a list of the attendees.

52. See J. W. Kirklin, "Open-Heart Surgery at the Mayo Clinic: The 25th Anniversary," *Mayo Clin. Proc.*, 1980, *55*: 339–341.

53. T. Thompson, "The Texas Tornado vs. Dr. Wonderful," *Life*, April 10, 1970, 62B–62D. See also R. Bailey and A. Kerr, "A Patient's Gift to the Future of Heart Repair," *Life*, May 6, 1966, 84–93; T. Thompson, *Hearts: Of Surgeons and Transplants, Miracles and Disasters along the Cardiac Frontier* (New York: McCall Publishing, 1971), 211–219; and L. K. Altman, "The Feud," *New York Times*, November 27, 2007.

54. M-C Wrenn, "The Artificial Heart is Here," *Life*, September 1981, 28–33.

55. J. Salter, "Two Surgical Teams Race for the Man-Made Heart," *Life*, September 1981, 34–36.

56. Ibid., 34.

57. M. J. Strauss, "The Political History of the Artificial Heart," *N. Engl. J. Med.*, 1984, *310*: 332–336, quotation from 332. See also J. R. Hogness and M. VanAntwerp, eds., *The Artificial Heart: Prototypes, Policies, and Patients* (Washington, DC: National Academy Press, 1991); and B. H. Lerner, "Hero or Victim? Barney Clark and the Technological Imperative," in *When Illness Goes Public: Celebrity Patients and How We Look at Medicine* (Baltimore: Johns Hopkins University Press, 2006), 180–200.

58. See M. W. Shaw, ed., *After Barney Clark: Reflections on the Utah Artificial Heart Program* (Austin: University of Texas Press, 1984). The number of heartbeats is from xi. See also W. C. DeVries, J. L. Anderson, L. D. Joyce, F. L. Anderson, E. H. Hammond, R. K. Jarvik et al., "Clinical Use of the Total Artificial Heart," *N. Engl. J. Med.*, 1984, *310*: 273–278.

59. J. Wheelwright, "Bill's Heart: The Troubling Story behind a Historic Experiment," *Life*, May 1985, 33–43. Schroeder lived for 620 days with an artificial heart. See also The Schroeder Family with Martha Barnette, *The Bill Schroeder Story* (New York: William Morrow, 1987).

60. W. C. DeVries, "The Physician, the Media, and the 'Spectacular' Case," *JAMA*, 1988, *259*: 886–890, quotations from 886 and 889.

61. R. L. Van Citters, C. B. Bauer, L. K. Christopherson, R. C. Eberhart, D. M. Eddy, R. L. Frye et al., "Artificial Heart and Assist Devices: Directions, Needs, Costs, Societal and Ethical Issues," *Artificial Organs*, 1985, *9*: 375–415.

62. T. E. Kottke, D. G. Pesch, R. L. Frye, D. C. McGoon, C. A. Warnes, and L. T. Kurland, "The Potential Contribution of Cardiac Replacement to the Control of Cardiovascular Diseases: A Population-Based Estimate," *Arch. Surg.*, 1990, *125*: 1148–1151.

63. Van Citters et al., "Artificial Heart and Assist Devices," 375.

64. Hogness and VanAntwerp, eds., *Artificial Heart*, 209–210.

65. H. C. Smith to Donald C. McIlrath, June 26, 1985, with attachment "Cardiac Transplantation/Artificial Heart Program, Mayo Clinic," MCA. For the context, see D. K. C. Cooper and R. P. Lanza, eds., *Heart Transplantation: The Present Status of Heterotopic Heart Transplantation* (Hingham, MA: MTP Press, 1984).

66. "Cardiac Transplantation/Artificial Heart Program, Mayo Clinic."

67. Quadrennial Review, Research, CV Division, January 10, 1986, MCA. See also N. O. Gentile, P. Jolly, G. S. Levey, and T. H. Dial, *Research Activity of Full-Time Faculty in Departments of Medicine* (Washington, DC: Association of American Medical Colleges, 1987).

68. J. H. Chesebro, "Cardiac Failure: Medical Management," in *Cardiology: Fundamentals and Practice*, ed. R. O. Brandenburg, V. Fuster, E. R. Giuliani, and D. C. McGoon (Chicago: Year Book Medical Publishers, 1987), 666–688.

69. R. H. Anderson, Review of Brandenburg et al., *Cardiology: Fundamentals and Practice*, *Int. J. Cardiol.*, 1988, *21*: 365–366, quotations from 365.

70. J. I. Mertz, J. C. Burnett Jr., and F. N. Knox, "Diuretic Therapy in Congestive Heart Failure," in Brandenburg et al., *Cardiology: Fundamentals and Practice*, 560–565.

71. J. C. Burnett Jr., P. C. Kao, D. C. Hu, D. W. Heser, D. Heublein, J. P. Granger et al., "Atrial Natriuretic Peptide Elevation in Congestive Heart Failure in Humans," *Science*, 1986, *231*: 1145–1147. See also T. Fried, "Atrial Natriuretic Factor: A Historic Perspective," *Am. J. Med. Sci.*, 1987, *294*: 134–138.

72. B. S. Edwards to W. B. Fye, February 13, 2013, e-mail. See also T. R. Schwab, B. S. Edwards, W. C. DeVries, R. S. Zimmerman, and J. C. Burnett Jr., "Atrial Endocrine Function in Humans with Artificial Hearts," *N. Engl. J. Med.*, 1986, *315*: 1398–1401; and B. S. Edwards, R. S. Zimmerman, and J. C. Burnett Jr., "Atrial Natriuretic Factor: Physiologic Actions and Implications in Congestive Heart Failure," *Cardiovasc. Drugs Ther.*, 1987, *1*: 89–100.

73. "Heart Transplant Program to Resume in 1988," *Mayovox*, October 1987. See also C. G. A. McGregor, P. E. Oyer, and N. E. Shumway, "Heart and Heart-Lung Transplantation," *Prog. Allergy*, 1986, *38*: 346–365; and C. G. A. McGregor, "Evolution of Heart Transplantation," *Cardiol. Clin.*, 1990, *8*: 3–10.

74. The author reviewed the patient's Mayo record.

75. L. J. Olson and W. L. Miller, "Pharmacotherapy of Congestive Heart Failure," in *Mayo Clinic Practice of Cardiology*, ed. E. R. Giuliani, B. J. Gersh, M. D. McGoon, D. L. Hayes, and H. V. Schaff (St. Louis: Mosby, 1996), 588–622. See also J. B. Young, "Evolution of Heart Failure Treatment: Considering Adrenergic Blocking Agents and Amiodarone," in *Management of End-Stage Heart Disease*, ed. E. A. Rose and L. W. Stevenson (Philadelphia: Lippincott-Raven, 1998), 73–89.

76. F. A. Willius, "The Prevention of Heart Disease," *Minn. Med.*, 1929, *12*: 355–359, quotations from 355, 356, and 359.

77. A. B. Davis, "Life Insurance and the Physical Examination: A Chapter in the Rise of American Medical Technology," *Bull. Hist. Med.*, 1981, *55*: 392–406.

78. R. W. Wilkins, "Recent Experiences with the Pharmacologic Treatment of Hypertension," in *Hypertension: A Symposium Held at the University of Minnesota on September 18, 19, and 20, 1950*, ed. E. T. Bell (Minneapolis: University of Minnesota Press, 1951), 492–501, quotation from 492.

79. E. V. Allen, N. W. Barker, E. A. Hines Jr., W. F. Kvale, R. M. Shick, R. W. Gifford Jr. et al., "Medical Treatment of Essential Hypertension," *Proceedings of the Staff Meetings of the Mayo Clinic* (hereafter *PSMMC*), 1954, *29*: 459–478, quotations from 459.

80. R. W. Gifford Jr., "Three Decades of Antihypertensive Therapy," *Clin. Pharmacol. Ther.*, 1980, *28*: 1–5, quotation from 1. See also Gifford, "Chlorothiazide in the Treatment of Hypertension," *Postgrad. Med.*, 1959, *25*: 559–571; and J. A. Greene, "Releasing the Flood Waters: Diuril and the Reshaping of Hypertension," *Bull. Hist Med.*, 2005, *79*: 749–794.

81. E. A. Hines Jr. Section Report to MC BOG for 1958, MCA. For a perspective by the head of Mayo's other vascular section, see J. E. Estes, "Hypertension in 1958: A Tale of Pills, Philosophy, and Perplexity," *Med. Clin. North Am.*, July 1958, 899–915.

82. "Hypertension Clinic Proves Worth in Services to Patients and Staff," *Mayovox*, October 12, 1963.

83. See W. A. Rocca, B. P. Yawn, J. L. St Sauver, B. R. Grossardt, and L. J. Melton III, "History of the Rochester Epidemiology Project: Half a Century of Medical Records Linkage in a US Population," *Mayo Clin. Proc.*, 2012, *87*: 1202–1213; and P. D. Stolley and T. Lasky, *Investigating Disease Patterns: The Science of Epidemiology* (New York: Scientific American Library, 1995).

84. "Hypertension: Conquering the Quiet Killer," *Time*, January 13, 1975, 60–64, quotation from 60.

85. S. G. Sheps, C. G. Strong, and R. C. Northcutt, "Evaluation and Treatment of Hypertension," in Brandenburg, ed., *Office Cardiology*, 45–59, quotation from 45. See also E. D. Frohlich, "Achievements in Hypertension: A 25 Year Overview," *J. Am. Coll. Cardiol.*, 1983, *1*: 225–239. For the perspective of a Mayo preventive medicine specialist who focused on hypertension, see I. Krishan, "Public Health Education and the Control of Hypertension in the United States," *Mayo Clin. Proc.*, 1979, *54*: 794–801.

86. W. B. Kannel, T. R. Dawber, A. Kagan, N. Revotskie, and J. Stokes III, "Factors of Risk in the Development of Coronary Heart Disease: Six-Year Follow-up Experience. The Framingham Study," *Ann. Intern. Med.*, 1961, *55*: 33–50. See also D. Levy and S. Brink, *A Change of Heart: How the Framingham Heart Study Helped Unravel the Mysteries of Cardiovascular Disease* (New York: Knopf, 2005); S. S. Mahmood, D. Levy, R. S. Vasan, and T. J. Wang, "The Framingham Heart Study and the Epidemiology of Cardiovascular Disease: A Historical Study," *Lancet*, 2014, *383*: 999–1008; and W. G. Rothstein, *Public Health and the Risk Factor: A History of an Uneven Medical Revolution* (Rochester, NY: University of Rochester Press, 2003).

87. "The Fat of the Land," *Time*, January 13, 1961, 48–52. quotations from 48 and 49. See also A. Keys, *Seven Countries: A Multivariate Analysis of Death and Coronary Heart Disease* (Cambridge, MA: Harvard University Press, 1980).

88. "Fat of the Land," 52.

89. M. Clark, "Pills That Will," *Newsweek*, June 16, 1958, 61–65, quotations from 61 and 62. See also P. B. Beeson, "Changes in Medical Therapy during the Past Half Century," *Medicine*, 1980, *59*: 79–99.

90. "Fat of the Land," 52.

91. K. G. Berge, G. W. Morrow Jr., M. I. Lindsay, and R. D. Hurt, *A History of Community Internal Medicine, Mayo Clinic Rochester* (Rochester, MN: Mayo Clinic, 1996), MCA. Kenneth G. Berge, interview by W. B. Fye, Rochester, MN, January 26, 2011.

92. W. B. Parsons Jr., R. W. P. Achor, K. G. Berge, B. F. McKenzie, and N. W. Barker, "Changes in Concentration of Blood Lipids following Prolonged Administration of Large Doses of Nicotinic Acid to Persons with Hypercholesterolemia: Preliminary Observations," *PSMMC*, 1956, *31*: 377–390, quotation from 378.

93. R. W. P. Achor, "Brief Survey of the Cholesterol Problem with Clinical Applications," *Minn. Med.*, 1960, *43*: 684–692, quotation from 684.

94. "Leukemia Fatal to Dr. Achor, 40. Mayo Consultant was Sick 18 Months," *Rochester Post-Bulletin*, November 26, 1962.

95. Minutes, MC Personnel Committee, October 8, 1963 with Minutes, MC BOG, MCA. See also J. Wittes, "A Tale of Three Species—Rabbits, Chickens and Humans: An Interview with Clinical Trials Pioneer Jeremiah Stamler," *Clin. Trials*, 2006, *3*: 320–334.

96. See W. J. Zukel, "Evolution and Funding of the Coronary Drug Project," *Controlled Clin. Trials*, 1983, *4*: 281–312; and P. L. Canner, "Brief Description of the Coronary Drug Project and Other Studies," *Controlled Clin. Trials*, 1983, *4*: 273–280.

97. A. Cooke, "The Patient Has the Floor," in *The Patient Has the Floor* (New York: Knopf, 1986), 5–17, quotations from 7 and 8, lecture delivered in Rochester on May 28, 1965.

98. See M. F. Oliver, "Pioneer Research in Britain into Atherosclerosis and Coronary Heart Disease: An Historical Review," *Atherosclerosis*, 2000, *150*: 1–12; A. La Berge, "How the Ideology of Low Fat Conquered America," *J. Hist. Med. Allied Sci.*, 2008, *63*: 139–177; D. Steinberg, *The Cholesterol Wars: The Skeptics vs. the Preponderance of Evidence* (New York: Academic Press, 2007); and A. S. Truswell, *Cholesterol and Beyond: The Research on Diet and Coronary Heart Disease 1900–2000* (New York: Springer, 2010). For a recent example of lingering questions regarding the relationship of dietary saturated fat and coronary disease, see R. Chowdhury, S. Warnakula, S. Kunutsor, F. Crowe, H. A. Ward, L. Johnson et al., "Association of Dietary, Circulating, and Supplementary Fatty Acids with Coronary Risk: A Systematic Review with Meta-analysis," *Ann. Intern. Med.*, 2014, *160*: 398–406.

99. *Smoking and Health: Report of the Advisory Committee to the Surgeon General of the Public Health Service* (Washington, DC: Government Printing Office, 1964), 317.

100. J. P. English, F. A. Willius, and J. Berkson, "Tobacco and Coronary Disease," *JAMA*, 1940, *115*: 1327–1329.

101. O. Paul and R. J. Bing, "Coronary Artery Disease," in *Cardiology: The Evolution of the Science and the Art*, ed. R. J. Bing (New Brunswick, NJ: Rutgers University Press, 1992), 133–153. See also A. M. Brandt, *The Cigarette Century: The Rise, Fall, and Deadly Persistence of the Product That Defined America* (New York: Basic Books, 2007).

102. *Smoking and Health*, 322 and 327. For the development of a smoke-free environment at Mayo, see R. D. Hurt, K. G. Berge, K. P. Offord, D. A. Leonard, D. K. Gerlach, C. L. Renquist et al., "The Making of a Smoke-free Medical Center," *JAMA*, 1989, *261*: 95–97.

103. J. L. Juergens, "Welcome," in *The Minnesota Symposium on Prevention in Cardiology: Reducing the Risk of Coronary and Hypertensive Disease*, ed. H. Blackburn and J. Willis, reprinted from *Minn. Med.*, August 1969, symposium held in Rochester, May 2–3, 1968.

104. H. Blackburn, "Introduction," *Minnesota Symposium on Prevention*, 5.

105. H. Blackburn, *If It Isn't Fun… A Memoir from a Different Sort of Medical Life: Volume 1. The First 30 Years, 1942–72* (Minneapolis: Privately printed, 2001), 334.

106. A. Keys, "Cardiology: The Essentiality of Prevention," *Minn. Med.*, 1969, *52*: 1191–1196, quotations from 1191 and 1196.

107. J. F. Fairbairn Section Report to MC BOG for 1966, MCA.

108. S. L. Nunn, J. L. Juergens, R. D. Ellefson, and K. G. Berge, "A Lipid Clinic: Preliminary Observations," *Minn. Med.*, 1969, *52*: 1253–1255.

109. J. Stamler, "Reducing Cardiovascular Risk: The Basis and Feasibility," *Minn. Med.*, 1969, *52*: 1342–1345, quotation from 1342.

110. R. O. Brandenburg to R. J. Reitemeier, May 5, 1971, MCA.

111. "Clinic Gets $2.1-Million Grant for Arteries Project," *Rochester Post-Bulletin*, July 16, 1971, MCA. For background on the SCOR program, see T. Cooper, "Arteriosclerosis: Policy, Polity, and Parity," *Circulation*, 1972, *45*: 433–440.

112. "$2.1 Million Grant Will Aid Research in Atherosclerosis," *Mayovox*, July 23, 1971. For an example of a publication that resulted from Mayo's SCOR grant, see B. A. Kottke and M. T. R. Subbiah, "Pathogenesis of Atherosclerosis: Concepts Based on Animal Models," *Mayo Clin. Proc.*, 1978, *53*: 35–48.

113. R. L. Frye to J. C. Hunt, February 9, 1978, MCA. See also W. C. Roberts, "Valentin Fuster, MD, PhD: A Conversation with the Editor," *Am. J. Cardiol.*, 2000, *86*: 182–197.

114. H. K. Hellerstein, "The Effects of Physical Activity: Patients and Normal Coronary Prone Subjects," *Minn. Med.*, 1969, *52*: 1335–1341, quotation from 1335.

115. "You've Had a Coronary? Maybe You Can Join the 'Club,'" *Mayovox*, October 27, 1972.

116. Ibid.

117. "Psychiatry Plays New Role in Coronary Care," *Mayovox*, February 1974.

118. Ralph Spiekerman and Malcolm Lindsay Jr., joint interview by W. B. Fye, Rochester, MN, February 2, 2011.

119. R. W. Squires and G. T. Gau, "Cardiac Rehabilitation and Cardiovascular Health Enhancement," in Brandenburg et al., *Cardiology: Fundamentals and Practice*, 1944–1960. See also R. W. Squires, G. T. Gau, T. D. Miller, T. G. Allison, and C. J. Lavie, "Cardiovascular Rehabilitation: Status, 1990," *Mayo Clin. Proc.*, 1990, *65*: 731–755; and F. J. Pashkow, "Issues in Contemporary Cardiac Rehabilitation: A Historical Perspective," *J. Am. Coll. Cardiol.*, 1993, *21*: 822–834.

120. G. M. Gura, "Cardiovascular Fitness Clinic for the Apparently Healthy and for the Coronary-Prone Adult," with Minutes, MC Cardiovascular Practice Committee, March 9, 1979, MCA.

121. Minutes, MC Cardiovascular Practice Committee, February 8, 1980, MCA.

122. "Cardiac Program Expands," *Mayovox*, August 1981.

123. The test numbers are from R. O. Brandenburg to R. J. Reitemeier, March 16, 1972, MCA, and R. L. Frye to R. E. Weeks with CV Annual Report for 1978, May 29, 1979, MCA. See also J. P. Naughton and H. K. Hellerstein, eds., *Exercise Testing and Exercise Training in Coronary Heart Disease* (New York: Academic Press, 1973).

124. H. T. Mankin, "Value and Limitations of Exercise Testing," in Brandenburg, ed., *Office Cardiology*, 61–81, quotations from 64 and 75.

125. "Eleventh Bethesda Conference: Prevention of Coronary Heart Disease," *Am. J. Cardiol.*, 1980, *47*: 713–776.

126. J. Stamler, "Opening Statement," *Am. J. Cardiol.*, 1980, *47*: 717.

127. P. B. Beeson, "The Natural History of Medical Subspecialties," *Ann. Intern. Med.*, 1980, *93*: 624–626, quotation from 625. See also T. Dormandy, *The White Death: A History of Tuberculosis* (New York: New York University Press, 2000). For the Mayo Clinic's major role in the early development of antibiotic therapy for tuberculosis, see W. H. Feldman, "Streptomycin: Some Historical Aspects of Its Development as a Chemotherapeutic Agent in Tuberculosis," *Am. Rev. Tuberc.*, 1954, *69*: 859–868; H. C. Hinshaw, "Historical Notes on Earliest Use of Streptomycin in Clinical Tuberculosis," *Am. Rev. Tuberc.*, 1954, *70*: 9–14; and F. Ryan, "First Cures," in *Tuberculosis: The Greatest Story Never Told* (Bromsgrove, England: Swift Publishers, 1992), 224–241. For the other diseases that Beeson mentioned, see P. C. English, *Rheumatic Fever in America and Britain: A Biological, Epidemiological, and Medical History* (New Brunswick, NJ: Rutgers University Press, 2004); and J. Parascandola, *Sex, Sin, and Science: A History of Syphilis in America* (Westport, CT: Praeger, 2008). Medical oncology is a compelling example of the emergence of a new medical subspecialty. It was stimulated by the development of drugs designed to treat cancer after World War II. See P. Keating and A. Cambrosio, *Cancer on Trial: Oncology as a New Style of Practice* (Chicago: University of Chicago Press, 2012).

128. Beeson, "Natural History of Medical Subspecialties," 626.

129. D. C. McGoon, "Reflections on the Future," in Brandenburg et al., *Cardiology: Fundamentals and Practice*, 1985–1986, quotation from 1986. For insight into McGoon's reference to "traumatized hearts," see V. Alexi-Meskishvili and W. Böttcher, "Suturing of Penetrating Wounds to the Heart in the Nineteenth Century: The Beginnings of Heart Surgery," *Ann. Thorac. Surg.*, 2011, *92*: 1926–1931.

130. A. Endo, "A Historical Perspective on the Discovery of Statins," *Proc. Jpn. Acad.*, 2010, *Ser. B, 86*: 484–493. See also J. J. Li, *Triumph of the Heart: The Story of Statins* (New York: Oxford University Press, 2009).

131. Scandinavian Simvastatin Survival Study Group, "Randomised Trial of Cholesterol Lowering in 444 Patients with Coronary Heart Disease: The Scandinavian Simvastatin

Survival Study (4S)," *Lancet*, 1994, *344*: 1383–1389, quotation from 1383. For an assessment of factors that limited cardiologists' enthusiasm for treating elevated cholesterol levels before the 4S trial results were published, see W. C. Roberts, "Getting Cardiologists Interested in Lipids," *Am. J. Cardiol.*, 1993, *72*: 744–745; and H. J. C. Swan, "Why Cardiologists Must Be Interested in Lipids," *Am. J. Cardiol.*, 1995, *75*: 1067–1068.

132. W. C. Roberts, "The Underused Miracle Drugs: The Statin Drugs Are to Atherosclerosis What Penicillin Was to Infectious Disease," *Am. J. Cardiol.*, 1996, *78*: 377–378, quotation from 377.

133. B. J. Gersh, ed., *Mayo Clinic Heart Book*, 2nd ed. (New York: William Morrow, 2000), 157.

134. R. Kornfield, J. Donohue, E. R. Berndt, and G. C. Alexander, "Promotion of Prescription Drugs to Consumers and Providers, 2001–2010," *PLoS ONE*, 2013, *8*: 1–7. See also J. A. Greene and D. Herzberg, "Hidden in Plain Sight: Marketing Prescription Drugs to Consumers in the Twentieth Century," *Am. J. Public Health*, 2011, *100*: 793–803; and J. G. Murphy, R. S. Wright, and T. G. Allison, "Lipid-Lowering Clinical Trials and Medications," in *Mayo Clinic Cardiology: Concise Textbook*, 4th ed., ed. J. G. Murphy and M. A. Lloyd (New York: Oxford University Press, 2013), 558–570. Two changes in Medicare had implications for identifying high cholesterol in older patients and for the cost of statins. Medicare began paying for cholesterol screening in 2005. The following year, the Medicare Modernization Prescription Drug Benefit (Part D) was launched. See P. B. Bach and M. B. McClellan, "The First Months of the Prescription-Drug Benefit: A CMS Update," *N. Engl. J. Med.*, 2006, *354*: 2312–2314.

135. Y. Gerber, S. J. Jacobsen, R. L. Frye, S. A. Weston, J. M. Killian, and V. L. Roger, "Secular Trends in Deaths from Cardiovascular Diseases: A 25-Year Community Study," *Circulation*, 2006, *113*: 2285–2292, quotation from 2289.

136. E. S. Ford, U. A. Ajani, J. B. Croft, J. A. Critchley, D. R. Labarthe, T. E. Kottke et al., "Explaining the Decrease in U.S. Deaths from Coronary Disease, 1980–2000," *N. Engl. J. Med.*, 2011, *356*: 2388–2398, quotation from 2395–2396. See also D. S. Jones and J. A. Greene, "The Contributions of Prevention and Treatment to the Decline in Cardiovascular Mortality: Lessions from a Forty-Year Debate," *Health Aff.*, 2012, *31*: 2250–2258.

137. A. S. Go, D. Mozaffarian, V. L. Roger et al., "Executive Summary: Heart Disease and Stroke Statistics, 2013 Update, A Report from the American Heart Association," *Circulation*, 2013, *127*: 143–152.

138. V. L. Roger, "Epidemiology of Heart Failure," *Circ. Res.*, 2013, *113*: 646–659.

139. R. J. Rodeheffer, "Hypertension and Heart Failure: The ALLHAT Imperative," *Circulation*, 2011, *124*: 1803–1805, quotation from 1803. See also A. F. Hernandez, "Preventing Heart Failure," *JAMA*, 2013, *310*: 44–45; and E. Braunwald, "Research Advances in Heart Failure," *Circ. Res.*, 2013, *113*: 633–645.

Chapter 20

1. For perspectives on health care policy in the United States (especially during the past half-century), see R. A. Stevens, C. E. Rosenberg, and L. R. Burns, eds., *History and Health Policy in the United States: Putting the Past Back In* (New Brunswick, NJ: Rutgers University Press, 2006); R. Stevens, *The Public-Private Health Care State: Essays on the History of American Health Care Policy* (New Brunswick, NJ: Transaction, 2007); C. K. Barsukiewicz, M. W. Raffel and N. K. Raffel, *The U.S. Health System: Origins and Functions*, 6th ed. (Clifton Park, NY: Delmar, 2011); and P. Starr, *Remedy and Reaction: The Peculiar American Struggle over Health Care Reform*, rev. ed. (New Haven, CT: Yale University Press, 2013).

2. "1983 Approaches Most Successful Year Ever for Mayo," *Mayovox*, December 1983.

3. W. E. Mayberry, "The Mayo Clinic in 1984," *Postgrad. Med.*, 1984, *76*: 13–15, quotation from 14. See also V. Johnson, *Mayo Clinic: Its Growth and Progress* (Bloomington, MN: Voyageur

Press, 1984); and J. T. Shepherd, *Inside the Mayo Clinic: A Memoir* (Afton, MN: Afton Historical Society, 2003).

4. "Press Release: Mayo Clinic, Saint Marys Hospital, Rochester Methodist Hospital Agree to Merge," March 3, 1986, Mayo Clinic Archives, Mayo Historical Unit, Rochester, MN (hereafter MCA). See also P. K. Strand, *A Century of Caring, 1889–1989: Saint Marys Hospital of Rochester, Minnesota* (Rochester, MN: Saint Marys Hospital, 1988), 103–122; and K. M. Swetz, M. E. Crowley, and T. D. Maines, "What Makes a Catholic Hospital 'Catholic' in an Age of Religious-Secular Collaboration? The Case of Saint Marys Hospital and the Mayo Clinic," *HEC Forum*, 2013, *25*: 95–107.

5. W. Parker, "Famous Clinic Faces Future as It Remains True to Tradition," *St. Paul Pioneer Press Dispatch*, July 13, 1986, MCA. Mayo Medical Ventures was created in response to the Bayh-Dole Act of 1980, which encouraged universities and teaching hospitals to commercialize technologies and intellectual property that had resulted from federal research grants. See also "'The Future Is Unlimited': Using Quality and Teamwork as Watchwords, Mayo Medical Ventures Charts Bold New Courses," *Mayovox*, April 1987; and H. Markel, "Patients, Profits, and the American People: The Bayh-Dole Act of 1980," *N. Engl. J. Med.*, 2013, *369*: 794–796.

6. M. Freudenheim, "Mayo Clinic Prescription: Growth," *New York Times*, July 4, 1988.

7. L. Sunshine and J. W. Wright, *The Best Hospitals in America* (New York: Henry Holt, 1987), quotations from 185 and 179. See also J. Christianson, B. Dowd, J. Kralewski, S. Hayes, and C. Wisner, "Managed Care in the Twin Cities: What Can We Learn?" *Health Aff.*, 1995, *14*: 114–130; R. L. Reece, *And Who Shall Care for the Sick? The Corporate Transformation of Medicine in Minnesota* (Minneapolis: Media Medicus, 1988); and J. Coombs, *The Rise and Fall of HMOs: An American Health Care Revolution* (Madison: University of Wisconsin Press, 2005).

8. H. C. Smith, "CV Division Quadrennial Review: 1985–1988," July 1989, MCA.

9. Mayo had launched an outreach computerized (trans-telephonic) electrocardiography service on July 1, 1973. See "Mayo ECG Service Links Clinic Facilities to Out-of-City Hospital," *Mayovox*, August 1973. See also D. R. Holmes, "Mobile Cardiac Catheterization Laboratory Proposal, Cardiovascular Division, Mayo Foundation," [January 1991], MCA. The program was discontinued in 1997, mainly because of low demand at the sites. See also G. Gilman, C. A. Lutzi, B. K. Daniels, R. F. Springer, and W. B. Fye, "The Architecture of a Mobile Outreach Echocardiography Service," *J. Am. Soc. Echocardiogr.*, 2006, *19*: 1526–1528.

10. R. L. Frye and D. L. Wood, "The Business of Medicine," *Circulation*, 1997, *95*: 546–547, quotation from 546.

11. H. C. Smith to R. Waller and R. L. Frye, April 5, 1988, with "Appendix 1, Cardiovascular Executive Committee Action on Recommendations from the Ad Hoc Task Force on the Floor [Outpatient]/Hospital Practice," MCA.

12. See J. L. Graner, "The Frye Administration," in *A History of the Department of Internal Medicine at the Mayo Clinic*, ed. Graner (Rochester, MN: Mayo Foundation, 2013), 88–122; and C. Lundstrom, "The Division of General Internal Medicine," in Graner, ed., *Department of Internal Medicine*, 249–255. See also C. C. Booth, "What Has Technology Done to Gastroenterology?" *Gut*, 1985, *26*: 1088–1094.

13. Smith, Quadrennial Review: 1985–1988, emphasis in the original. See also J. O. Goodman, *Cardiology in Transition* (Torrance, CA: John Goodman, 1989); and P. R. Kletke, W. D. Marder, and S. L. Thran, *Socioeconomic Characteristics of Cardiology Practice* (Chicago: American Medical Association, 1988).

14. T. M. Habermann, R. E. Ziemer, and J. L. Graner, *The Internal Medicine Heritage of the Mayo Clinic* (Rochester, MN: Mayo Foundation, 2002), 142–145.

15. L. Scott, "Mayo Builds Primary-Care Muscle," *Mod. Healthcare*, October 2, 1995, 66. See also P. W. Carryer and S. Sterioff, "Mayo Health System: A Decade of Achievement," *Mayo Clin. Proc.*, 2003, *78*: 1047–1053.

16. S. M. Shortell, R. R. Gillies, and K. J. Devers, "Reinventing the American Hospital," *Milbank Q*, 1995, *73*: 131–160, quotation from 131. For the Clinton administration's attempts

to reform health care, see T. Skocpol, *Boomerang: Clinton's Health Security Effort and the Turn Against Government in U.S. Politics* (New York: W. W. Norton, 1996); and H. Johnson and D. S. Broder, *The System: The American Way of Politics at the Breaking Point* (Boston: Little, Brown, 1996).

17. "Department of Internal Medicine, Mayo Clinic, Business Plan," May 1995, MCA.

18. See A. N. DeMaria, T. H. Lee, D. F. Leon, D. J. Ullyot, M. J. Wolk, P. S. Mills et al., "Effect of Managed Care on Cardiovascular Specialists: Involvement, Attitudes and Practice Adaptations," *J. Am. Coll. Cardiol.*, 1996, *28*: 1884–1895; and W. B. Fye, "Managed Care and Patients with Cardiovascular Disease," *Circulation*, 1998, *97*: 1895–1896.

19. W. B. Fye, *American Cardiology: The History of a Specialty and Its College* (Baltimore: Johns Hopkins University Press, 1996), 317. See also L. P. Casalino, H. Pham, and G. Bazzoli, "Growth of Single-Specialty Medical Groups," *Health Aff.*, 2004, *23*: 82–90.

20. *Mayo Clinic Facts, Highlights 2000* (Rochester, MN: Mayo Foundation, 2001).

21. *Lessons in Care: 2000 Mayo Foundation Annual Report*, quotation from 36, MCA.

22. *Mayo Clinic Model of Care* (Rochester, MN: Mayo Clinic, 2000), MCA. The 1910 address was reprinted, see W. J. Mayo, "The Necessity of Cooperation in Medicine," *Mayo Clin. Proc.*, 2010, *75*: 553–556.

23. M. B. Wood, "Mayo Foundation at the Turn of the 21st Century: Adapting to Change but Consistent in Values," *Mayo Clin. Proc.*, 2000, *75*: 333–334, quotation from 334, ellipsis points in the original. For recent articles on these themes by Mayo authors, see T. R. Viggiano, W. Pawlina, K. D. Lindor, K. D. Olsen, and D. A. Cortese, "Putting the Needs of the Patient First: Mayo Clinic's Core Value, Institutional Culture, and Professionalism Covenant," *Acad. Med.*, 2007, *82*: 1089–1093; and H. H. Ting, S. R. Ommen, D. A. Foley, F. K. Timimi, and D. L. Hayes, "Perfecting Patient-Centered Care: The Needs of the Patient Come First," *J. Cardiovasc. Trans. Res.*, 2008, *1*: 295–300.

24. See R. A. Nishimura, J. A. Linderbaum, J. M. Naessens, B. Spurrier, M. B. Koch, and K. A. Gaines, "A Nonresident Cardiovascular Inpatient Service Improves Residents' Experiences in an Academic Medical Center: A New Model to Meet the Challenges of the New Millennium," *Acad. Med.*, 2004, *79*: 426–431. See also J. Fairman, *Making Room in the Clinic: Nurse Practitioners and the Evolution of Modern Health Care* (New Brunswick, NJ: Rutgers University Press, 2008); K. M. Ludmerer, *Time to Heal: American Medical Education from the Turn of the Century to the Era of Managed Care* (New York: Oxford University Press, 1999); and W. B. Fye and J. W. Hirshfeld Jr., eds., "35th Bethesda Conference: Cardiology's Workforce Crisis, A Pragmatic Approach," *J. Am. Coll. Cardiol.*, 2004, *44*: 216–275.

25. Frye and Wood, "Business of Medicine," 546. See also R. Mayes, "Pursuing Cost Containment in a Pluralistic Payer Environment: From the Aftermath of Clinton's Failure at Health Care Reform to the Balanced Budget Act of 1997," *Health Economics, Policy & Law*, 2006, *1*: 237–261.

26. T. H. Lee, *Eugene Braunwald and the Rise of Modern Medicine* (Cambridge, MA: Harvard University Press, 2013), 117.

27. E. Braunwald, M. R. Bristow, C. H. Hennekens, S. Izumo, and D. P. Zipes, "Report of the Review Committee: Research Program, Cardiovascular Division, Mayo Clinic," December 22, 1999, MCA. Division chair A. Jamil Tajik requested this external review.

28. See E. Braunwald, "Cardiovascular Medicine at the Turn of the Millennium: Triumphs, Concerns, and Opportunities," *N. Engl. J. Med.*, 1997, *337*: 1360–1369; and W. N. Kelley and J. K. Stross, "Faculty Tracks and Academic Success," *Ann. Intern. Med.*, 1992, *116*: 654–659. Valentin Fuster, a leading academic cardiologist who had spent the 1970s at the clinic, explained in an interview: "At Mayo I had witnessed first-hand the best physician-patient integrated system anywhere." See W. C. Roberts, "Valentin Fuster, MD, PhD: A Conversation with the Editor," *Am. J. Cardiol.*, 2000, *86*: 182–197, quotation from 189.

29. Braunwald et al., "Report of the Review Committee."

30. See V. L. Roger, "CV Division Strategic Planning Retreat on Research," March 13, 2003, MCA; *Cardiovascular Research 2008* (Rochester, MN: Mayo Foundation, 2008), MCA; For Mayo's focus on patient-oriented research, see J. C. Burnett Jr., "Biomedical Research at Mayo Clinic: A Tradition of Collaboration and a Vision for the Year 2000 and Beyond," *Mayo Clin. Proc.*, 2000, *75*: 337–339; and J. L. Goldstein and M. S. Brown, "The Clinical Investigator: Bewitched, Bothered, and Bewildered—But Still Beloved," *J. Clin. Invest.*, 1997, *99*: 2803–2812. Mayo has been perceived as a national leader in addressing some thorny issues relating to clinical research. See R. L. Frye, R. D. Simari, B. J. Gersh, J. C. Burnett, S. Brumm, K. Myerle et al., "Ethical Issues in Cardiovascular Research Involving Humans," *Circulation*, 2009, *120*: 2113–2121; and M. Camilleri, G. L. Gamble, S. L. Kopecky, M. B. Wood, and M. L. Hockema, "Principles and Process in the Development of Mayo Clinic's Individual and Institutional Conflict of Interest Policy," *Mayo Clin. Proc.*, 2005, *80*: 1340–1346.

31. Eugene Braunwald, interview by W. B. Fye, Rochester, MN, May 3, 2005.

32. Ibid.

33. W. C. Roberts, "Bernard John Gersh, MD: A Conversation with the Editor," *Am. J. Cardiol.*, 1998, *82*: 1087–1104, quotation from 1097.

34. B. J. Gersh, quoted in B. Shurlock, "The Mayo Clinic, Rochester: 'Only the Best Need Apply,'" *Eur. Heart J.*, 2009, *30*: 1017–1026, quotation from 1018. See also J. A. Kastor, *Selling Teaching Hospitals and Practice Plans: George Washington and Georgetown Universities* (Baltimore: Johns Hopkins University Press, 2008). For tensions at other institutions, see J. A. Kastor, *Mergers of Teaching Hospitals in Boston, New York, and Northern California* (Ann Arbor: University of Michigan Press, 2001); J. A. Kastor, *Governance of Teaching Hospitals: Turmoil at Penn and Hopkins* (Baltimore: Johns Hopkins University Press, 2004); and J. A. Kastor, *Specialty Care in the Era of Managed Care: Cleveland Clinic versus University Hospitals of Cleveland* (Baltimore: Johns Hopkins University Press, 2005).

35. F. L. Lucas, A. Stewers, D. C. Goodman, D. Wang, and D. E. Wennberg, "New Cardiac Surgery Programs Established from 1993 to 2004 Led to Little Increased Access, Substantial Duplication of Services," *Health Aff.*, 2011, *30*: 1569–1574, quotation from 1569.

36. T. W. Concannon, J. Nelson, J. Goetz, and J. L. Griffith, "A Percutaneous Coronary Intervention Lab in Every Hospital?" *Circ. Cardiovasc. Qual. Outcomes*, 2012, *5*: 14–20.

37. Minutes, CV Executive Committee, July 6, 1999, MCA. There was also an initiative to promote Mayo's pioneering program in vascular medicine. See J. W. Hallett, T. W. Rooke, and M. Koch, "The Mayo Vascular Center Experience," *Cardiovasc. Surg.*, 1998, *6*: 333–336.

38. See, for example, M. A. Konstam, "Heart Failure Society of America: A Society with a Mission," *J. Cardiac Failure*, 2002, *8*: 275–278. The American Heart Association, the American College of Cardiology, and the European Society of Cardiology introduced several cardiology subspecialty journals around 2010. See J. Loscalzo, "A Bold New Initiative for *Circulation*: A Family of Subspecialty Journals," *Circulation*, 2008, *117*: 4–5; and A. N. DeMaria, "Steve Jobs and *JACC*: Heart Failure," *J. Am. Coll. Cardiol.*, 2012, *59*: 1810–1811. See also C. K. Cassel and D. B. Reuben, "Specialization, Subspecialization, and Subsubspecialization in Internal Medicine," *N. Engl. J. Med.*, 2011, *364*: 1169–1173. Mayo staff members have been president (or board chair) of several national cardiovascular organizations: American Association of Cardiovascular and Pulmonary Rehabilitation: Randal J. Thomas (2009–2010); American Association for Thoracic Surgery: Stuart Harrington (1921–1922), O. Theron Clagett (1961–1962), Dwight C. McGoon (1983–1984), and Hartzell V. Schaff (2011–2012); American College of Cardiology: Robert O. Brandenburg (1980–1981), Robert L. Frye (1991–1992), W. Bruce Fye (2002–2003), and David R. Holmes Jr. (2011–2012); American Heart Association: Arlie R. Barnes (1947–1948), Edgar V. Allen (1956–1957), John T. Shepherd (1975–1976), and Raymond J. Gibbons (2006–2007); American Society for Preventive Cardiology: Stephen L. Kopecky (2012–2014); American Society of Echocardiography: Bijoy Khandheria (2005–2006) and Patricia A. Pellikka (2011–2012); Heart Rhythm Society: David L. Hayes (1998–1999), Stephen

C. Hammill (2004–2005), and Douglas L. Packer (2010–2011); Pulmonary Hypertension Association: Michael D. McGoon (2006–2008); and Society for Cardiovascular Angiography and Interventions: David R. Holmes Jr. (1995–1996).

39. R. J. Glasscock, J. A. Benson Jr., R. B. Copeland, H. A. Godwin Jr., W. G. Johanson Jr., W. Point et al., "Time-Limited Certification and Recertification: The Program of the American Board of Internal Medicine," *Ann. Intern. Med.*, 1991, *114*: 59–62. The program has continued to become more demanding and controversial. See H. H. Ting, E. R. Bates, M. E. Beliveau, J. P. Drozda Jr., J. G. Harold, H. M. Krumholz et al., "Update on the American Board of Internal Medicine Maintenance of Certification Program," *J. Am. Coll. Cardiol.*, 2014, *63*: 92–100.

40. W. W. Parmley, Review of *Mayo Clinic Cardiology Review*, ed. J. G. Murphy (Armonk, NY: Futura, 1997) in *Mayo. Clin. Proc.* 1998, *73*: 100–101.

41. "Special Cardiovascular Division Meeting, February 28, 2001," MCA. Courses were held in various locations in the United States as well as Austria, Canada, Germany, Mexico, and Spain. Eight courses were part of a series of teleconferences marketed as *Cardiology: Today and Tomorrow*. Launched in 1995, this satellite broadcast was beamed to more than 2,000 sites worldwide.

42. In 2013 Mayo sponsored or cosponsored more than thirty courses with more than 5,500 registrants. J. A. McAdams to W. B. Fye, September 26, 2013, e-mail.

43. D. S. Jones and J. A. Greene, "The Contributions of Prevention and Treatment to the Decline in Cardiovascular Mortality: Lessons from a Forty-Year Debate," *Health Aff.*, 2012, *31*: 2250–2258, quotations from 2250.

44. "LBJ Declares War on 3 Killer Diseases," *Boston Globe*, December 10, 1964.

45. The President's Commission on Heart Disease, Cancer and Stroke, *Report to the President: A National Program to Conquer Heart Disease, Cancer and Stroke*, 2 vols. (Washington, DC: Government Printing Office, 1965), 1: 88–89. See also C. G. Lasby, "The War on Disease," in *The Johnson Years*, Vol. 2: *Vietnam, the Environment, and Science*, ed. R. A. Divine (Lawrence: University Press of Kansas, 1987), 183–216.

46. J. S. Alpert, "The 10 Most Important Advances in Cardiovascular Medicine during the Past 50 Years, with Apologies to David Letterman," *Curr. Cardiol. Rep.*, 2001, *3*: 433–435. See also N. J. Mehta and I. A. Khan, "Cardiology's 10 Greatest Discoveries of the 20th Century," *Texas Heart Inst. J.*, 2002, *29*: 164–171; and M. E. Silverman, "A View from the Millennium: The Practice of Cardiology Circa 1950 and Thereafter," *J. Am. Coll. Cardiol.*, 1999, *33*: 1141–1151.

47. V. R. Fuchs and H. C. Sox Jr., "Physicians' Views of the Relative Importance of Thirty Medical Innovations," *Health Aff.*, 2001, *20*: 30–42, quotation from 41.

48. D. M. Cutler, A. B. Rosen, and S. Vijan, "The Value of Medical Spending in the United States, 1960–2000," *N. Engl. J. Med.*, 2006, *355*: 920–927. See also S. Capewell and M. O'Flaherty, "Trends in Cardiovascular Disease: Are We Winning the War?" *Can. Med. Assoc. J.*, 2009, *180*: 1285–1286; G. B. Faguet, *The War on Cancer: An Anatomy of Failure, A Blueprint for the Future* (Dordrecht, The Netherlands: Springer, 2005); D. M. Cutler, "Are We Finally Winning the War on Cancer?" *J. Econ. Perspect.*, 2008, *22*: 3–26; D. Cantor, ed., *Cancer in the Twentieth Century* (Baltimore: Johns Hopkins University Press, 2008); S. Mukherjee, *The Emperor of All Maladies: A Biography of Cancer* (New York: Scribner, 2010); and P. Keating and A. Cambrosio, *Cancer on Trial: Oncology as a New Style of Practice* (Chicago: University of Chicago Press, 2012). See also F. J. Quevedo and R. G. Hahn, "The Beginnings of Medical Oncology at the Mayo Clinic in Rochester," *Mayo Clin. Proc.*, 2000, *75*: 666–668.

49. L. K. Altman, "Cheney File Traces Heart Care Milestones," *New York Times*, April 23, 2012.

50. Chapter 7 focuses on Franklin Roosevelt's cardiovascular disease. See also B. E. Park, *The Impact of Illness on World Leaders* (Philadelphia: University of Pennsylvania Press, 1986); J. M. Post and R. S. Robins, *When Illness Strikes the Leader: The Dilemma of the Captive King*

(New Haven, CT: Yale University Press, 1993); D. Blumenthal and J. A. Morone, *The Heart of Power: Health and Politics in the Oval Office* (Berkeley: University of California Press, 2009); and W. H. Frishman, F. H. Zimmerman, and R. G. Lerner, "Vascular and Heart Diseases in the Incumbent Presidents and Vice Presidents of the United States of America: A Medico-Historical Perspective," *Cardiology in Review*, 2012, *21*: 1–8.

51. D. Cheney, *In My Time: A Personal and Political Memoir* (New York: Threshold Editions, 2011), 292.

52. D. E. Sanger, "Cheney Gets Heart Device and Declares, 'I Feel Good,'" *New York Times*, July 1, 2001. See also M. H. Gollob and J. J. Seger, "Current Status of the Implantable Cardioverter-Defibrillator," *Chest*, 2001, *119*: 1210–1221; and K. Jeffrey, *Machines in Our Hearts: The Cardiac Pacemaker, the Implantable Defibrillator, and American Health Care* (Baltimore: Johns Hopkins University Press, 2001).

53. D. Cheney and J. Reiner, *Heart: An American Odyssey* (New York: Simon & Schuster, 2013), 183.

54. Cheney, *In My Time*, 524.

55. Cheney and Reiner, *Heart*, 245.

56. Ibid., 266.

57. Ibid., 246–247. See also L. K. Altman, "A New Pumping Device Brings Hope for Cheney," *New York Times*, July 19, 2010. The average LVAD implantation cost (including the device and all hospital and professional service costs) is about $200,000. But Cheney's five-week hospitalization was about ten days longer than average, so the hospital costs would have been higher. See J. G. Rogers, R. R. Bostic, K. B. Tong, R. Adamson, M. Russo, and M. S. Slaughter, "Cost-Effectiveness Analysis of Continuous-Flow Left Ventricular Assist Devices as Destination Therapy," *Circ. Heart Fail.*, 2012, *5*: 10–16. For a video of the HeartMate II LVAD (the type that was implanted in Cheney), see http://www.youtube.com/watch?v=YBxDhUzSrsk.

58. D. Brown and L. H. Sun, "Cheney Doing 'Exceedingly Well' after Heart Transplant," *Washington Post*, March 25, 2012.

59. D. Grady, "From a Prominent Death, Some Painful Truths," *New York Times*, June 24, 2008.

60. A. Johnson, J. Yang, and K. Strickland, "NBC's Tim Russert Dies of Heart Attack at 58," June 14, 2008, http://www.nbcnews.com/id/25145431/

61. D. Grady, "A Search for Answers in Tim Russert's Death," *New York Times*, June 17, 2008. See also R. J. Myerburg and J. Junttila, "Sudden Cardiac Death Caused by Coronary Heart Disease," *Circulation*, 2012, *125*: 1043–1052.

62. J. Brody, "The Treadmill's Place in Evaluating Hearts," *New York Times*, July 29, 2008. See also T. D. Miller, "The Exercise Treadmill Test: Estimating Cardiovascular Prognosis," *Cleve. Clin. J. Med.*, 2008, *75*: 424–430.

63. G. Keillor, "I Just Needed a Valve Job," *Time*, August 13, 2001, 72.

64. See D. C. McGoon, "Repair of Mitral Insufficiency Due to Ruptured Chordae Tendineae," *J. Thorac. Cardiovasc. Surg.*, 1960, *39*: 357–362; N. S. Braunwald, "It Will Work: The First Successful Mitral Valve Replacement," *Ann. Thorac. Surg.*, 1989, *48*: S1–S3; and W. R. Chitwood Jr., "Mitral Valve Repair: An Odyssey to Save the Valves!" *J. Heart Valve Dis.*, 1998, *7*: 255–261.

65. See D. Cosgrove, "View from North America's Cardiac Surgeons," *Eur. J. Cardio-thoracic Surg.*, 2004, *26*: S27–S31; L. H. Lieng, M. Enriquez-Sarano, J. B. Seward, A. J. Tajik, H. V. Schaff, K. R. Bailey et al., "Clinical Outcome of Mitral Regurgitation Due to Flail Leaflet," *N. Engl. J. Med.*, 1996, *335*: 1417–1423.

66. A. Comarow, "Higher Volume, Fewer Deaths: For a Risky Operation Head for a Hospital That Does It Regularly," *U.S. News & World Report*, July 17, 2000, 68–70, quotation from 70. See also C. T. Wilson, E. S. Fisher, H. G. Welch, A. E. Siewers, and F. L. Lucas, "U.S. Trends in CABG Hospital Volume: The Effect of Adding Cardiac Surgery Programs," *Health*

Aff., 2007, *26*: 162–168; and A. Kilic, A. S. Shah, J. V. Conte, W. A. Baumgartner, and D. D. Yuh, "Operative Outcomes in Mitral Valve Surgery: Combined Effect of Surgeon and Hospital Volume in a Population-Based Analysis," *J. Thorac. Cardiovasc. Surg.*, 2013, *146*: 638–646.

67. S. Brink, "To Get Top Care: Get Pushy," *U.S. News & World Report*, July 17, 2000, 72–73, quotation from 73.

68. See W. B. Fye, N. F. Goldschlager, J. V. Messer, and S. A. Rubenstein, "Referral Guidelines and the Collaborative Care of Patients with Cardiovascular Disease," *J. Am. Coll. Cardiol.*, 1997, *29*: 1162–1170; and R. Mayes, "Medicare and America's Healthcare System in Transition: From the Death of Managed Care to the Medical Modernization Act of 2003 and Beyond," *J. Health Law*, 2005, *38*: 391–422.

69. V. R. Fuchs, "The Gross Domestic Product and Health Care Spending," *N. Engl. J. Med.*, 2013, *369*: 107–109.

70. S. Goodell and P. B. Ginsburg, "High and Rising Health Care Costs: Demystifying U.S. Health Care Spending," Robert Wood Johnson Foundation, October 2008, http://www.rwjf. org/content/dam/farm/reports/issue_briefs/2008/rwjf32704. See also H. Moses III, D. H. M. Matheson, E. R. Dorsey, B. P. George, D. Sadoff, and S. Yoshimura, "The Anatomy of Health Care in the United States," *JAMA*, 2013, *310*: 1947–1963.

71. See S. H. Altman and R. Blendon, eds., *Medical Technology: The Culprit behind Health Care Costs?* (Washington, DC: US Dept. of Health, Education, and Welfare, 1979); A. C. Gelijns, ed., *Technology and Health Care in an Era of Limits* (Washington, DC: National Academy Press, 1992); A. B. Cohen and R. S. Hanft, *Technology in American Health Care: Policy Directions for Effective Evaluation and Management* (Ann Arbor: University of Michigan Press, 2004); and D. Callahan, *Taming the Beloved Beast: How Medical Technology Costs Are Destroying Our Health Care System* (Princeton, NJ: Princeton University Press, 2009).

72. A. Gawande, "The Cost Conundrum," *New Yorker*, June 1, 2009, 36–44, quotations from 36.

73. Ibid., 38–39.

74. Ibid., 39.

75. Ibid., 42–43. See also L. L. Berry and K. D. Seltman, *Management Lessons from Mayo Clinic: Inside One of the World's Most Admired Service Organizations* (New York: McGraw Hill, 2008).

76. Timothy Penny quoted in R. Willsher, "Meeting of the Minds: Mayo Clinic Hosts a National Symposium on Health Care Reform to Jump-Start Discussions on Real Reform," *Mayo Today*, July–August, 2006, 12. See also D. A. Cortese and R. K. Smoldt, "Healing America's Ailing Health Care System," *Mayo Clin. Proc.*, 2006, *81*: 492–496.

77. "President Obama Outlines Goals for Health Care Reform," June 6, 2009, http://www.white-house.gov/the_press_office/WEEKLY-ADDRESS-President-Obama-Outlines-Goals-for-Heal th-Care-Reform/.

78. A. MacGillis and R. Stein, "Is the Mayo Clinic a Model or a Mirage: Jury Is Still Out, Duplication Won't Be Easy, Critics Say," *Washington Post*, September 20, 2009. See also M. Grunwald, "More Data + Less Care = Lower Cost + Better Health," *Time*, June 29, 2009, 36–40; and T. H. Lee and J. J. Mongan, *Chaos and Organization in Health Care* (Cambridge, MA: MIT Press, 2009).

79. E. A. Hall, "Echoes from St. Mary's Clinic, Rochester, Minn," *Canada Lancet*, 1906, *40*: 289–303.

80. C. R. Rorem, *Private Group Clinics*, reprint of 1931 ed. with a new preface (New York: Milbank Memorial Fund, 1971).

81. I. S. Falk, C. R. Rorem, and M. D. Ring, *The Costs of Medical Care* (Chicago: University of Chicago Press, 1933), 582. See also I. S. Falk, "Some Lessons from the Fifty Years Since the CCMC Final Report, 1932," *J. Pub. Health Policy*, 1983, *4*: 135–161; and J. Engel, *Doctors and*

Reformers: Discussion and Debate over Health Policy, 1925–1950 (Columbia: University of South Carolina Press, 2002).

82. I. S. Falk, "Group Practice is Pattern of the Future," *Mod. Hosp.*, 1963, *101*: 117–120, 203. See also D. L. Madison and T. R. Konrad, "Large Medical Group-Practice Organizations and Employed Physicians: A Relationship in Transition," *Milbank Q.*, 1988, *66*: 240–282.

83. See J. B. Sterns, "Quality, Efficiency, and Organizational Structure," *J. Health Care Finance*, 2007, *34*: 100–107; W. B. Weeks, D. J. Gottlieb, D. J. Nywelde, J. M. Sutherland, J. Bynum, L. P. Casalino et al., "Higher Health Care Quality and Bigger Savings Found at Large Multispecialty Medical Groups," *Health Aff.*, 2010, *29*: 991–997; and J. D. Ketcham, L. C. Baker, and D. MacIsaac, "Physician Practice Size and Variations in Treatments and Outcomes: Evidence from Medicare Patients with AMI [Acute Myocardial Infarction]," *Health Aff.*, 2007, *26*: 195–205.

84. "Destination Medical Center," *Mayo Alumni*, 2013, no. 3: 2–5.

85. "Destination Medical Center (DMC)," 2013, http://www.mayoclinic.org/ destination-medical-center/. See also J. Crosby, "Mayo Offers $6 Billion Vision to Remake Rochester," *Star Tribune*, January 30, 2013; and "Mission Accomplished: Lawmakers, Locals Praise Passage of DMC," *Rochester Post-Bulletin*, May 23, 2013.

86. E. Lucas, "The Domestic Medical Tourist," *Delta Sky Magazine*, July 2013, 103–112, quotations from 103–104. See also M. Hathaway and K. Seltman, "International Market Research at the Mayo Clinic," *Marketing Health Services*, Winter 2001, 19–23; and S. J. Swensen, J. A. Dilling, C. M. Harper Jr., and J. H. Noseworthy, "The Mayo Clinic Value Creation System," *Am. J. Med. Qual.* 2012, *27*: 58–65.

87. "Best Hospitals: Cardiology & Heart Surgery," *U.S. News & World Report Best Hospitals*, 2014 ed., 104–106.

88. A. Comarow, "A Guide to the Rankings." *U.S. News & World Report Best Hospitals*, 2014 ed., 97–98, quotation from 97. A study of the role of reputation in the 2009 rankings of the top fifty hospitals for cardiology and heart surgery revealed a significant relationship between subjective reputations and objective measures of hospital quality. This was not true for several other specialties, however. See A. R. Sehgal, "The Role of Reputation in *U.S. News & World Report's* Rankings of the Top 50 American Hospitals," *Ann. Intern. Med.*, 2010, *152*: 521–525.

89. T. M. Ziedalski, R. S. Liebowizt, and J. G. Copeland, "The Oldest Patient to Undergo Aortic Valve Replacement," *Cardiology*, 1999, *92*: 282–283.

90. Ibid., 283. See also T. Langanay, E. Flécher, O. Fouquet, V. G. Ruggieri, B. De La Tour, C. Félix et al., "Aortic Valve Replacement in the Elderly: The Real Life," *Ann. Thorac. Surg.*, 2012, *93*: 70–78.

91. Ziedalski et. al., "The Oldest Patient," 282. For life expectancy in 1900, see "Mortality and Life Expectancy," chapter 12 in *Life Insurers Fact Book 2013*, https:www.acli.com/Tools/ Industry%20Facts/Life%20Insurers%20Fact%20Book/Documents/FB13%20Chapter%2012_ Mortality.pdf. The 2000 US census reported that just 0.1 percent of the population (337,238 persons) was 95 years of age and older. See L. Hetzel and A, Smith, "The 65 Years and Over Population: 2000," Census Brief Issued October 2001, http://www.census.gov/prod/2001pubs/ c2kbr01-10.pdf.

92. V. R. Fuchs, "The Growing Demand for Medical Care," *N. Engl. J. Med.*, 1968, *279*: 190–195, quotations from 192. See also B. A. Koenig, "The Technological Imperative in Medical Practice: The Social Creation of a 'Routine' Treatment," in *Biomedicine Examined*, ed. M. Lock and D. Gordon (Boston: Kluwer Academic Publishers, 1988), 465–496; D. J. Rothman, *Beginnings Count: The Technological Imperative in American Health Care* (New York: Oxford University Press, 1997); M. L. Eaton and D. Kennedy, *Innovation in Medical Technology: Ethical Issues and Challenges* (Baltimore: Johns Hopkins University Press, 2007); and S. J. Reiser, *Technological Medicine: The Changing World of Doctors and Patients* (New York: Cambridge University Press, 2009).

93. V. R. Fuchs, *Who Shall Live? Health, Economics and Social Choice*, 2nd ed. (Hackensack, NJ: World Scientific, 2011), xix. See also D. Rowland and A. Shartzer, "America's Uninsured: The Statistics and Back Story," *J. Law Med. Ethics*, 2008, *36*: 618–628.

94. See M. Stefik and B. Stefik, *Breakthrough: Stories and Statgies of Radical Innovation* (Cambridge, MA: MIT Press, 2004); A. S. Brett, "Addressing Requests by Patients for Nonbeneficial Interventions," *JAMA*, 2012, *307*: 149–150; and S. H. Woolf, "The Price of False Beliefs: Unrealistic Expectations as a Contributor to the Health Care Crisis," *Ann. Fam. Med.*, 2012, *10*: 491–494.

95. G. Cowley and A. Underwood, "New Heart, New Hope," *Newsweek*, June 25, 2001, 42–49, quotations from 44. But the public had been reading or hearing encouraging reports about artificial hearts for more than two decades. See M.-C. Wrenn, "The Artificial Heart is Here," *Life*, September 1981, 28–33; and J. R. Hogness and M. VanAntwerp, eds., *The Artificial Heart: Prototypes, Policies, and Patients* (Washington, DC: National Academy Press, 1991).

96. See A. Cribier, "Development of Transcatheter Aortic Valve Implantation (TAVI): A 20-Year Odyssey," *Arch. Cardiovasc. Dis.*, 2012, *105*: 146–152; and C. R. Smith, M. B. Leon, M. J. Mack, D. C. Miller, J. W. Moses, L. G. Svensson et al., "Transcatheter versus Surgical Aortic-Valve Replacement in High-Risk Patients," *N. Engl. J. Med.*, 2011, *364*: 2187–2198.

97. "Less Invasive Heart Valve Replacement Is Approved," *New York Times*, November 3, 2011. See also M. Gössl and D. R. Holmes Jr., "An Update on Transcatheter Aortic Valve Replacement," *Curr. Probl. Cardiol.*, 2013, *38*: 245–283; and M. L. Stone, J. A. Kern, and R. M. Sade, "Transcatheter Aortic Valve Replacement: Clinical Aspects and Ethical Considerations," *Ann. Thorac. Surg.*, 2012, *94*: 1791–1795. By the end of 2013, the valves were being implanted at more than 250 sites in the United States. See J. D. Carroll, F. H. Edwards, D. Marinac-Dabic, R. G. Brindis, F. L. Grover, E. D. Peterson et al., "The STS-ACC Transcatheter Valve Therapy National Registry," *J. Am. Coll. Cardiol.*, 2013, *62*: 1026–1034. Other catheter-based procedures have been developed as an alternative to open-heart surgery for severe mitral regurgitation. See F. Maisano, G. La Canna, A. Colombo, and O. Alfieri, "The Evolution from Surgery to Percutaneous Mitral Valve Intervention," *J. Am. Coll. Cardiol.*, 2011, *58*: 2174–2182. For the evolving concept of personalized or individualized medicine, which emphasizes the potential of genomics to improve medical treatments and prevention strategies, see E. J. Topol, "Individualized Medicine from Prewomb to Tomb," *Cell*, 2014, *157*: 241–253.

98. A. Hartocollis, "Rise Seen in Medical Efforts to Improve Very Long Lives," *New York Times*, July 18, 2008. Clinical trial results regarding the therapy this patient received were appearing, but there were no data demonstrating benefit in nonogenarians. See A. E. Epstein, G. N. Kay, V. J. Plumb, H. T. McElderry, H. Doppalapudi, T. Yamada et al., "Implantable Cardioverter-Defibrillator Prescription in the Elderly," *Heart Rhythm*, 2009, 6: 1136–1143; I. A. Scott and G. H. Guyatt, "Cautionary Tales in the Interpretation of Clinical Studies Involving Older Persons," *Arch. Intern. Med.* 2010, *170*: 587–595; M. Jessup, "MADIT-CRT: Breathtaking or Time to Catch Our Breath?" *N. Engl. J. Med.*, 2009, *361*: 1394–1396; and S. R. Kaufman, P. S. Mueller, A. L. Ottenberg, and B. A. Koenig, "Ironic Technology: Old Age and the Implantable Cardioverter Defibrillator in US Health Care," *Soc. Sci. Med.*, 2011, *72*: 6–14.

99. A. Hartocollis, "Remembering Hazel, and Her Moment in the Spotlight," *New York Times*, March 25, 2010. See also B. Thorsteinsdottir, K. M. Swetz, and J. C. Tilburt, "Dialysis in the Frail Elderly: A Current Ethical Problem, An Impending Ethical Crisis," *J. Gen. Intern. Med.*, 2013, *28*: 1511–1516.

100. G. B. Shaw, "Preface on Doctors," in *The Doctor's Dilemma, Getting Married, & The Shewing-up of Blanco Posnet* (London: Constable, 1911), xiii–xciv, quotation from xciv. See also R. Boxill, *Shaw and the Doctors* (New York: Basic Books, 1969).

101. M. J. Mack, "In-Hospital Outcomes of Very Elderly Patients (85 Years and Older) Undergoing Percutaneous Coronary Intervention," *Cathet. Cardiovasc. Intervent.*, 2011, *77*: 642.

102. See T. R. Cole, *The Journey of Life: A Cultural History of Aging in America* (New York: Cambridge University Press, 1992); P. S. Mueller, C. Hook, and K. C. Fleming, "Ethical Issues in Geriatrics: A Guide for Clinicians," *Mayo Clin. Proc.*, 2004, *79*: 554–562; S. R. Kaufman, J. K. Shim, and A. J. Russ, "Revisiting the Biomedicalization of Aging: Clinical Trends and Ethical Challenges," *Gerontologist*, 2004, *44*: 731–738; M. R. Gillick, "The Technological Imperative and the Battle for the Hearts of America," *Perspect. Biol. Med.*, 2007, *50*: 276–294; J. K. Shim, A. J. Russ, and S. R. Kaufman, "Late-Life Cardiac Interventions and the Treatment Imperative," *PLoS Med.*, 2008, *5*: 344–346; and M. D. Neuman and C. L. Bosk, "The Redefinition of Aging in American Surgery," *Milbank Q.*, 2013, *91*: 288–315. For trends and some earlier predictions about the future, see J. Flower, L. S. Dreifus, A. A. Bove, and W. S. Weintraub, "Technological Advances and the Next 50 Years of Cardiology," *J. Am. Coll. Cardiol.*, 2000, *35*: 1082–1091; D. K. Foot, R. P. Lewis, T. A. Pearson, and G. A. Beller, "Demographics and Cardiology, 1950–2050," *J. Am. Coll. Cardiol.*, 2000, *35*: 1067–1081; and D. M. Steinwachs, R. L. Collins-Nakai, L. H. Cohn, A. Garson Jr., and M. J. Wolk, "The Future of Cardiology: Utilization and Costs of Care," *J. Am. Coll. Cardiol.*, 2000, *35*: 1092–1099.

103. H. Spiro, "An Old Doctor Grows Older," *Perspect. Biol. Med.*, 2009, *52*: 604–611, quotation from 609. See also H. Spiro, M. G. M. Curnen, and L. P. Wandel, eds., *Facing Death: Where Culture, Religion, and Medicine Meet* (New Haven, CT: Yale University Press, 1996); S. B. Nuland, *How We Die: Reflections on Life's Final Chapter* (New York: Alfred A. Knopf, 1994); and M. J. Lewis, *Medicine and the Care of the Dying* (New York: Oxford University Press, 2007).

104. V. R. Fuchs, "The Doctor's Dilemma: What Is 'Appropriate' Care?" *N. Engl. J. Med.*, 2011, *365*: 585–587, quotation from 585. For perspectives by Mayo internists, see P. S. Mueller and C. C. Hook, "Technological and Treatment Imperatives, Life-Sustaining Technologies, and Associated Ethical and Social Challenges," *Mayo Clin. Proc.*, 2013; *88*: 641–644; and K. M. Swetz and J. K. Mansel, "Ethical Issues and Palliative Care in the Cardiovascular Intensive Care Unit," *Cardiol. Clin.*, 2013; *31*: 657–668.

105. See, for example, R. M. Antiel, F. A. Curlin, K. M. James, and J. C. Tilburt, "The Moral Psychology of Rationing among Physicians: The Role of Harm and Fairness Intuitions in Physician Objections to Cost-Effectiveness and Cost-Containment," *Philos. Ethics Humanit. Med.*, 2013, *8*: 0.

106. J. C. Tilburt and C. K. Cassel, "Why the Ethics of Parsimonious Medicine Is Not the Ethics of Rationing," *JAMA*, 2013, *309*: 773–774, quotation from 773. See also C. K. Cassel and J. A. Guest, "Choosing Wisely: Helping Physicians and Patients Make Smart Decisions about Their Care," *JAMA*, 2012, *307*: 1801–1802; J. S. Blumenthal-Barby, "'Choosing Wisely' to Reduce Low-Value Care: A Conceptual and Ethical Analysis," *J. Med. Philo.*, 2013, *38*: 559–580; and L. Snyder, "American College of Physicians Ethics Manual," 6th ed., *Ann. Intern. Med.*, 2012, *156*: 73–104. For the controversial issue of rationing health care, see D. Callahan, *Setting Limits: Medical Goals in an Aging Society* (New York: Simon & Schuster, 1987); D. Callahan, "Must We Ration Health Care for the Elderly," *J. Law Med. Ethics*, 2012, *40*: 10–16; and A. B. Cohen, "The Debate over Health Care Rationing: Déjà Vu All over Again," *Inquiry*, 2012, *49*: 90–100. For a study of health care rationing in Britain, see H. J. Aaron and W. B. Schwartz, *Can We Say No? The Challenge of Rationing Health Care* (Washington, DC: Brookings Institution Press, 2005).

107. R. L. Frye, "President's Page: Does It Really Make a Difference?" *J. Am. Coll. Cardiol.*, 1992, *19*: 468–470.

108. Tilburt and Cassel, "Ethics of Parsimonious Medicine," 773.

109. "Choosing Wisely: Consumer Reports is Working with Doctors to Help Patients Avoid Unnecessary and Potentially Harmful Medical Care," September 2013, http://consumerreports.org/cro/ChoosingWisely.htm. See also R. M. Veatch, *Patient, Heal Thyself: How the New Medicine Puts the Patient in Charge* (New York: Oxford University Press, 2009).

110. D. E. Wood, J. D. Mitchell, D. S. Schmitz, S. C. Grondin, J. S. Ikonomidis, F. G. Bakaeen et al., "Choosing Wisely: Cardiothoracic Surgeons Partnering with Patients to Make Good Health Care Decisions," *Ann. Thorac. Surg.*, 2013, *95*: 1130–1135, quotation from 1135.

111. E. M. Firebaugh, *The Story of a Doctor's Telephone: Told by His Wife* (Boston: Roxburgh, 1912), 5.

112. R. Rozenblum and D. W. Bates, "Patient-Centered Healthcare, Social Media and the Internet: The Perfect Storm?" *BMJ Qual. Saf.*, 2013, *22*: 183–186.

113. J. H. Noseworthy, "Foreword," in Mayo Clinic Center for Social Media, *Bringing the Social Media #Revolution to Health Care* (Rochester, MN: Mayo Foundation, 2012), viii. See also F. Griffiths, J. Cave, F. Boardman, J. Ren, T. Pawlikowska, R. Ball et al., "Social Networks: The Future of Health Care Delivery," *Soc. Sci. Med.*, 2012, *75*: 2233–2241.

114. http://mhadegree.org/top-50-most-social-media-friendly-hospitals-2013/.

115. F. K. Timimi, "The Shape of Digital Engagement: Health Care and Social Media," *J. Ambulatory Care Manage.*, 2013, *36*: 187–192.

116. E. Gardner, "Digital Access: Your Medical Records May Now Be Keystrokes Away." *U.S. News & World Report*, Best Hospitals, 2013 edition, 40–42. See also P. C. Carpenter, "The Electronic Medical Record: Perspective from Mayo Clinic," *Int. J. Biomed. Comput.*, 1994, *34*: 159–171; and D. L. Andreen, L. J. Dobie, J. C. Jasperson, T. A. Lucas, and C. L. Wubbenhorst, "The Conversion to Electronic Hospital Notes at Mayo Clinic: Overcoming Barriers and Challenges," *J. Healthc. Inf. Manag.*, 2010, *24*: 57–64.

117. http://www.mayoclinic.org/_portal/html/C/PatientOnlineServices.htm.

118. "Know Your Numbers, 8675309 Parody" (Mayo Clinic, 2011) http://www.youtube.com/watch?v=kkps4XwvxK4.

119. M. Grogan, ed., *Mayo Clinic Healthy Heart for Life!* (New York: Time Home Entertainment, 2012), 6.

120. P. A. Heidenreich, J. G. Trogdon, O. A. Khavjou, J. Butler, K. Dracup, M. D. Ezekowitz et al., "Forecasting the Future of Cardiovascular Disease in the United States," *Circulation*, 2011, *123*: 933–944. See also L. J. Laslett, P. Alagona Jr., B. A. Clark III, J. P. Drozda Jr., F. Saldivar, S. R. Wilson et al., "The Worldwide Environment of Cardiovascular Disease: Prevalence, Diagnosis, Therapy, and Policy Issues: A Report from the American College of Cardiology," *J. Am. Coll. Cardiol.*, 2013, *60 (suppl. S)*: S1–S49.

{ INDEX }

Page numbers followed by an *f* or a *t* indicate figures and tables respectively.